MARRIOTT'S

Practical Electrocardiography

SOUTH ASIAN EDITION

MARRIOTT'S Practical Electrocardiography

SOUTH ASIAN EDITION

David G. Strauss, MD, PhD[1]

Director, Division of Applied Regulatory Science
U.S. Food and Drug Administration
Silver Spring, Maryland

[1]*This work was completed outside of Dr. Strauss's duties at the U.S. Food and Drug Administration (FDA). This book reflects the views of the authors and should not be construed to represent FDA's views or policies.*

Douglas D. Schocken, MD

Professor, Division of Cardiology
Department of Medicine
Duke University School of Medicine
Durham, North Carolina

SAE Editor

Raja J Selvaraj, MD, DNB, FCE

Professor, Department of Cardiology
Jawaharlal Institute of Postgraduate Medical Education and Research
Puducherry, India

This work is an adaptation of the *Marriott's Practical Electrocardiography, thirteenth edition.* Authorized for sale only in South Asia.

Wolters Kluwer

Publishing Manager: Saravanan S.
Commissioning Editor: Chandan Kumar
Production Editor: Megha Saini
Assistant Manager Manufacturing: Sumit Johry

10th Floor, Tower C, Building No. 10, Phase - II, DLF Cyber City
Gurgaon, Haryana - 122002

First South Asian Edition
ISBN: 978-93-90612-26-0

Published by Wolters Kluwer (India) Pvt. Ltd., New Delhi
Compositor: Chennai Publisher Services

Printed and bound at Nutech Print Services - India
For product enquiry, please contact–
Marketing Department (marketing@wolterskluwerindia.co.in) or log on to our website www.wolterskluwerindia.co.in.

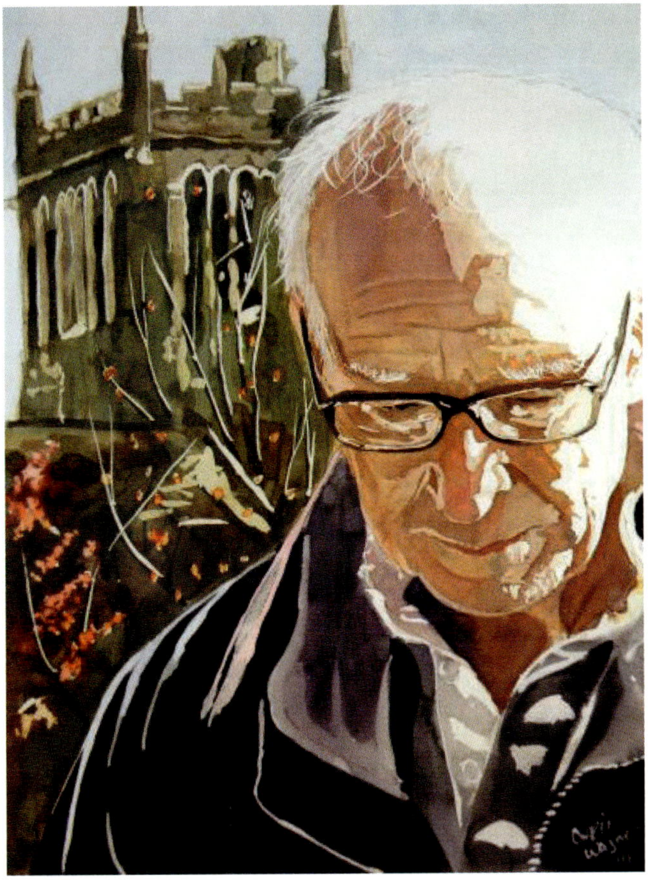

Galen S. Wagner watercolor by Chris Wagner. Courtesy of Marilyn Wagner.

This Thirteenth edition is dedicated to Galen S. Wagner, MD, who after assisting Henry Marriott, MD, with the 8th edition in 1988, took over as the author of the book from Ninth, Tenth, Eleventh, and Twelfth editions before passing away in 2016.

Preface to the International Edition

Barney Marriott created *Practical Electrocardiography* in 1954 and nurtured it through eight editions. After assisting him with the 8th edition, Galen S. Wagner enthusiastically accepted the challenge of writing subsequent editions up through the 12th edition. For the 12th edition, David G. Strauss joined Galen as coauthor, adding digital content in the form of animated figures and videos, and multiple chapters were added or significantly enhanced. With the passing of Galen S. Wagner in 2016, David G. Strauss took on the torch to create the 13th edition, combining with Douglas D. Schocken to coauthor the new edition. Doug had been a friend, mentee, and colleague of both Barney Marriott and Galen S. Wagner.

One of the strengths of *Marriott's Practical Electrocardiography* through its more than 65-year history has been its lucid foundation for understanding the basis for electrocardiogram (ECG) interpretation. Again, in this revision, we have attempted to retain the best of the Marriott tradition—emphasis on the concepts required for everyday ECG interpretation and the simplicities, rather than complexities, of the ECG recordings. In addition, quizzes have returned to the book as a learning tool that are available online.

The current edition underwent a major restructuring. With the exception of Section I (Basic Concepts) that remained in the same order, subsequent sections and chapters were reorganized. Section II covers chamber enlargement and conduction abnormalities with updates to both. Section III covers ischemia and infarction with advanced content contained in an online-only supplement. Section IV covers drugs, electrolytes, and miscellaneous conditions with a substantially updated chapter on drug effects and a completely new chapter on adult congenital heart disease. Sections I through IV are authored by combinations of David G. Strauss, Tobin H. Lim, and Douglas D. Schocken, with additional contributors to the chapters on interpretation of the ECG in 3D (Charles W. Olson, E. Harvey Estes Jr, Vivian P. Kamphuis, and Esben Andreas Carlson), chamber enlargement (Ljuba Bacharova), electrolytes and drugs (Robbert Zusterzeel and Jose Vicente Ruiz), and adult congenital heart disease (Sarah A. Goldstein and Richard Krasuski).

Section V on Abnormal Rhythms has undergone a complete reorganization with substantial updates and revisions by multiple members of the Duke Cardiology Division, Electrophysiology Section led by James Daubert. The chapters on ventricular preexcitation and inherited arrhythmia disorders had previously appeared earlier in the book but now appear in this section along with other core chapters on abnormal rhythms. This section of the book had last undergone a major update in the 9th edition of the book in 1994. With the acceleration of interventional electrophysiology over the past decades, we have learned so much more about abnormal rhythms. This section of the book now aims to leverage that knowledge to better understand and teach interpretation of the body-surface ECG, while maintaining simplicities, as championed by Barney Marriott and Galen S. Wagner. For this major revision of the section on arrhythmias, James Daubert did an outstanding job of recruiting contributors, shepherding them, and editing their work. He deserves a special note of appreciation. Thank you to all of the Duke Electrophysiology contributors: Zak Loring, James P. Daubert, Fredrik Holmqvist, Aimée Elise Hiltbold, Kevin P. Jackson, Jonathan P. Piccini, Tristram D. Bahnson, Albert Sun, Jason Koontz, Larry R. Jackson II, Camille Frazier-Mills, Francis Ugowe, Donald Hegland, Steve Gaeta, John Symmons, Brett D. Atwater, and Dan Friedman.

We thank the Wolters Kluwer teams for all of their support throughout the process to include ambitious updates to this edition; this includes Julie Kostelnik (Editorial Coordinator), Ashley Fischer (Senior Development Editor), Sharon Zinner (Executive Editor), Alicia Jackson (Senior Production Project Manager), and Don Famularcano (Project Manager, Absolute Service, Inc.).

Our goal for the 13th edition is to continue to preserve the spirit of Barney Marriott and Galen S. Wagner to teach electrocardiography through a fundamental understanding of why the waveforms and rhythms appear as they do rather than just memorizing patterns. David has written a new tribute to Galen S. Wagner that follows this preface, and the foreword written by Douglas from the 12th edition to honor Barney Marriott comes next.

We hope you enjoy the book!

David G. Strauss and Douglas D. Schocken
Washington, District of Columbia, and Durham, North Carolina

Contributors to the International Edition

Brett D. Atwater, MD

Associate Professor
Electrophysiology Section, Cardiology Division
Department of Medicine
Duke University School of Medicine
Durham, North Carolina

Ljuba Bacharova, MD, DSc, MBA

Senior Researcher
Biophotonics
International Laser Center
Bratislava, Slovakia

Tristram D. Bahnson, MD

Professor
Electrophysiology Section, Cardiology Division
Department of Medicine
Duke University School of Medicine
Durham, North Carolina

Esben Andreas Carlsen, MD, PhD student

Department of Clinical Physiology, Nuclear Medicine &
PET and Cluster for Molecular Imaging
Rigshospitalet
Department of Biomedical Sciences
University of Copenhagen
Copenhagen, Denmark

James P. Daubert, MD

Professor
Electrophysiology Section, Cardiology Division
Department of Medicine
Duke University School of Medicine
Durham, North Carolina

E. Harvey Estes, Jr., MD

Professor Emeritus
Department of Community and Family Medicine
Duke University School of Medicine
Durham, North Carolina

Camille Genise Frazier-Mills, MD, MHS
Associate Professor
Electrophysiology Section, Cardiology Division
Department of Medicine
Duke University School of Medicine
Durham, North Carolina

Daniel J. Friedman, MD
Assistant Professor, Attending Physician
Internal Medicine, Electrophysiology Section
Yale School of Medicine, Yale New Haven Hospital
New Haven, Connecticut

Stephen Gaeta, MD, PhD
Cardiac Electrophysiologist
Inova Medical Group—Arrhythmia
Inova Heart and Vascular Insitute
Fairfax, Virginia

Sarah A. Goldstein, MD
Adult Congenital Heart Disease Fellow
Department of Medicine
Duke University Medical Center
Durham, North Carolina

Donald D. Hegland, MD
Associate Professor
Electrophysiology Section, Cardiology Division
Department of Medicine
Duke University School of Medicine
Durham, North Carolina

Aimée Elise Hiltbold, MD
Fellow
Electrophysiology Section, Cardiology Division
Department of Medicine
Duke University School of Medicine
Durham, North Carolina

Fredrik Holmqvist, MD, PhD
Associate Professor
Department of Cardiology
Lund University
Lund, Sweden

Kevin P. Jackson, MD
Associate Professor
Electrophysiology Section, Cardiology Division
Department of Medicine
Duke University School of Medicine
Durham, North Carolina

Larry R. Jackson II, MD, MHS

Assistant Professor
Electrophysiology Section, Cardiology Division
Department of Medicine
Duke University School of Medicine
Durham, North Carolina

Vivian P. Kamphuis, MD, PhD

Resident
Department of Pediatrics
Erasmus University Medical Center
Rotterdam, The Netherlands

Jason Koontz, MD

Associate Professor
Electrophysiology Section, Cardiology Division
Department of Medicine
Duke University School of Medicine
Durham, North Carolina

Richard A. Krasuski, MD

Professor of Medicine
Director, Adult Congenital Heart Center
Department of Medicine
Cardiology
Duke University School of Medicine
Duke University Health System
Durham, North Carolina

Tobin H. Lim, MD

Associate Professor of Medicine
Texas A&M School of Medicine
Round Rock, Texas

Zak Loring, MD, MHS

Fellow
Electrophysiology Section, Cardiology Division
Department of Medicine
Duke University School of Medicine
Durham, North Carolina

Charles W. Olson, MSEE

Huntington Station, New York

Jonathan P. Piccini, MD, MHS

Associate Professor
Electrophysiology Section, Cardiology Division
Department of Medicine
Duke University School of Medicine
Durham, North Carolina

Douglas D. Schocken, MD

Professor
Division of Cardiology
Department of Medicine
Duke University School of Medicine
Durham, North Carolina

David G. Strauss, MD, PhD

Director
Division of Applied Regulatory Science
U.S. Food and Drug Administration
Silver Spring, Maryland

This work was completed outside of Dr. Strauss' duties at the U.S. Food and Drug Administration (FDA). This book reflects the views of the authors and should not be construed to represent FDA's views or policies.

Albert Y. Sun, MD

Associate Professor
Electrophysiology Section, Cardiology Division
Department of Medicine
Duke University School of Medicine
Durham, North Carolina

John Symons, MD

Assistant Professor
Department of Medicine
Uniformed Services University of Health Sciences
Bethesda, Maryland

Francis E. Ugowe, MD

Fellow
Division of Cardiology
Department of Medicine
Duke University School of Medicine
Durham, North Carolina

Jose Vicente Ruiz, PhD

Senior Staff Fellow
Center for Drug Evaluation and Research
U.S. Food and Drug Administration
Silver Spring, Maryland

Robbert Zusterzeel, MD, PhD, MPH

Director (Research Network)
National Evaluation System for Health Technology Coordinating Center (NESTcc)
Medical Device Innovation Consortium
Arlington, VA

Preface to the South Asian Edition

More than a century since its initial use as a clinical tool, the electrocardiogram (ECG), in an act of astounding tenaciousness, remains a vital diagnostic tool in the clinician's armamentarium even today. The information density in an ECG is very high and it takes years and thousands of ECGs before one acquires mastery in its interpretation. How best to transfer this knowledge of ECGs to newcomers in the field remains a vexing question and the number of books and online resources that exist for this purpose is a testament to the fact that this hasn't been satisfactorily answered.

Dr. Henry Marriott has been one of the most successful teachers to grapple with this question. There are multiple reasons behind the success of this book as a learning resource that is useful to wide range of readers. The first reason is that Dr. Marriott was a prolific teacher of ECGs who traveled and lectured frequently. This book is a distillation of the experience he garnered on how best to teach ECGs. The second is his teaching style that is original and highly engaging with many unique quotes. Reading the book gives an impression of listening to an enthusiastic teacher rather than just reading academic text. The last reason is the sheer amount of time that the book has been around. More than 60 years and multiple editions means that the content has evolved to optimally impart knowledge on ECGs to those still new to the field.

Participating in this evolution has been an honour for me and the other contributors to this edition. We have attempted to preserve the unique style of Dr. Marriott while improving the content and presentation to make the book more accessible and valuable to students of the South Asian region. This edition will be a valuable resource for undergraduates in Medicine, Nursing and Allied Sciences, postgraduates and all other students who wish to learn the interpretation of ECGs.

Raja J Selvaraj, MD, DNB, FCE
Puducherry, India

Reviewer and Contributors to the South Asian Edition

REVIEWER:

Johnson Francis, MD, DM
Senior Consultant Interventional Cardiologist
Baby Memorial Hospital
Calicut, Kerala

CONTRIBUTORS:

Ameya Udyavar, MD, DM, DNB
Consultant Cardiologist and Cardiac Electrophysiologist
P D Hinduja National Hospital
Mumbai, Maharashtra

Anand Manickavasagam, MD, DM
Assistant Professor, Department of Cardiology
Christian Medical College
Vellore, Tamil Nadu

Anandaraja Subramanian, MD, DM
Consultant in Cardiology and Electrophysiology
Indira Gandhi Government General Hospital & Post Graduate Institute (IGGGH & PGI)
Puducherry

Anindya Ghosh, MD, DM
Fellow in Clinical Cardiac Electrophysiology and Pacing
The Madras Medical Mission
Chennai, Tamil Nadu

Bhima Shankar P R, MD, DM
Consultant Cardiac Electrophysiologist
Lakeshore Hospital
Kochi, Kerala

Daljeet Kaur Saggu, MD, DM
Consultant Cardiologist and Electrophysiologist
AIG Hospitals
Hyderabad, Telangana

Debabrata Bera, MD, DM, DNB, PDF (EP)
Consultant Cardiology & Electrophysiology
Rabindranath Tagore International Institute of Cardiac Sciences (RTIICS)
Kolkata, West Bengal

Deepak Padmanabhan, DM
Fellowship in EP and Advanced Adult Cardiology
Sri Jayadeva Institute of Cardiovascular Sciences and Research
Bangalore, Karnataka

John Roshan, MD, DM, CEPS, CCDS
Professor, Department of Cardiology
Christian Medical College
Vellore, Tamil Nadu

Kartikeya Bhargava, MD, DNB
Director, Cardiac Electrophysiology and Pacing
Medanta-The Medicity
Gurugram, Haryana

Kumar Narayanan, MD, DM, FHRS, CEPS (A)
Consultant Electrophysiologist
Medicover Hospitals
Hyderabad, Telangana

Mukund Aravind Prabhu, MD, DM, PDF (EP and Pacing)
Associate Professor, Department of Cardiology
Kasturba Medical College Manipal
Manipal Academy of Higher Education
Manipal, Karnataka

Muralidharan T R, MD, DM, FRCP
Professor, Department of Cardiology
Sri Ramachandra Institute of Higher Education and Research
Chennai, Tamil Nadu

Narayanan Namboodiri K K, MD, DM
Professor, Department of Cardiology
Sree Chitra Tirunal Institute for Medical Sciences and Technology (SCTIMST)
Thiruvananthapuram, Kerala

Natarajan K U, MD, DNB, DM
Professor, Head of EP division
Amrita School of Medicine
Kochi, Kerala

Nischal Hegde, MD
Senior Resident, Department of Cardiology
Amrita School of Medicine
Kochi, Kerala

Preetam Krishnamurthy, MD, DM
Assistant Professor, Department of Cardiology
Sri Ramachandra Institute of Higher Education and Research
Chennai, Tamil Nadu

Ramalingam Vadivelu, MD, DM
Consultant Interventional Cardiologist & Electrophysiologist
Velammal Medical College Hospital and Research Institute
Madurai, Tamil Nadu

Sai Kiran Kakarla, MD
Senior Resident
Sree Chitra Tirunal Institute for Medical Sciences and Technology (SCTIMST)
Thiruvananthapuram, Kerala

Saurabh Deshpande, MD, DM, PDF (EP)
Consultant Electrophysiologist
Sri Jayadeva Institute of Cardiaovascular Sciences and Research
Bangalore, Karnataka

Shomu Bohora, MD, DM, PDF (EP)
Associate Professor, Department of Cardiology
U N Mehta Institute of Cardiology and Research Centre
Ahmedabad, Gujarat

Suchit Majumdar, MD, DM, PDF (Cardiac EP), CEPS-A
Consultant Cardiac Electrophysiologist
Apollo Gleneagles Hospital
Kolkata, West Bengal

Ulhas M Pandurangi, MD, DM
Chief, Department of Cardiac Electrophysiology and Pacing
The Madras Medical Mission
Chennai, Tamil Nadu

Contents

Digital Contents

This book contains quizzes, animated figures (animations) and videos accessible through lww.co.in. Please see the inside front cover for instructions.

The animations and videos are referenced within the chapters and a full list is noted below.

The quizzes are organized by topic. A complete list can be found at lww.co.in.

Chapter 6

Chapter 13

Chapter 15

Chapter 16

Chapter 17

Chapter 19

Topical Quizzes

SECTION I

Basic Concepts

1

Cardiac Electrical Activity

TOBIN H. LIM, DAVID G. STRAUSS, AND KUMAR NARAYANAN

The Book: *Marriott's Practical Electrocardiography*, 13th Edition

What Can This Book Do for Me?

This 13th edition of **Marriott's Practical Electrocardiography** has been specifically designed to provide you with a practical approach to reading *electrocardiograms (ECGs)*. This book has value for all learners. No previous text or experience is required. If you are most comfortable acquiring a basic understanding of a subject even before you encounter a need to use the subject information, you probably want to read the first section (Basic Concepts) carefully. If you have found that this approach is not really helpful, you probably want to quickly scan this first section.

Many medical terms are defined in a glossary at the end of each chapter. Each individual "practical concept" is presented in a "Learning Unit." The Learning Units are listed in the Table of Contents for easy reference.

Because ECG reading is a visual experience, most of the book's illustrations are typical examples of the various clinical situations for which ECGs are recorded.

To understand better the basic concepts the ECG provides, we have added summary illustrations in each chapter and quizzes online along with additional digital content including animations and video content.

While updates have been made throughout the book, substantial revisions were made to the abnormal rhythms section of the book.

What Can I Expect From Myself When I Have "Completed" This Book?

This book is not intended for you to "complete." Rather, it is intended as both a learning tool and as a reference for the ECG problems you encounter. Through your experience with this book, you should develop confidence in identifying a "normal" ECG and be able to accurately diagnose the many common ECG abnormalities. You should also have an understanding of the practical aspects of the pathophysiologic basis for most of these common ECG abnormalities.

The Electrocardiogram

What Is an Electrocardiogram?

An ECG is the recording (gram) of the electrical activity (electro) generated by the cells of the heart (cardio) that reaches the body surface. This electrical activity initiates the heart's muscular contraction that pumps the blood to the body. Each ECG recording *electrode* provides one of the poles of a *lead*, which gives the view of this electrical activity that it "sees" from its particular position on the body surface. In other words, a pair of electrodes makes up a lead. Observation of the 12 views provided by the 12 leads of the routine clinical ECG allows you to see the heart's electrical activity from various aspects. Reversal of the poles of each lead provides a reciprocal view.

What Does an Electrocardiogram Actually Measure?

The ECG recording plots voltage on its vertical axis and time on its horizontal axis. Measurements along the horizontal axis indicate the overall heart rate, regularity, and the time intervals during electrical activation that moves throughout the heart. Measurements along the vertical axis indicate the voltage measured on the body surface. This voltage represents the "summation" of the electrical activation of all of the cardiac cells at that time. Some abnormalities can be detected by measurements on a single ECG recording, but other abnormalities become apparent only by observing serial recordings over time.

What Medical Problems Can Be Diagnosed With an Electrocardiogram?

Many cardiac abnormalities can be diagnosed by ECG interpretation, including enlargement of heart muscle, electrical conduction delay or blocks, insufficient blood flow, and death of heart muscle due to a coronary occlusion. The ECG can even identify which of the heart's coronary arteries is occluded when it is still only threatening to destroy a region of heart muscle. The ECG is also the primary method for identifying problems with heart rate and regularity. In addition to its value for understanding cardiac problems, the ECG can be used to aid in diagnosing medical conditions throughout the body. For example, the ECG can provide clues to abnormal levels of ions in the blood, such as potassium and calcium, and abnormal function of glands such as the thyroid. It can also help diagnose potentially dangerous levels of certain drugs.

Anatomic Orientation of the Heart

The position of the heart within the body determines the "view" of the cardiac electrical activity that can be observed from any site on the body surface. A frontal plane magnetic resonance image of the heart within the thorax is seen in **Figure 1.1A**. The atria are located in the top or *base* of the heart, and the *ventricles* taper toward the bottom or *apex*. The long axis of the heart, which extends from base to apex, is tilted to the left at its apical end in the schematic drawing of this frontal plane view (**Figure 1.1B**).

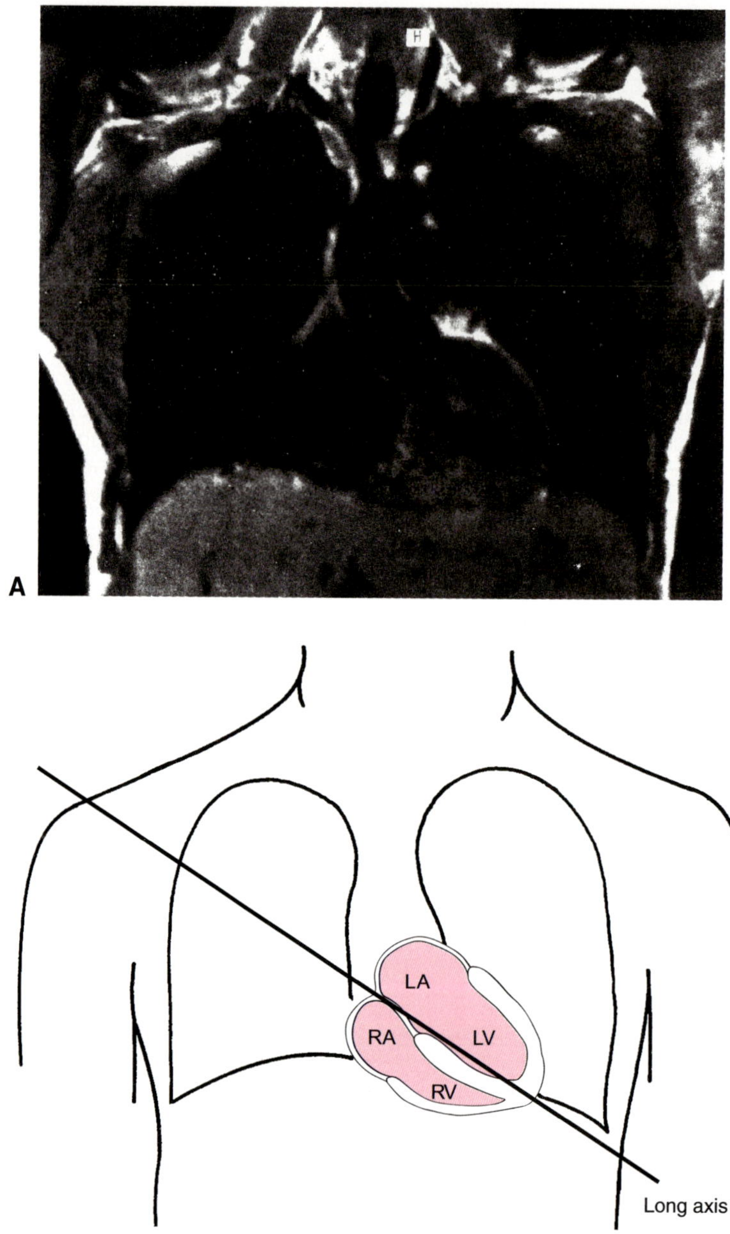

FIGURE 1.1. **A.** Frontal plane magnetic resonance image. **B.** Chambers of the heart. LA, left atrium; LV, left ventricle; RA, right atrium; RV, right ventricle.

The right *atrium*/right ventricle and left atrium/left ventricle, however, are not directly aligned with the right and left sides of the body as viewed in the transverse plane magnetic resonance image of the heart within the thorax (**Figure 1.2A**). The schematic drawing shows how the right-sided chambers of the heart are located *anterior* to the left-sided chambers, with the result that the interatrial and interventricular septa form a diagonal in this transverse plane view (**Figure 1.2B**).

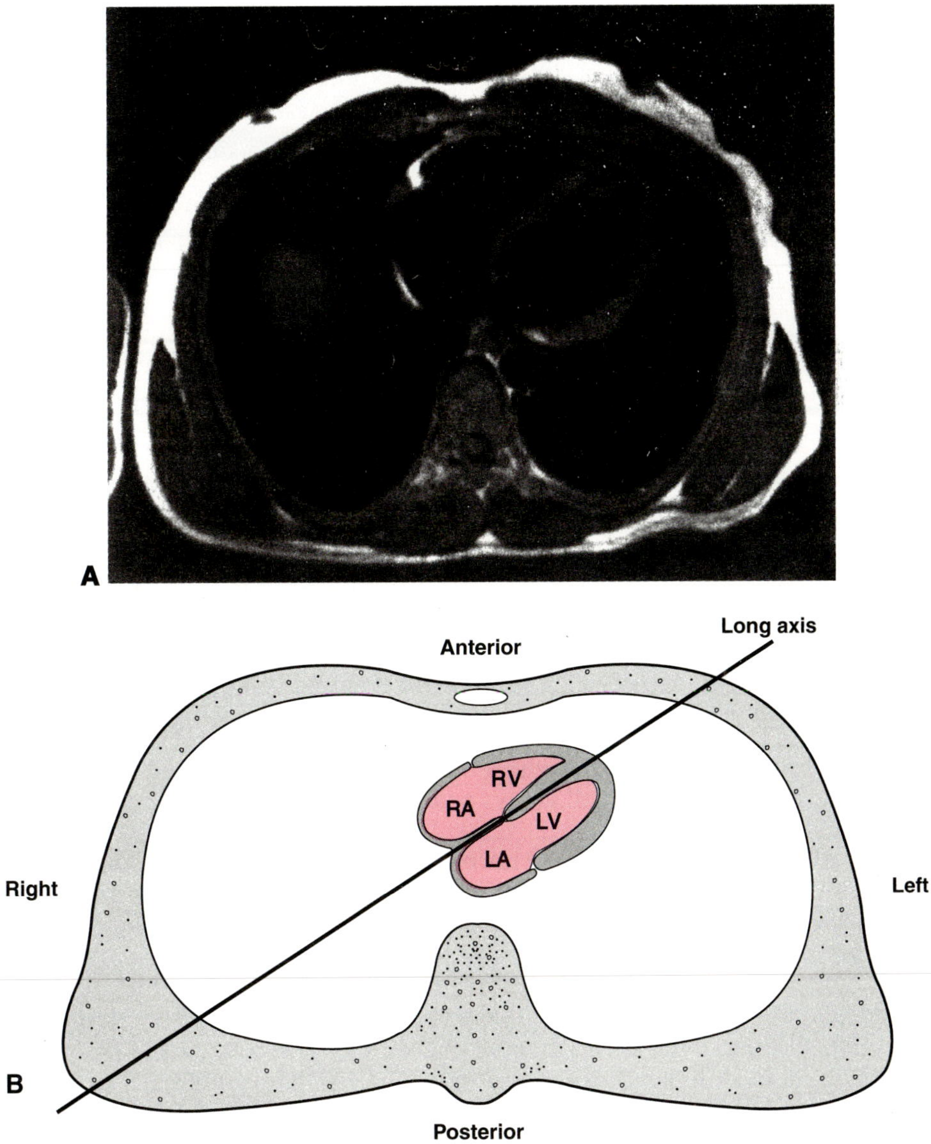

FIGURE 1.2. **A.** Transverse plane magnetic resonance image, as viewed from below. **B.** Chambers of the heart. LA, left atrium; LV, left ventricle; RA, right atrium; RV, right ventricle.

The Cardiac Cycle

The mechanical pumping action of the heart is produced by cardiac muscle ("myocardial") cells that contain contractile proteins (actin and myosin). The timing and synchronization of contraction of these myocardial cells are controlled by noncontractile cells of the pacemaking and conduction system. Impulses generated within these specialized cells create a rhythmic repetition of events called *cardiac cycles*. Each cycle includes electrical and mechanical activation (*systole*) and recovery (*diastole*). The terms commonly applied to these components of the cardiac cycle are listed in **Table 1.1**. Because the electrical events initiate the mechanical events, there is a brief delay between the onsets of electrical and mechanical systole and of electrical and mechanical diastole.

Table 1.1.

Terms Describing Cardiac Cycle

Systole	Diastole
Electrical	
Activation	Recovery
Excitation	Recovery
Depolarization	Repolarization
Mechanical	
Shortening	Lengthening
Contraction	Relaxation
Emptying	Filling

The electrical recording from inside a single myocardial cell as it progresses through a cardiac cycle is illustrated in **Figure 1.3** and in **Animation 1.1**. During electrical diastole, the cell has a *baseline* negative electrical potential and is also in mechanical diastole, with separation of the contractile proteins. At top (**Figure 1.3A**), a single cardiac cell is shown at three points in time, during which it is relaxed, contracted, and relaxed again. An electrical impulse arriving at the cell allows positively charged ions to cross the cell membrane, causing its *depolarization*. This movement of ions initiates "electrical systole," which is characterized by an *action potential*. This electrical event then initiates mechanical systole, in which the contractile proteins within the myocardial cell engage with one another and slide over each other, thereby shortening the cell. Electrical systole continues until the positively charged ions are pumped out of the cell, causing its *repolarization*. Below the cell is a representation of an internal electrical recording that begins at resting, undergoes depolarization, and then returns to its negative resting level (**Figure 1.3B**). The repolarization process begins with an initial brief component that is followed by a "plateau" that varies among myocardial cells. Repolarization is completed by a rapid component. This return of "electrical diastole" causes the contractile proteins within the cell to uncouple. The cell is then capable of being reactivated when another electrical impulse arrives at its membrane.

To view the animation(s) and video(s) associated with this chapter please access lww.co.in. Instructions are located on the inside front cover.

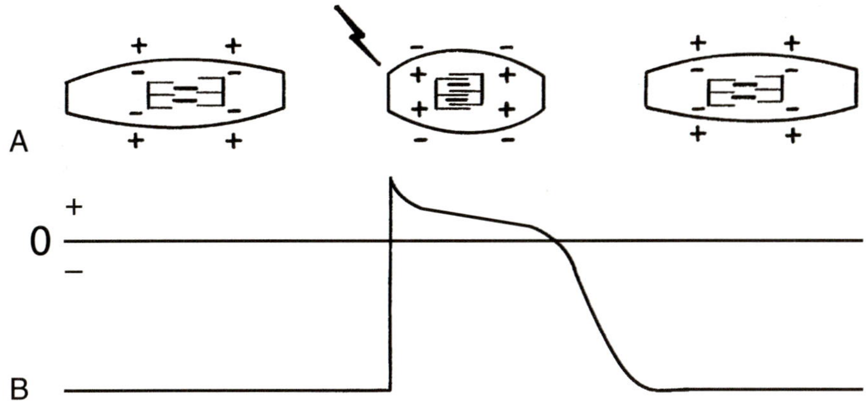

FIGURE 1.3. Cardiac cycle in a single myocardial cell. **A**, lightning bolt: electrical impulse; +, positive ions; –, negative ions. **B**, horizontal line: level of zero (0) potential, with positive (+) values above and negative (–) values beneath the line. (Modified with permission from Thaler MS. *The Only EKG Book You'll Ever Need*. Philadelphia, PA: JB Lippincott; 1988:11.) See **Animation 1.1**.

The electrical and mechanical changes in a series of myocardial cells (aligned end to end) as they progress through a cardiac cycle are illustrated in **Figure 1.4**. In **Figure 1.4A**, the four representative cells are in their resting or repolarized state. Electrically, the cells have negative charges. Mechanically, their contractile proteins are separated. An electrical stimulus arrives at the second myocardial cell in **Figure 1.4B**, causing electrical and then mechanical systole. The wave of depolarization in **Figure 1.4C** spreads throughout all the myocardial cells. In **Figure 1.4D**, the recovery or repolarization process begins in the second cell, which was the first to depolarize. Finally, in **Figure 1.4E**, the wave of repolarization spreads throughout all of the myocardial cells; they then await the coming of another electrical stimulus.[1,2] See **Animation 1.2**.

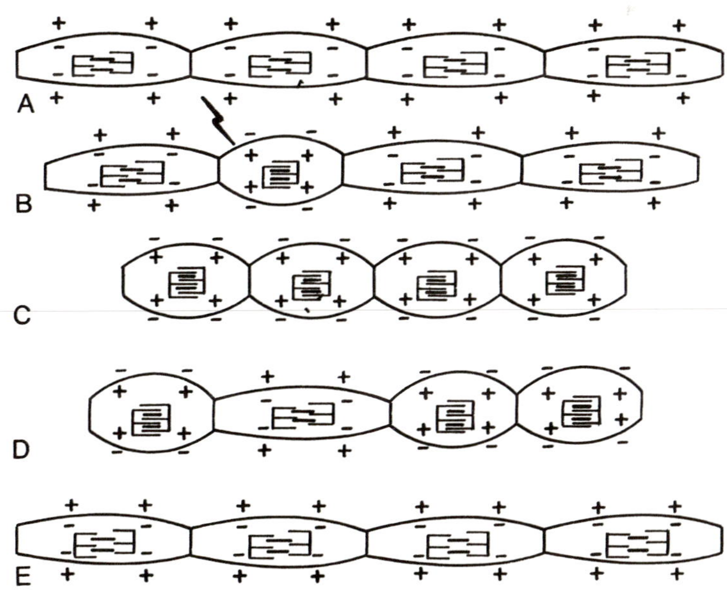

FIGURE 1.4. Cardiac cycle in a series of myocardial cells. The symbols are the same as in Figure 1.3. (Modified with permission from Thaler MS. *The Only EKG Book You'll Ever Need*. Philadelphia, PA: JB Lippincott; 1988:9.) See **Animation 1.2**.

In **Figure 1.5** and **Animation 1.3**, the relationship between the intracellular electrical recording from a single myocardial cell presented in **Figure 1.3** is combined with an ECG recording on a "lead" that has its positive and negative electrodes on the body surface. The ECG recording is the summation of electrical signals from all of the myocardial cells. There is a flat baseline in two very different situations: (1) when the cells are in their resting state electrically and (2) when the summation of cardiac electrical activity is directed perpendicular to a line between the positive and negative electrodes. The depolarization of the cells produces a high-frequency ECG *waveform*. Between the initial transient and final complete phases of repolarization, the ECG returns to the baseline. Completion of repolarization of the myocardial cells is represented on the ECG by a lower frequency waveform in the opposite direction from that representing depolarization.

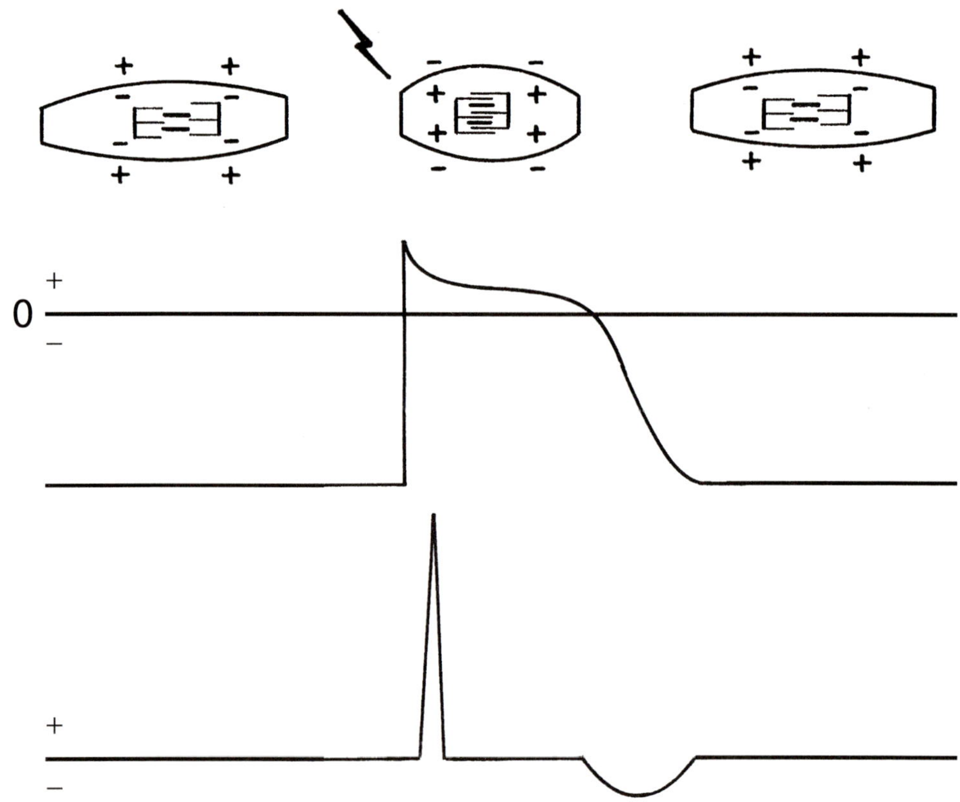

FIGURE 1.5. Single-cell recording combined with an electrocardiogram. The symbols are the same as in Figure 1.3. (Modified with permission from Thaler MS. *The Only EKG Book You'll Ever Need.* Philadelphia, PA: JB Lippincott; 1988:11.) See **Animation 1.3**.

In **Figure 1.6** and **Animation 1.3**, a lead with its positive and negative electrodes has been placed on the body surface and connected to a single-channel ECG recorder. The process of production of the ECG recording by waves of depolarization and repolarization spreading from the negative toward the positive electrode is illustrated. In **Figure 1.6A**, the first of the four cells shown is electrically activated, and the activation then spreads into the second cell. This spread of depolarization toward the positive electrode produces a positive (upward) *deflection* on the ECG. In **Figure 1.6B**, all of the cells are in their depolarized state, and the ECG recording returns to its baseline level. In **Figure 1.6C**, repolarization begins in the same cell in which depolarization was initiated, and the wave of repolarization spreads into the adjoining cell. This repolarization produces the oppositely directed negative (downward) waveform on the ECG recording.

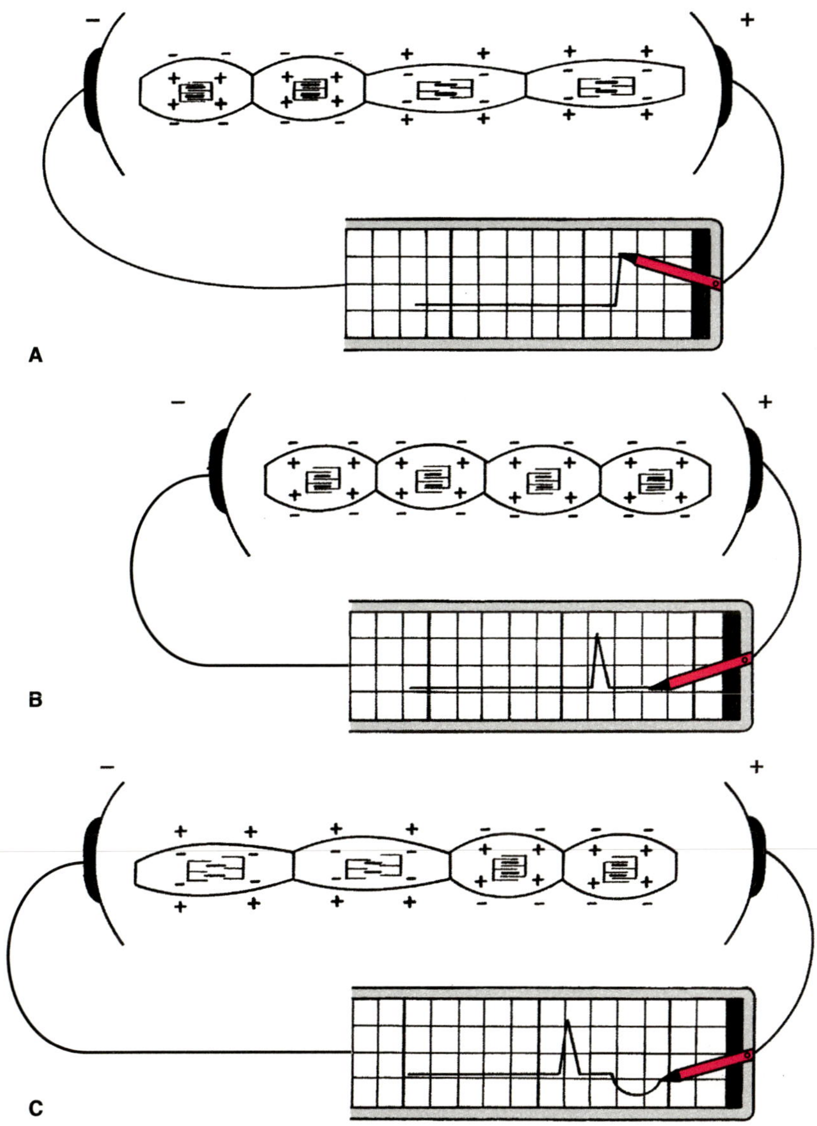

FIGURE 1.6. Single-channel electrocardiogram recording. The symbols are the same as in Figure 1.3. Black semiovals represent the electrodes. (Modified with permission from Thaler MS. *The Only EKG Book You'll Ever Need*. Philadelphia, PA: JB Lippincott; 1988:29,31.) See **Animation 1.3**.

Cardiac Impulse Formation and Conduction

The electrical activation of a single cardiac cell or a small group of cells does not produce enough voltage to be recorded on the body surface. Clinical electrocardiography is made possible by the activation of large groups of atrial and ventricular myocardial cells, whose collective electrical activity can be recorded on the body surface.

Myocardial cells normally lack the ability for either spontaneous formation or rapid conduction of an electrical impulse. They depend on special cells of the *cardiac pacemaking and conduction system* that are located strategically in groups through the heart for these functions (**Figure 1.7**). These cells are arranged in nodes, bundles, *bundle branches*, and branching networks of *fascicles*. The cells that form these structures lack contractile capability, but they can generate spontaneous electrical impulses (act as pacemakers) and alter the speed of electrical conduction throughout the heart. The intrinsic pacemaking rate is fastest in the specialized cells in the atria and slowest in the ventricles. This intrinsic pacemaking rate is altered by the balance between the sympathetic and parasympathetic components of the autonomic nervous system.[3]

Figure 1.7 illustrates three different anatomic relationships between the cardiac pumping chambers and the specialized pacemaking and conduction system: anterior precordium with less tilt (**Figure 1.7A**), right anterior precordium looking at the interatrial and interventricular septa through the right atrium and ventricle (**Figure 1.7B**), and left posterior thorax looking at the septa through the left atrium and ventricle (**Figure 1.7C**). The *sinoatrial (SA) or sinus node* is an epicardial structure, located high in the right atrium, posteriorly and laterally, near its junction with the *superior vena cava*. The SA node is the predominant cardiac pacemaker, and its highly developed capacity for response to autonomic input controls the heart's pumping rate to meet the changing needs of the body during various states such as rest and exercise. The *atrioventricular (AV) node* is an endocardial structure, located low in the right atrium, adjacent to the interatrial *septum*. Its primary function is to delay electrical conduction sufficiently to allow adequate ventricular filling and synchronize the atrial contribution to ventricular pumping. Normally, the AV node is the only structure that can conduct impulses from the atria to the ventricles because these chambers are otherwise separated by nonconducting fibrous and fatty tissue at the atrioventricular junction.[4,5]

In the atria, the electrical impulse generated by the SA node spreads through the myocardium without needing to be carried by any specialized conduction bundles. Electrical impulses reach the AV node where the impulse slows before reaching the intraventricular conduction pathways.

The intraventricular conduction pathways include a *common bundle (bundle of His)* that leads from the AV node to the summit of the interventricular septum as well as the right and left bundle branches of the bundle of His, which proceed along the septal surfaces of their respective ventricles. The left bundle branch fans out into fascicles (smaller bundles) that course along the left septal endocardial surface and toward the two papillary muscles of the mitral valve. The right bundle branch remains compact until it reaches the right *distal* septal surface, where it branches into many smaller groups of conducting cells along the interventricular septum and toward the free wall of the right ventricle. These intraventricular conduction pathways are composed of fibers of *Purkinje cells*, which have specialized capabilities for both pacemaking and rapid conduction of electrical impulses.

Fascicles composed of Purkinje fibers form networks that extend just beneath the surface of the right and left ventricular *endocardium*. After reaching the ends of these Purkinje fascicles, the impulses then travel more slowly from endocardium to *epicardium* throughout the right and left ventricles.[6] This synchronization process allows activation of the myocardium at the upper region (base) to be delayed until the apical region has been activated. This sequence of electrical activation is necessary to achieve the most efficient cardiac pumping because the pulmonary and aortic outflow valves are located at the ventricular bases.

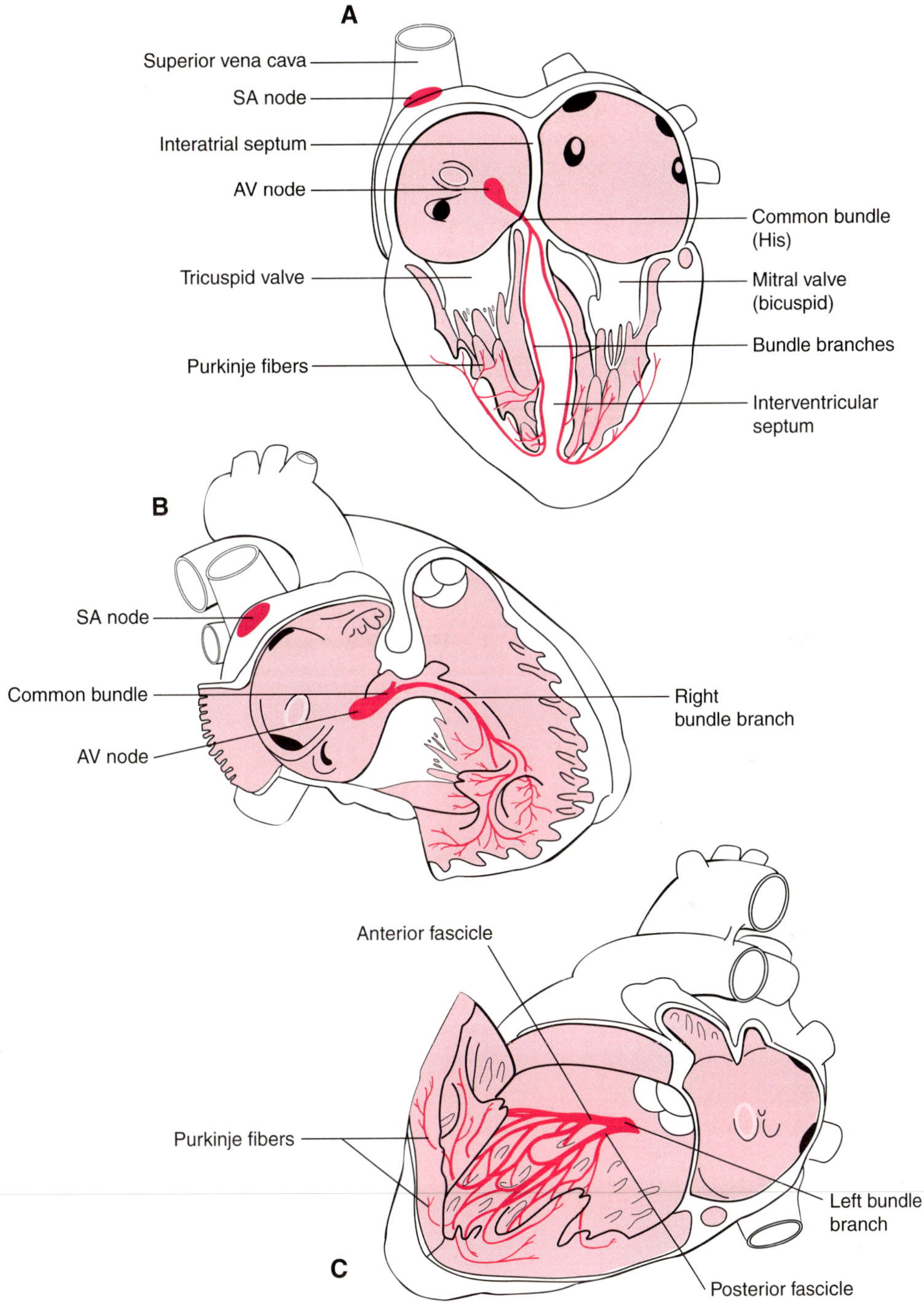

FIGURE 1.7. Special cells of the cardiac pacemaking and conduction system. In **A**, the anterior aspect of all chambers has been removed to reveal the entire AV and ventricular conduction system. In **B**, the lateral aspect of the right atrium and ventricle has been removed. In **C**, the lateral aspect of the left atrium and ventricle has been removed to reveal the right and left bundle branches, respectively. AV, atrioventricular; SA, sinoatrial. (Modified from Netter FH. In: Yonkman FF, ed. *The Ciba Collection of Medical Illustrations*. Vol 5: *Heart*. Summit, NJ: Ciba–Geigy; 1978:13,49.)

Recording Long-Axis (Base-Apex) Cardiac Electrical Activity

The schematic frontal plane view of the heart in the thorax is shown in **Figure 1.1B**, with the negative and positive electrodes located where the long axis of the heart intersects with the body surface. The optimal body surface sites for recording long-axis (base-apex) cardiac electrical activity are located where the extensions of the long axis of the heart intersect with the body surface (**Figure 1.8** and **Animation 1.4**). The negative electrode on the right shoulder and the positive electrode on the left lower chest are aligned from the cardiac base to apex parallel to the interatrial and interventricular septa. This long-axis "ECG lead" is oriented similarly to a lead termed *aVR* on the standard 12-lead ECG (see Chapter 2). However, the lead in **Figure 1.8** would actually be lead −aVR because, for lead aVR, the positive electrode is placed on the right arm. Both the positive and negative electrodes are attached to a single-channel ECG recorder that produces predominantly upright waveforms on the ECG, as explained later in this unit (see also Chapter 2).

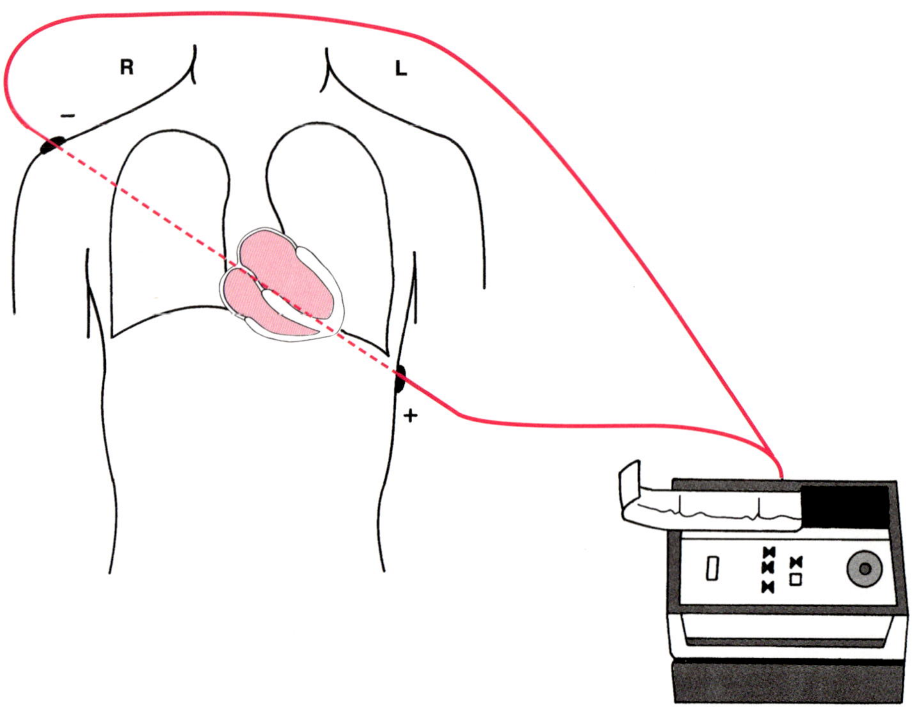

FIGURE 1.8. Optimal sites for recording long-axis cardiac electrical activity. Black semiovals represent the electrodes. L, left; R, right. See **Animation 1.4**.

The long-axis recording in **Figure 1.8** has been magnified to illustrate the sequence of activation in structures of the pacemaking and conduction system (**Figure 1.9** and **Animation 1.5**). This figure contains vital information and for emphasis is repeated elsewhere. The initial wave of a cardiac cycle represents activation of the atria and is called the *P wave*. Because the SA node is located in the right atrium, the first part of the P wave represents the activation of this chamber. The middle section of the P wave represents completion of right-atrial activation and initiation of left-atrial activation. The final section of the P wave represents completion of left-atrial activation. Activation of the AV node begins by the middle of the P wave and proceeds slowly during the final portion of the P wave and PR segment. The wave representing electrical recovery of the atria is usually too small to be seen on the ECG, but it may appear as a distortion of the *PR segment*. The bundle of His and bundle branches are activated during the PR segment but do not produce waveforms on the body surface ECG.

The next group of waves recorded is termed the *QRS complex*, representing the simultaneous activation of the right and left ventricles. On this long-axis recording, the P wave is entirely positive and the QRS complex is predominantly positive.

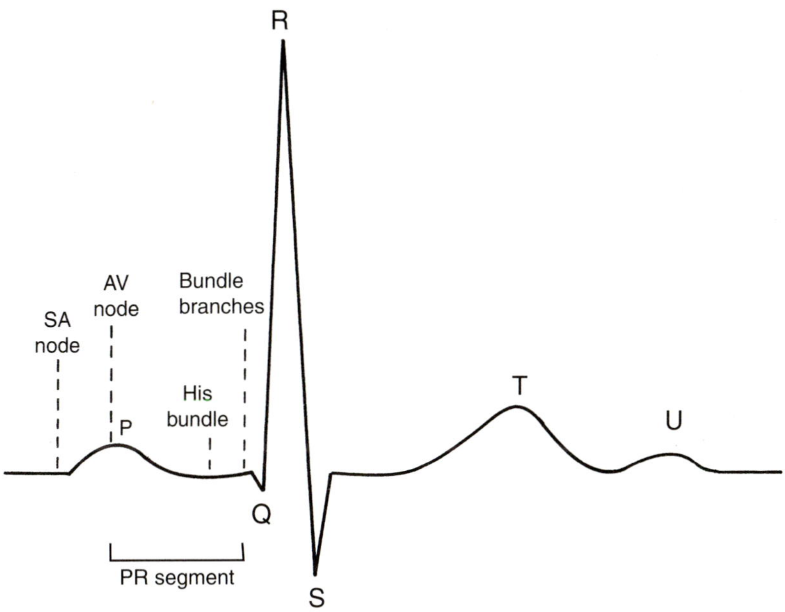

FIGURE 1.9. Waveforms. P, atrial activation; Q, R, and S, ventricular activation; T and U, ventricular recovery. AV, atrioventricular; SA, sinoatrial. See **Animation 1.5**.

The QRS complex may normally appear as one (*monophasic*), two (*diphasic*), or three (*triphasic*) individual waveforms (**Figure 1.10** and **Animation 1.5**). By convention, a negative wave at the onset of the QRS complex is called a *Q wave*. The predominant portion of the QRS complex recorded from this long-axis viewpoint is normally positive and is called the *R wave*, regardless of whether or not it is preceded by a Q wave. A negative deflection following an R wave is called an *S wave*. When a second positive deflection occurs, it is termed *R′* (R prime). A monophasic negative QRS complex should be termed a *QS wave* (see **Figure 1.10**, left). Biphasic complexes are either RS or QR (see **Figure 1.10**, center), and triphasic complexes are RSR′ or QRS (see **Figure 1.10**, right). Occasionally, more complex patterns of QRS waveforms occur (see Chapter 3).

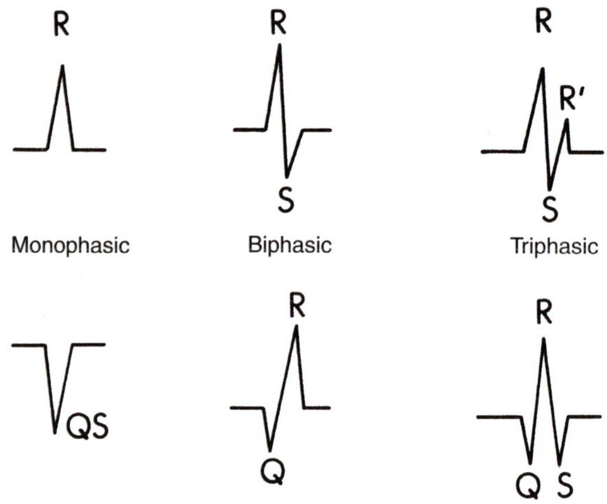

FIGURE 1.10. QRS complex waveforms and their alphabetical terms. (From Selvester RH, Wagner GS, Hindman NB. The development and application of the Selvester QRS scoring system for estimating myocardial infarct size. *Arch Intern Med*. 1985;145:1879, with permission. Copyright 1985, American Medical Association.) See **Animation 1.5**.

The wave in the cardiac cycle that represents recovery of the ventricles is called the *T wave*. The frontal plane view of the right and left ventricles (as in **Figure 1.7A**) is presented along with schematic recordings from left-ventricular myocardial cells on the endocardial and epicardial surfaces (**Figure 1.11** and **Animation 1.6**). The numbers below the recordings refer to the time (in seconds) required for these sequential electrical events. The Purkinje fibers provide electrical activation of the endocardium, initiating a "wavefront" of *depolarization* that spreads through the myocardial wall to the cells on the epicardial surface (*endocardium to epicardium*). Because recovery of the ventricular cells (repolarization) causes an ion flow opposite to that of depolarization, one might expect the T wave to be inverted in relation to the QRS complex, as shown in **Figures 1.5** and **1.6**. However, epicardial cells repolarize earlier than endocardial cells, thereby causing the wave of *repolarization* to spread in the direction opposite to that of depolarization (*epicardium to endocardium*; **Figure 1.11A**). This results in the long-axis body surface ECG waveform (as in **Figure 1.9**) with the T wave deflected in a similar direction as the QRS complex (**Figure 1.11B**). The T wave is sometimes followed by another small upright wave (the source of which is uncertain), called the *U wave*, as seen in **Figure 1.9**.

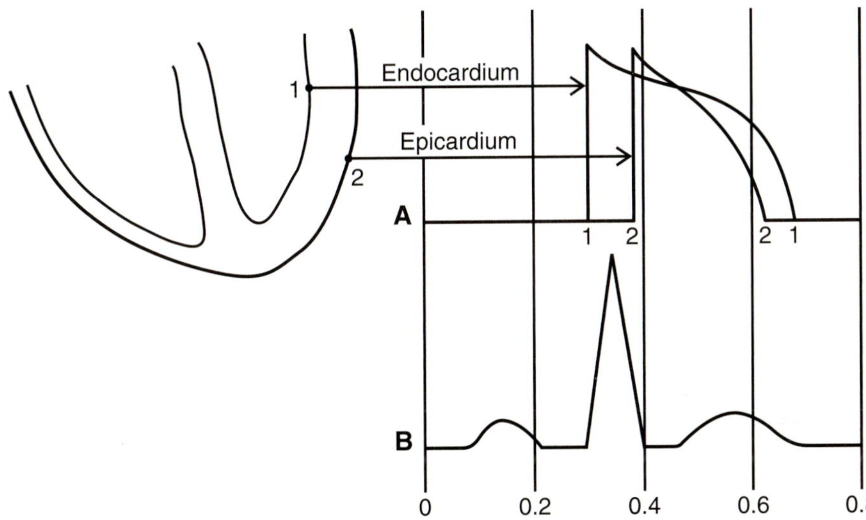

FIGURE 1.11. **A**, action potential of left-ventricular myocardial cells; **B**, long-axis body surface ECG waveforms. See **Animation 1.6**.

The magnified recording from **Figure 1.9** is again presented with the principal ECG segments (P-R and S-T) and time intervals (P-R, QRS, Q-T, and T-P) as displayed in **Figure 1.12** and **Animation 1.7**. The time from the onset of the P wave to the onset of the QRS complex is called the *PR interval*, regardless of whether the first wave in this QRS complex is a Q wave or an R wave. This interval measures the time between the onset of activation of the atrial and ventricular myocardium. The designation PR segment refers to the time from the end of the P wave to the onset of the QRS complex. The *QRS interval* measures the time from the beginning to the end of ventricular activation. Because activation of the thick left-ventricular free wall and interventricular septum requires more time than does activation of the right-ventricular free wall, the terminal portion of the QRS complex represents the balance of forces between the basal portions of these thicker regions.

The ST segment is the interval between the end of ventricular activation and the beginning of ventricular recovery. The term *ST segment* is used regardless of whether the final wave of the QRS complex is an R or an S wave. The junction of the QRS complex and the ST segment is called the *J point*. The interval from the onset of ventricular activation to the end of ventricular recovery is called the *QT interval*. This term is used regardless of whether the QRS complex begins with a Q or an R wave.

At low heart rates in a healthy person, the PR, ST, and TP segments are at approximately the same level (*isoelectric*). The TP segment between the end of the T or U wave and beginning of the P wave is typically used as the baseline for measuring the amplitudes of the various waveforms.

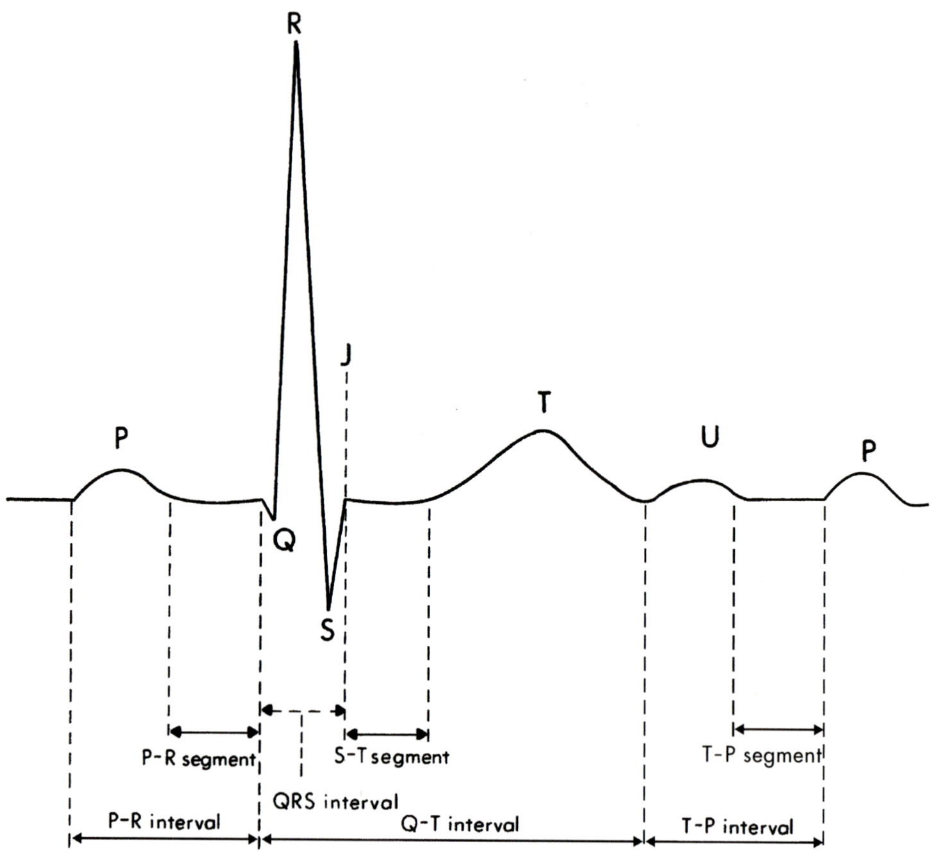

FIGURE 1.12. Magnified cardiac long-axis viewpoint of electrocardiogram segments and time intervals. See **Animation 1.7**.

Recording Short-Axis (Left Versus Right) Cardiac Electrical Activity

It is often important to determine whether an abnormality originates from the left or right side of the heart. The optimal sites for recording left- versus right-sided cardiac electrical activity are located where the extensions of the short axis of the heart intersect with the body surface as illustrated in the schematic transverse plane view (**Figure 1.13** and **Animation 1.8**). The negative electrode on the left posterior thorax (back) and the positive electrode on the right anterior thorax (right of sternum) are aligned perpendicular to the interatrial and interventricular septa, and they are attached to a single-channel ECG recorder. This short-axis "ECG lead" is oriented similarly to a lead termed V_1 on the standard 12-lead ECG (see Chapter 2). The positive electrode for lead V_1 is placed on the anterior thorax in the fourth intercostal space at the right edge of the sternum. The typically diphasic P and T waves and the predominantly negative QRS complex recorded by electrodes at these positions are indicated on the ECG recording.

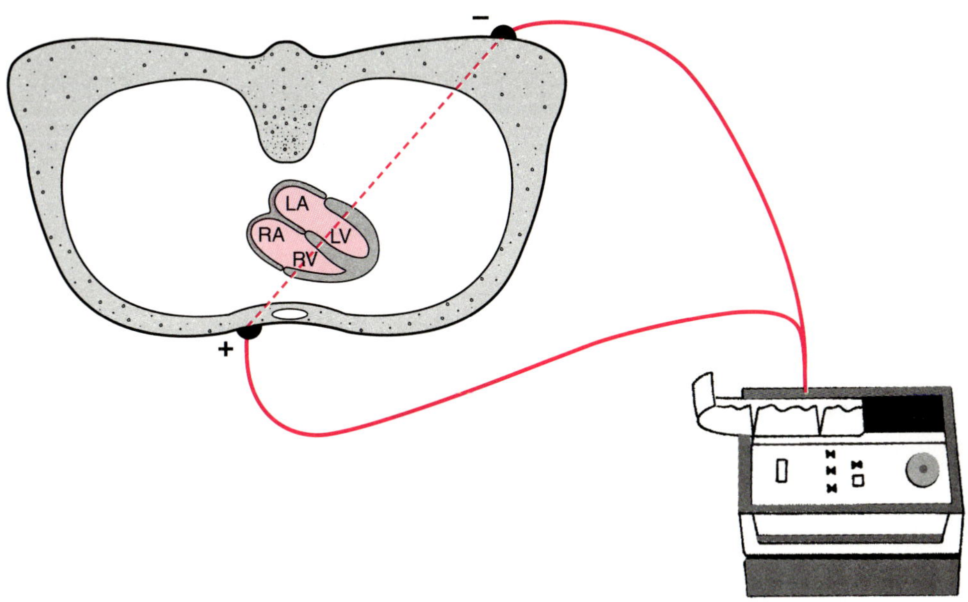

FIGURE 1.13. Optimal recording sites for left- versus right-sided cardiac electrical activity, as viewed from above. Black semiovals represent the electrodes. LA, left atrium; LV, left ventricle; RA, right atrium; RV, right ventricle. See **Animation 1.8**.

The ECG waveforms from the cardiac short-axis viewpoint (see **Figure 1.13**) are magnified in **Figure 1.14** and **Animations 1.9-1.10**), with the principal ECG segments and time intervals indicated. The initial part of the P wave, representing only right-atrial activation, appears positive at this site because of the progression of electrical activity from the interatrial septum toward the right-atrial free wall and the positive electrode. The final part of the P wave, representing only left-atrial activation, appears negative because of progression of electrical activity from the interatrial septum toward the left-atrial free wall and the negative electrode. This activation sequence produces a diphasic P wave.

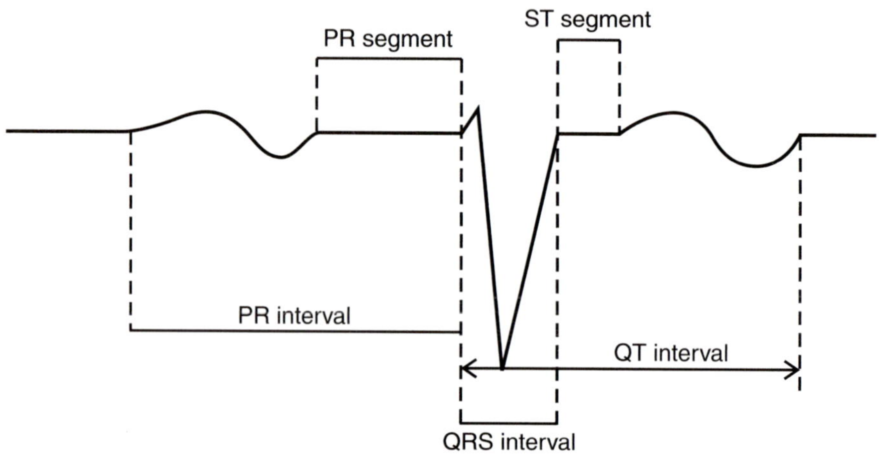

FIGURE 1.14. Magnified cardiac short-axis viewpoint of electrocardiogram segments and time intervals. See **Animations 1.9 and 1.10**.

The initial part of the QRS complex represents the progression of activation in the interventricular septum. This movement is predominantly from the left toward the right side of the septum, producing a positive (R wave) deflection at this left- versus right-sided recording site. The midportion of the QRS complex represents progression of electrical activation through the left- and right-ventricular myocardium. Because the posteriorly positioned left-ventricular free wall is much thicker than the anteriorly placed right-ventricular free wall, its activation predominates over that of the latter, resulting in a deeply negative deflection (S wave). The final portion of the QRS complex represents the completion of activation of the left-ventricular free wall and interventricular septum. This posteriorly directed excitation is represented by the completion of the S wave. The T wave is typically biphasic in this short-axis view, and there is no U wave.

CHAPTER 1 SUMMARY ILLUSTRATION

Electrical activation from the SA node to the ventricular Purkinje fibers

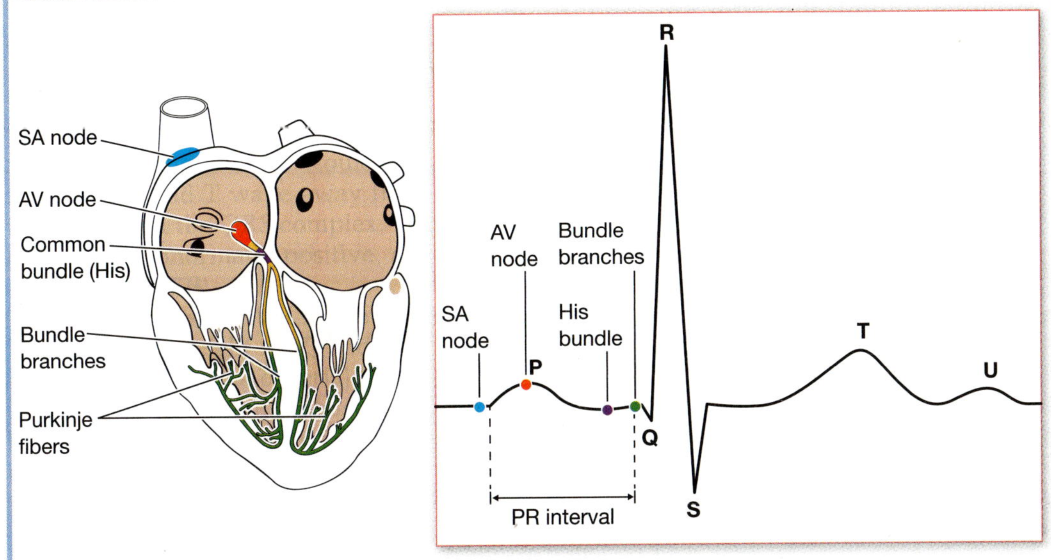

Depolarization/Repolarization and the ECG

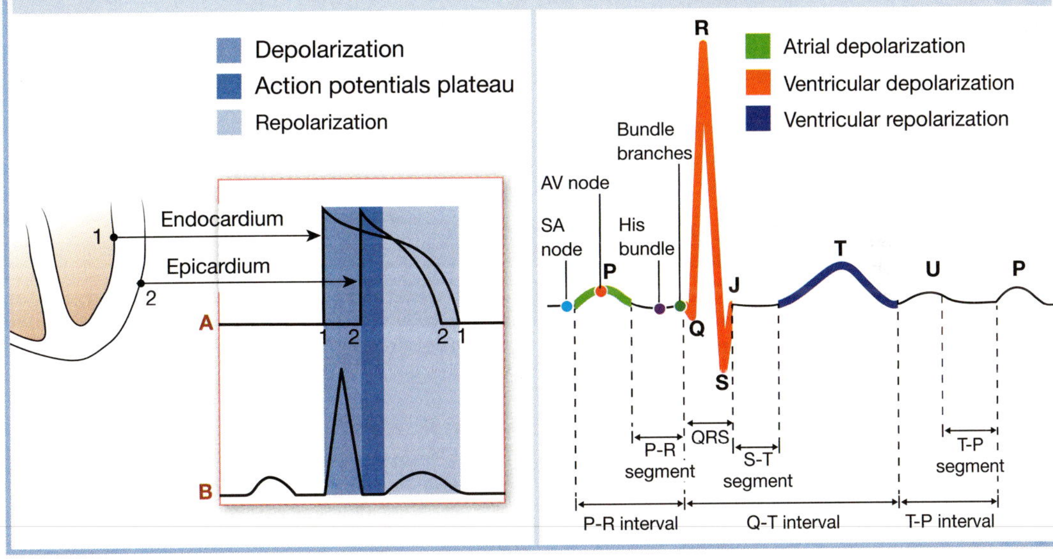

Abbreviations: AV, atrioventricular; SA, sinoatrial.

Glossary

Action potential: the electrical potential recorded from within a cell as it is activated by an electrical current or impulse.

Anterior: located toward the front of the body.

Apex: the region of the heart where the narrowest parts of the ventricles are located. The anatomic "tip" of the heart.

Atrioventricular (AV) node: a small mass of tissue situated in the inferior aspect of the right atrium, adjacent to the septum between the right and left atria. Its function is to slow impulses traveling from the atria to the ventricles, thereby synchronizing atrial and ventricular pumping.

Atrium: a chamber of the heart that receives blood from the veins and passes it along to its corresponding ventricle.

Base: the broad top of the heart where the atria are located.

Baseline: see **Isoelectric line**.

Bundle branches: groups of Purkinje fibers that emerge from the common bundle (of His); the right bundle branch rapidly conducts electrical impulses to the right ventricle, whereas the left bundle branch conducts impulses to the left ventricle.

Cardiac cycle: a single episode of electrical and mechanical activation and recovery of a myocardial cell or of the entire heart.

Cardiac pacemaking and conduction system: groups of modified myocardial cells strategically located throughout the heart and capable of forming an electrical impulse and/or of conducting impulses particularly slowly or rapidly.

Common bundle (of His): a compact group of Purkinje fibers that originates at the AV node and rapidly conducts electrical impulses to the right and left bundle branches.

Deflection: a waveform on the ECG; its direction may be either upward (positive) or downward (negative).

Depolarization: electrical activation of the cell, during which the difference between the electrical charge and potential on the inside versus the outside of the cell becomes minimal. In the resting state, the cell is polarized, with the inside of the cell markedly negative in comparison to the outside. Depolarization is initiated by a current that alters the permeability of the cell membrane, allowing positively charged ions to cross into the cell.

Diastole: the period in which the electrical and mechanical aspects of the heart are in their baseline or resting state: Electrical diastole is characterized by repolarization and mechanical diastole by relaxation. During mechanical diastole, the cardiac chambers are filling with blood.

Diphasic: consisting of two components.

Distal: situated away from the point of attachment or origin; the opposite of proximal.

Electrocardiogram (ECG): the recording made by the electrocardiograph, depicting the electrical activity of the heart.

Electrode: an electrical contact that is placed on the skin and is connected to an ECG recorder.

Endocardium: the inner aspect of a myocardial wall, adjacent to the blood-filled cavity of the corresponding chamber.

Epicardium: the outer aspect of a myocardial wall, adjacent to the pericardial lining that closely envelops the outer surface of the heart.

Fascicle: a small bundle of Purkinje fibers that emerges from a bundle or a bundle branch to rapidly conduct impulses to the endocardial surfaces of the ventricles.

Isoelectric line: a horizontal line on an ECG recording that forms a baseline; representing neither a positive nor a negative electrical potential.

J point: junction of the QRS complex and the ST segment.

Lateral: situated toward either the right or left side of the heart or of the body as a whole.

Monophasic: consisting of a single component, being either positive or negative.

P wave: the first wave depicted on the ECG during a cardiac cycle; it represents atrial activation.

PR interval: the time from onset of the P wave to onset of the QRS complex. This interval represents the time between the onsets of activation of the atrial and the ventricular myocardium.

PR segment: the time from the end of the P wave to the onset of the QRS complex.

Purkinje cells or fibers: modified myocardial cells that are found in the distal aspects of the pacemaking and conduction system, consisting of the common bundle, the bundle branches, the fascicles, and individual strands.

Q wave: a negative wave at the onset of the QRS complex.

QRS complex: the second wave or group of waves depicted on the ECG during a cardiac cycle; it represents ventricular activation (depolarization).

QRS interval: the time from the beginning to the end of the QRS complex, representing the duration required for activation of the ventricular myocardial cells.

QS: a monophasic negative QRS complex.

QT interval: the time from the onset of the QRS complex to the end of the T wave. This interval represents the time from the beginning of ventricular activation to the completion of ventricular recovery.

R wave: the first positive wave appearing in a QRS complex; it may appear at the onset of the QRS complex or following a Q wave.

R′ wave: the second positive wave appearing in a QRS complex.

Repolarization: the transition in which the inside of the cell becomes markedly negative in relation to the outside. This condition is maintained by a pump in the cell membrane, and it is disturbed by the arrival of an electrical current.

Septum: a dividing wall between the atria or between the ventricles.

Sinoatrial (SA) node: a small mass of tissue situated in the superior aspect of the right atrium, adjacent to the entrance of the superior vena cava. It functions as the dominant pacemaker, which forms the electrical impulses that are then conducted throughout the heart.

ST segment: the interval between the end of the QRS complex and the beginning of the T wave.

Superior: situated above and closer to the head than another body part.

Superior vena cava: one of the large veins that empties into the right atrium.

Systole: the period in which the electrical and mechanical aspects of the heart are in their active state: Electrical systole is characterized by depolarization and mechanical systole by contraction. During mechanical systole, blood is being pumped out of the heart.

T wave: the final major wave depicted on the ECG during a cardiac cycle; it represents ventricular recovery.

Triphasic: consisting of three components.

U wave: a wave on the ECG that follows the T wave in some individuals; it is typically small, and its source is uncertain.

Ventricle: a chamber of the heart that receives blood from its corresponding atrium and pumps the blood it receives out into the corresponding great artery.

Waveform: electrocardiographic representation of either the activation or recovery phase of electrical activity of the heart.

Acknowledgment

We gratefully acknowledge the past contributions of the previous edition's author, Dr. Galen S. Wagner, as portions of that chapter were retained in this revision.

References

1. Hoffman BF, Cranefield PF. *Electrophysiology of the Heart*. New York, NY: McGraw-Hill; 1960.
2. Guyton AC. Heart muscle: the heart as a pump. In: Guyton AC, ed. *Textbook of Medical Physiology*. Philadelphia, PA: WB Saunders; 1991.
3. Rushmer RF. Functional anatomy and the control of the heart and electrical activity of the heart, part I. In: Rushmer RF, ed. *Cardiovascular Dynamics*. Philadelphia, PA: WB Saunders; 1976:76-104.
4. Truex RC. The sinoatrial node and its connections with the atrial tissue. In: Wellens HJJ, Lie KI, Janse MJ, eds. *The Conduction System of the Heart*. The Hague, The Netherlands: Martinus Nijhoff; 1978.
5. Becker AE, Anderson RH. Morphology of the human atrioventricular junctional area. In: Wellens HJJ, Lie KI, Janse MJ, eds. *The Conduction System of the Heart*. The Hague, The Netherlands: Martinus Nijhoff; 1978.
6. Guyton AC. Rhythmic excitation of the heart. In: Guyton AC, ed. *Textbook of Medical Physiology*. Philadelphia, PA: WB Saunders; 1991.

2 Recording the Electrocardiogram

DAVID G. STRAUSS, TOBIN H. LIM,
DOUGLAS D. SCHOCKEN, AND
KUMAR NARAYANAN

The Standard 12-Lead Electrocardiogram

Frontal Plane

The standard electrocardiogram (ECG) uses the two viewpoints presented in Chapter 1 (see **Figures 1.8** and **1.13**): base-apex (long axis) and left-right (short axis) plus 10 other viewpoints for recording cardiac electrical activity. Each view is provided by recording the electrical potential difference between a positive and a negative pole, referred to as a *lead*. Six of these leads provide views in the *frontal plane* of the body and six provide views in the transverse (horizontal) plane of the body. A single recording electrode on the body surface serves as the positive pole of each lead; the negative pole of each lead is provided either by a single recording electrode or by a *central terminal* that averages the input from multiple recording electrodes. The device used for recording the ECG, called the *electrocardiograph*, contains the circuitry that creates the "central terminal," which serves as the negative electrode for the nine standard leads that are termed *V leads*.

More than 100 years ago, Einthoven et al[1] placed recording electrodes on the right and left arms and the left leg and called the recording an elektrokardiogramme (EKG), which is replaced by the anglicized ECG throughout this book. Einthoven's work produced three leads (I, II, and III), each produced by a pair of the limb electrodes, with one electrode of the pair serving as the positive and the other as the negative pole of the lead (**Figure 2.1** and **Animation 2.1**). The positive poles of these leads were positioned on the body surface to the left and inferiorly so that the cardiac electrical waveforms would appear primarily upright on the ECG. This waveform direction results because the summations of both the atrial and ventricular electrical forces are generally directed toward the apex of the heart. For lead I, the left arm electrode provides the positive pole and the right arm electrode provides the negative pole. Lead II, with its positive electrode on the left leg and its negative electrode on the right arm, provides a long-axis view of the cardiac electrical activity only slightly different from that presented in Chapter 1 (see **Figures 1.8**, **1.9**, and **1.12**). Lead III has its positive electrode on the left leg and its negative electrode on the left arm. An electrode placed on the right leg is used to ground the system.

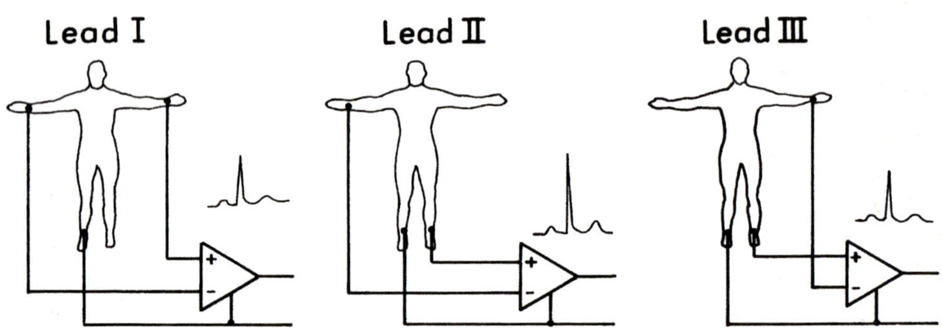

FIGURE 2.1. Einthoven's three original limb leads: (+) positive and (−) negative electrode pairs on distal limb sites. (Modified from Netter FH, ed. *The CIBA Collection of Medical Illustrations*. Summit, NJ: Ciba-Geigy; 1978:51. *Heart*; vol 5, with permission.) See **Animation 2.1**.

To view the animation(s) and video(s) associated with this chapter please access lww.co.in. Instructions are located on the inside front cover.

The three ECG leads (I, II, and III) form an equiangular (60 degree) and, therefore, equilateral triangle known as the *Einthoven triangle* (**Figure 2.2A** and **Animation 2.2**). Picture these three leads so that they intersect in the center of the cardiac electrical activity. Keep their original spatial orientation. You now have a triaxial reference system for viewing the cardiac electrical activity (**Figure 2.2B**). These are the only leads in the standard 12-lead ECG that are recorded using only two body surface electrodes. They are typically called "bipolar leads." Indeed, the other nine leads are also bipolar. Their negative poles are provided by the central terminal.

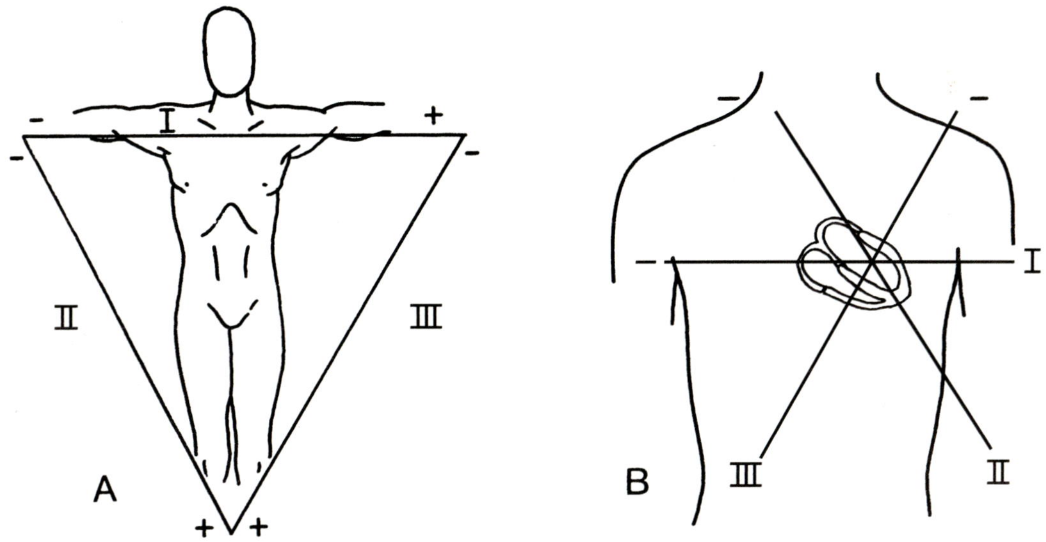

FIGURE 2.2. Leads I, II, and III with positive and negative electrode poles. **A.** Einthoven triangle. **B.** Einthoven triangle in relation to the schematic heart. See **Animation 2.2**.

The 60-degree angles between leads I, II, and III create wide gaps among the three views of the cardiac electrical activity. Wilson and coworkers[2] developed a method for filling these gaps without additional body surface electrodes: They created a central terminal by connecting the three limb electrodes on the right and left arms and the left leg. An ECG lead using this central terminal as its negative pole and a recording electrode on the body surface as its positive pole is termed a *V lead*, as stated earlier.

When the central terminal, however, is connected to a recording electrode on a limb to produce an additional frontal plane lead, the resulting electrical signals are small. These small signals occur because the electrical signal from the recording electrode is partially cancelled when both the positive electrode and one of the three elements of the negative electrode are located on the same extremity. The amplitude of these signals may be increased or "augmented" by disconnecting the central terminal from the electrode on the limb serving as the positive pole. Such an augmented V lead is termed an *aV lead*. The "wavy" lines in the figure indicate resistors on the connections between two of the recording electrodes that produce the negative poles for each of the aV leads. For example, lead aVR fills the gap between leads I and II by recording the potential difference between the right arm and the average of the potentials on the left arm and left leg (**Figure 2.3** and **Animation 2.3**). Lead aVR, like lead II, provides a long-axis viewpoint of the cardiac electrical activity but with the opposite orientation from that provided by lead II, as presented in Chapter 1, **Figure 1.8**. The gap between leads II and III is filled by lead aVF, and the gap between leads III and I is filled by lead aVL. The three aV frontal plane leads were introduced by Goldberger.[3]

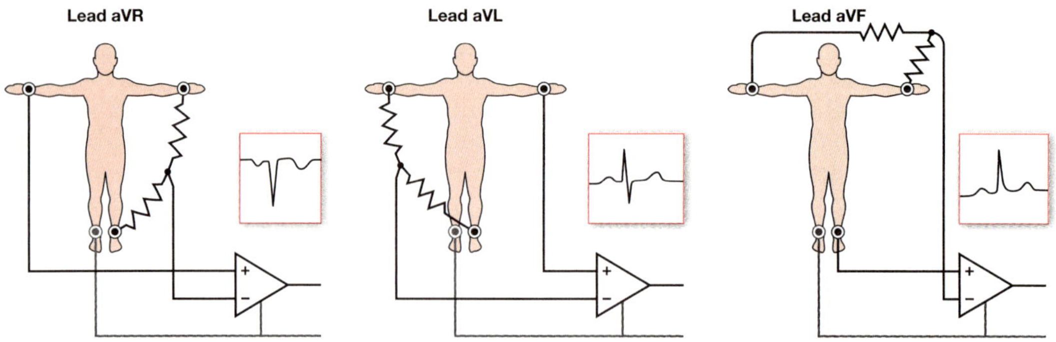

FIGURE 2.3. Positive (+) and negative (−) poles for each of the augmented V leads. See **Animation 2.3**.

Figure 2.2B is reproduced with the addition of the three aV leads to the triaxial reference system, producing a hexaxial system (**Figure 2.4** and **Animation 2.4**) for viewing the cardiac electrical activity in the frontal plane. Five of the six leads of this system are separated by angles of only 30 degrees. The exception is lead aVR because its positive electrode on the right arm is oriented to −150 degrees.

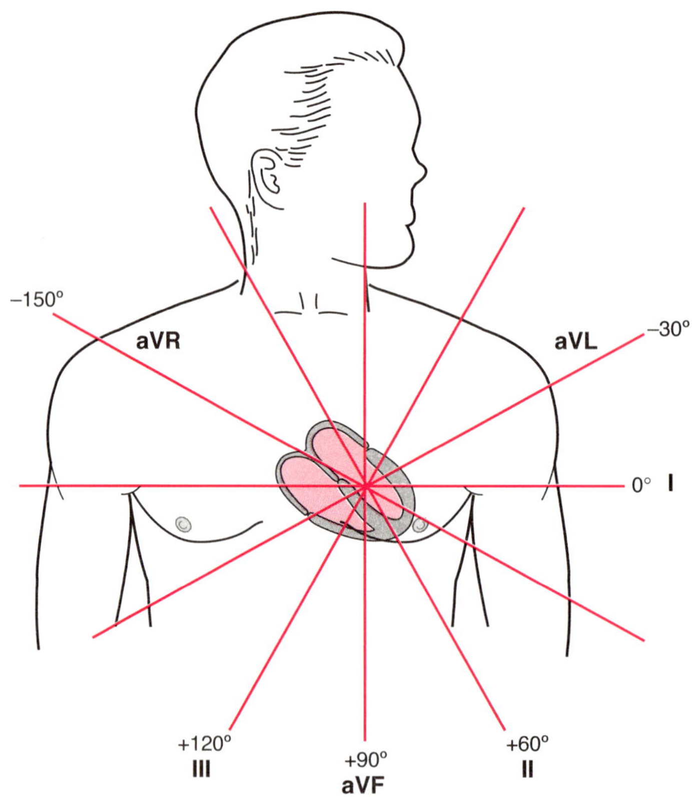

FIGURE 2.4. Frontal plane limb leads that are named according to the locations of their positive electrodes. See **Animation 2.4**.

This arrangement of leads provides a 360-degree perspective of the frontal plane similar to the positions of the 2, 3, 5, 6, 7, and 10 on the face of a clock. By convention, the degrees are arranged as shown. With lead I (located at 0 degrees) used as the reference lead, positive designations increase in 30-degree increments in a clockwise direction to +180 degrees, and negative designations increase by the same increments in a counterclockwise direction to −180 degrees. Lead II appears at +60 degrees, lead aVF at +90 degrees, and lead III at +120 degrees. Leads aVL and aVR have designations of −30 and −150 degrees, respectively. The negative poles of each of these leads complete the "clock face." (See also **Figure 2.11** later in this chapter.)

Modern electrocardiographs, using digital technology, record leads I and II only and then calculate the voltages in the remaining limb leads in real time on the basis of Einthoven law: I + III = II.[1] The algebraic outcome of the formulas for calculating the voltages in aV leads from leads I, II, and III are the following:

$$aVR = -\tfrac{1}{2}(I + II)$$
$$aVL = I - \tfrac{1}{2}(II)$$
$$aVF = II - \tfrac{1}{2}(I)$$

Thus,

$$aVR + aVL + aVF = 0$$

Transverse Plane

The standard 12-lead ECG includes the six frontal plane leads of the hexaxial system and six additional leads relating to the *transverse plane* of the body. These additional leads, introduced by Wilson et al,[4] are produced by using the central terminal of the hexaxial system as the negative pole and electrodes placed at various positions on the anterior and left lateral chest wall as positive poles.[4-7] Because the positions of these latter leads are immediately in front of the heart, they are termed *precordial*. Because the positive poles of these leads are provided from an electrode that is not included in the central terminal, no "augmentation" of the recorded waveforms is required. The six additional leads used to produce the 12-lead ECG are labeled V_1 through V_6.

Figure 2.5 shows lead V_1, with its positive pole on the right anterior precordium and its negative pole in the center of the cardiac electrical activity. Therefore, this lead provides a short-axis view of cardiac electrical activity that is useful for distinguishing left versus right location of various abnormal conditions as described (see **Figure 1.13**). The wavelike lines in the figure indicate resistors in the connections between the recording electrodes on the three limb leads that produce the negative poles for each of the V leads.

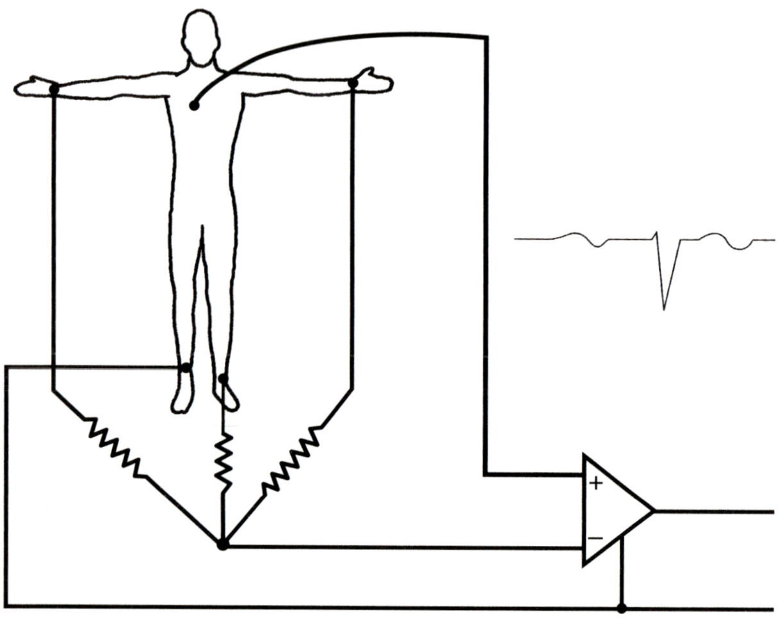

FIGURE 2.5. Positive (+) and negative (−) poles for precordial lead V_1 (right anterior precordium) (+) and negative pole (−) in the center of the cardiac electrical activity.

The body surface positions of each of these electrodes are determined by bony landmarks on the thorax (**Figure 2.6**). The clavicles should be used as a reference for locating the first rib. The space between the first and second ribs is called the *first intercostal space*, the space between the second and third ribs is called the *second intercostal space*, and so on. The V_1 electrode is placed in the *fourth* intercostal space just to the right of the *sternum*. The V_2 electrode is placed in the fourth intercostal space just to the left of the sternum (directly anterior to the center of cardiac electrical activity), and electrode V_4 is placed in the fifth intercostal space on the *midclavicular line*. Placement of electrode V_3 is then halfway along a straight line between electrodes V_2 and V_4. Electrodes V_5 and V_6 are positioned directly lateral to electrode V_4, with electrode V_5 in the *anterior axillary line* and electrode V6 in the *midaxillary line*. In women, electrodes V_4 and V_5 should be positioned on the chest wall beneath the breast.

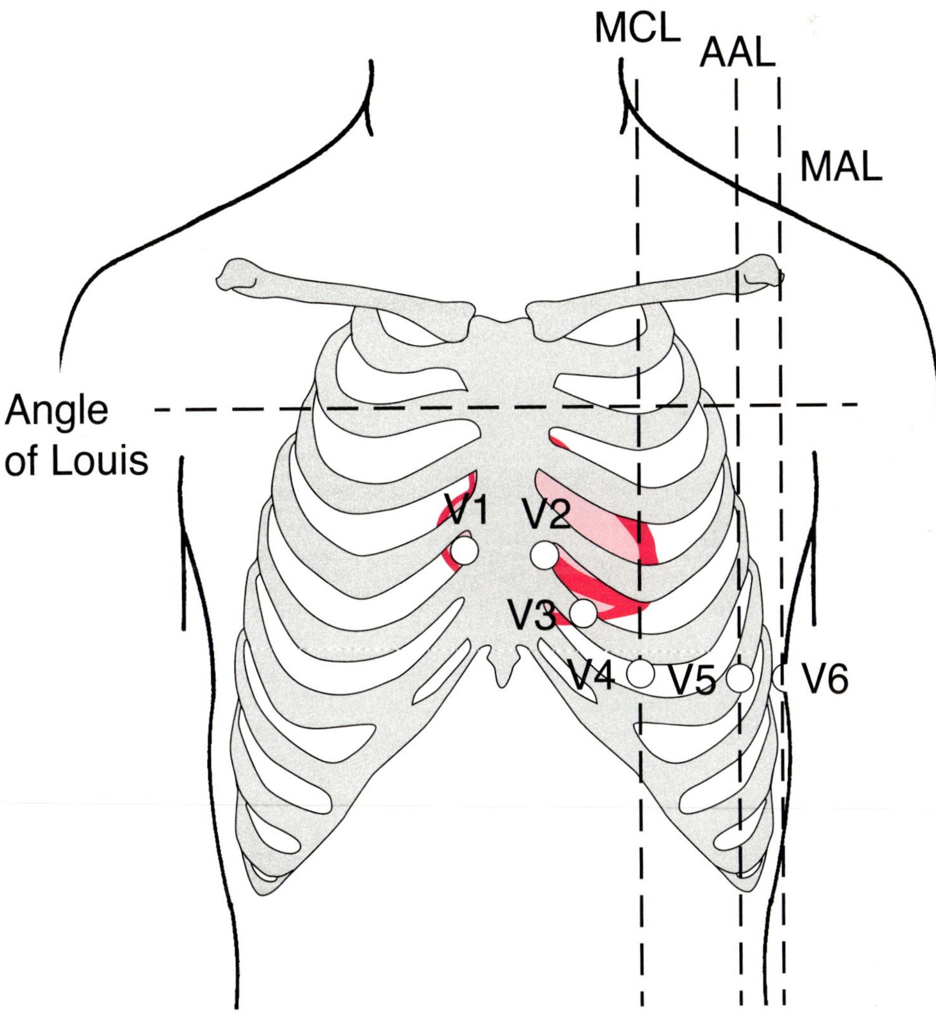

FIGURE 2.6. Bony landmarks for electrode positions. Open circles and semicircle are electrodes. Dashed vertical lines are the midclavicular (MCL) (through lead V_4), anterior axillary (AAL) (through lead V_5), and midaxillary (MAL) (through lead V_6). Dashed horizontal line is along the angle of Louis (costochondral junction of the second ribs). (Modified with permission from Thaler MS, ed. *The Only EKG Book You'll Ever Need*. Philadelphia, PA: JB Lippincott; 1988:41.)

Placement of V Leads on the Precordium (see **Figure 2.6**)

- V_1 fourth ICS to the right of the sternum
- V_2 fourth ICS to the left of the sternum
- V_3 midway between V_2 and V_4
- V_4 fifth ICS at MCL
- V_5 lateral to V_4 in AAL
- V_6 lateral to V_5 in MAL

Abbreviations: AAL, anterior axillary line; ICS, intercostal space; MAL, midaxillary line; MCL, midclavicular line.

Figure 2.7 (**Animation 2.5**) shows the orientation of the six chest leads from each of their positive electrode sites through the approximate center of cardiac electrical activity. The angles between the six transverse plane leads are approximately 30 degrees as in the frontal plane (see **Figure 2.4**). Lead positions when viewed from above are at 11, 12, 1, 2, 3, and 4 on the face of a clock. Extension of these lines through the chest indicates the opposite positions on the chest that would complete the clock face, which can be considered the locations of the negative poles of the six precordial leads. The same format as in **Figure 2.4** indicates the angles on the clock face.

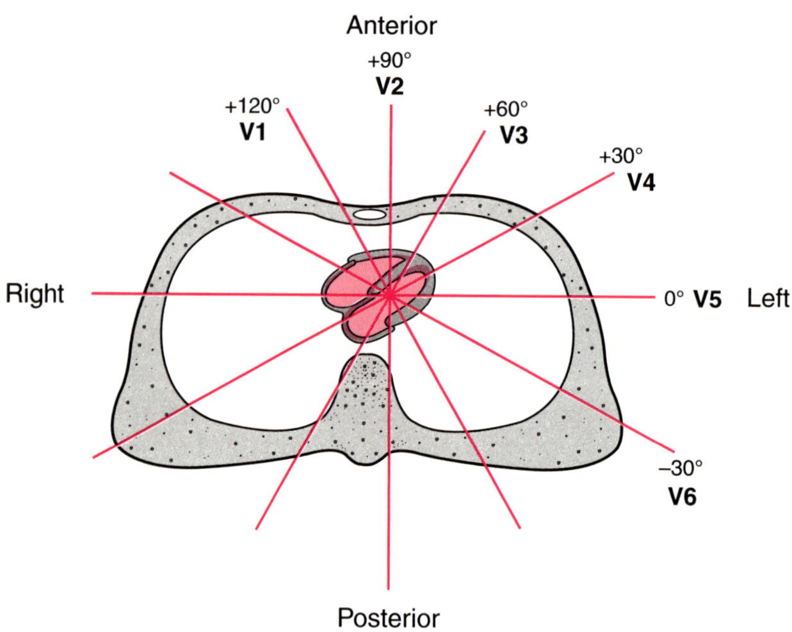

FIGURE 2.7. Transverse plane chest leads as viewed from below. Solid red lines represent the six precordial leads that are named according to the locations of their positive electrodes. See **Animation 2.5**.

Correct and Incorrect Electrode Placements

A single cardiac cycle from each of the standard 12 ECG leads of a healthy individual, recorded with all nine recording electrodes positioned correctly, is shown in **Figure 2.8A**. An accurate electrocardiographic interpretation is possible only if the recording electrodes are placed in their proper positions on the body surface. The three frontal plane electrodes (right arm, left arm, and left leg) used for recording the six limb leads should be placed at distal positions on the designated extremity. It is important to note that when more proximal positions are used, particularly on the left arm,[6] marked distortion of the QRS complex may occur. The distal limb positions provide "clean" recordings when the individual maintains the extremities in "resting" positions.

There can be many errors in the placement of the nine ECG electrodes. This includes reversal of any pair of the six chest electrodes. Reversal of the positions of the V_1 and V_2 electrodes produces the recording shown in **Figure 2.8B**.

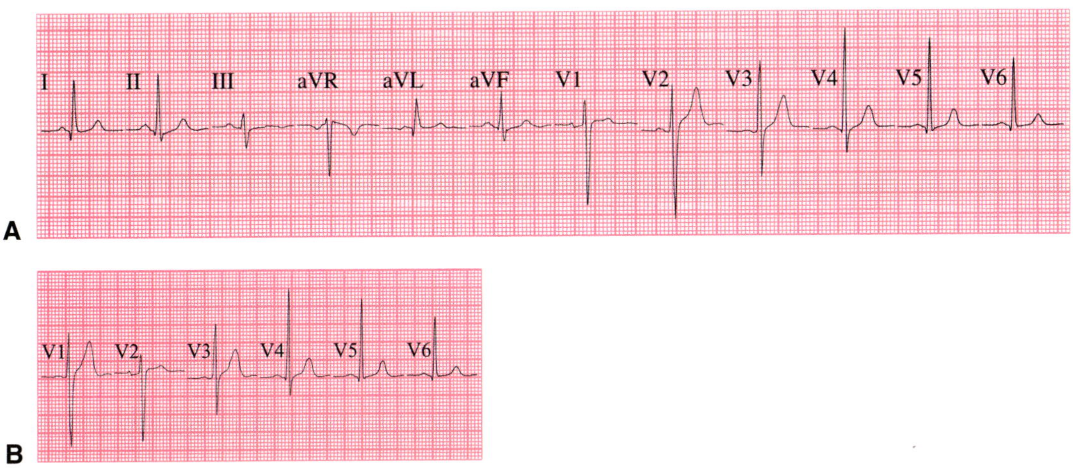

FIGURE 2.8. **A.** Normal electrocardiogram. **B.** Precordial lead reversal. *(continued)*

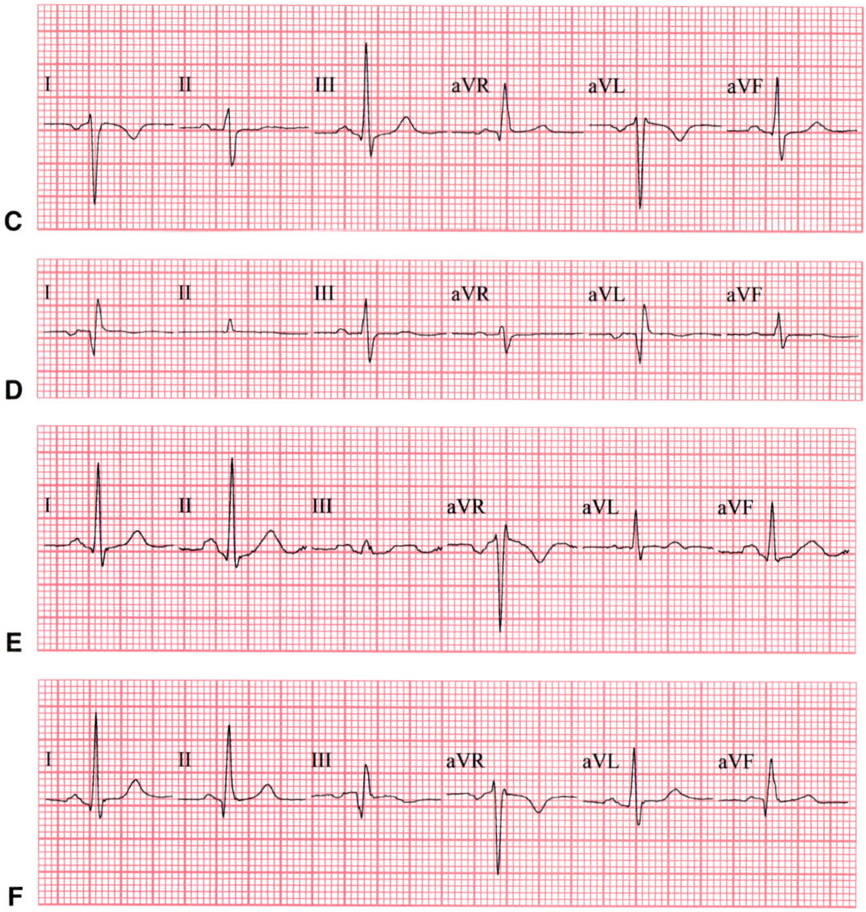

FIGURE 2.8. *(continued)* **C–F.** Limb lead reversals.

Figures 2.8C through **2.8F** present examples of ECG recordings produced by incorrect placement of a limb electrode on the same individual, as described. The most common error in frontal plane recording results from reversal of two of the electrodes. One example of this is reversal of the right and left arm electrodes (see **Figure 2.8C**). In this instance, lead I is inverted, leads II and III are reversed, leads aVR and aVL are reversed, and lead aVF is correct. Another example that produces a characteristic ECG pattern is reversal of the right leg grounding electrode with one of the arm electrodes. Extremely low amplitudes of all waveforms appear in lead II when the right arm electrode is on the right leg (see **Figure 2.8D**) and in lead III when the left arm electrode is on the right leg (see **Figure 2.8E**). These amplitudes are so low because the potential difference between the two legs is almost zero. Left arm and leg electrode reversal is the most difficult to detect; lead III is inverted and leads I and II and aVL and aVF are reversed (see **Figure 2.8F**).

However, a more common error in transverse plane recording involves failure to place the individual electrodes according to their designated landmarks (see **Figure 2.6**). Precise identification of the bony landmarks for proper electrode placement may be difficult in women, obese individuals, and persons with chest wall deformities. Even slight alterations of the position of these electrodes may significantly distort the appearance of the cardiac waveforms. Comparison of serial ECG recordings relies on precise electrode placement.

Figure 2.9 shows a screen shot of ECG simulation software that allows the user to interchange and misplace electrodes. **Video 2.1** available with the online version of the book demonstrates the effects of misplacement of precordial and limb electrodes.

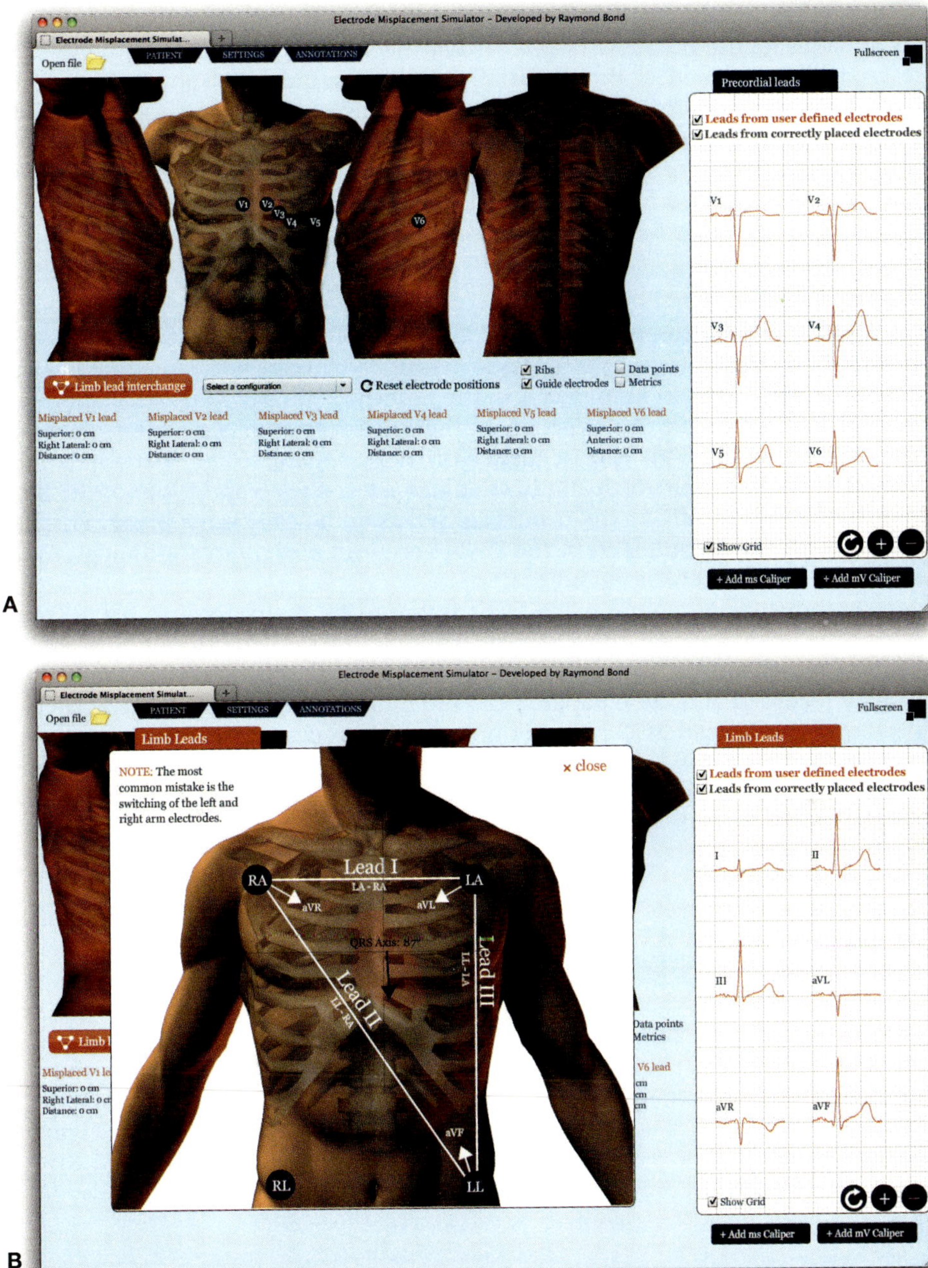

FIGURE 2.9. Screenshot of ECG simulation software that allows the user to interchange and misplace electrodes. **Video 2.1** available with the online version of the book demonstrates how to use the software and discusses typical electrode misplacements and how they appear on the precordial (**A**) or limb (**B**) leads. After viewing **Video 2.1**, the software can be downloaded at http://goo.gl/zlZoCe for further exploration of electrode misplacements. LA, left arm; LL, left leg; RA, right arm; RL, right leg.

Alternative Displays of the 12 Standard Electrocardiogram Leads

Alternative displays of the 12-lead electrocardiogram (ECG) may help improve ECG diagnostic capability and the ability of the ECG to display different waveform morphologies. Each lead provides its unique view of the cardiac electrical activity, but only the six chest leads are typically displayed in their spatially ordered sequence. The six limb leads are displayed in their two classical sequences (two columns of three leads—I, II, and III and aVR, aVL, and aVF; **Figure 2.10A**). This limitation in the standard display becomes most clinically important for the diagnosis of acute myocardial *ischemia* and infarction; ST-segment elevation in two or more spatially adjacent leads is the cornerstone for an ST-segment elevation myocardial infarction (see Chapters 7 and 8).

Cabrera Sequence

Only in Sweden and scattered other places are the six frontal plane leads integrated into the single orderly sequence from aVL to III, as described by Cabrera.[8] Note that lead aVR in the classical sequence is inverted to −aVR in the orderly sequence to provide another long-axis orientation as lead II. The "10" position on the clock face of lead aVR is replaced by the "4" position of lead −aVR. This lead sequence provides six individual spatially contiguous leads (aVL to III) and five pairs of spatially contiguous leads (aVL and I; I and −aVR; −aVR and II; II and aVF; aVF and III) in the frontal as well as in the transverse plane. This alternative limb lead display was endorsed in the 2000 European Society of Cardiology/American College of Cardiology consensus guidelines.[9]

The orderly sequence of frontal plane leads followed by the transverse plane leads provides a panoramic display[10] of cardiac electrical activity proceeding from left (aVL) to right (III) and then from right (V1) to left (V6; **Figure 2.10B**). The Swedish version of the panoramic display recorded at double paper speed (50 mm/s) is shown in **Figure 2.10C**.

This display of the 12-lead ECG provides orderly views covering a 150-degree arc in both frontal and transverse planes, which encompasses views of a majority of the left-ventricular myocardium. However, there are some left-ventricular walls in which ischemia and infarction can occur that lie outside these arcs, as presented in Chapter 6.

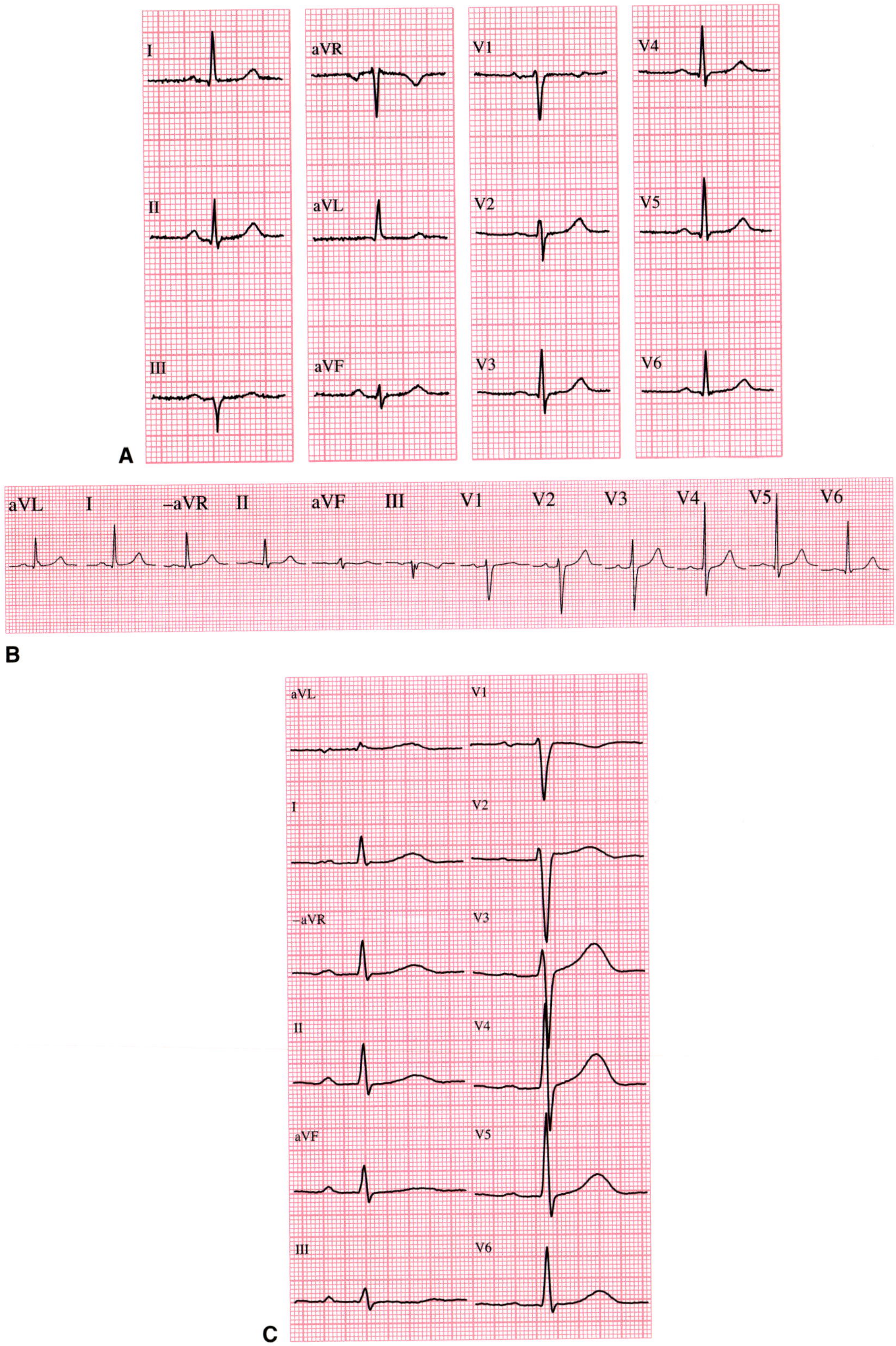

FIGURE 2.10. **A.** Classical display. **B.** Single horizontal display. **C.** Parallel vertical displays.

Twenty-four–Lead Electrocardiogram

Just as lead −aVR in the Cabrera sequence provides an alternative to lead aVR in the classical sequence, the remaining inverted leads provide 11 additional views of the cardiac electrical activity. Thus, the "12-lead ECG" can potentially serve as a "24-lead ECG." **Figures 2.4** and **2.7** are reproduced with all 24 positive and negative leads of an ECG positioned around the frontal and transverse plane clock faces (**Figure 2.11** and **Animation 2.6**). When a schematic view of the heart in its anatomic position is displayed in the center of the clock, all 24 views provide complete panoramic displays in each of the planes.

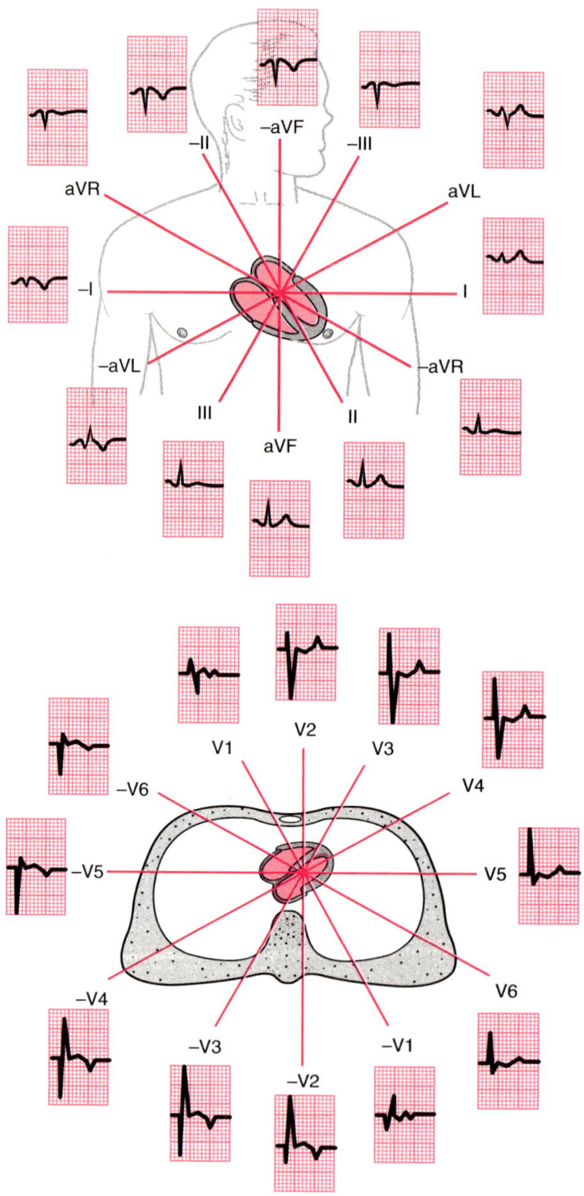

FIGURE 2.11. Clock faces. Top. Frontal plane, as seen from the front. Bottom. Transverse plane, as seen from below. See **Animation 2.6**.

Continuous Monitoring

The standard electrode placement sites are not ideal for continuous monitoring of cardiac electrical activity (eg, standard sites produce a recording obscured by skeletal muscle potentials and *artifacts*, especially during ambulatory monitoring). Monitoring may be performed at the bedside, during routine activity, or during exercise stress testing.

Monitoring

There is currently a transition from replacing electrodes for each ECG recording to keeping the electrodes in place for serial recordings. Such "monitoring" has been routine for surveillance in cardiac arrhythmias and during stress testing. However, monitoring is now being adopted for ischemic surveillance. Indeed, the term diagnostic monitoring is now used, requiring multiple views of the cardiac electrical activity. Either 3 orthogonal leads or all 12 standard leads are used for ischemia monitoring. The ECG waveforms are somewhat altered by all monitoring methods. Movement of limb electrodes to torso positions produces altered views for all limb leads, and an altered central terminal produces altered negative pole for all chest leads. In many monitoring methods, the number of chest leads is reduced for efficiency of recording. The missing leads are derived from those recorded, creating further waveform alterations. Therefore, changes observed during monitoring should be viewed in relation to a baseline recording using these leads rather than the standard leads.

Clinical Situation

BEDSIDE. When monitoring for disturbances of cardiac *rhythm*, electrodes should be placed outside the left parasternal area to allow easy access for clinical examination of the heart and possible use of an external defibrillator. A modified lead, modified chest lead V_1 (*MCL_1*), with the positive electrode in the same position as lead V_1 and the negative electrode near the left shoulder, typically provides good visualization of atrial activity (**Figure 2.12**, specifically **Figure 2.12C**) and differentiation of left versus right cardiac activity (see **Figures 1.13** and **1.14**).

When monitoring for evidence of ischemia, a complete set of 12 leads may be preferred for recording the ECG. Krucoff and associates[11] described the usefulness of continuous ST-segment monitoring with 12 leads during various unstable coronary syndromes. Some of the major applications of this technique include detection of reoccluded coronary arteries after percutaneous coronary interventions, detection of *reperfusion* and *reocclusion* during acute myocardial infarction,[12,13] and surveillance during acute coronary syndrome.

ROUTINE AMBULATORY ACTIVITY. The method of continuous monitoring and recording of cardiac electrical activity is referred to as Holter monitoring[14] after its developer. Originally, only one lead was used. In monitoring for abnormalities of cardiac rhythm, the American Heart Association recommends use of a "V_1-type" lead, with the positive electrode in the fourth right intercostal space 2.5 cm from the sternum and the negative electrode below the left clavicle. Currently, three relatively orthogonal leads are used to provide views in all three dimensions (left-right, superior-inferior, and anterior-posterior). This provides the redundancy for electrocardiographic information should one or more leads fail. The EASI lead system method (see **Figure 2.12**) results in a derived 12-lead ECG.

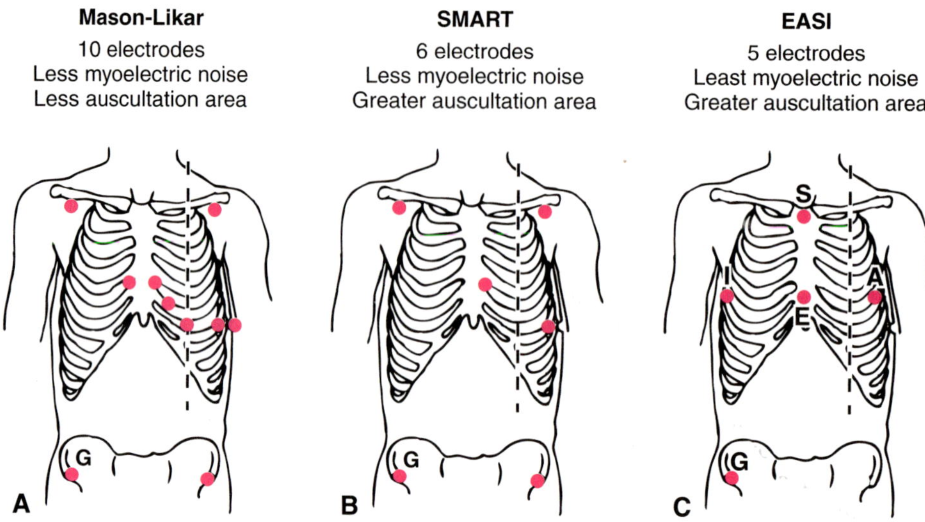

FIGURE 2.12. Electrode placement methods for electrocardiogram monitoring. Circles represent the electrode positions. **A.** Mason-Likar system—standard 12-lead ECG precordial leads with limb electrodes moved proximally. **B.** SMART (Simon Meij Algorithm Reconstruction) system—proximal limb electrodes as with Mason-Likar but only precordial electrodes for V_2 and V_5 (others are derived). **C.** EASI system—E, A, S, and I are the "EASI" system electrode placements, where E, A and I are the position of the Frank vectorcardiographic lead system and S is for sternum. Electrode placement G indicates position of the ground electrode.

EXERCISE STRESS TESTING. The ECG monitoring during exercise stress testing is typically performed to diagnose or evaluate cardiac ischemia owing to increased metabolic demand. Typically, all 12 leads are monitored with the limb leads in the torso sites, as originally described by Mason and Likar.[15]

Bony landmarks on the torso provide alternative sites for the right and left arm and leg electrodes that are required for continuous monitoring. Ideally, these sites (1) avoid skeletal muscle artifact, (2) provide stability for the recording electrodes, and (3) record waveforms similar to those from the limb sites. The Mason-Likar[15] system (see **Figure 2.3A**) and modified Mason-Likar[16] system have been used for continuous ST-segment monitoring. The resultant recordings from both, however, have some features that differ from the standard 12-lead recording.[16,17]

Methods other than the original or modified Mason-Likar method for continuous 12-lead ECG monitoring using alternative electrode placement and reduced electrode sites have emerged: (1) reduced electrode sets and (2) EASI. Both are alternative methods of ECG reconstruction based on bipolar orthogonal leads measured through both space and time, called vectorcardiography. Transformation of the vectorcardiogram to a 12-lead ECG[18] has shown that the 12-lead ECG can be reconstructed with good approximation using a mathematical transformation matrix.

Reduced electrode sets from the standard 12-lead ECG eliminate excessive electrodes and electrode wires that interfere with precordial examination. This method is based on systematically removing precordial leads that provide redundant information. These fewer, selectively chosen leads contain sufficient diagnostic information for 12-lead reconstruction. Removed precordial leads are reconstructed from existing limb and precordial leads based on general and specific patient coefficients calculated from the patient's existing 12-lead ECG.[19] The Simon Meij Algorithm Reconstruction (SMART) method[19] uses Mason-Likar torso sites and the six electrodes required for leads I, II, V_2, and V_5 for reconstructing precordial leads V_1, V_3, V_4, and V_6 (**Figure 2.12**).

The EASI system, introduced by Dower et al,[18] uses five electrodes (see **Figure 2.12C**). Through mathematical transformations, a reconstructed 12-lead ECG is produced.[18,20] Positions I, E, and A are incorporated from the Frank vectorcardiographic system. The E is placed on the inferior most aspect of the sternal body. The I and A are placed on the left and right midaxillary lines, respectively, in the same transverse plane as E. The S is placed on the superiormost aspect of the sternal manubrium.

Advantages in using the reconstructive lead placement method (EASI or Simon Meij Algorithm Reconstruction) over the Mason-Likar are listed in **Figure 2.12B,C**. Other advantages include continuous monitoring, clear anatomic landmarks for electrode placement (EASI), reproducibility, and time and cost savings (by using fewer electrodes). Thus, it is likely that both reconstructive lead placement methods can be used for diagnostic ECG monitoring of myocardial ischemia and cardiac rhythm abnormalities.

Alternative Electrode Placement

Clinical Indications

Several reasons exist for selecting alternative sites for placement of ECG electrodes: unavailable standard site(s), specific cardiac abnormalities, and continuous monitoring. These sites should be prominently noted on the recording. If the standard lead locations are not used, the recording should be prominently so annotated.

Standard Site(s) Unavailable

Standard electrode placement sites may be unavailable because of patient pathology (eg, amputation or burns) or other impediments (eg, bandages). In these instances, the electrodes should be positioned as closely as possible to the standard sites and the lead or leads affected by the nonstandard electrode placement clearly designated.

Specific Cardiac Abnormalities

The standard electrode placement sites may not be in the optimal position to detect a particular cardiac waveform or abnormality (eg, P waves obscured within T waves or *situs inversus dextrocardia*). Detection of P waves requires sufficient time between cardiac cycles to provide a baseline between the end of the T wave and the beginning of the next QRS complex. In the presence of a rapid cardiac rate (*tachycardia*), alternative electrode placement may produce a lead that reveals recognizable atrial activity (**Figure 2.13A**). Alternative lead placement methods include (1) moving the positive V_1 electrode one intercostal space above its standard site, (2) using this site for the positive V_1 electrode and the *xiphoid process* of the sternum for the negative V_1 electrode, or (3) using a transesophageal site for the positive V_1 electrode.

When the congenital position of the heart is rightward (situs inversus dextrocardia), the right and left arm electrodes should be reversed (and the precordial leads should be recorded from rightward-oriented positive electrodes progressing from V_1R [V_2] to V_6R) (**Figure 2.13B**). Right-ventricular *hypertrophy* and infarction may best be detected via an electrode in the V_3R or V_4R position. In infants, in whom the right ventricle is normally more prominent, standard lead V_3 is often replaced by lead V_4R.

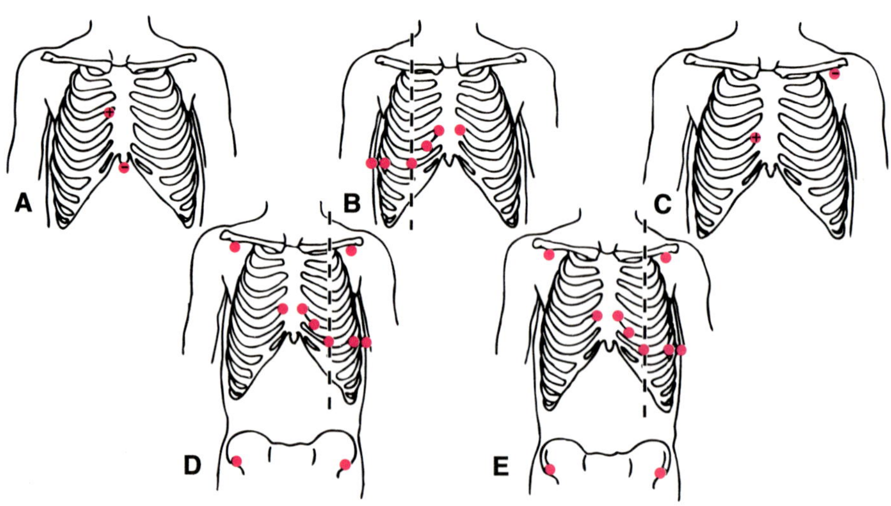

FIGURE 2.13. Positive and negative poles of a single electrocardiogram lead are shown in **A** and **C**. Precordial V electrode locations are shown in **B**, **D**, and **E**. Torso locations of positive electrodes are shown in **D** and **E**. The vertical dashed lines indicate the midclavicular line in **B**, **D**, and **E**.

Experimental studies have used body surface maps with multiple rows of electrodes on the anterior and posterior torso to identify specific cardiac abnormalities. This technique improves the ability to diagnose clinical problems such as left-ventricular hypertrophy or various locations of myocardial infarction.[7]

Other Practical Points for Recording the Electrocardiogram

Care should be taken to ensure that technique is uniform from one ECG recording to another.

Key Points

The following points are important to consider when preparing to record an ECG.

1. Electrodes should be selected for maximum adhesiveness and minimum discomfort, electrical noise, and skin-electrode impedance. The standards for electrodes published by the American Association for the Advancement of Medical Instrumentation[21] should be followed.
2. Effective contact between electrode and skin is essential. Sites with skin irritation or skeletal abnormalities should be avoided. The skin should be cleaned with only a dry wipe. Poor electrode contact or slight body movement may produce instability of the baseline recording termed *baseline wander*, when the instability occurs gradually, or shifting baseline, when the instability occurs abruptly (**Figure 2.14A** shown at half scale for illustrative purposes).
3. Calibration of the ECG signal is typically 1 mV = 10 mm. When large QRS waveform amplitudes require that calibration be reduced to 1 mV = 5 mm, this should be noted to facilitate interpretation.
4. The ECG paper speed is typically 25 mm per second, and variations used for particular clinical purposes should be noted. A faster speed may be used to provide a clearer depiction of waveform morphology, and a slower speed may be used to provide visualization of a greater number of cardiac cycles to facilitate rhythm analysis.

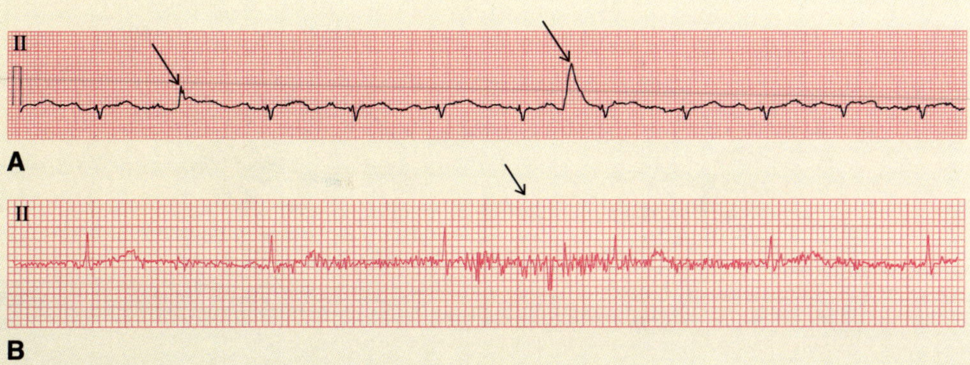

FIGURE 2.14. **A.** Shifting baseline. Arrows show movement during the second cycle and between the sixth and seventh cycles. **B.** Noisy baseline. Arrow shows the area of maximal baseline deformity.

(continued)

Key Points (continued)

5. Electrical artifacts in the ECG may be external or internal. External artifacts introduced by line current (50 or 60 Hz) may be minimized by straightening the lead wires so that they are aligned with the patient's body. Internal artifacts may result from muscle tremors, shivering, hiccups, or other factors, producing a "noisy baseline" (**Figure 2.14B**).
6. It is important that the patient remain supine during recording of the ECG. If another position is clinically required, notation of the altered position should be made. Lying on either side or elevation of the torso may change the position of the heart within the chest. A change in body position may affect the accuracy of an ECG recording[22] similar to a change in electrode placement.

CHAPTER 2 SUMMARY ILLUSTRATION

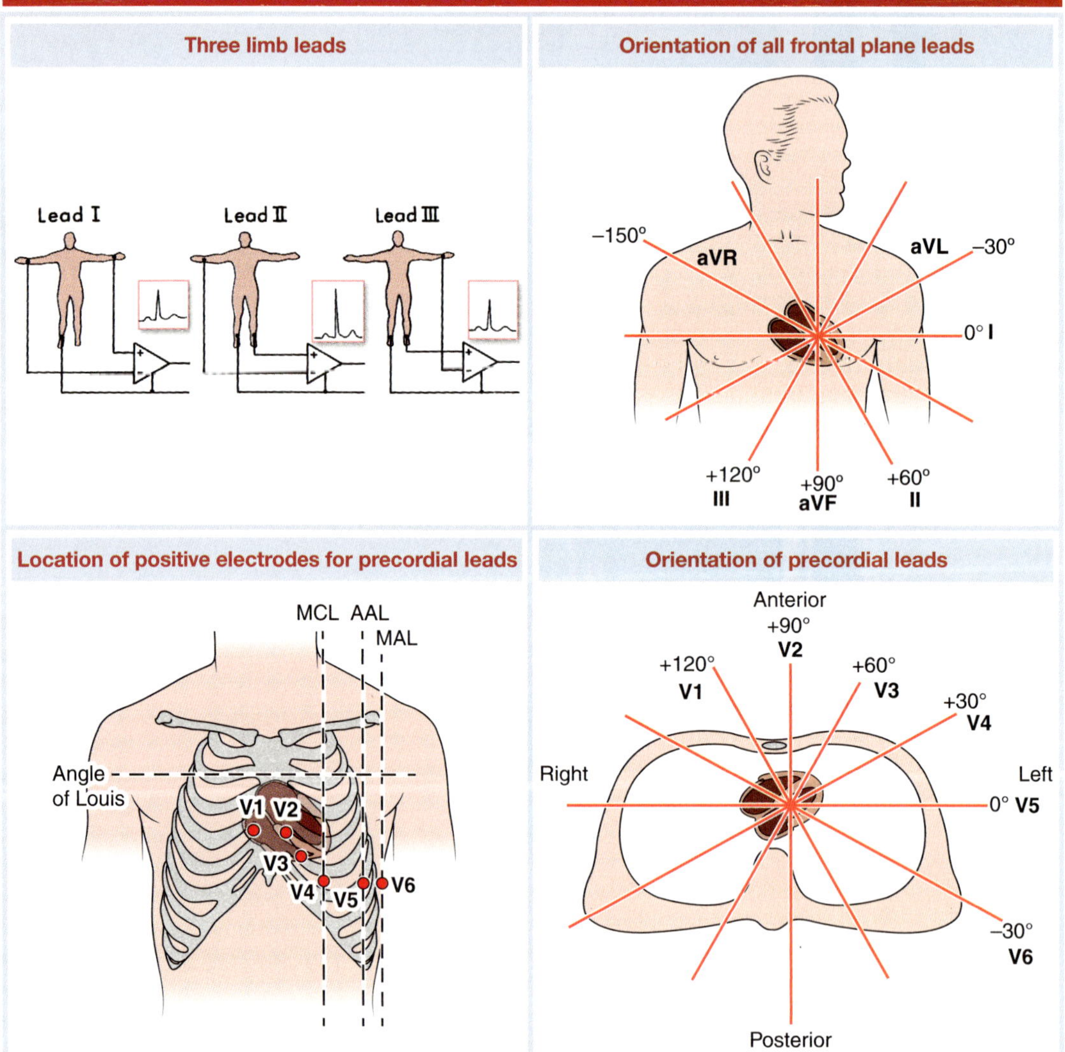

Abbreviations: AAL, anterior axillary line; MAL, midaxillary line; MCL, midclavicular line.

Glossary

Anterior axillary line: a vertical line on the thorax at the level of the anterior aspect of the axilla, which is the area where the arm joins the body.

Artifact: an electrocardiographic waveform that arises from sources other than the myocardium.

aV lead: an augmented V lead (see following text) that uses a modified central terminal with inputs from the electrode on the designated limb (R for right arm, L for left arm, and F for left foot) as its positive pole and the average of the potentials from the leads on the other two limbs as its negative pole.

Baseline wander: a back-and-forth movement of the isoelectric line or baseline, interfering with precise measurement of the various ECG waveforms; sometimes termed *baseline shift* when it is abrupt.

Central terminal: a terminal created by Wilson and colleagues[2] that connects all three limb electrodes through a 5000 Ω resistor so that it can serve as the negative pole for an exploring positive electrode to form a V lead.

Einthoven triangle: an equilateral triangle composed of limb leads I, II, and III that provides an orientation for electrical information from the frontal plane.

Electrocardiograph: a device used to record the ECG.

Frontal plane: a vertical plane of the body (also called the *coronal plane*) that is perpendicular to both the horizontal and sagittal planes.

Hypertrophy: an increase in muscle mass; it most commonly occurs in the ventricles when they are compensating for a pressure (systolic) overload.

Infarct: an area of necrosis in an organ resulting from an obstruction in its blood supply.

Intercostal: situated between the ribs.

Ischemia: an insufficiency of blood flow to an organ that is so severe that it disrupts the function of the organ; in the heart, ischemia is often accompanied by precordial pain and diminished contraction.

Lead: a recording of the electrical potential difference between a positive and a negative body surface electrode. The negative electrode can originate from a combination of two or three electrodes (see **V lead** and **aV lead**).

MCL_1: a modified lead V_1 used to enhance visualization of atrial activity.

Midaxillary line: a vertical line on the thorax at the level of the midpoint of the axilla, which is the area where the arm joins the body.

Midclavicular line: a vertical line on the thorax at the level of the midpoint of the clavicle or collarbone.

Precordial: situated on the thorax, directly overlying the heart.

Reocclusion: a recurrence of a complete obstruction to blood flow.

Reperfusion: the restoration of blood circulation to an organ or tissue upon reopening of a complete obstruction to blood flow.

Rhythm: the pattern of recurrence of the cardiac cycle.

Situs inversus dextrocardia: an abnormal condition in which the heart is situated on the right side of the body and the great blood vessels of the right and left sides are reversed.

Sternum: the narrow, flat bone in the middle of the anterior thorax; breastbone.

Tachycardia: a rapid heart rate with a frequency above 100 beats/min.

Transverse plane: the horizontal plane of the body; it is perpendicular to both the frontal and sagittal planes.

V lead: an ECG lead that uses a central terminal with inputs from leads I, II, and III as its negative pole and an exploring electrode as its positive pole.

Xiphoid process: the lower end of the sternum; it has a triangular shape.

Acknowledgment

We gratefully acknowledge the past contributions of the previous edition's author, Dr. Galen S. Wagner, as portions of that chapter were retained in this revision.

References

1. Einthoven W, Fahr G, de Waart A. Uber die richtung und die manifeste grosse der potentialschwankungen im menschlichen herzen und uber den einfluss der herzlage auf die form des elektrokardiogramms. *Pfluegers Arch.* 1913;150:275-315.
2. Wilson FN, Macloed AG, Barker PS. The interpretation of the initial deflections of the ventricular complex of the electrocardiogram. *Am Heart J.* 1931;6:637-664.
3. Goldberger E. A simple, indifferent, electrocardiographic electrode of zero potential

and a technique of obtaining augmented, unipolar, extremity leads. *Am Heart J.* 1942;23:483-492.

4. Wilson FN, Johnston FD, Macloed AG, Barker PS. Electrocardiograms that represent the potential variations of a single electrode. *Am Heart J.* 1934;9:447-458.
5. Kossmann CE, Johnston FD. The precordial electrocardiogram: I. The potential variations of the precordium and of the extremities in normal subjects. *Am Heart J.* 1935;10:925-941.
6. Joint Recommendations of the American Heart Association and the Cardiac Society of Great Britain and Ireland. Standardization of precordial leads. *Am Heart J.* 1938;15:107-108.
7. Barnes AR, Pardee HEB, White PD, Wilson FN, Wolferth CC; and Committee of the American Heart Association for the Standardization of Precordial Leads. Standardization of precordial leads: supplementary report. *Am Heart J.* 1938;15:235-239.
8. Cabrera E. *Bases Electrophysiologiques de l'Electrocardiographie: ses Applications Clinique*. Paris, France: Masson; 1948.
9. The Joint European Society of Cardiology/American College of Cardiology Committee. Myocardial infarction redefined—a consensus document of The Joint European Society of Cardiology/American College of Cardiology Committee for the redefinition of myocardial infarction. *J Am Coll Cardiol.* 2000;36:959-969 and *Eur Heart J.* 2000;21:1502-1513.
10. Anderson ST, Pahlm O, Selvester RH, et al. Panoramic display of the orderly sequenced 12-lead ECG. *J Electrocardiol.* 1994;27:347-352.
11. Krucoff MW, Parente AR, Bottner RK, et al. Stability of multilead ST-segment "fingerprints" over time after percutaneous transluminal coronary angioplasty and its usefulness in detecting reocclusion. *Am J Cardiol.* 1988;61:1232-1237.
12. Krucoff MW, Wagner NB, Pope JE, et al. The portable programmable microprocessor-driven real-time 12-lead electrocardiographic monitor: a preliminary report of a new device for the noninvasive detection of successful reperfusion or silent coronary reocclusion. *Am J Cardiol.* 1990;65:143-148.
13. Krucoff MW, Croll MA, Pope JE, et al. Continuously updated 12-lead ST-segment recovery analysis for myocardial infarct artery patency assessment and its correlation with multiple simultaneous early angiographic observations. *Am J Cardiol.* 1993;71:145-151.
14. Holter NJ. New method for heart studies. *Science.* 1961;134:1214-1220.
15. Mason RE, Likar I. A new system of multiple-lead exercise electrocardiography. *Am Heart J.* 1966;71:196-205.
16. Sevilla DC, Dohrmann ML, Somelofski CA, Wawrzynski RP, Wagner NB, Wagner GS. Invalidation of the resting electrocardiogram obtained via exercise electrode sites as a standard 12-lead recording. *Am J Cardiol.* 1989;63:35-39.
17. Pahlm O, Haisty WK, Edenbrandt L, et al. Evaluation of changes in standard electrocardiographic QRS waveforms recorded from activity-compatible proximal limb lead positions. *Am J Cardiol.* 1992;69:253-257.
18. Dower GE, Yakush A, Nazzal SB, Jutzy RV, Ruiz CE. Deriving the 12-lead electrocardiogram from four (EASI) electrodes. *J Electrocardiol.* 1988;21(suppl):S182-S187.
19. Nelwan SP, Kors JA, Meij SH, Bemmel JH, Simoons ML. Reconstruction of the 12-lead electrocardiogram from reduced lead sets. *J Electrocardiol.* 2004;37:11-18.
20. Dower GE. *EASI 12-Lead Electrocardiography*. Washington, DC: Totemite Inc; 1996.
21. Mirvis DM, Berson AS, Goldberger AL, et al. Instrumentation and practice standards for electrocardiographic monitoring in special care units. A report for health professionals by a Task Force of the Council on Clinical Cardiology, American Heart Association. *Circulation.* 1989;79:464-471.
22. Sutherland DJ, McPherson DD, Spencer CA, Armstrong CS, Horacek BM, Montague TJ. Effects of posture and respiration on body surface electrocardiogram. *Am J Cardiol.* 1983;52:595-600.

To view digital content associated with this chapter please access lww.co.in. Instructions are located on the inside front cover.

3 Interpretation of the Normal Electrocardiogram

DAVID G. STRAUSS, TOBIN H. LIM,
DOUGLAS D. SCHOCKEN, AND
MUKUND ARAVIND PRABHU

Electrocardiographic Features

Systematic Approach to Electrocardiogram Interpretation

1. Rate and regularity
2. P-wave morphology
3. PR interval
4. QRS complex morphology
5. ST-segment morphology
6. T-wave morphology
7. U-wave morphology
8. QTc interval
9. Rhythm

Rate, *regularity*, and *rhythm* are commonly grouped together. To assess rhythm accurately, it is necessary to consider not only rate and regularity but also the various waveforms and intervals.

Describing the electrocardiogram (ECG) features requires understanding of the grid markings provided on the ECG paper (**Figure 3.1**). The paper shows thin lines every 1 mm and thick lines every 5 mm. The thin lines, therefore, form small (1 mm) squares and the thick lines form large (5 mm) squares. The vertical lines facilitate measurements of the various intervals and determination of cardiac rate. At the standard paper speed of 25 mm/s, the thin lines occur at 0.04-second (40-ms) intervals and thick lines occur at 0.20-second (200-ms) intervals. The horizontal lines facilitate measurements of waveform amplitudes. At the standard calibration of 10 mm/mV, the thin lines are at 0.1-mV increments, and the thick lines are at 0.5-mV increments. Therefore, each small square is 0.04 second × 0.1 mV, and each large square is 0.20 second × 0.5 mV.

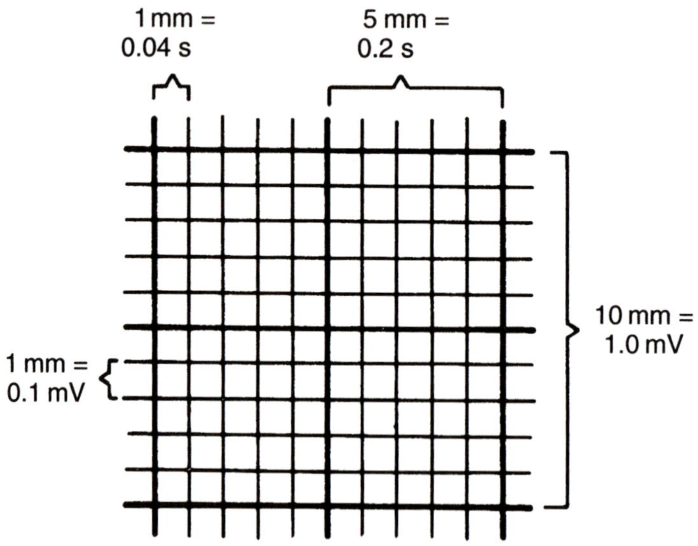

FIGURE 3.1. Grid lines on standard electrocardiogram paper.

Much of the information provided by the ECG is contained in the morphologies of three principal waveforms: (1) the P wave, (2) the QRS complex, and (3) the T wave. It is helpful to develop a systematic approach to the analysis of these waveforms.

Electrocardiogram Waveform Morphologies

1. General *contours*
2. *Durations*
3. Positive and negative *amplitudes*
4. *Axes* in the frontal and transverse planes

The guidelines for measuring and estimating these four parameters for each of the three principal ECG waveforms are presented in this chapter. The definitions of the various waveforms and intervals were presented in Chapter 1.

Rate and Regularity

The cardiac rhythm is rarely precisely regular. Even when electrical activity is initiated normally in the sinus node, the rate is affected by the *autonomic nervous system*. When an individual is at rest, minor variations in autonomic balance are produced by the phases of the respiratory cycle. A glance at the sequence of cardiac cycles is sufficient to determine whether the cardiac rate is essentially regular or irregular. Normally, there are equal numbers of P waves and QRS complexes. Either of these may be used to determine cardiac rate and regularity. With certain abnormal cardiac rhythms, the number of P waves and QRS complexes are not the same. Atrial and ventricular rates and regularities must be determined separately.

If there is essential regularity in the cardiac rhythm, cardiac rate can easily be determined by counting the number of large squares between cycles. Because each square indicates one-fifth of a second and there are 300 fifths of a second in a minute (5 × 60), it is necessary only to determine the number of large squares between consecutive cycles and divide this number by 300. It is most convenient to select the peak of a prominent ECG waveform that occurs on a thick line and then count the number of large squares until the same waveform recurs in the following cycle. When this interval is only one-fifth of a second (0.2 s), the cardiac rate is 300 beats/min; if the interval is two-fifths of a second (0.4 s), the cardiac rate is 150 beats/min; if the interval is three-fifths of a second (0.6 s), the cardiac rate is 100 beats/min, and so forth. Lead II is displayed in **Figure 3.2** with the second QRS complex following the onset of the initial QRS complex after four large squares (heart rate = 75 beats/min).

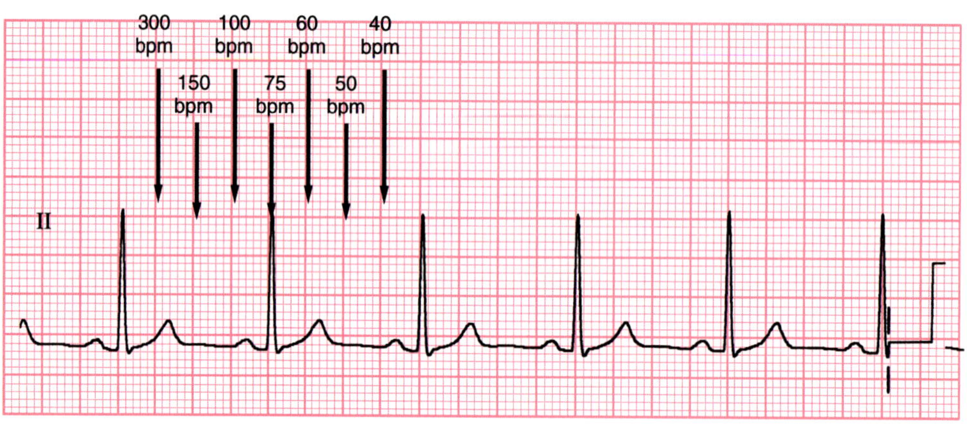

FIGURE 3.2. Lead II. bpm, beats per minute.

When the cardiac rate is <100 beats/min, rate can be easily determined by examining intervals between complexes as a function of large (200 ms) blocks. When the rate is >100 beats/min (*tachycardia*), however, small differences in the observed rate may alter the assessment of the underlying cardiac rhythm, and the number of small squares must also be considered (**Figure 3.3**). This illustrates the importance of considering the small squares (0.04 s or 40 ms) rather than the large squares (0.2 s or 200 ms) for estimating rates in the tachycardic range, where small differences in the number of intervals between cardiac cycles result in large differences in the estimated rate. Because there are five small squares in each large square, the number of small squares between successive waveforms of the same type must be divided into 1500 (6 squares = 250 beats/min, 7 squares = 214 beats/min, etc.).

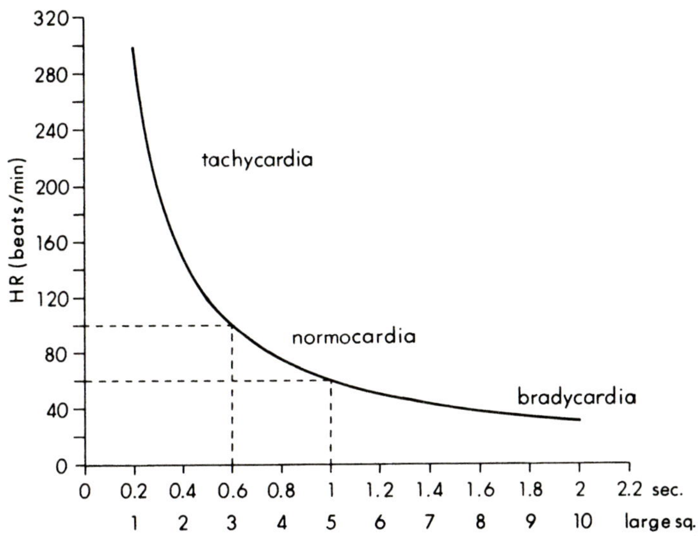

FIGURE 3.3. Intervals between electrocardiogram waveforms can be used to estimate cardiac rate.

P-wave Morphology

At either slow or normal heart rates, the small, rounded P wave is clearly visible just before the taller, more peaked QRS complex. At more rapid rates, however, the P wave may merge with the preceding T wave and become difficult to identify. Four steps should be taken to define the morphology of the P wave, as follows.

General Contour

The P-wave contour is normally smooth and is either entirely positive or entirely negative (see **Figure 1.9**; monophasic) in all leads except V_1 and possibly V_2. In the short-axis view provided by lead V_1, which best distinguishes left- versus right-sided cardiac activity, the separation of right- and left-atrial activation often produces a biphasic P wave (see **Figure 1.14**). The contributions of right- and left-atrial activation to the beginning, middle, and end of the P wave are indicated in **Figure 3.4**. Typical appearances of a normal P wave in a long-axis lead such as II (**Figure 3.4A**) and a short-axis lead such as V_1 (**Figure 3.4B**) are illustrated.

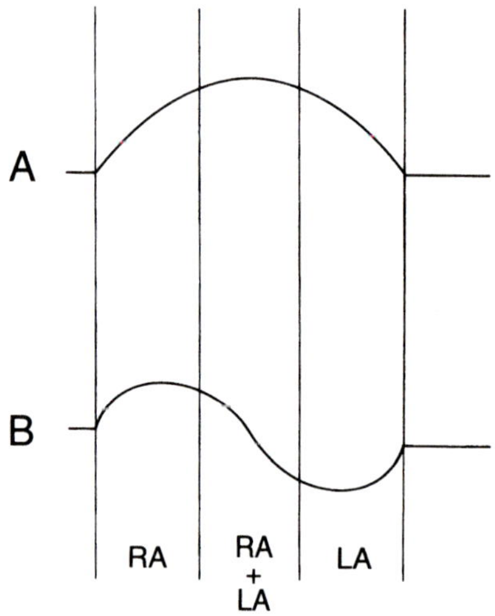

FIGURE 3.4. Typical normal P wave. **A.** Long axis (frontal plane, lead II). **B.** Short axis (transverse plane, lead V_1). LA, left atrium; RA, right atrium.

P-wave Duration

The P-wave duration is normally <0.12 second. Displayed in **Figure 3.4**, the P-wave duration is divided into thirds (vertical lines) to indicate the relative times of activation in the right and left atria.

Positive and Negative Amplitudes

The maximal P-wave amplitude is normally no more than 0.2 mV in the frontal plane leads and no more than 0.1 mV in the transverse plane leads.

Axis in the Frontal and Transverse Planes

The P wave normally appears entirely upright in leftward and inferiorly oriented leads such as I, II, aVF, and V_4 to V_6. It is negative in aVR because of the rightward orientation of that lead and is variable in other standard leads. The direction of the P wave, or its axis in the frontal plane, should be determined according to the method for determining the axis of an ECG waveform presented later in the section "Morphology of the QRS Complex." The normal limits of the P-wave axis are between 0 and +75 degrees.[1]

The atrial repolarization wave (Ta wave)

The Ta wave represents the repolarization of the atria and is usually not evident in the normal electrocardiogram since it is of low (0.1–0.2 mV) amplitude. It has an axis opposite to that of the P wave and hence is usually an inverted, shallow saucer-like depression following the P wave. It is usually obscured by the QRS complex, but may be evident when there is second- or third-degree atrioventricular (AV) block or prolonged PR interval (**Figure 3.5**: Ta wave). Its duration (around 300 ms) is 2–3 times that of the P wave, and starting from the end of the wave, it can extend beyond the QRS complex, especially at faster heart rates.[A]

Identifying the Ta wave can be of clinical importance in multiple scenarios. The PR segment depression seen in acute pericarditis is the most striking example of Ta wave becoming prominent. Similarly, the PR segment elevation seen in atrial infarction is due to the elevated Ta wave. More common and familiar is the setting of exercise testing where the Ta wave can mimic ST depression. At faster heart rates, the P wave as well as the Ta wave becomes more prominent, and the Ta wave can fall on the ST segment resulting in ST depression. A steep slope of the PR segment and the more prominent ST depression seen in inferior leads such as aVF and the up-sloping morphology of the ST depression are the clues toward the prominent Ta wave as the cause for the ST depression. Finally, the Ta wave is more prominent when the P wave is inverted and is directed superiorly resulting in ST elevation that can mimic inferior wall myocardial infarction.[B]

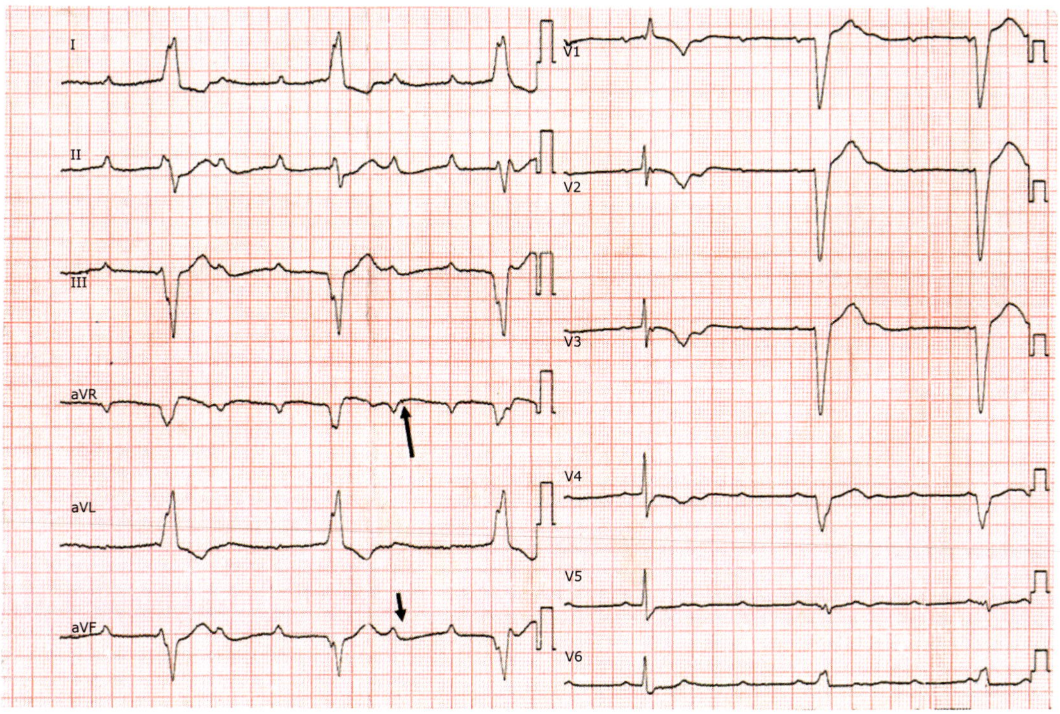

FIGURE 3.5. The electrocardiogram shows advanced atrioventricular conduction block with a wide QRS escape rhythm. The Ta waves are seen after the blocked P waves as a subtle low voltage deflection causing the baseline to dip after the P wave (downward arrow) in aVF and rise above it in aVR (upward arrow).

The PR Interval

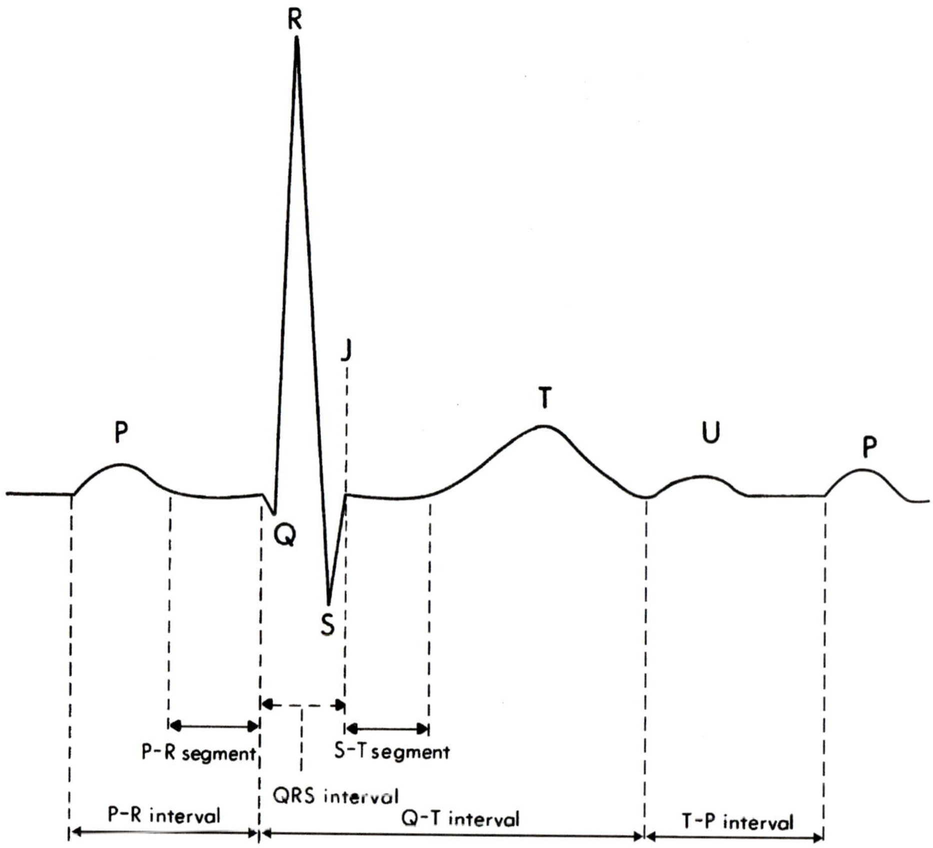

Magnified cardiac long-axis viewpoint of electrocardiogram segments and time intervals.

The PR interval measures the time required for an electrical impulse to travel from the atrial myocardium adjacent to the sinoatrial (SA) node to the ventricular myocardium adjacent to the fibers of the Purkinje network (see **Figure 1.12**, repeated above). This duration is normally from 0.10 to 0.21 second. A major portion of the PR interval reflects the slow conduction of an impulse through the atrioventricular (AV) node, which is controlled by the balance between the sympathetic and parasympathetic divisions of the autonomic nervous system. Therefore, the PR interval varies with the heart rate: shorter at faster rates when the sympathetic component predominates and longer at slower rates when the parasympathetic component predominates. The PR interval tends to increase with age[2]:

In childhood: 0.10 to 0.12 second
In adolescence: 0.12 to 0.16 second
In adulthood: 0.14 to 0.21 second

Morphology of the QRS Complex

In developing a systematic approach to waveform analysis, the following steps should be taken to determine the morphology of the QRS complex.

General Contour

The QRS complex is composed of higher frequency signals than are the P and T waves, thereby causing its contour to be peaked rather than rounded. Positive and negative components of the P and T waves are simply termed positive and negative deflections, whereas those of the QRS complex are assigned specific labels, such as "Q wave" (see **Figure 1.10**).

Q waves

In some leads (V_1, V_2, and V_3), the presence of any Q wave should be considered abnormal, whereas in all other leads (except rightward-oriented leads III and aVR), a "normal" Q wave is very small. The upper limit of normal for such Q waves in each lead is illustrated in **Figure 3.6** and indicated in **Table 3.1**.[3]

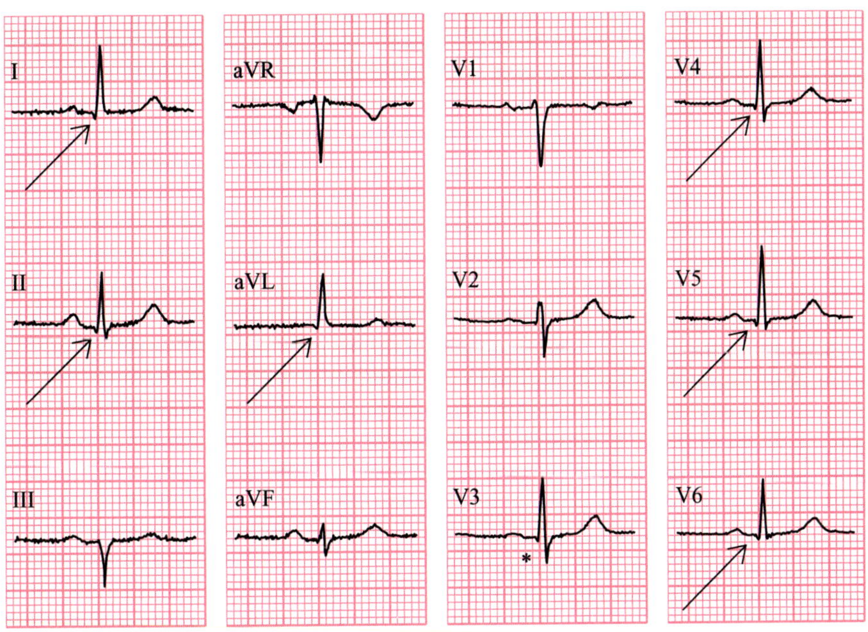

FIGURE 3.6. Normal 12-standard electrocardiogram presented in the classical format. Arrows, small Q waves; asterisk, minute Q wave.

Table 3.1.

Normal Q-wave Duration Limits[a]

Limb Leads		Precordial Leads	
Lead	Upper Limit(s)	Lead	Upper Limit(s)
I	<0.03	V_1	Any Q[b]
II	<0.03	V_2	Any Q[b]
III	None	V_3	Any Q[b]
aVR	None	V_4	<0.02
aVL	<0.03	V_5	<0.03
aVF	<0.03	V_6	<0.03

[a]Modified with permission from Wagner GS, Freye CJ, Palmeri ST, et al. Evaluation of a QRS scoring system for estimating myocardial infarct size. I. Specificity and observer agreement. *Circulation*. 1982;65:345.

[b]In these leads, any Q wave is abnormal.

The absence of small Q waves in leads V_5 and V_6 should be considered abnormal. A Q wave of any size is normal in leads III and aVR because of their rightward orientations (see **Figure 2.4**). Q waves may be enlarged in conditions with local loss of myocardial tissue (infarction), enlargement (hypertrophy or dilatation) of the ventricular myocardium, or abnormalities of ventricular conduction.

R waves

Because the precordial leads provide a panoramic view of the cardiac electrical activity progressing from the thinner right ventricle across the thicker left ventricle, the positive R wave normally increases in amplitude and duration from lead V_1 to V_4 or V_5 (**Figure 3.7**). Larger R waves in leads V_1 and V_2 can be produced by right-ventricular hypertrophy, and accentuation of this sequence, with larger R waves in leads V_5 and V_6, can be produced by left-ventricular hypertrophy. Loss of normal R-wave progression from lead V_1 to V_4 may indicate loss of left-ventricular myocardium, as occurs with myocardial infarction (see Chapter 9).

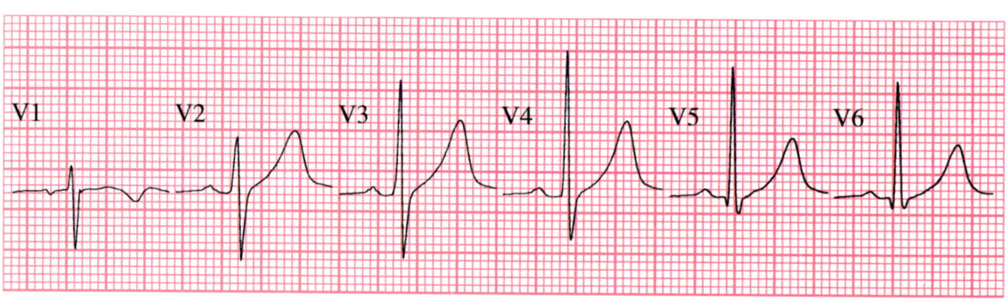

FIGURE 3.7. Panoramic display of the precordial leads.

S waves

The S wave also has a normal sequence of progression in the precordial leads. It should be large in V_1, larger in V_2, and then progressively smaller from V_3 through V_6 (see **Figure 3.6**). As with the R wave, this sequence could be altered by hypertrophy of one of the ventricles, myocardial infarction, or disorders of ventricular conduction.

QRS Complex Duration

The duration of the QRS complex is termed the QRS interval, and it normally ranges from 0.07 to 0.11 second (see **Figure 1.12**). The duration of the complex tends to be slightly longer in males than in females.[4] The QRS interval is measured from the beginning of the first-appearing Q or R wave to the end of the last-appearing R, S, R′, or S′ wave. **Figure 3.8** illustrates the use of three simultaneously recorded limb leads (I, II, and III) to identify the true beginning and end of the QRS complex. An isoelectric period of approximately 0.02 second is apparent in lead II at the beginning of the QRS complex, and an isoelectric period of approximately 0.01 second is apparent in lead III at the end of the QRS complex. Note that only lead I reveals the true QRS duration (0.12 s).

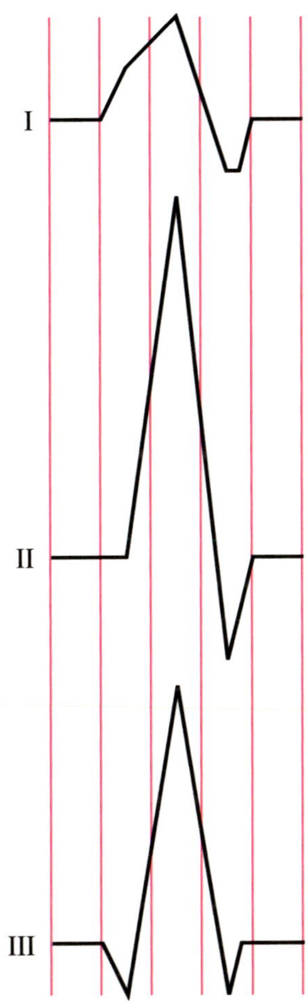

FIGURE 3.8. QRS complexes. Vertical grid lines, 0.04-second time intervals.

Such multilead comparison is necessary; either the beginning or the end of the QRS complex may be isoelectric (neither positive nor negative) in a particular lead, causing an apparently shorter QRS duration. This isoelectric appearance occurs whenever the summation of ventricular electrical forces is perpendicular to the involved lead. The onset of the QRS complex is usually quite apparent in all leads, but its ending at the junction with the ST segment (termed the J point) is often indistinct, particularly in the precordial leads. The QRS interval has no lower limit that indicates abnormality. Prolongation of the QRS interval may be caused by left-ventricular hypertrophy, an abnormality in intraventricular impulse conduction, or a ventricular site of origin of the cardiac impulse.

The duration from the beginning of the earliest appearing Q or R wave to the peak of the R wave in several of the precordial leads has been termed the *intrinsicoid deflection* (**Figure 3.9**). Electrical activation of the myocardium begins at the endocardial insertions of the Purkinje network. The end of the intrinsicoid deflection represents the time at which the electrical impulse arrives at the epicardial surface as viewed by that particular lead. The deflection is called an intrinsic deflection when the electrode is on the epicardial surface and an intrinsicoid deflection when the electrode is on the body surface.[5]

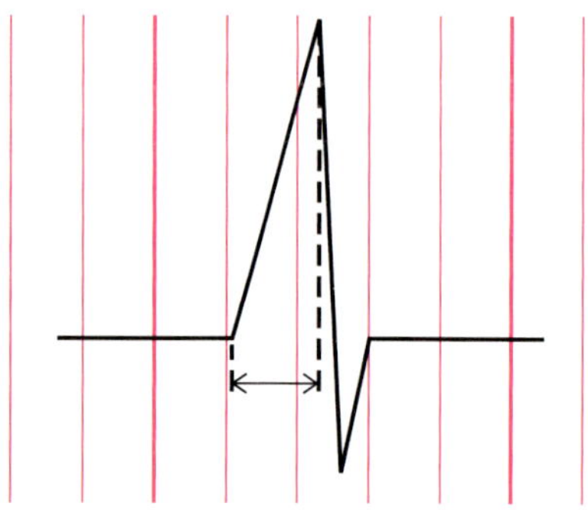

FIGURE 3.9. Magnified QRS complex. Vertical grid lines, 0.04-second time intervals. Double-headed arrow, length indicates the duration (0.05 s of intrinsicoid deflection).

Positive and Negative Amplitudes

The amplitude of the overall QRS complex has wide normal limits. Amplitude varies with age, increasing until about age 30 years and then gradually decreasing. The amplitude is generally larger in males than in females. Overall QRS amplitude is measured between the peaks of the tallest positive and negative waveforms in the complex. It is difficult to set an arbitrary upper limit for normal voltage of the QRS complex; peak-to-peak amplitudes as high as 4 mV are occasionally seen in normal individuals. Factors that contribute to higher amplitudes include youth, physical fitness, slender body build, intraventricular conduction abnormalities, and ventricular enlargement.

An abnormally low QRS amplitude occurs when the overall amplitude is no more than 0.5 mV in any of the limb leads and no more than 1.0 mV in any of the precordial leads. The QRS amplitude is decreased by any condition that increases the distance between the myocardium and the recording electrode, such as a thick chest wall or various intrathoracic conditions that decrease the electrical signal that reaches the electrode such as hypothyroidism, amyloidosis, or other infiltrative processes.

Axis in the Frontal and Transverse Planes

The QRS axis represents the average direction of the total force produced by right- and left-ventricular depolarization. Although the Purkinje network facilitates the spread of the depolarization wavefront from the apex to the base of the ventricles (see Chapter 1), the QRS axis is normally in the positive direction in the frontal plane leads (except aVR) because of the endocardial-to-epicardial spread of depolarization in the thicker walled left ventricle.

In the frontal plane, the full 360-degree circumference of the hexaxial reference system is provided by the positive and negative poles of the six limb leads (see **Figure 2.4**); in the transverse plane, it is provided by the positive and negative poles of the six precordial leads (see **Figure 2.7**). It should be noted that the leads in both planes are not separated by precisely 30 degrees. In the frontal plane, the scalene Burger triangle has been shown more applicable then the equilateral Einthoven triangle.[6] Of course, body shape and electrode placement determine the spacing between contiguous leads.

Identification of the frontal plane axis of the QRS complex would be easier if the six leads were displayed in their orderly sequence (see **Figure 2.10B,C**) than in their typical classical sequence. A simple method for identifying the QRS complex frontal plane axis with the limb leads in orderly sequence is illustrated in **Figure 3.10**.[7] Note that there is no truly *transitional lead* in **Figure 3.10A**, indicating that the QRS transition is located between leads aVF and III.

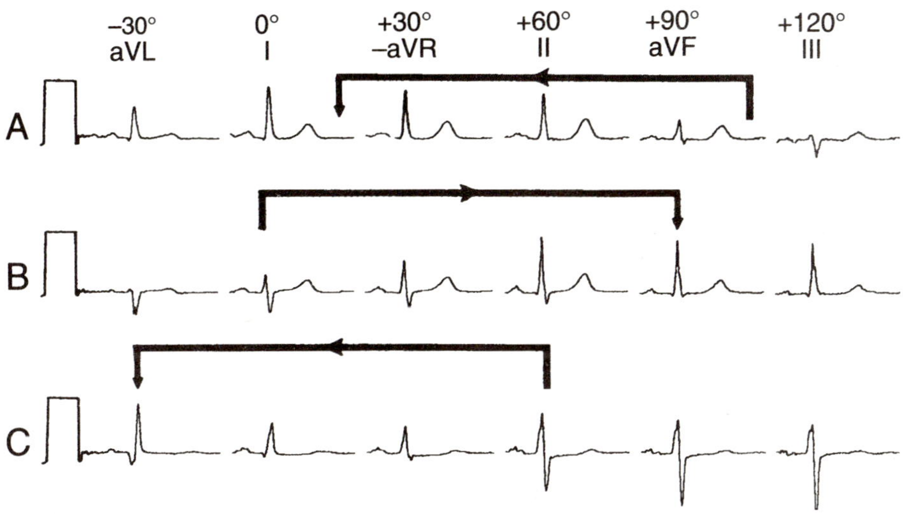

FIGURE 3.10. Identifying the QRS complex frontal plane axis. The vertical line without an arrow indicates the location of the frontal plane QRS transitional lead. Note that there is no transitional lead in **A**, indicating that the QRS transition is located between leads aVF and III. The long horizontal line contains an arrow indicating movement to 90 degrees away from the transitional lead in the direction of the tallest R wave. The vertical line with an arrow indicates the location of the axis: +15 degrees in **A**, +90 degrees in **B**; and −30 degrees in **C**.

Determining QRS Axis in the Frontal Plane

1. Identify the transitional lead (the lead perpendicular to the waveform axis) by locating the lead in which the QRS complex has the most nearly equal positive and negative components. These positive and negative components may vary from miniscule to quite prominent.
2. Identify the lead that is oriented perpendicular to the transitional lead by using the hexaxial reference system (**Figure 3.11**, top left).
3. Consider the predominant direction of the QRS complex in the lead identified in step 2. If the direction is positive, the axis is the same as the positive pole of that lead. If the direction is negative, the axis is the same as the negative pole of the lead. Note that the positive poles of each lead are labeled with the lead name in **Figure 3.11**.

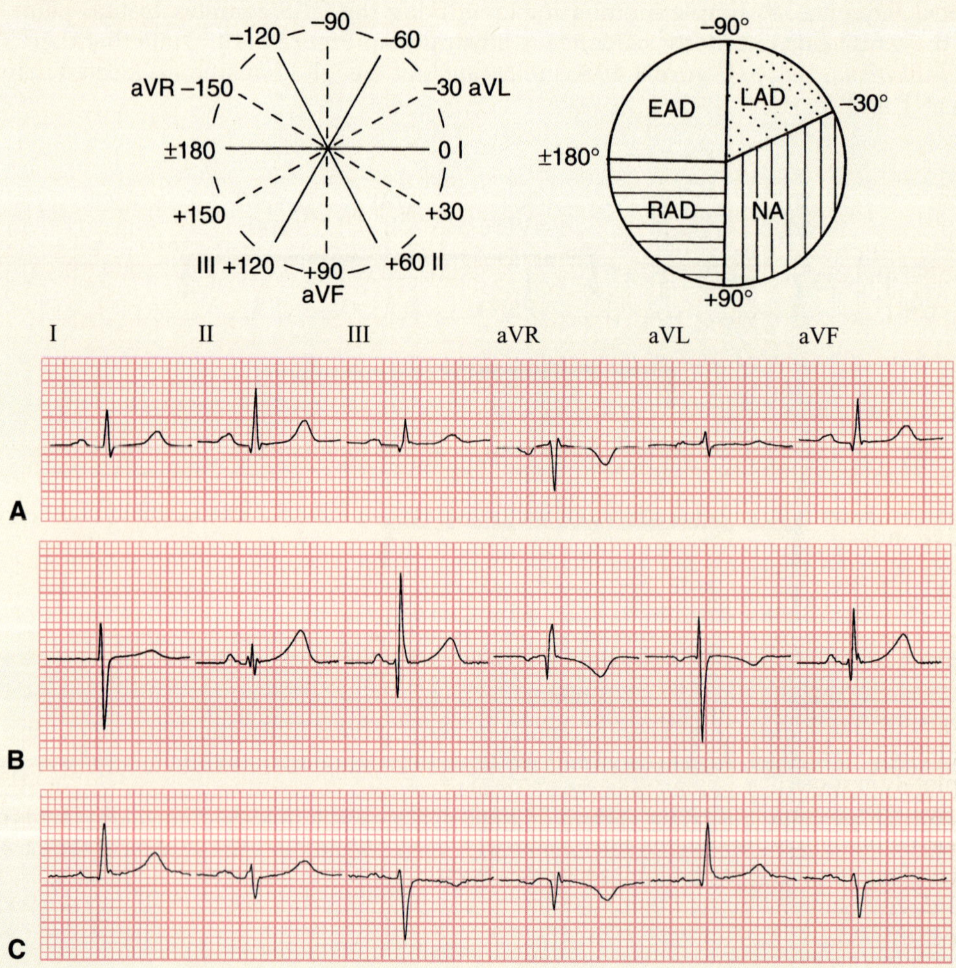

FIGURE 3.11. **A.** +60 degrees. **B.** +150 degrees. **C.** −30 degrees. *(continued)*

(continued)

Determining QRS Axis in the Frontal Plane (continued)

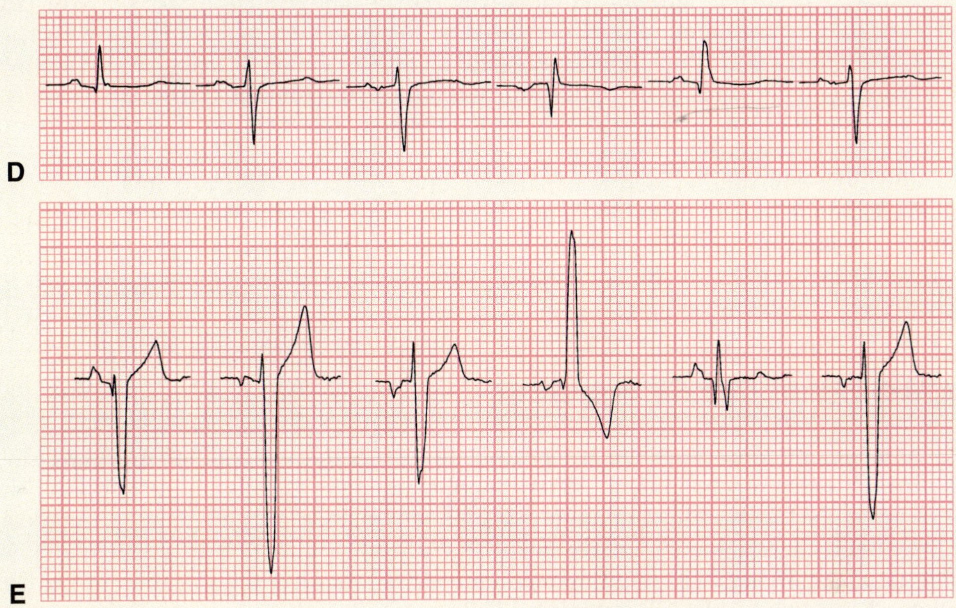

FIGURE 3.11 *(continued)* **D.** −60 degrees. **E.** −120 degrees. EAD, extreme axis deviation; LAD, left axis deviation; NA, normal axis; RAD, right axis deviation.

The frontal plane axis of the QRS complex is normally directed leftward and either slightly superiorly or inferiorly in the region between −30 and +90 degrees (see **Figure 3.11**, top right). Therefore, the QRS complex is normally predominantly positive in both leads I and II (see **Figure 3.11A**). A very useful shortcut method follows: If the net amplitude is positive in lead I and positive in lead aVF, then the frontal plane mean QRS axis must lie between 0 and +90 degrees, therefore, normal for most of the adult population. If the QRS complex is negative in lead I but positive in lead II, its axis is deviated rightward, to the region between +90 and ±180 degrees (*right-axis deviation*; see **Figure 3.11B**). If the QRS complex is positive in lead I but negative in lead II, its axis is deviated leftward to the region between −30 and −120 degrees (*left-axis deviation*; see **Figure 3.11C,D**). Right-ventricular enlargement may produce right-axis deviation, and left-ventricular enlargement may produce left-axis deviation of the QRS complex. The axis of the QRS complex is rarely directed completely opposite to its normal direction (−90 to ±180 degrees) with a predominantly negative QRS orientation in both leads I and II (*extreme axis deviation*; see **Figure 3.11E**).

Using this method for determining the direction of the axis of the QRS complex in the frontal plane permits no more than a "rounding" of the direction to the nearest multiple of 30 degrees. Although automated ECG analysis provides axis designation to the nearest degree, the manual method described here is sufficient for clinical purposes.

The normal frontal plane axis of the QRS complex is rightward in the neonate, moves to a vertical position during childhood, and then moves to a more leftward position during adulthood.[8] In normal adults, the electrical axis of the QRS complex is almost parallel to the anatomic base-to-apex axis of the heart in the direction of lead II. However, these axes are more vertical in thin individuals and more horizontal in heavy individuals. This same normal growth-dependent rightward-to-leftward movement of the QRS axis that is seen in the frontal plane is also apparent in the transverse plane, but the transverse plane shows the anterior-to-posterior movement of the axis that is not visible in the frontal plane. In the adult, the transitional lead is usually V_3 or V_4, and the lead oriented perpendicular to this transitional lead is therefore lead V_6 or V_1, respectively. Because the normal predominant direction of the QRS complex is positive in lead V_6 and negative in lead V_1, the axis of the QRS complex in the transverse plane in the adult is typically between 0 and −60 degrees.

Morphology of the ST Segment

The ST segment represents the period during which the ventricular myocardium proceeds through early repolarization. At its junction with the QRS complex (J point), the ST segment typically forms a distinct angle with the downslope of the R wave or upstroke of the S wave and then proceeds nearly horizontally until it curves gently into the T wave. The length of the ST segment is influenced by factors that alter the duration of ventricular activation. Points along the ST segment are designated with reference to the number of milliseconds beyond the J point, such as "J + 20," "J + 40," and "J + 60."

The first section of the ST segment is normally located at the same horizontal level as the baseline formed by the TP segment that fills the space between electrical cardiac cycles (**Figure 3.12A**). Slight upsloping, downsloping, or horizontal depression of the ST segment may occur as a normal variant (**Figure 3.12B**). Another variant of the ST segment appears when there is altered early repolarization within the ventricles and was previously considered a normal variant.[9] Early repolarization causes displacement of the ST segment by as much as 0.1 mV in the direction of the ensuing T wave (**Figure 3.12C**). Early repolarization pattern can be diagnosed when the J-point is elevated ≥1 mm in ≥2 contiguous inferior and/or lateral leads, whereas in the setting of ventricular fibrillation or sudden death, it is termed early repolarization syndrome.[C] Occasionally, the ST segment in young males may show even greater elevation in leads V_2 and V_3 (**Figure 3.12D**).[9] The appearance of the ST segment may also be altered when there is an abnormally prolonged QRS complex (**Figure 3.12E**).

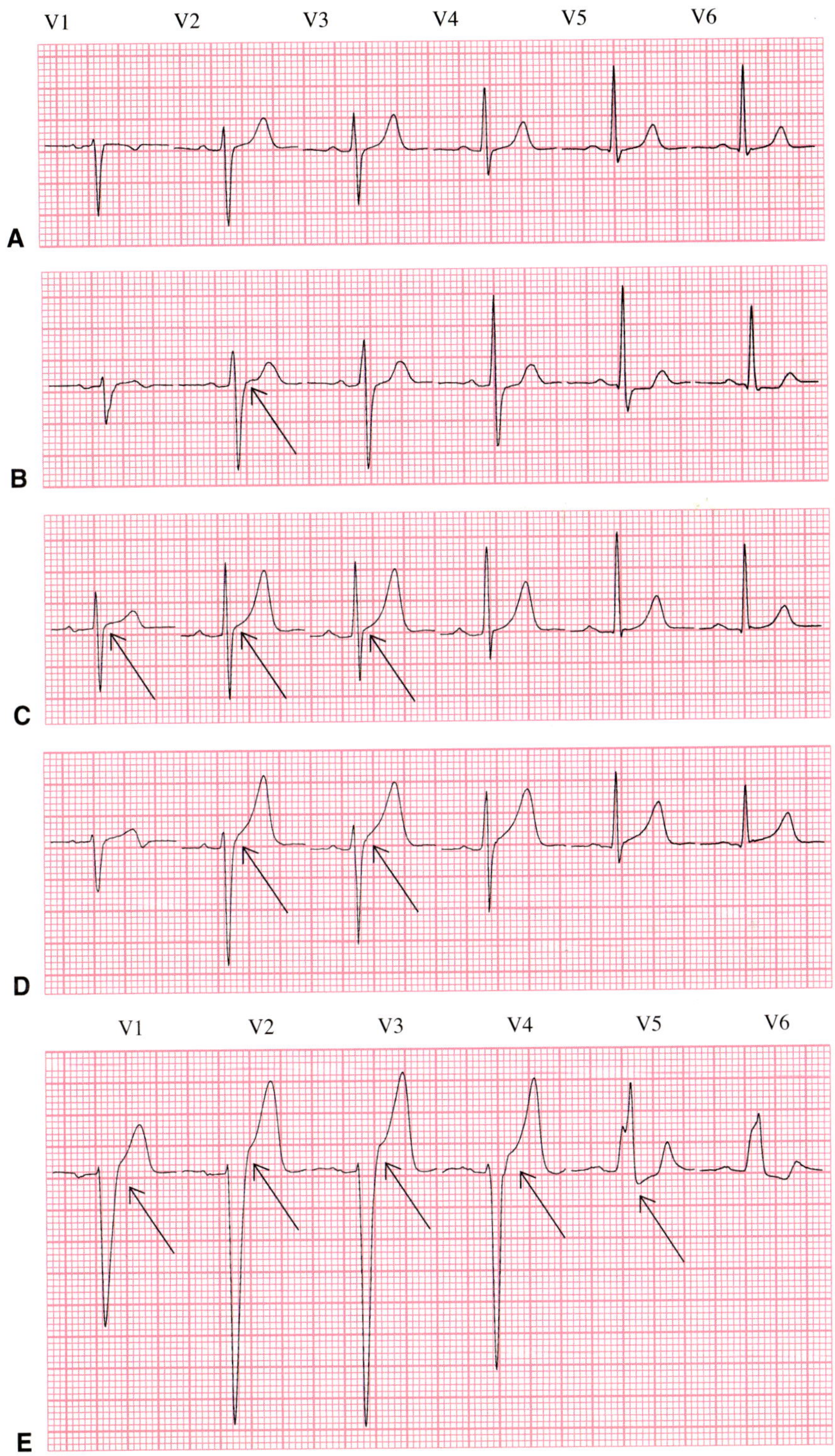

FIGURE 3.12. **A.** Normal electrocardiogram (ECG). **B–D.** Normal variant ECGs. **E.** Abnormal ECG. Arrows, ST-segment deviations in precordial leads.

T-wave Morphology

In continuing the systematic approach to waveform analysis, the steps taken in examining the morphology of the T wave are as follows.

General Contour

Both the shape and axis of the normal T wave resemble those of the P wave (see **Figures 1.9** and **1.14**). The waveforms in both cases are smooth and rounded and are positively directed in all leads except aVR, where they are negative, and V_1, where they may be biphasic (initially positive and terminally negative) or may be entirely negative.

T-wave Duration

The duration of the T wave itself is not usually measured, but it is instead included in the QT interval discussed in Chapter 10.

Positive and Negative Amplitudes

The amplitude of the T wave, like that of the QRS complex, has wide normal limits. It tends to diminish with age and is larger in males than in females. T-wave amplitude tends to vary with QRS amplitude and should always be greater than that of the U wave if the latter is present. T-wave amplitudes do not normally exceed 0.5 mV in any limb lead or 1.5 mV in any precordial lead. In females, the upper limits of T-wave amplitude are about two-thirds of these values. The T-wave amplitude tends to be lower at the extremes of the panoramic views (see **Figure 2.10B**) of both the frontal and transverse planes. The amplitude of the wave at these extremes does not normally exceed 0.3 mV in leads aVL and III or 0.5 mV in leads V_1 and V_6.[8]

Axis in the Frontal and Transverse Planes

The axis of the T wave should be evaluated in relation to that of the QRS complex. The rationale for the similar directions of the waveforms of these two ECG features, despite their representing the opposite myocardial electrical events of activation and recovery, has been presented in Chapter 1. The methods presented earlier for determining the axis of the QRS complex in the two ECG planes should be applied for determining the axis of the T wave. The term *QRS-T angle* is used to indicate the number of degrees between the axes of the QRS complex and the T wave in the frontal and transverse planes.[10] This angle has clinical utility in the presence of ventricular hypertrophy, myocardial infarction, or conduction abnormalities.

The axis of the T wave in the frontal plane tends to remain constant throughout life, whereas the axis of the QRS complex moves from a vertical toward a horizontal position, as shown at the top of **Figure 3.13**.[8] Therefore, during childhood, the T-wave axis is more horizontal than that of the QRS complex, but during adulthood, the T-wave axis becomes more vertical than that of the QRS complex. Despite these changes, the QRS-T angle in the frontal plane does not normally exceed 45 degrees.[10]

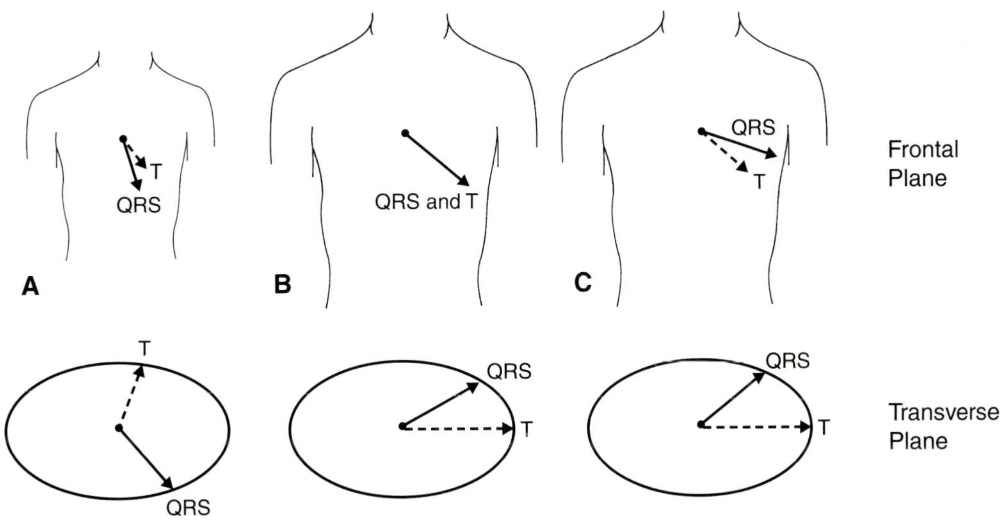

FIGURE 3.13. **A.** Young child. **B.** Young adult. **C.** Elderly adult. Solid arrows, directions of QRS axis and T axes in frontal plane; dashed line arrows, directions of QRS and T axes in transverse plane.

In the normal young child, the T-wave axis in the transverse plane may be so posterior that the T waves may be negative in even the most leftward precordial leads V_5 and V_6 (see **Figure 3.13**, bottom). During childhood, the T-wave axis moves anteriorly, toward the positive pole of lead V_5, and the QRS axis moves posteriorly, toward the negative pole of lead V_1, where these two axes typically remain throughout life. The QRS-T angle in the transverse plane normally does not exceed 60 degrees in the adult.[10]

U-wave Morphology

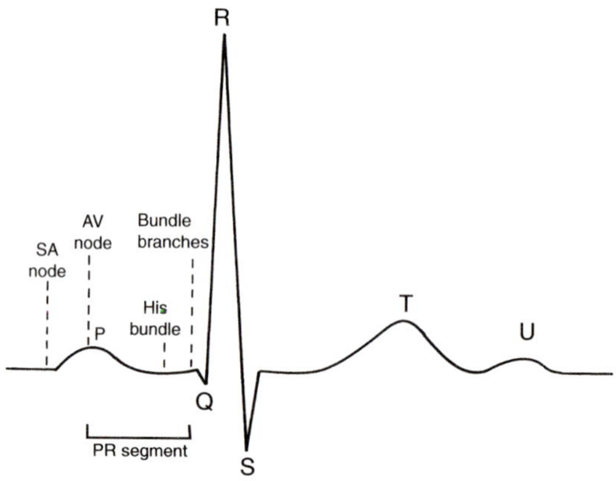

Waveforms. P, atrial activation; Q, R, and S, ventricular activation; T and U, ventricular recovery. AV, atrioventricular; SA, sinoatrial.

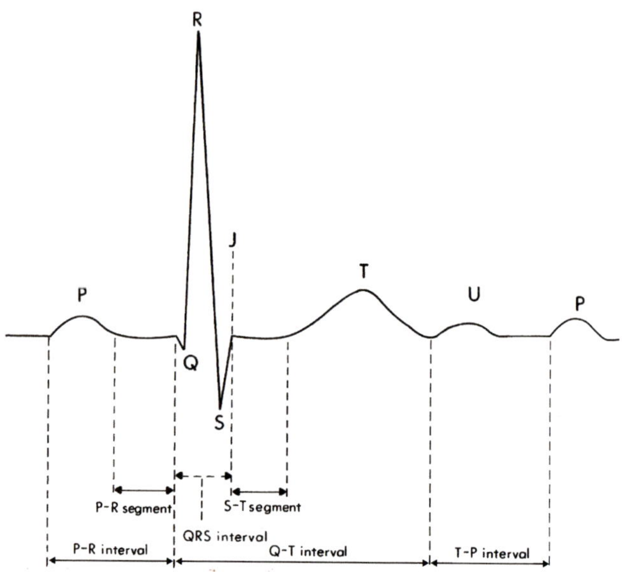

Magnified cardiac long-axis viewpoint of electrocardiogram segments and time intervals.

The U wave is normally either absent from the ECG or present as a small, rounded wave following the T wave (see **Figures 1.9** and **1.12**, repeated here). It is normally oriented in the same direction as the T wave, has approximately 10% of the amplitude of the latter, and is usually most prominent in leads V_2 or V_3. The U wave is larger at slower heart rates, and both the U wave and the T wave diminish in size and merge with the following P wave at faster heart rates. The U wave is usually separated from the T wave, with the *TU junction* occurring along the baseline of the ECG. There may be *fusion* of the T and U waves, making measurement of the QT interval more difficult. The source of the U wave is uncertain. Three possible theories regarding its origin are (1) tardy repolarization of the subendocardial Purkinje fibers, (2) prolonged repolarization of the midmyocardium ("M cells"), and (3) afterpotentials resulting from mechanical forces in the ventricular wall.[11]

QT and QTc Intervals

The QT interval measures the duration of electrical activation and recovery of the ventricular myocardium. Currently used in determining the end of the T wave for QT interval measuring is the tangential method. This is defined as a tangent line that is drawn at the end of the T wave's steepest portion of its terminal point crossing the isoelectric line (**Figure 3.14**).[12] In addition, the QT interval varies inversely with the cardiac rate. To ensure complete recovery from one cardiac cycle before the next cycle begins, the duration of recovery must decrease as the rate of activation increases. Therefore, the "normality" of the QT interval can be determined only by correcting for the cardiac rate. The corrected QT interval (*QTc interval*) rather than the measured QT interval is included in routine ECG analysis. Bazett[13] developed the following formula for performing this correction:

$$QTc = QT / \sqrt{RR}$$

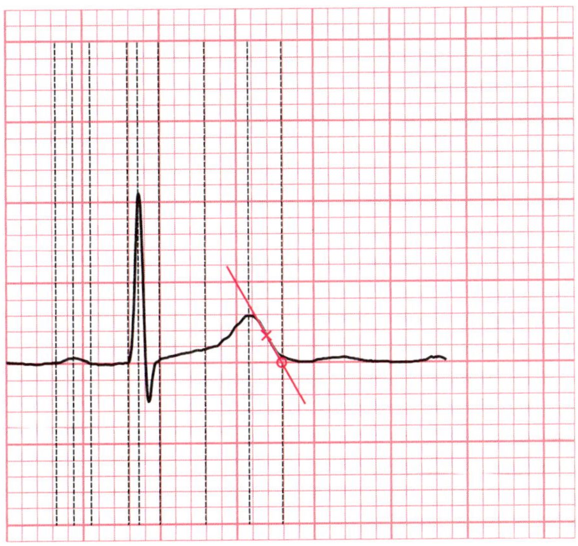

FIGURE 3.14. Tangential method used for determining end of the T wave. The end of the T wave is the point where a line fit through the steepest part of the descending T wave intersects the baseline.

RR is defined as the interval duration between two consecutive R waves measured in seconds. The modification of Bazett's formula by Hodges and coworkers,[14,15] as follows, corrects more completely for high and low heart rates:

$$QTc = QT + 0.00175 \times (\text{ventricular rate} - 60)$$

The upper limit of QTc interval duration is approximately 0.46 second (460 ms). The QTc interval is slightly longer in adult females than males and increases slightly with age, many physiologic states, and medications (see Chapter 10). Adjustment of the duration of electrical recovery to the rate of electrical activation does not occur immediately, but it requires several cardiac cycles. Thus, an accurate measurement of the QTc interval can be made only after a series of regular, equal cardiac cycles.

Cardiac Rhythm

Assessment of the final electrocardiographic feature named at the beginning of this chapter, the cardiac rhythm, requires consideration of all eight other electrocardiographic features. Certain irregularities of cardiac rate and regularity, P-wave morphology, and the PR interval may in themselves indicate abnormalities in cardiac rhythm, and certain irregularities of the remaining five electrocardiographic features may indicate the potential for development of abnormalities in cardiac rhythm. Disturbances in rhythm are addressed in Section III of this book. The following paragraphs provide a very brief introduction to this important topic.

Cardiac Rate and Regularity

The normal cardiac rhythm is called *sinus rhythm* because it is produced by electrical impulses formed within the SA node. The rate of sinus rhythm is normally between 60 and 100 beats/min during wakefulness and at rest. When <60 beats/min, the rhythm is called sinus bradycardia, and when >100 beats/min it is called sinus tachycardia. However, the designation of "normal" requires consideration of the individual's activity level: Sinus bradycardia with a rate as low as 40 beats/min may be normal during sleep, and sinus tachycardia with a rate as rapid as 200 beats/min may be normal during exercise. Indeed, a rate of 90 beats/min would be "abnormal" during either sleep or vigorous exercise. Sinus rates in the bradycardic range may occur normally during wakefulness, especially in well-trained athletes whose resting heart rates range at 30 beats/min and often <60 beats/min even with moderate exertion.

As indicated, normal sinus rhythm is essentially but not absolutely regular because of continual variation of the balance between the sympathetic and parasympathetic divisions of the autonomic nervous system. Loss of this normal *heart rate variability* may be associated with significant underlying autonomic or cardiac abnormalities.[16] The term *sinus arrhythmia* describes the normal variation in cardiac rate that cycles with the phases of respiration; sinus rate accelerates with inspiration and slows with expiration (**Figure 3.15**). Occasionally, sinus arrhythmia produces such marked irregularity that it can be confused with clinically important arrhythmias.

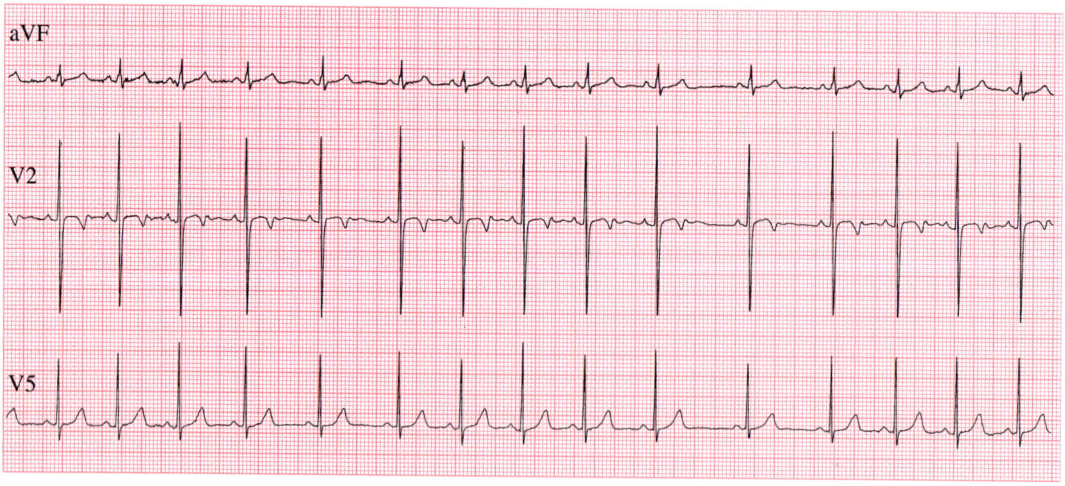

FIGURE 3.15. Sinus arrhythmia.

P-wave Axis

The normal frontal plane axis of the P wave was discussed in the section on "P-wave Morphology." Alteration of this axis to either <+30 *or* >+75 degrees may indicate that the cardiac rhythm is being initiated from a site low in the right atrium, AV node, or left atrium.

PR Interval

The normal relationship between the P wave and QRS complex (the PR interval) is presented schematically in **Figure 3.16A** and **Animation 3.1**, and various abnormal relationships between the P wave and QRS complex are illustrated in **Figure 3.16B–F**. An abnormal P-wave axis is often accompanied by an abnormally short PR interval because the site of impulse formation has moved from the SA node to a position closer to the AV node (see **Figure 3.16B**). However, a short PR interval in the presence of a normal P-wave axis (see **Figure. 3.16C**) suggests either an abnormally rapid conduction pathway within the AV node or the presence of an abnormal bundle of cardiac muscle connecting the atria to the bundle of His (an unusual source of *ventricular preexcitation*; see Chapter 19). This short PR is not in itself an abnormality of the cardiac rhythm; however, the pathway either within or bypassing the AV node that is responsible for the preexcitation creates the potential for electrical *reactivation* or *reentry* into the atria, thereby producing a tachyarrhythmia.

An abnormally long PR interval in the presence of a normal P-wave axis indicates delay of impulse transmission at some point along the normal pathway between the atrial and ventricular myocardium (see **Figure 3.16D**). When a prolonged PR interval is accompanied by an abnormal P-wave contour, it should be considered that the P wave may actually be associated with the preceding rather than with the following QRS complex because of reverse (retrograde) activation from the ventricles to the atria (see **Figure. 3.16E**). This retrograde activation occurs when the cardiac impulse originates from the ventricles rather than

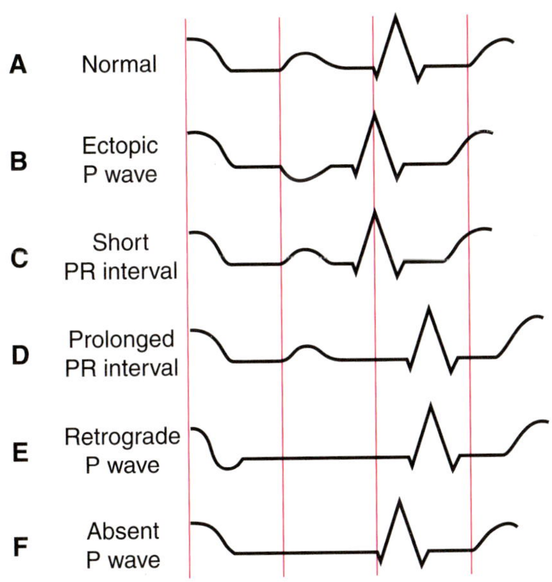

FIGURE 3.16. Vertical grid lines, 0.2-second time intervals. Note that in **A**, the PR interval is 0.2 second (the upper limit of normal). See **Animation 3.1**.

To view the animation(s) and video(s) associated with this chapter please access lww.co.in. Instructions are located on the inside front cover.

the atria. In this case, the P wave might only be identified as a distortion of the T wave. When the PR interval cannot be determined because of the absence of any visible P wave, there is obvious abnormality of the cardiac rhythm (see **Figure 3.16F**). Therefore, it is incumbent on the ECG reader to locate the P wave, if present.

Morphology of the QRS Complex

Figure 3.16A is presented again as **Figure 3.17A** and **Animation 3.2** for reference to atypical, normally appearing QRS complex with Q, R, and S waves present. Various causes of abnormal QRS-complex morphology are presented in **Figure 3.17B–D**.

A normal P-wave axis with an abnormally short PR interval is accompanied by a normal morphology of the QRS complex when there is no AV nodal bypass directly into the ventricular myocardium (see **Figure 3.16C**). When such a bypass directly enters the ventricular myocardium, it creates abnormality in the morphology of the QRS complex (see **Figure 3.17B**). This ventricular "preexcitation" eliminates the isoelectric PR segment and creates a fusion between the P wave and the QRS complex. The initial Q or R wave begins slowly (in what is termed a delta wave), prolonging the duration of the QRS complex.

Abnormally slow impulse conduction within the normal intraventricular conduction pathways also produces abnormalities of QRS complex morphology (see **Figure 3.17C**). The cardiac rhythm remains normal when the conduction abnormality is confined to either the right or left bundle branch. However, if the process responsible for the slow conduction spreads to the other bundle branch, the serious rhythm abnormality of partial or even total failure of AV conduction could suddenly occur.

An abnormally prolonged QRS duration in the absence of a preceding P wave suggests that the cardiac rhythm may be originating from the ventricles rather than from the atria (see **Figure 3.17D**).

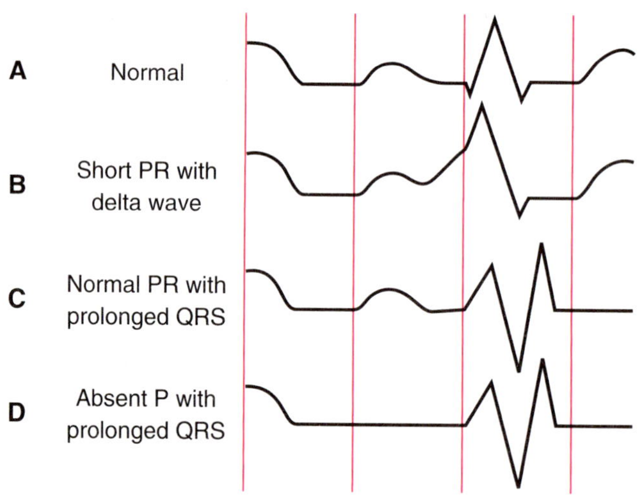

FIGURE 3.17. **A.** Normal. **B–D.** Abnormal. Vertical grid lines, 0.2-second time intervals. See Animation 3.2.

ST Segment, T wave, U wave, and QTc Interval

Figure 3.18A shows a normal waveform. Marked elevation of the ST segment (**Figure 3.18B**), an increase or decrease in T-wave amplitude (**Figure 3.18C,E**), prolongation of the QTc interval (**Figure 3.18D**), or an increase in U-wave amplitude (see **Figure 3.18E**) may be an indication of underlying cardiac conditions that may produce serious abnormalities of cardiac rhythm. Each example begins with the completion of a TP segment and ends with the initiation of the following TP segment. These abnormal QRS-to-T relationships are discussed in Chapters 8 (see **Figure 3.18B,C**) and 13 (see **Figure 3.18C–E**). See **Animation 3.3**.

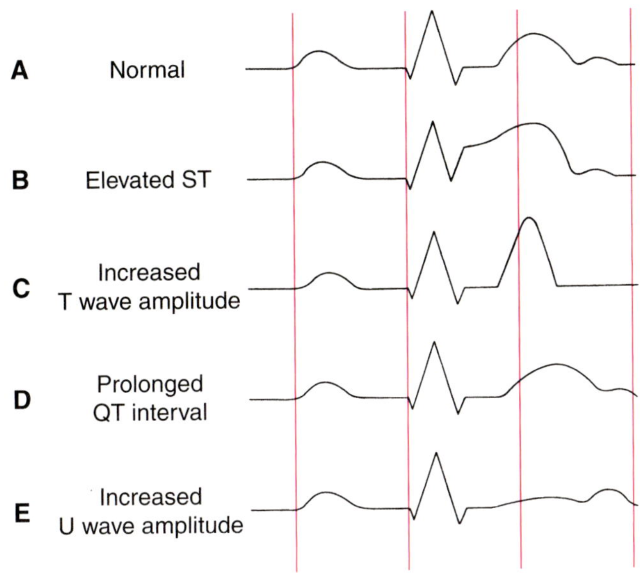

FIGURE 3.18. QRS-to-T relationship. **A.** Normal. **B–E.** Abnormal. See **Animation 3.3**.

A Final Word

No discussion of the systematic protocol for interpretation of ECGs could be complete without one of the most important features of all, comparison to prior tracings. The ECGs capture a moment in time. The physiology and electrical activity of the heart are highly dynamic and may change from moment to moment. Comparing the current ECG to immediate prior and even further past remote tracings can provide vital information about evolving disease processes and response to therapy. Locating prior tracings and comparing them with the current ECG is one of the most important tasks for ECG readers and can be the critical element in patient care diagnosis and management decisions.

CHAPTER 3 SUMMARY ILLUSTRATION

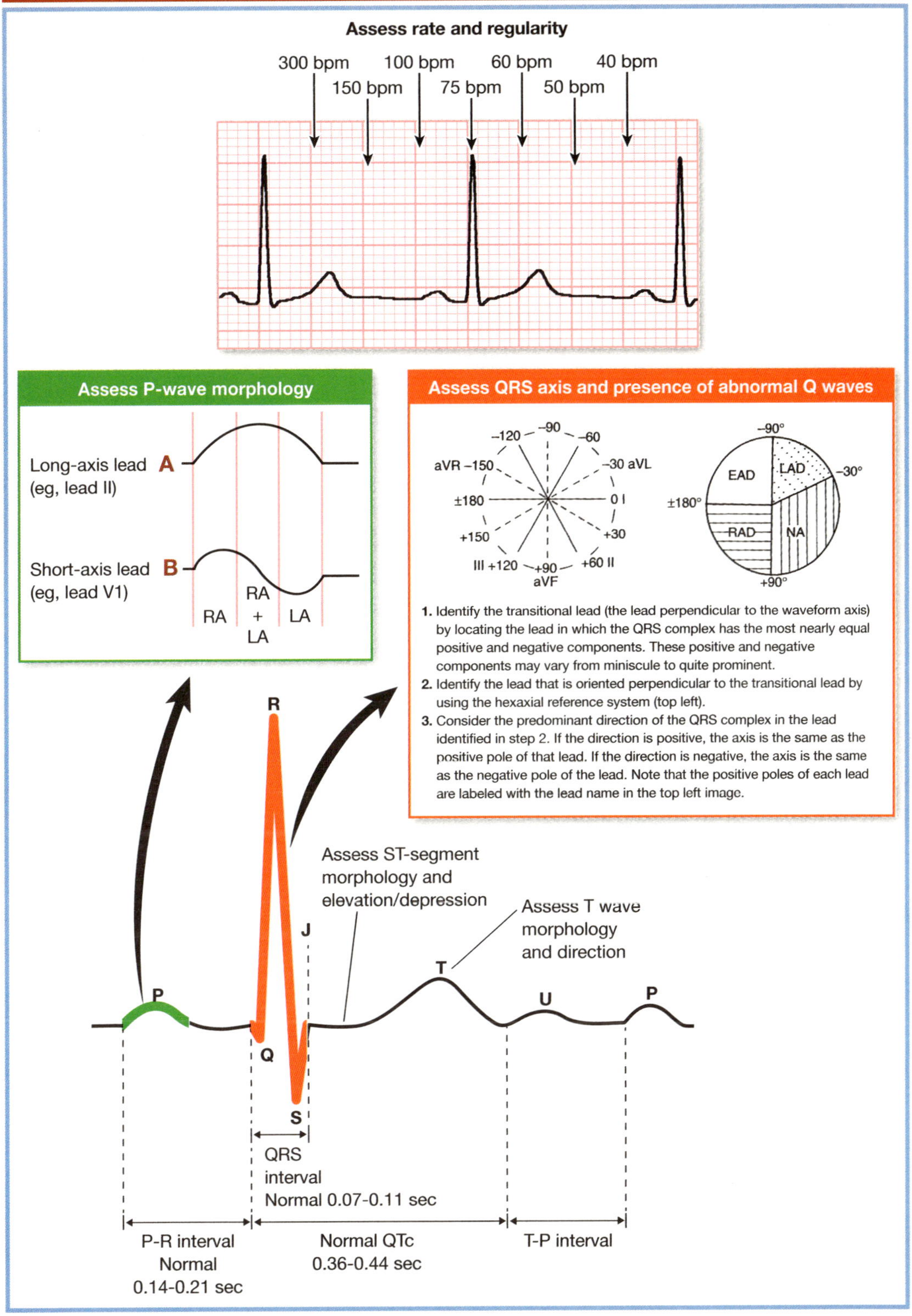

Abbreviations: bpm, beats per minute; EAD, extreme axis deviation; LA, left atrium; LAD, left axis deviation; NA, normal axis; RA, right atrium; RAD, right axis deviation.

Glossary

Amplitude: the vertical magnitude of a waveform extending from the isoelectric baseline to the waveform peak.

Autonomic nervous system: the nervous system that spontaneously controls involuntary bodily functions; it innervates glands, smooth-muscle tissue, blood vessels, and the heart.

Axis: direction of an ECG waveform in the frontal or horizontal plane, measured in degrees.

Bradycardia: a slow heart rate, <60 beats/min.

Contour: the general shape of a waveform—peaked or flat.

Deflections: ECG waveforms moving either upward (positive deflection) or downward (negative deflection) with respect to the baseline.

Duration: the interval in milliseconds between the onset and offset of a waveform. Because the apparent duration may vary in an individual lead because either the initial or terminal portion of the wave is perpendicular to that lead and is therefore isoelectric, the true waveform duration extends from the earliest onset to the latest offset in multiple simultaneously recorded ECG leads.

Extreme axis deviation: deviation of the frontal-plane QRS axis from normal, with the axis located between −90 and ±180 degrees.

Fusion: merging together of waveforms (ie, P and T waves).

Heart rate variability: the normal range of variability of heart rates observed while an individual is in the resting state.

Intrinsicoid deflection: the time interval between the beginning of the QRS complex and the peak of the R wave; this represents the time required for the electrical impulse to travel from the endocardial to the epicardial surfaces of the ventricular myocardium.

Left-axis deviation: deviation of the frontal plane QRS axis from normal, with the axis located between −30 and −90 degrees.

QRS-T angle: the number of degrees between the QRS complex and T-wave axes in the frontal and horizontal planes.

QTc interval: the corrected QT interval; it represents the duration of activation and recovery of the ventricular myocardium; the correction is applied by using a formula that takes into consideration the ventricular rate.

Rate: a measure of the frequency of occurrence of cardiac cycles; it is expressed in beats per minute.

Reentry or reactivation: passage of the cardiac electrical impulse for a second time or an even greater number of times through a structure such as the AV node or the atrial or ventricular myocardium, as the result of a conduction abnormality in that area of the heart. Normally, the cardiac electrical impulse, after its initiation in specialized pacemaking cells, spreads through each area of the heart only once.

Regularity: an expression for the consistency of the cardiac rate over a period of time.

Right-axis deviation: deviation of the frontal plane QRS axis from normal, with the axis located between +90 and ±180 degrees.

Sinus arrhythmia: the normal variation in sinus rhythm that occurs during the inspiratory and expiratory phases of respiration.

Sinus rhythm: the normal cardiac rhythm originating via impulse formation in the SA or sinus node.

Tachycardia: a rapid heart rate of >100 beats/min.

TP junction: the merging point of the T and P waves that occurs at faster heart rates.

Transitional lead: the lead in which the positive and negative components of an ECG waveform are of almost equal amplitude, indicating that lead is perpendicular to the direction of the waveform.

TU junction: the point of merging of the T and U waves; it is sometimes on and sometimes off of the isoelectric line.

Ventricular preexcitation: an event that occurs when a cardiac activating impulse bypasses the AV node and Purkinje system owing to an abnormal bundle of muscle fibers connecting the atria and ventricles. Normally, the electrical impulse must spread through the slowly conducting AV node and rapidly conducting Purkinje system to travel from the atrial to the ventricular myocardium.

Acknowledgment

We gratefully acknowledge the past contributions of the previous edition's author, Dr. Galen S. Wagner, as portions of that chapter were retained in this revision.

References

1. Grant RP. *Clinical Electrocardiography: The Spatial Vector Approach*. New York, NY: McGraw-Hill; 1957.
2. Beckwith JR. *Grant's Clinical Electrocardiography*. New York, NY: McGraw-Hill; 1970:50.
3. Wagner GS, Freye CJ, Palmeri ST, et al. Evaluation of a QRS scoring system for estimating myocardial infarct size. I. Specificity and observer agreement. *Circulation*. 1982;65:342-347.
4. Macfarlane PW, Lawrie TDV, eds. *Comprehensive Electrocardiology*. Vol 3. New York, NY: Pergamon Press; 1989:1442.
5. Beckwith JR. *Basic Electrocardiography and Vectorcardiography*. New York, NY: Raven Press; 1982:46.
6. Macfarlane PW, Lawrie TDV, eds. *Comprehensive Electrocardiology*. Vol 1. New York, NY: Pergamon Press; 1989:296-305.
7. Anderson ST, Pahlm O, Selvester RH, et al. Panoramic display of the orderly sequenced 12-lead ECG. *J Electrocardiol*. 1994;27:347-352.
8. Macfarlane PW, Lawrie TDV, eds. *Comprehensive Electrocardiology*. Vol 3. New York, NY: Pergamon Press; 1989:1459.
9. Surawicz B. STT abnormalities. In: Macfarlane PW, Lawrie TDV, eds. *Comprehensive Electrocardiology*. Vol 1. New York, NY: Pergamon Press; 1989:515.
10. Beckwith JR, ed. *Grant's Clinical Electrocardiography*. New York, NY: McGraw-Hill; 1970:59-63.
11. Ritsema van Eck HJ, Kors JA, van Herpen G. The U wave in the electrocardiogram: a solution for a 100-year-old riddle. *Cardiovasc Res*. 2005;67:256-262.
12. Castellanos A, Inerian A Jr, Myerburg RJ. The resting electrocardiogram. In: Fuster V, Alexander RW, O'Rourke RA, et al, eds. *Hurst's The Heart*. 11th ed. New York, NY: McGraw-Hill; 2004: 295-324.
13. Bazett HC. An analysis of the time-relations of electrocardiograms. *Heart*. 1920;7: 353-370.
14. Hodges M, Salerno D, Erlien D. Bazett's QT correction reviewed. Evidence that a linear QT correction for heart is better. *J Am Coll Cardiol*. 1983;1:69.
15. Macfarlane PW, Lawrie TDV, eds. The normal electrocardiogram and vectorcardiogram. In: *Comprehensive Electrocardiology*. Vol 1. New York, NY: Pergamon Press; 1989:451-452.
16. Kleiger RE, Miller JP, Bigger JT Jr, Moss AJ. Decreased heart rate variability and its association with increased mortality after acute myocardial infarction. *Am J Cardiol*. 1987;59:256-262.

References to the South Asian Edition

A. Slavich G, Tuniz D, Fregolent R, Slavich M. Pseudoischemic ST-segment due to atrial repolarization during exercise test. Review of the literature, diagnostic criteria and personal experience. *Giornale Italiano Di Cardiologia*. 2006;7(10):670-674.

B. Childers R. Atrial repolarization: its impact on electrocardiography. *Journal of Electrocardiology*. 2011;44:635-640.

C. Priori SG, Wilde AA, Horie M, Cho Y, Behr ER, Berul C, et al. HRS/EHRA/APHRS expert consensus statement on the diagnosis and management of patients with inherited primary arrhythmia syndromes: document endorsed by HRS, EHRA, and APHRS in May 2013 and ACCF, AHA, PACES, and AEPC in June 2013. *Heart Rhythm*. 2013;10:1932-1963. 10.1016/j.hrthm.2013.05.014

To view digital content associated with this chapter please access lww.co.in.
Instructions are located on the inside front cover.

SECTION II

Chamber Enlargement and Conduction Abnormalities

4 Chamber Enlargement

DOUGLAS D. SCHOCKEN,
LJUBA BACHAROVA, DAVID G. STRAUSS,
AND RAMALINGAM VADIVELU

Chamber enlargement refers to the increase in size of cardiac chambers—atria and ventricles. This enlargement can be due to hemodynamic overload (pressure or volume) or due to structural changes (cardiomyopathy). Measurement of the chamber size is the domain of imaging methods. Chamber enlargement (**Figure 4.1**) is, however, accompanied by and can be even preceded by electrocardiogram (ECG) changes. Thus, the ECG provides additional complementary diagnostic and prognostic information.[1]

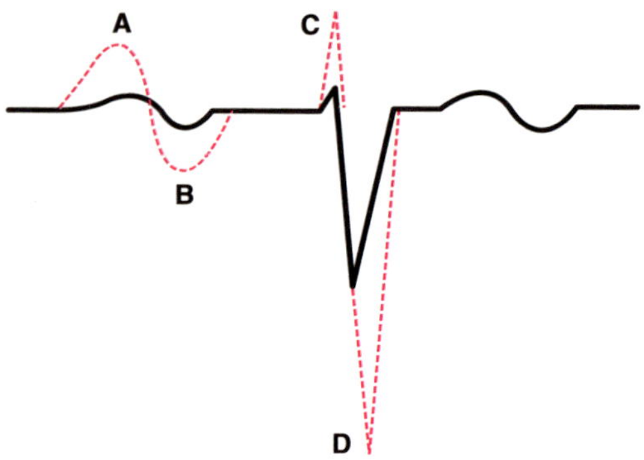

FIGURE 4.1. Schematic cartoon of how chamber enlargement affects the ECG as shown in a short-axis oriented lead (V_1). Black solid line is normal ECG and dashed line represents chamber enlargement for **A**, right atrium; **B**, left atrium; **C**, right ventricle; **D**, left ventricle.

Atrial Enlargement

The thinner wall atrial chambers generally respond to both pressure and volume overload with characteristic changes in the ECG. The usual terms for enlargement of the atria are *right-atrial enlargement* (RAE) and *left-atrial enlargement* (LAE). The term overload rather than *enlargement* might be a more accurate term for the ECG changes seen with enlargement, but the latter term prevails in clinical use. Electrical effects may occur before measurable increase in size of the affected atria (as can be seen by echocardiography).[2] These changes reflect the changes in electrical properties of the atrial myocardium preceding the anatomic enlargement.

The ECG evaluation of RAE and LAE is aided by the differing onset timing of initiation of activation of the two atria and by the differing directional spread of activation in each atrium. Right-atrial activation begins first from the sinoatrial node and proceeds in an inferior and anterior direction to produce the initial deflection of the P wave, which has a positive direction in all leads except aVR. Left-atrial activation begins later and proceeds from high in the interatrial septum in a leftward, inferior, and posterior direction. This electrical activation path produces the final deflection of the P wave, which is positive in the lead II but negative in the lead V_1 (**Figure 4.2A**). Therefore, RAE is characterized by an increase in the initial deflection (**Figures 4.2B** and **4.3A**), seen as a prominent positive deflection (*P pulmonale*) and LAE by widening of the P wave in lead II often with M-shaped morphology (*P mitrale*). An increase in the final deflection of the P wave is seen in lead V_1 in the presence of LAE as a deeper negative terminal part (**Figures 4.2C** and **4.3B**). An increase in both the initial and final aspects of the P wave suggests biatrial enlargement (**Figures 4.2D** and **4.3C**).

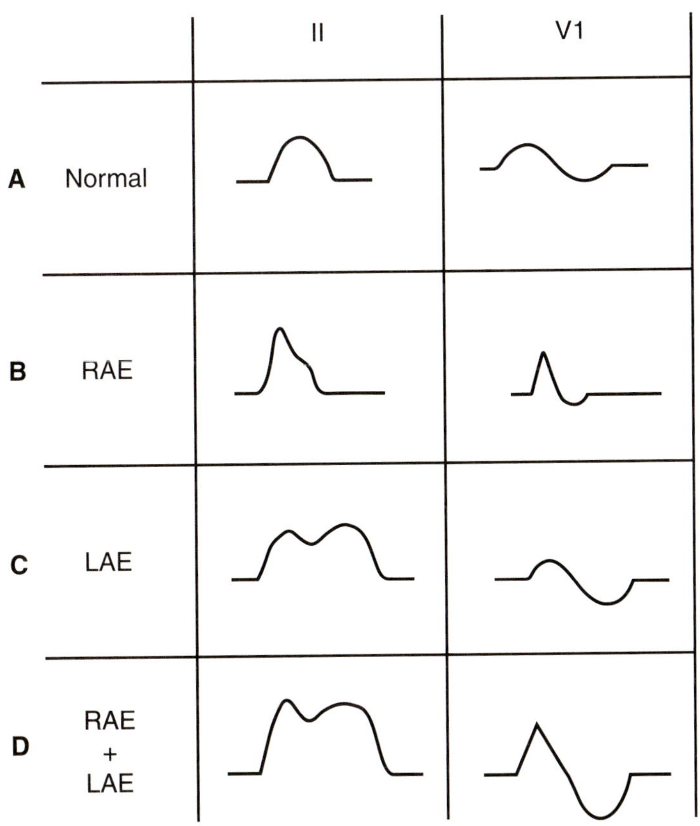

FIGURE 4.2. Schematic cartoon of key ECG features of P-wave morphology in leads II and V_1 in the presence of atrial enlargement. LAE, left-atrial enlargement; RAE, right-atrial enlargement; RAE + LAE, biatrial enlargement.

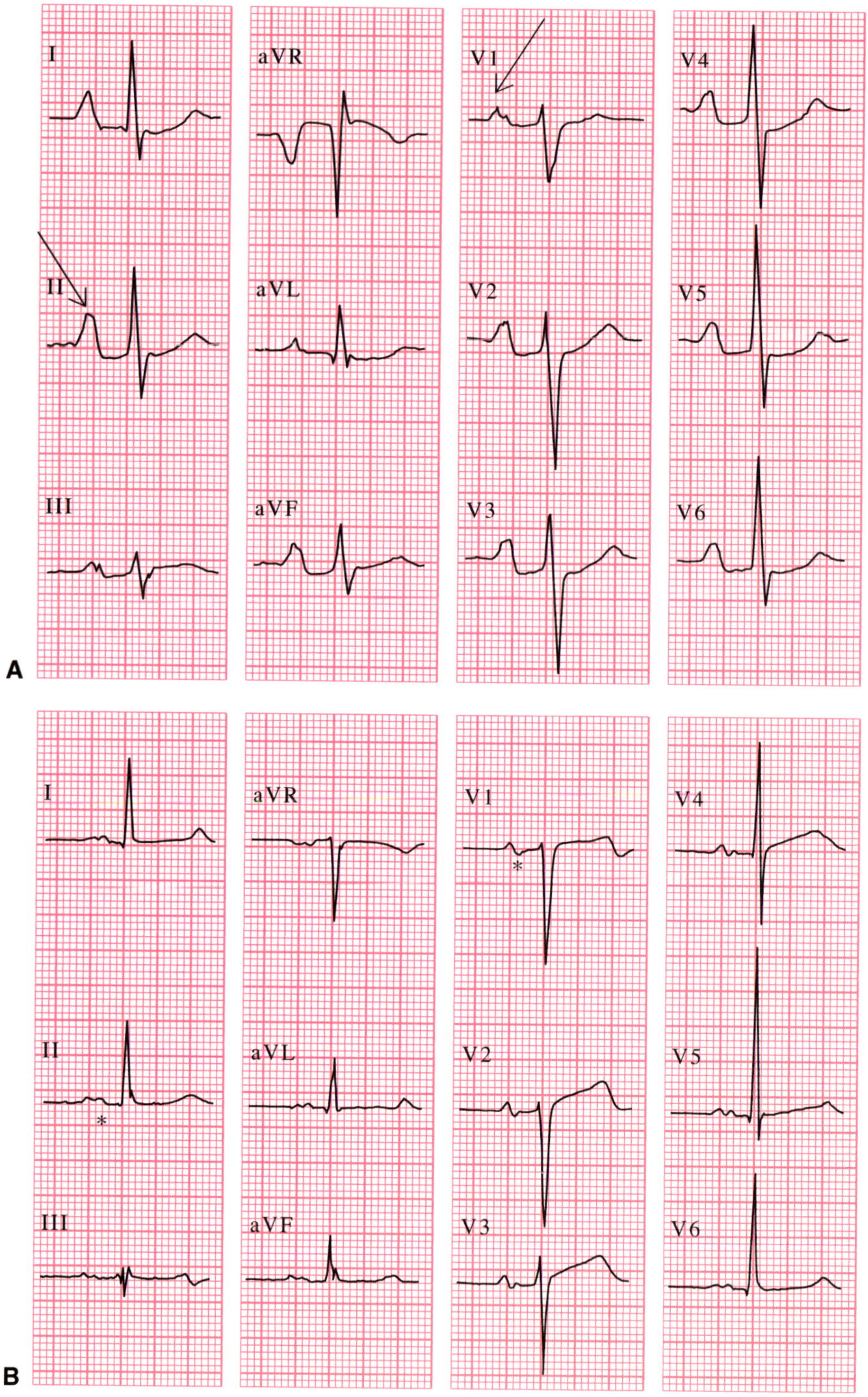

FIGURE 4.3. ECGs demonstrating atrial enlargement. Note the prolonged PR interval (0.28 s in **A**). **A.** Right-atrial enlargement. **B.** Left-atrial enlargement. *(continued)*

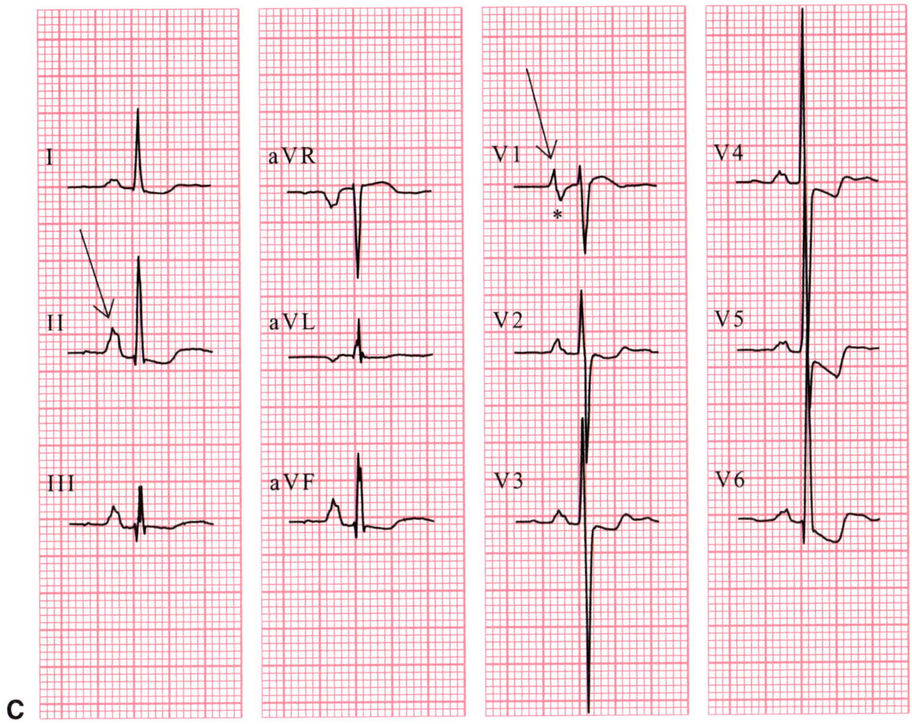

FIGURE 4.3 *(continued)* **C.** Biatrial enlargement. Arrows indicate key features of these diagnoses.

Electrocardiogram Pattern With Atrial Enlargement

General Contour

The smooth, rounded contour of the P wave is changed by RAE, which gives the wave a peaked appearance. Colloquially, "You wouldn't want to sit there." LAE causes a notch in the middle of the P wave, followed by a second "hump." In leads such as II, the P waves of RAE have a "peaked" appearance (termed *P pulmonale*) (taller than 0.20 mV), and the changes of LAE have an M-like appearance (termed *P mitrale*).

P-wave Duration

RAE does not affect the duration of the P wave. LAE prolongs the total P-wave duration in lead II to >0.12 second. LAE also prolongs the duration of the terminal, negatively directed portion of the P wave in lead V_1 to >0.04 second.

Positive and Negative Amplitudes

RAE increases the maximal amplitude of the P wave to >0.20 mV in leads II and aVF and to >0.10 mV in leads V_1 and V_2. Usually, LAE does not increase the overall amplitude of the P wave but increases only the amplitude of the terminal, negatively directed portion of the wave in lead V_1 to >0.10 mV.

Axis in the Frontal and Transverse Planes

Estimate the axes of the P wave in the two electrocardiographic planes. RAE may cause a slight rightward shift and LAE may cause a slight leftward shift in the P-wave axis in the frontal plane. However, in the absence of atrial enlargement, axis usually remains within the normal limits of 0 to +75 degrees.

With extreme RAE, the P wave may be inverted in lead V_1, creating the illusion of LAE. With extreme LAE, the P-wave amplitude may increase and the terminal portion of the wave may become negative in leads II, III, and aVF. Biatrial enlargement produces characteristics of both RAE and LAE (see **Figures 4.2D** and **4.3C**).

Munuswamy and colleagues,[2] using echocardiography as the standard for determining LAE, evaluated the percentage of patients with true-positive and true-negative ECG criteria for LAE (**Table 4.1**). They found that the most *sensitive* criterion for LAE is an increased duration (>0.04 s) of the terminal, negative portion of the P wave in lead V_1. The most *specific* criterion for LAE is a wide, notched P wave that resembles the P wave seen in the case of an *intra-atrial block, P mitrale*.

Table 4.1.

Comparison of ECG Criteria for Left-Atrial Enlargement and the Echocardiographic Measurements[a]

ECG Criteria	% True Positive[b]	% True Negative[c]
Duration of terminal negative P-wave deflection in lead V_1 >0.04 s	83	80
Amplitude of terminal negative P-wave deflection in lead V_1 >0.10 mV	60	93
Duration between peaks of P-wave notches >0.04 s	15	100
Maximal P-wave duration >0.11 s	33	88
Ratio of P-wave duration to PR-segment duration >1:1.6	31	64

[a]Modified from Munuswamy K, et al.[2] Copyright © 1984 Elsevier. With permission.

[b]Percentage of patients with left-atrial enlargement (LAE) by echocardiogram who meet the ECG criterion for LAE.

[c]Percentage of patients without LAE by echocardiogram who do not meet the ECG criterion for LAE.

Ventricular Enlargement

Ventricular Enlargement due to Hemodynamic Overload

Ventricular enlargement may occur because of either an increase in the volume of blood within the chamber or an increase in the resistance to blood flow out of the chamber. The former condition is termed *volume overload* or *diastolic overload*, and the latter is termed *pressure overload* or *systolic overload*. The increase in blood volume causes *dilation* of the ventricle, and the increase in resistance to outflow causes thickening of the myocardial wall of the ventricle (hypertrophy).

The thick-walled ventricles dilate in response to receiving an excess volume of blood during diastole, and they become hypertrophied in response to exerting excess pressure in ejecting the blood during systole (**Figure 4.4**). Volume overload in the ventricles may be caused by regurgitation of blood through a leaking valve back into the partially emptied chamber (**Figure 4.4A**).

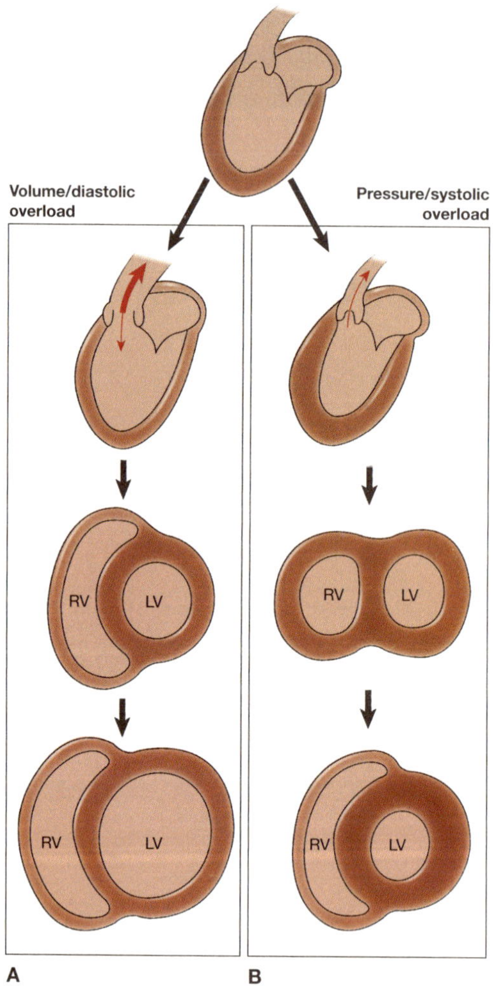

FIGURE 4.4. **A.** Volume load. Thick upward arrow, direction of blood flow; thin downward arrow, regurgitant blood. **B.** Pressure load. Thin upward arrow, direction of blood flow through narrowed outflow valve. LV, left ventricle; RV, right ventricle. (Adapted from Rushmer RF. Cardiac compensation, hypertrophy, myopathy and congestive heart failure. In: Rushmer RF, ed. *Cardiovascular Dynamics*. 4th ed. Philadelphia, PA: WB Saunders; 1976:532-565. Copyright © 1984 Elsevier. With permission.)

Pressure overload caused by obstruction to ejection through a narrowed outflow valve is displayed in **Figure 4.4B**. Enlargement of the right or left ventricle is commonly accompanied by enlargement of its corresponding atrium. Therefore, ECG findings that meet the criteria for atrial enlargement should be considered suggestive of ventricular enlargement.

Ventricular Enlargement Primarily due to Structural Changes (Cardiomyopathy)

In contrast to the concept of pressure overload response to systemic hypertension or obstruction to ventricular outflow and volume overload response to valvular regurgitation or intracardiac shunting, primary disease of the cardiac muscle (cardiomyopathy) occurs directly, thereby influencing ability of the ventricles both to contract and to relax. These pathophysiologic processes often end in heart failure. In some cases, heart failure occurs because of a decrease in cardiac output due to loss of myocytes with resulting fall in contractility. In other circumstances, the decline in output is due to diastolic dysfunction producing failure of ventricular relaxation. In the former situation, myocytes may be lost due to infarction or scarring from inflammatory processes such as myocarditis. In other circumstances, myocytes are displaced by abnormal infiltration of the heart muscle by any of a number of pathologic conditions such as sarcoidosis or abnormal protein infiltration such as amyloidosis (see Chapter 11). Diastolic dysfunction is most commonly encountered in elderly individuals, especially females with hypertension. In each of these scenarios, as ventricular (and atrial) enlargement takes place, the ECG provides a cost-efficient, readily available, noninvasive means of assessing cardiac chamber enlargement.

Electrocardiogram QRS Changes With Ventricular Enlargement

Typical changes in the QRS waveforms that occur with enlargement of the ventricles are shown schematically in **Figure 4.5**. In the absence of either right- or left-ventricular enlargement, a predominantly positive QRS complex appears in lead I and a predominantly negative QRS complex appears in lead V_1 (**Figure 4.5A**). With left-ventricular enlargement, the QRS complexes increase in amplitude but do not change in direction (**Figure 4.5B**). With right-ventricular enlargement, however, the directions of the overall QRS waveform reverse to predominantly negative in lead I and predominantly positive in lead V_1 (**Figure 4.5C**). With both right- and left-ventricular enlargement, a combination of these waveform abnormalities occurs (**Figure 4.5D**).

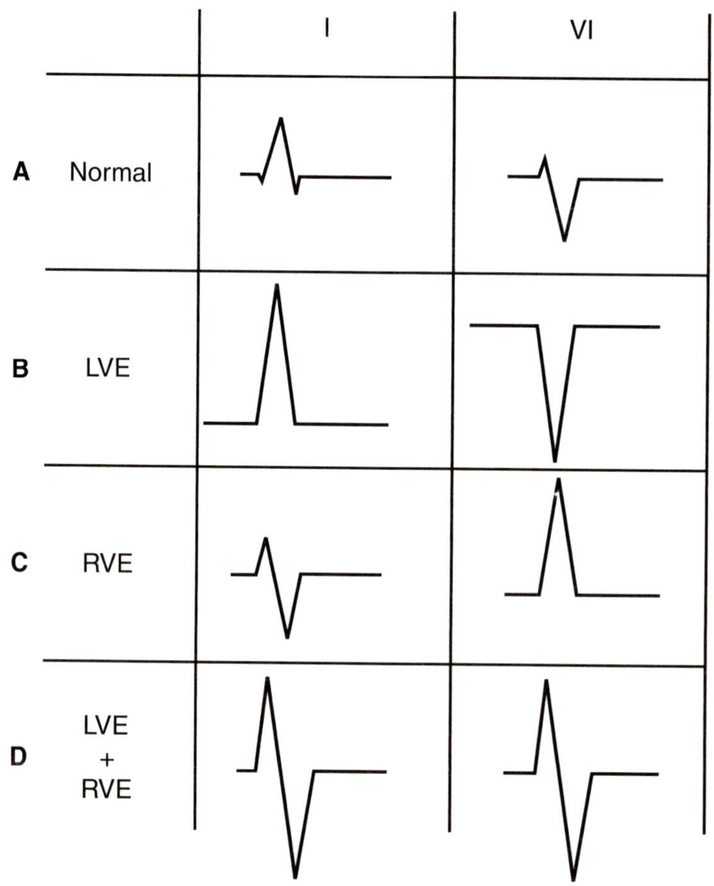

FIGURE 4.5. Schematic cartoon of QRS complex typical of ventricular enlargement in leads I and V_1. LVE, left-ventricular enlargement; LVE + RVE, biventricular enlargement; RVE, right-ventricular enlargement.

Left-Ventricular Dilation

The left ventricle dilates due to maladaptive pathophysiologic responses to pressure or volume overload or by loss of myocytes to infarction or displacement by infiltration of myocardial tissue with foreign proteins (amyloid), cells (sarcoidosis), or noncellular matter such as iron (hemochromatosis). Two factors affect the resultant ECG patterns in left-ventricular dilation: the change in size and anatomic shape of the left ventricle and the alteration in the impulse propagation velocity in the left ventricle.[3-5] The longer time required for the spread of an electrical impulse across the dilated left ventricle may produce an ECG pattern similar to that of *incomplete left-bundle-branch block* (LBBB; see Chapter 5). The duration of the QRS complex may become so prolonged that the ECG changes in left-ventricular dilation mimic those in complete LBBB (see Chapter 5).[6]

Dilation enlarges the area of the activation front in the left ventricle, which increases the amplitudes of leftward and posteriorly directed QRS waveforms (**Figure 4.6**).[3] The S-wave amplitudes are increased in leads V_2 and V_3, and the R-wave amplitudes are increased in leads I, aVL, V_5, and V_6 (**Figure 4.6A**). The T-wave amplitudes may also be increased in the same direction as the amplitudes of the QRS complex (**Figure 4.6A**).[7,8] T waves may be directed away from the QRS complex, indicating left-ventricular "strain" pattern (**Figure 4.6B**).[7-9] **Figure 4.6A** illustrates ECG changes indicating mild to moderate left-ventricular dilation, and **Figure 4.6B** shows more severe changes, including abnormally prominent Q waves in many leads and left-ventricular strain.

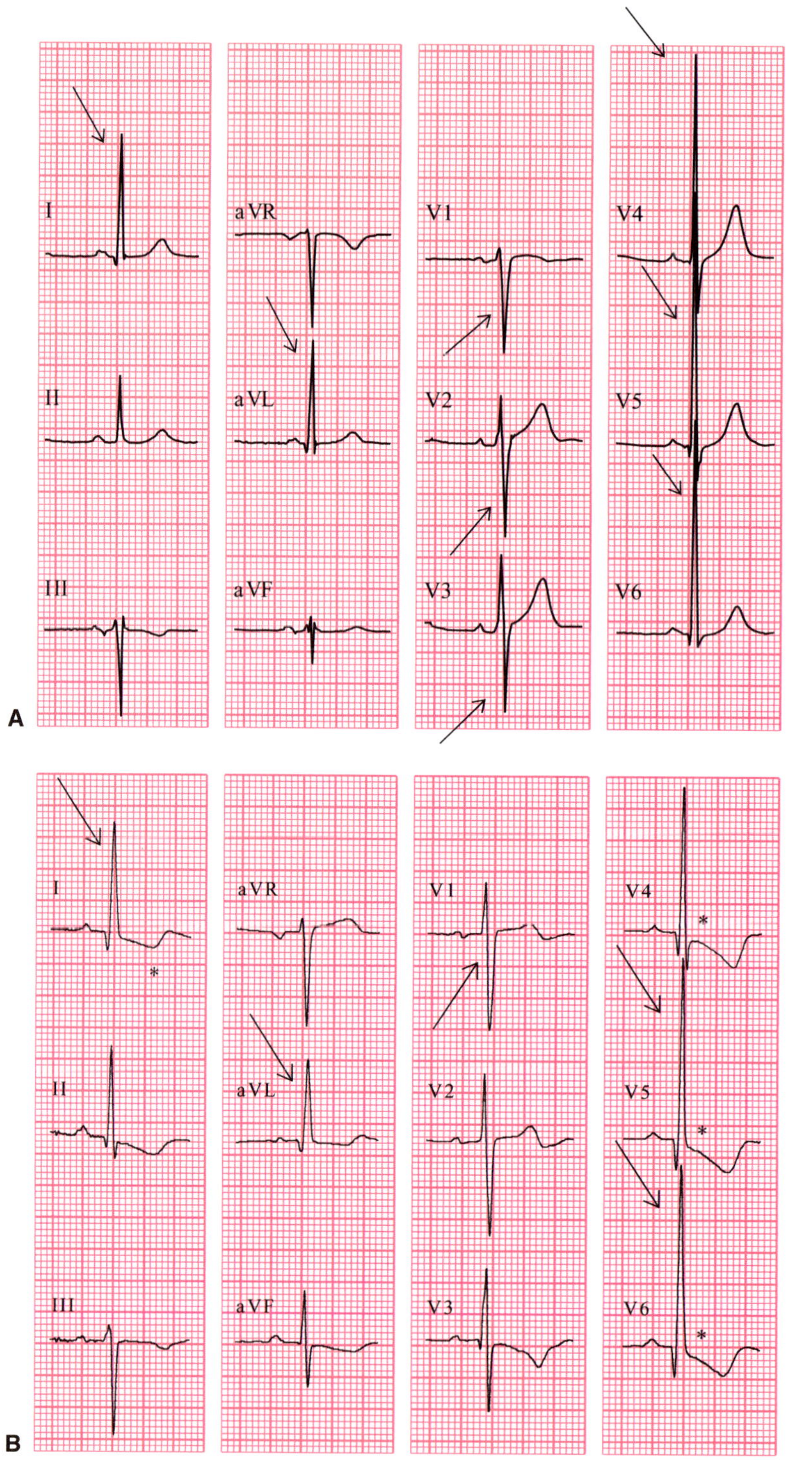

FIGURE 4.6. **A** and **B**. ECGs of patients with left-ventricular dilation. Arrows, increased leftward posterior and upward QRS waveforms; asterisks, ST-segment and T-wave changes in left-ventricular strain.

Left-Ventricular Hypertrophy

The left ventricle normally becomes larger than the right ventricle after the neonatal period. Abnormal hypertrophy, which occurs in response to a pressure overload, produces exaggeration of the normal ECG pattern of left-ventricular predominance. Like dilation, hypertrophy enlarges the area of the activation front in the left ventricle, which increases the voltages of leftward and posteriorly directed QRS waveforms, thereby causing similar shifts in the frontal and transverse plane axes, leftward and posterior.

As in left-ventricular dilation, two factors affect the resultant ECG patterns with left-ventricular hypertrophy (LVH): the change in size and anatomic shape of the left ventricle and the alteration in the impulse propagation velocity in the left ventricle.[3,7,8] Thus, with LVH, a longer period is required for spread of electrical activation from the endocardial to the epicardial surfaces of the hypertrophied myocardium, prolonging the intrinsicoid deflection (time to peak of the R wave) (see **Figure 3.9**) as well as for total left-ventricular activation. Because of the disproportion between the activation of the left and right ventricles, an interventricular conduction delay mimicking incomplete or even complete LBBB may occur with LVH as with left-ventricular dilation (**Figure 4.7A**).[6]

Pressure overload also affects repolarization and causes sustained delayed repolarization of the left ventricle, producing a negative ST segment and T wave in leads with leftward orientation (ie, V_5-V_6); this condition is termed *left-ventricular strain* (**Figure 4.7B**).[8,9] The epicardial cells no longer repolarize early, reversing the spread of recovery so that it proceeds from endocardium to epicardium. The mechanism responsible for this "strain" pattern is uncertain, but "strain" is related to the increased pressure (overload) in the left-ventricular cavity. Computer simulation studies show that the delayed depolarization of the left ventricle can also contribute to the repolarization changes in ST segment and T wave referred to as "strain."[7]

Although the two varieties of right- and left-ventricular enlargement—dilation and hypertrophy—have somewhat different effects on ECG waveforms as discussed, no specific sets of criteria for dilation versus hypertrophy have been developed. The term *enlargement* has currently been accepted with regard to the atria. For a number of reasons beyond the scope of this book, for practical purposes, the term *hypertrophy* is still used in ECG parlance instead of "enlargement" with regard to the ventricles. Additionally, the term enlargement refers to the increase in size. The term *hypertrophy* is more complex, encompassing underlying changes at tissue and cellular levels accompanying hypertrophic growth of myocardial intracellular and extracellular elements. Therefore, the systematic approach to waveform analysis introduced in Chapter 3 is applied here to "ventricular hypertrophy."

Electrocardiogram Pattern With Left-Ventricular Hypertrophy

General Contour

Prolongation of the intrinsicoid deflection by the hypertrophied ventricular myocardium diminishes the slope of the initial waveforms of the QRS complex. As activation of the ventricular myocardium spreads, the smooth contour of the mid-QRS waveforms may be disrupted by indentations or notches (**Figure 4.7A**). The terminal portions of the prolonged QRS complexes have low-frequency, smooth waveforms.

The contour of the ECG baseline may be altered. Ventricular hypertrophy shifts the J point off the horizontal baseline formed by the PR and TP segments and causes the ST segment to slope in the direction of the T wave (see **Figure 4.7B**; **Figure 4.8C**). When this change occurs in the rightward precordial leads, it is referred to as right-ventricular strain; in the left precordial leads, it is referred to as left-ventricular strain.

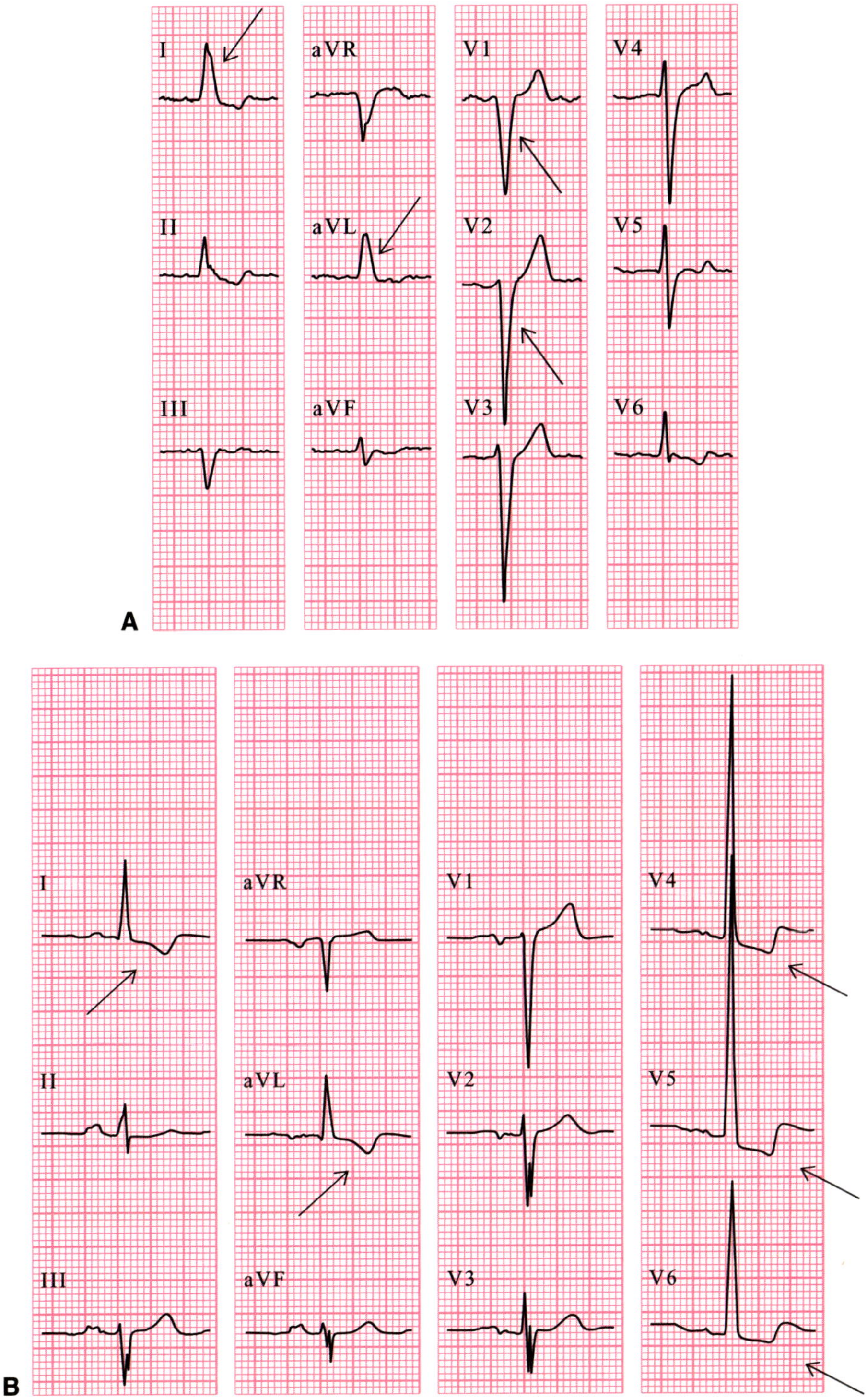

FIGURE 4.7. **A** and **B**. ECGs of patients with left-ventricular hypertrophy. Arrows in **A**, intraventricular conduction delay; arrows in **B**, ST-segment depression and T-wave inversion.

QRS Complex Duration

Hypertrophy of the left ventricle may cause prolongation of the QRS complex beyond its normal limit of 0.07 to 0.11 second, above 0.10 second indicates the beginning of delayed depolarization (intraventricular conduction delay). Hypertrophy of the right ventricle usually does *not* significantly prolong the duration of the QRS complex. Right-ventricular hypertrophy (RVH) can cause slight prolongation of the QRS complex when there is marked right-ventricular dilation. Hypertrophy of the left ventricle, however, even without dilation, may prolong the duration of the QRS complex to 0.13 or 0.14 second (a slowing of conduction often classified as bundle-branch block if its characteristic morphology fits that diagnosis but otherwise referred to as nonspecific intraventricular conduction delay if the term bundle-branch block does not apply).

Positive and Negative Amplitudes

The amplitude of the QRS complex is normally maximal in the left posterior downward direction. The left posterior direction is accentuated by LVH (and opposed by RVH). The electrical axis of the heart in frontal plane is shifted to the left with LVH (ie, upward). The criteria for LVH reflect these changes. The Sokolow-Lyon criteria (**Table 4.2**)[10] consider transverse plane leads (V_1, V_5/V_6), that is, the left and posterior waveform amplitudes, whereas the Cornell criteria (**Table 4.3**)[11] and the Romhilt-Estes criteria (**Table 4.4**)[12] consider both transverse plane leads and frontal plane leads (aVL, electrical axis), that is, the left-axis (upward) deviation. New criteria for ECG diagnosis of left-ventricular hypertrophy have been proposed by Peguero and colleagues using S wave amplitudes.[13] While promising, these criteria await further application and validation.

Table 4.2.

Sokolow-Lyon Criteria for Left-Ventricular Hypertrophy[a]

S wave in lead V_1 + R wave in lead V_5 or V_6 ≥3.50 mV
or
R wave in lead V_5 or V_6 >2.60 mV

[a]Modified from Sokolow M, Lyon TP.[10] Copyright © 1949 Elsevier. With permission.

Table 4.3.

Cornell Voltage Criteria for Left-Ventricular Hypertrophy[a]

Females	R wave in lead aVL + S wave in lead V_3 >2.00 mV
Males	R wave in lead aVL + S wave in lead V_3 >2.80 mV

[a]Modified with permission from Casale PN, Devereux RB, Alonso DR, et al.[11]

Table 4.4.

Romhilt-Estes Scoring System for Left-Ventricular Hypertrophy (LVH)[a,b]

	Points
1. R or S wave in any limb ≥2 mV	3
Or S in lead V_1 or V_2	
Or R in lead V_5 or V_6 ≥3 mV	
2. Left-ventricular strain	
ST segment and T wave in opposite direction to QRS complex	
Without digitalis	3
With digitalis	1
3. Left-atrial enlargement	
Terminal negativity of the P wave in lead V_1 is ≥0.10 mV in depth and ≥0.04 s in duration.	3
4. Left-axis deviation ≥−30 degrees	2
5. QRS duration ≥0.09 s	1
6. Intrinsicoid deflection in lead V_5 or V_6 ≥0.05 s	1
Maximally attainable	13

[a]Modified with permission from Romhilt DW, Bove KE, Norris RJ, et al.[12]

[b]5 points = definite LVH; 4 points = probable LVH.

Right-Ventricular Hypertrophy

The right ventricle dilates either during compensation for volume overload or after its hypertrophy eventually fails to compensate for pressure overload. Because of this dilation, the right ventricle takes longer to activate than is normally the case. Instead of completing its activation during the midportion of the QRS complex (see Chapter 1), the dilated right ventricle contributes anterior and rightward forces during the time of completion of left-ventricular activation. Thus, the frontal plane QRS axis shifts rightward and an RSR′ pattern appears in leads V_1 and V_2, with an appearance similar to that in *incomplete right-bundle-branch block* (see Chapter 5). The duration of the QRS complex may become so prolonged that the ECG changes occurring in right-ventricular dilation mimic those in *complete right-bundle-branch block*. These ECG changes may appear during the early or compensatory phase of volume overload or during the advanced or failing phase of pressure overload.[3]

The right ventricle hypertrophies because of compensation for pressure overload. The final third of the QRS complex is normally produced solely by activation of the thicker walled left ventricle and interventricular septum. As the right ventricle hypertrophies, it provides an increasing contribution to the early portion of the QRS complex and also begins to contribute to the later portion of the complex.

In distinction from criteria relating to LVH, the Sokolow-Lyon criteria for RVH (**Table 4.5**)[14] contain thresholds for rightward and anterior amplitudes in the transverse plane (chest) leads. Butler-Leggett criteria for RVH (**Table 4.6**)[15] require that the combination of maximal anterior and maximal rightward amplitudes exceeds the maximal leftward posterior amplitude by a threshold voltage difference.

Table 4.5.

Sokolow-Lyon Criteria for Right-Ventricular Hypertrophy[a]

R wave in lead V_1 + S wave in lead V_5 or V_6 ≥1.10 mV

[a]Modified from Sokolow M, Lyon TP.[14] Copyright © 1949 Elsevier. With permission.

Table 4.6.

Butler-Leggett Formula for Right-Ventricular Hypertrophy (RVH)[a]

Directions	Anterior	Rightward	Posterior Leftward
Amplitude	Tallest R or R′ in lead V_1 or V_2	Deepest S in lead V_1 or V_6	S in lead V_1
RVH formula	A + R − PL ≥0.70 mV		

[a]Modified from Butler PM, Leggett SI, Howe CM, Freye CJ, et al.[15] Copyright © 1986 Elsevier. With permission.

Axis in the Frontal and Transverse Planes

RVH shifts the frontal plane QRS axis rightward, to a vertical or rightward position, and shifts the transverse plane QRS axis anteriorly (see **Figure 4.8C**). LVH shifts the frontal plane QRS axis leftward and the transverse plane QRS axis posteriorly (see **Figure 4.3C**).

Lead V_1, with its left-to-right orientation, provides the optimal view of the competition between the two ventricles for electrical predominance. As shown in **Figure 4.5A**, the normal QRS complex in the adult is predominantly negative in lead V_1, with a small R wave followed by a prominent S wave. When the right ventricle hypertrophies in response to pressure overload, this negative predominance may be lost, producing a prominent R wave and a small S wave (see **Figure 4.5C**).

In mild RVH, the left ventricle retains predominance, and there is either no ECG change or the QRS axis moves rightward (see **Figure 4.8A**). Note the $S > R$ amplitude in lead I, indicating that the frontal plane axis is slightly $>+90$ degrees, meeting the threshold presented in Chapter 3 for right-axis deviation.

With moderate RVH, the initial QRS forces are predominantly anterior (with an increased R wave in lead V_1), and the terminal QRS forces may or may not be predominantly rightward (**Figure 4.8B**). These changes could also be indicative of myocardial infarction in the lateral wall of the left ventricle (see Chapter 9).

With severe RVH, the QRS complex typically becomes predominantly negative in lead I and positive in lead V_1, and the delayed repolarization of the right-ventricular myocardium may produce negativity of the ST segment and a T-wave pattern indicative of so-called right-ventricular *strain* in leads such as V_1 to V_3 (see **Figure 4.8C**).[7]

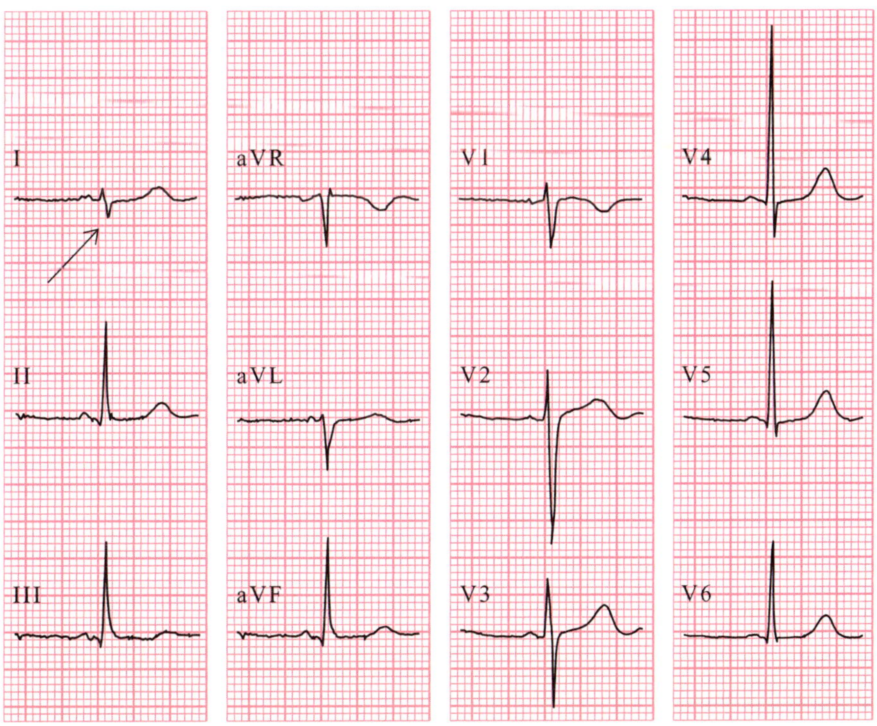

A

FIGURE 4.8. **A–C.** ECGs of patients with right-ventricular hypertrophy. Arrows, right-ventricular hypertrophy in the QRS complex; asterisk, ST and T wave in right-ventricular strain. *(continued)*

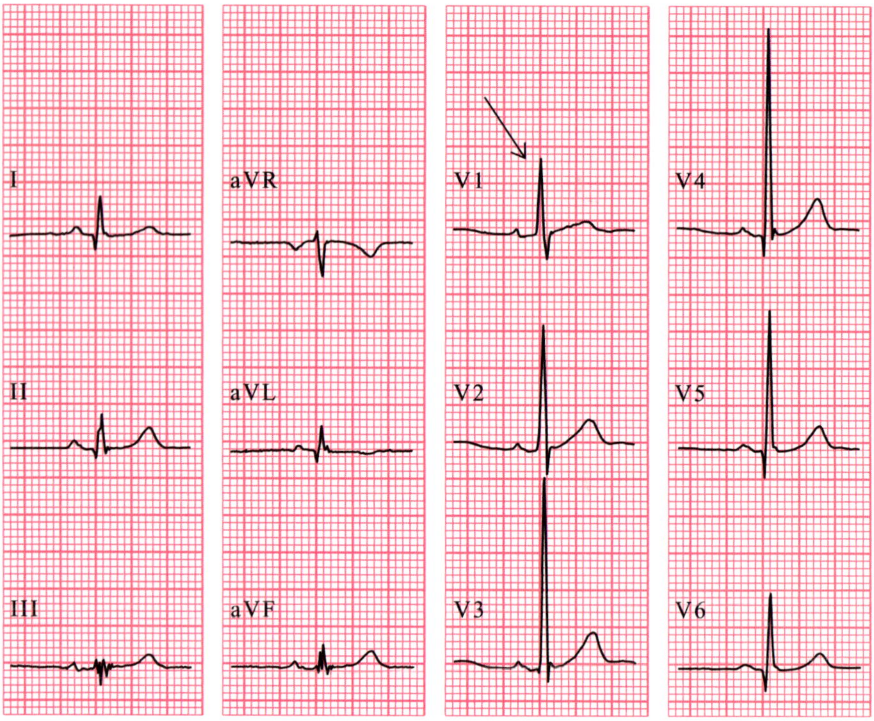

B

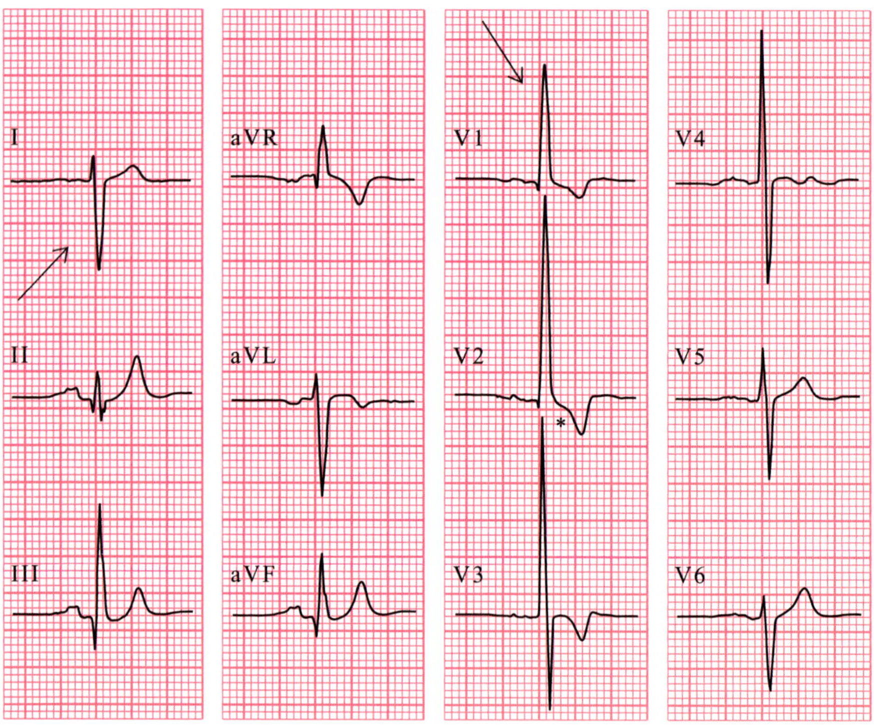

C

FIGURE 4.8. *(continued)*

In the neonate, the right ventricle is more hypertrophied than the left because there is greater resistance in the pulmonary circulation than in the systemic circulation during fetal development (**Figure 4.9**). Right-sided resistance is greatly diminished when the lungs fill with air, and left-sided resistance is greatly increased when the placenta is removed.[16] From this time onward, the ECG evidence of right-ventricular predominance is gradually lost as the left ventricle becomes hypertrophied in relation to the right. Therefore, hypertrophy, like dilation, may be a compensatory rather than a pathologic condition.[6] Pressure overload of the right ventricle may recur in later years because of increased resistance to blood flow through the pulmonary valve, the pulmonary circulation, or the left side of the heart.

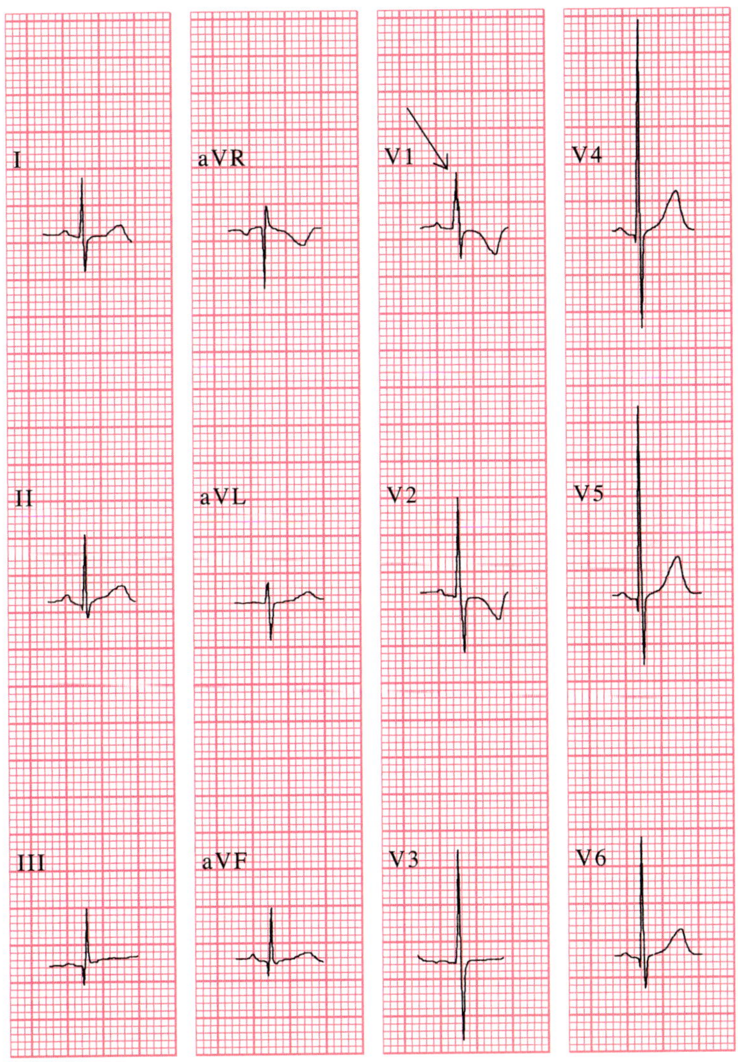

FIGURE 4.9. Healthy neonatal ECG. Arrow, normal right-ventricular predominance.

Most criteria for LVH and RVH are based on voltage measures. Elevated anterior and rightward forces are generally consistent with RVH because the right ventricle is the most anterior chamber. Other ECG features make one think of RVH. Some of these features are listed in **Table 4.7**.

Table 4.7.

Electrocardiogram Clues Suggesting Right-Ventricular Hypertrophy

1.	Right-axis deviation (+90 degrees or more)
2.	RV1 = 7 mm or more
3.	RV1 + SV5 or SV6 = 10 mm or more
4.	R/S ratio in V_1 = 1.0 or more
5.	S/R ratio in V_6 = 1.0 or more
6.	Late intrinsicoid deflection in V_1 (>0.035 s)
7.	Incomplete right-bundle-branch block pattern
8.	ST-T "strain" in leads II, III, and aVF
9.	P pulmonale or *P congenitale*
10.	SI, SII, SIII pattern (in children)

Biventricular Hypertrophy

In many circumstances, both ventricles will enlarge. An old aphorism, now somewhat out of date but with retained validity, is that the leading cause of right-ventricular failure is left-ventricular failure. The process of the development of biventricular enlargement or hypertrophy is in keeping with the concept that pressure or volume overload leads to the final common pathway of nonischemic cardiomyopathy. On the ECG, biventricular hypertrophy will manifest itself as a combination of the various diagnostic criteria for both LVH and RVH. **Figure 4.10A-C** demonstrates some of the variable characteristics of the ECG encountered in these patients.

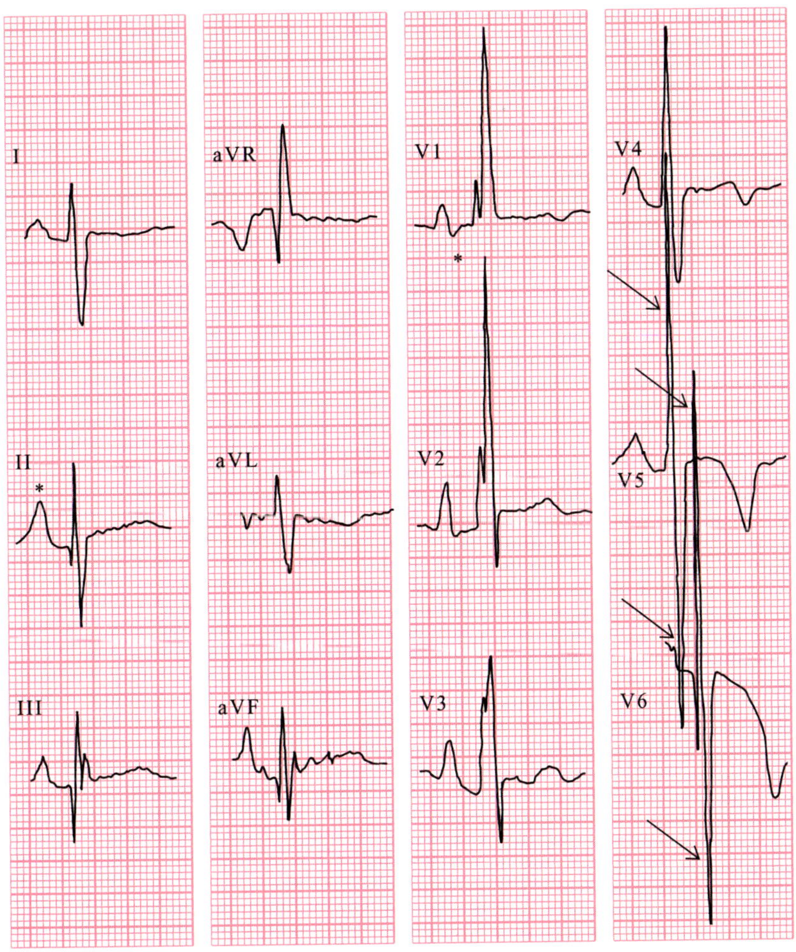

A

FIGURE 4.10. **A–C.** ECGs of patients with biventricular hypertrophy. Arrows in **A** and **B**, S > R in lead I, prominent R in lead V_1, and increased S in lead V_3; arrows in **C**, prominent R precordial leads; asterisks in **A**, typical P-wave abnormalities of right-atrial enlargement and left-atrial enlargement; asterisks in **B**, typical P-wave abnormalities of right-atrial enlargement. *(continued)*

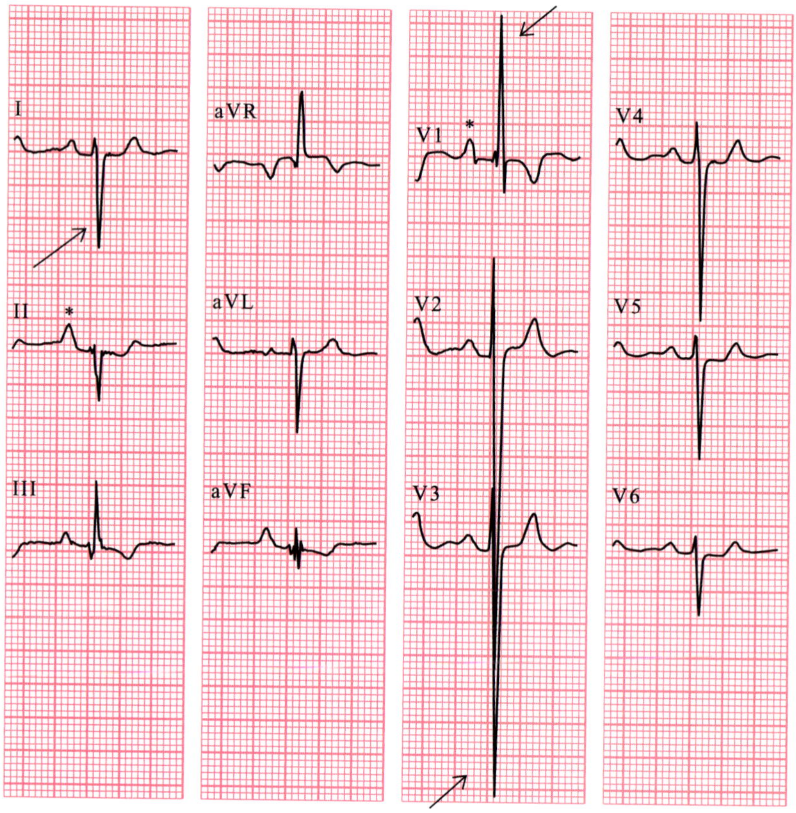

B

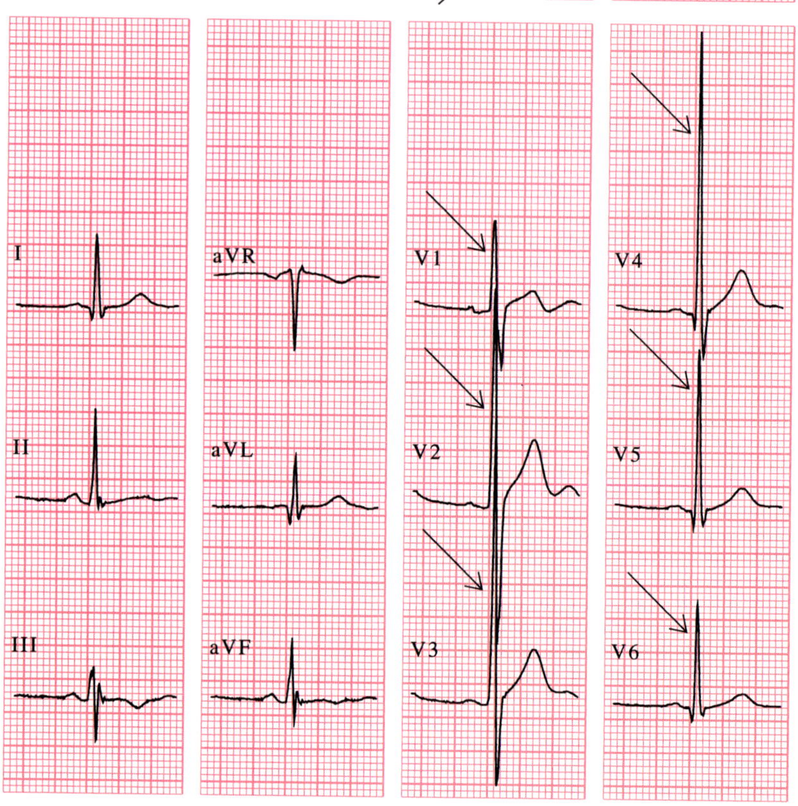

C

FIGURE 4.10. *(continued)*

Scoring Systems for Assessing LVH and RVH

Three sets of criteria for LVH (see **Tables 4.2-4.4**) and two of criteria for RVH (see **Tables 4.5** and **4.6**) are presented in this chapter. As stated, there is no distinction between dilation and hypertrophy.

RVH shifts the direction of both the ST segment and the T wave away from the right ventricle, opposite to the shift that such hypertrophy produces in the QRS complex. Typically, in rightward leads such as V_1, the QRS complex would be abnormally positive, whereas the ST segment and T wave would be abnormally negative (see **Figure 4.8C**). LVH shifts the ST segment and T wave away from the left ventricle in the direction opposite to the shift it produces in the QRS complex. Therefore, in leftward leads such as aVL and V_5, the QRS complex is abnormally positive, and the ST segment and T wave are abnormally negative (see **Figure 4.7B**).

The diagnosis of RVH in the presence of complete RBBB is suggested by the presence of R of >15 mm height in V_1 and >10 mm height in V_1 in the presence of incomplete RBBB (Barker and Valencia criteria).[A]

The presence of tall diphasic QRS complexes >50 mm in height in V_2-V_4 is suggestive of biventricular hypertrophy (Katz-Wachtel phenomenon) and is usually seen in the presence of congenital heart diseases.

CHAPTER 4 SUMMARY ILLUSTRATION

Salient Features of Chamber Enlargement

Lead II

Right atrial enlargement

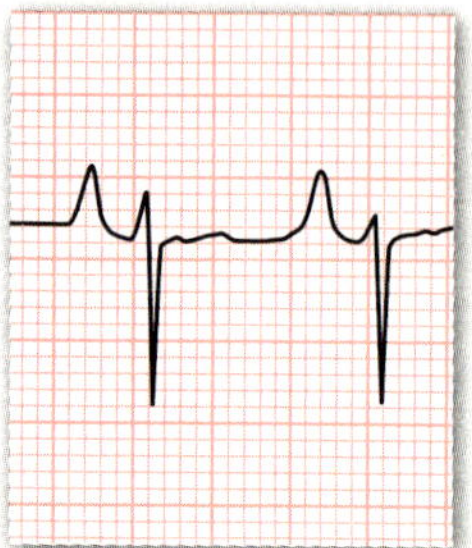

Lead V1

Right ventricular enlargement

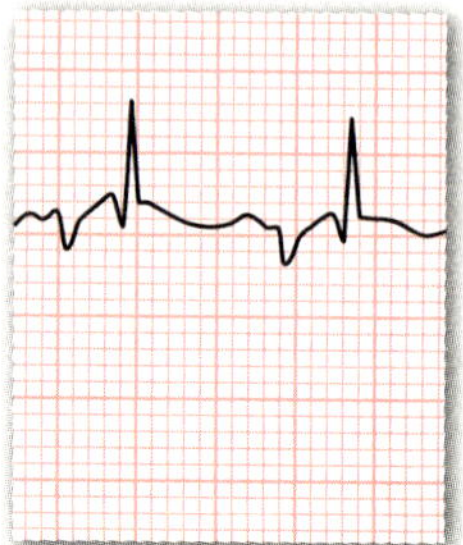

Lead V1

Right ventricular enlargement with repolarization abnormality ("strain")

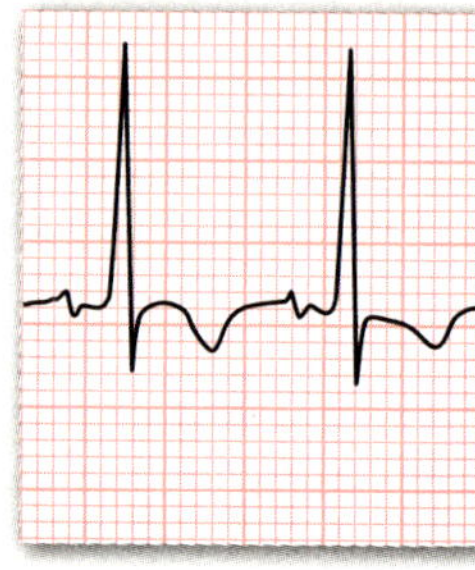

Lead V1

Left atrial enlargement

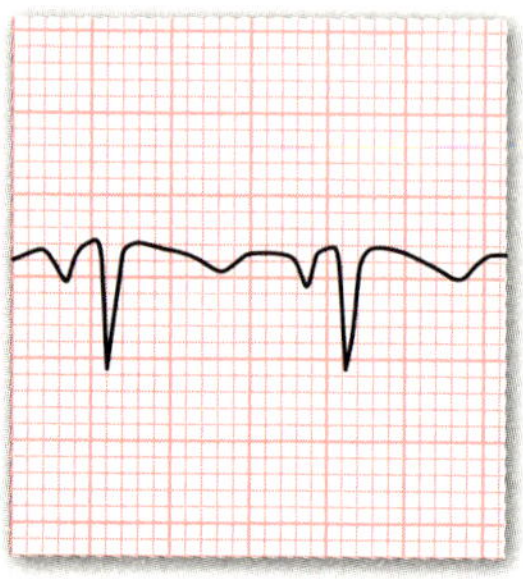

Lead aVL

Left ventricular enlargement

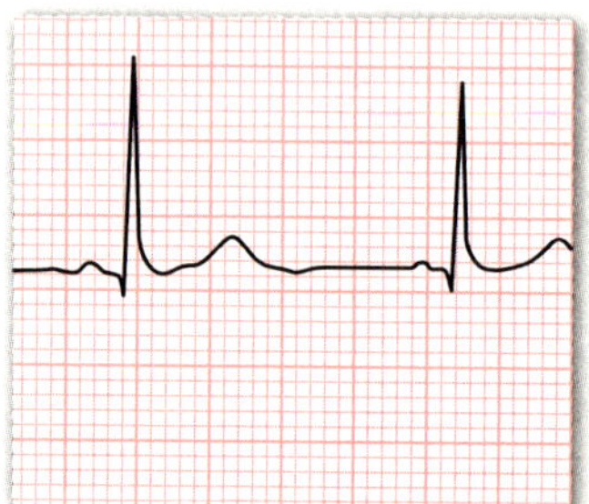

Lead aVL

Left ventricular enlargement with repolarization abnormalities ("strain")

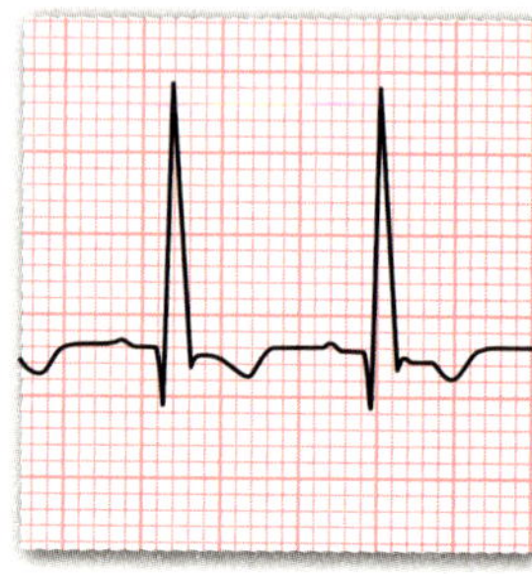

Glossary

Dilation: increase in the internal diameter of the ventricle beyond its normal dimensions.

Enlargement: dilation or hypertrophy of a cardiac chamber.

Hypertrophy: (noun) an increase in mass of a cardiac chamber, caused by the thickening of myocardial fibers, addition of sarcomeres; (verb) to increase in mass.

Incomplete bundle-branch block: partial failure of conduction in the right or left bundle branch.

Intra-atrial block: a conduction delay within the atria.

Left-atrial enlargement (LAE): dilation of the left atrium to accommodate an increase in blood volume or due to resistance to outflow.

Left-bundle-branch block (LBBB): failure of conduction in the left bundle branch of the ventricular Tawara system.

Left-ventricular strain: an ECG pattern characteristic of marked LVH, which is accompanied by ST-segment and T-wave changes (negativity of the ST segment and T wave) in addition to changes in the QRS complex.

P congenitale: appearance of P wave in RAE, most commonly associated with congenital heart disease, with tall, peaked P waves in leads I and II and in right-sided precordial leads but with frontal plane P-wave axis less rightward than with P pulmonale (see following text).

P mitrale: appearance of the P wave in LAE; named for its common occurrence in mitral valve disease. Characterized by P wave prolongation (>120 ms wide), usually seen in lead II, often with a notch in the midportion producing an overall "M"-shaped appearance and with deepening of the terminal negative portion (>0.01 mV deep), best seen in the lead V_1.

P pulmonale: appearance of the P wave in RAE; named for its common occurrence in chronic pulmonary disease. Characterized by increased P wave amplitude (>0.2 mV), best seen in the lead II and frontal plane P-wave axis +70 degrees or more.

Pressure or systolic overload: a condition in which a ventricle pumps against an increased resistance during systole, such as in the case of systemic hypertension (left ventricle) or pulmonary hypertension (right ventricle).

Right-atrial enlargement (RAE): dilation of the right atrium to accommodate an increase in blood volume or resistance to outflow.

Right-bundle-branch block (RBBB): failure of conduction in the right branch of the ventricular Tawara system.

Sensitive: a term referring to the ability (sensitivity) of a test to indicate the presence of a condition (ie, if the test is positive in every subject with the condition, it attains 100% sensitivity).

Specific: a term referring to the ability (specificity) of a test to indicate the absence of a condition (ie, if the test is negative in every control subject without the condition, it attains 100% specificity).

Strain: an ECG pattern characteristic of marked hypertrophy that is accompanied by ST-segment and T wave changes in addition to changes in the QRS complex.

Volume or diastolic overload: a condition in which a ventricle becomes filled with an increased amount of blood during diastole.

Acknowledgment

We gratefully acknowledge the past contributions of the previous edition's author, Dr. Galen S. Wagner, as portions of that chapter were retained in this revision.

References

1. Bacharova L, Chen H, Estes EH, et al. Determinants of discrepancies in detection and comparison of the prognostic significance of left ventricular hypertrophy by electrocardiogram and cardiac magnetic resonance imaging. *Am J Cardiol.* 2015;115(4):515-522.
2. Munuswamy K, Alpert MA, Martin RH, Whiting RB, Mechlin NJ. Sensitivity and specificity of commonly used electrocardiographic criteria for left atrial enlargement determined by M-mode echocardiography. *Am J Cardiol.* 1984;53(6):829-832.
3. Bacharova L, Szathmary V, Kovalcik M, Mateasik A. Effect of changes in left ventricular anatomy and conduction velocity on the QRS voltage and morphology in left ventricular hypertrophy: a model study. *J Electrocardiol.* 2010;43(3):200-208.
4. Maanja M, Wieslander B, Schlegel TT, et al. Diffuse myocardial fibrosis reduces electrocardiographic voltage measures of

left ventricular hypertrophy independent of left ventricular mass. *J Am Heart Assoc.* 2017;6(1):e003795.
5. Bacharova L, Estes EH, Schocken DD, et al. The 4th report of the working group on ECG diagnosis of left ventricular hypertrophy. *J Electrocardiol.* 2017;50(1):11-15.
6. Strauss DG, Selvester RH, Wagner GS. Defining left bundle branch block in the era of cardiac resynchronization therapy. *Am J Cardiol.* 2011;107(6):927-934.
7. Bacharova L, Szathmary V, Mateasik A. Primary and secondary T wave changes in LVH: a model study. *J Electrocardiol.* 2010;43(6):624-633.
8. Devereux RB, Reichek N. Repolarization abnormalities of left ventricular hypertrophy. Clinical, echocardiographic and hemodynamic correlates. *J Electrocardiol.* 1982;15(1):47-53.
9. Schocken DD. Electrocardiographic left ventricular strain pattern: everything old is new again. *J Electrocardiol.* 2014;47(5):595-598.
10. Sokolow M, Lyon TP. The ventricular complex in left ventricular hypertrophy as obtained by unipolar precordial and limb leads. *Am Heart J.* 1949;37(2):161-186.
11. Casale PN, Devereux RB, Alonso DR, Campo E, Kligfield P. Improved sex-specific criteria of left ventricular hypertrophy for clinical and computer interpretation of electrocardiograms: validation with autopsy findings. *Circulation.* 1987;75(3):565-572.
12. Romhilt DW, Bove KE, Norris RJ, et al. A critical appraisal of the electrocardiographic criteria for the diagnosis of left ventricular hypertrophy. *Circulation.* 1969;40(2):185-195.
13. Peguero JG, Presti SL, Perez J, et al. Electrocardiographic criteria for the diagnosis of left ventricular hypertrophy. *J Am Coll Cardiol.* 2017;69:1694-1703.
14. Sokolow M, Lyon TP. The ventricular complex in right ventricular hypertrophy as obtained by unipolar precordial and limb leads. *Am Heart J.* 1949;38(2):273-294.
15. Butler PM, Leggett SI, Howe CM, Freye CJ, Hindman NB, Wagner GS. Identification of electrocardiographic criteria for diagnosis of right ventricular hypertrophy due to mitral stenosis. *Am J Cardiol.* 1986;57(8):639-643.
16. Cabrera E, Monroy JR. Systolic and diastolic loading of the heart. II. Electrocardiographic data. *Am Heart J.* 1952;43(5):669-686.

Reference to the South Asian Edition

A. Barker JM, Valencia F. The precordial electrocardiogram in incomplete right bundle branch block. *Am Heart J.* 1949;38(3):376-406.

To view digital content associated with this chapter please access lww.co.in. Instructions are located on the inside front cover.

5 Intraventricular Conduction Abnormalities

DAVID G. STRAUSS, TOBIN H. LIM,
AND SUCHIT MAJUMDAR

Normal Conduction

Many cardiac conditions cause electrical impulses to be conducted abnormally through the ventricular myocardium, producing changes in QRS complexes and T waves. Therefore, it is important to understand the conditions that can mimic or complicate the diagnosis of bundle-branch block (BBB) or fascicular block (intraventricular conduction abnormalities). These are as follows:

Mimics and Complicating Conditions of Bundle Branch Block

1. Ventricular hypertrophy (right or left) (see Chapter 4)
2. Myocardial infarction or ischemia (see Chapters 6-9)
3. Delayed conduction through the His-Purkinje system (as discussed later in this chapter)
4. Accessory pathways from atria to ventricles (producing early, often aberrant ventricular conduction (see Chapter 19)
5. Myocardial infiltrative disorders—amyloidosis and sarcoidosis.
6. Electrolyte abnormalities—hyperkalemia.

Bundle-Branch and Fascicular Blocks

Because the activation of the ventricular Purkinje system is not represented on the surface electrocardiogram (ECG), abnormalities of the ventricular Purkinje system conduction must be detected indirectly by their effects on myocardial activation and recovery. The ECG waveforms (see **Figure 1.14**) are reproduced with the addition of specific QRS complex abnormalities in **Figure 5.1**. A conduction disturbance within the right bundle branch (RBB) causes right-ventricular activation to occur after left-ventricular activation is completed, producing an R′ deflection in lead V_1 (see **Figure 5.1**). A delay in conduction through the left bundle branch (LBB) markedly postpones left-ventricular activation, resulting in an abnormally prominent S wave in lead V_1 (see **Figure 5.1**). This difference in appearance in V_1 is due to the fact that the late activated RV being under the lead shows late positive deflection in RBBB, while in LBBB, the late activation of LV changes the net vector away from V_1 to produce the late negative deflection.

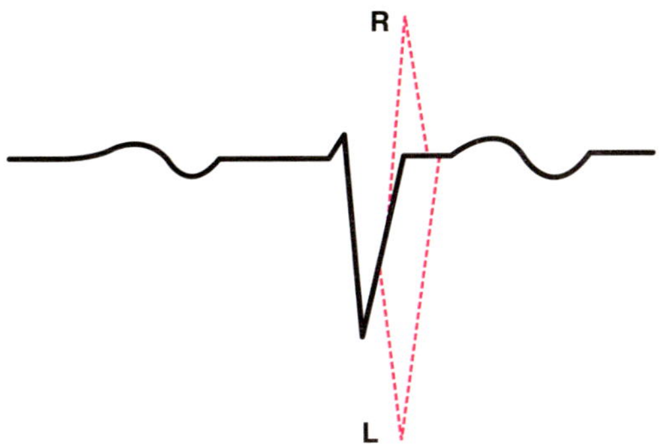

FIGURE 5.1. Dashed lines indicate right-sided (R) and left-sided (L) intraventricular conduction delays in this schematic recording from lead V_1 that provides the short-axis viewpoint.

Conduction delays in the left-bundle *fascicles* or between the Purkinje fibers and the adjacent myocardium may alter the QRS complex and T wave (**Figure 5.2**). A conduction disturbance in the common bundle (bundle of His) has similar effects on the entire distal Purkinje system and, therefore, does not alter the appearance of the QRS complex or T wave.

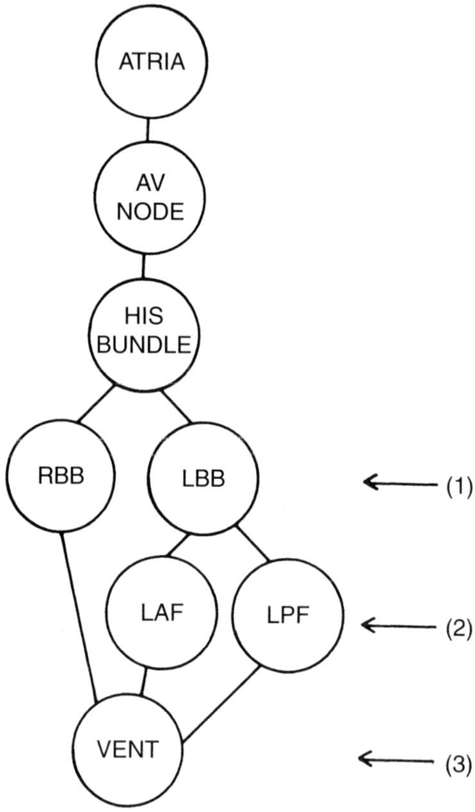

FIGURE 5.2. Possible locations of intraventricular conduction abnormalities causing QRS complex and T-wave alterations are indicated by numbers 1, 2, and 3. AV, atrioventricular; LAF, left anterior fascicle; LBB, left-bundle-branch block; LPF, left posterior fascicle; RBB, right-bundle-branch block; VENT, ventricle. (Modified from Wagner GS, Waugh RA, Ramo BW. *Cardiac Arrhythmias*. New York, NY: Churchill Livingstone; 1983:18. Copyright © 1983 Elsevier. With permission.)

Block of an entire bundle branch requires that its ventricle be activated by spread of electrical activity from the other ventricle, with prolongation of the overall QRS complex. Block of the entire RBB is termed complete right-bundle-branch block (RBBB). Block of the entire LBB is termed complete left-bundle-branch block (LBBB). In both of these conditions, the ventricles are activated successively instead of simultaneously. The other conditions in which the ventricles are activated successively occur when one ventricle is preexcited via an accessory atrioventricular (AV) pathway (see Chapter 19) and when there are independent ventricular rhythms (see Chapters 14 and 17). Under these conditions, there is a fundamental similarity in the distortions of the ECG waveforms. The duration of the QRS complex is prolonged and the ST segment slopes into the T wave in the direction away from the ventricle in which the abnormality is located. The difference between successive activation of ventricles due to bundle branch block and that due to accessory pathway conduction or a VT/paced rhythm lies in the fact that the initial part of QRS is sharp in BBB due to intact activation of the unaffected bundle, while in the other cases, it is slurred due to myocardial conduction. **Figure 5.3** compares QRS morphologies in lead V_1 when the two ventricles are activated successively rather than simultaneously.

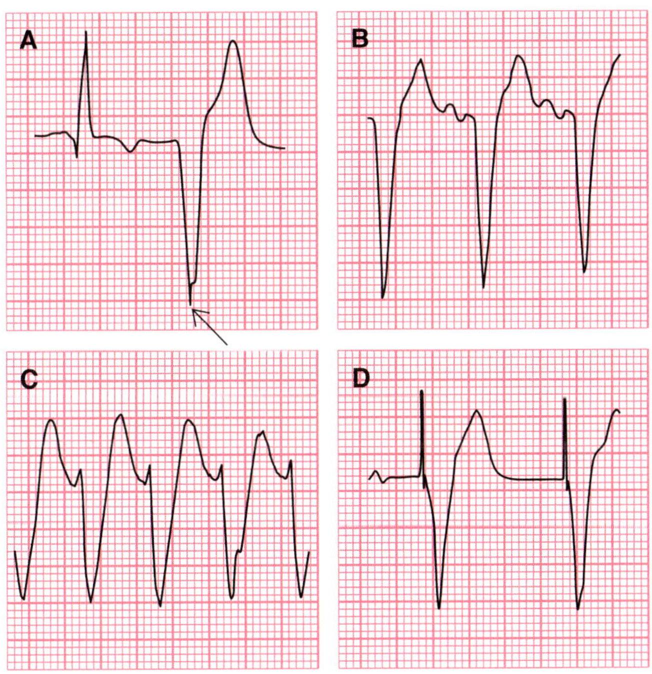

FIGURE 5.3. Comparison of patterns of QRS morphology in lead V_1 when the two ventricles are activated successively rather than simultaneously. **A.** Ventricular beat. **B.** Bundle-branch block. **C.** Ventricular tachycardia. **D.** Artificially paced ventricular rhythm.

A ventricular conduction delay with only slight prolongation of the QRS complex due to slowed conduction through the bundle branches could be termed incomplete RBBB or incomplete LBBB. It is important to remember from Chapter 4, however, that enlargement of the right ventricle may produce a distortion of the QRS complex that mimics incomplete RBBB (see **Figure 4.11A**). Enlargement of the left ventricle may produce a prolongation of the QRS complex that mimics incomplete LBBB (see **Figure 4.7A**). Because the LBB has multiple fascicles, another form of incomplete LBBB could be produced by a disturbance in either of its major fascicles.

The ventricular Purkinje system is considered trifascicular. It consists of the RBB and the anterior and posterior portions of the LBB. The proximal RBB is small and compact and may therefore be considered either a bundle branch or a fascicle. The proximal LBB is also compact but is too large to be considered a fascicle. It remains compact for 1 to 2 cm and then fans into its two fascicles.[1] As Demoulin and Kulbertus[2] have shown in humans, there are multiple individual anatomic variations in these fascicles. The left ventricle has been opened (**Figure 5.4**) to reveal the LBB and its fascicles as originally presented in **Figure 1.7C**. Note the anterior and posterior fascicles of the LBB are also designated superior and inferior, respectively, because these terms indicate their true anatomic positions. Based on their anatomic locations, the two fascicles are termed the left anterior fascicle (LAF) and left posterior fascicle (LPF; see **Figure 5.4**). The LAF of the LBB courses toward the anterosuperior papillary muscle, and the LPF of the LBB courses toward the postero-inferior papillary muscle. There are also Purkinje fibers that emerge from the LBB that proceed along the surface of the interventricular septum (sometimes termed the left septal fascicle) and initiate left-to-right spread of activation through the interventricular septum.

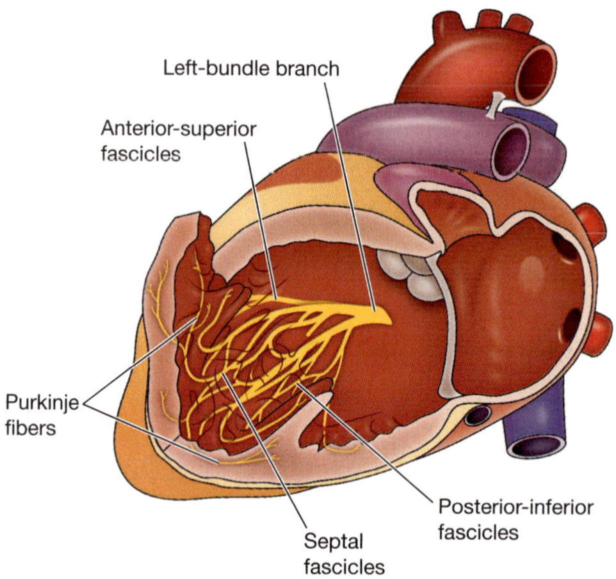

FIGURE 5.4. The left ventricle has been opened to reveal the left bundle branch (LBB) and its fascicles as originally presented in **Figure 1.7C**. Note that the anterior and posterior fascicles to the LBB are also designated superior and inferior, respectively, because these terms indicate their true anatomic positions. (From Netter FH, ed. *The CIBA Collection of Medical Illustrations*. Summit, NJ: Ciba-Geigy; 1978:13. *Heart*; vol 5, with permission.)

Rosenbaum and coworkers[3] described the concept of blocks in the fascicles of the LBB, which they termed left anterior and left posterior hemiblock. These two kinds of block are, however, more appropriately termed *left anterior fascicular block* (LAFB) and *left posterior fascicular block* (LPFB). Isolated LAFB, LPFB, or RBBB is considered unifascicular block. Complete LBBB or combinations of RBBB with LAFB or with LPFB are bifascicular blocks, and the combination of RBBB with both LAFB and LPFB is considered *trifascicular block*.

Unifascicular Blocks

The term *unifascicular block* is used when there is ECG evidence of blockage of only the RBB, LAF, or LPF. Isolated RBBB or LAFB occur commonly, whereas isolated LPFB is rare. Rosenbaum and coworkers[3] identified only 30 patients with LPFB, as compared with 900 patients with LAFB.

Right-Bundle-Branch Block

Because the right ventricle contributes minimally to the normal QRS complex, RBBB produces little distortion of the QRS complex during the time required for left-ventricular activation. **Figure 5.5** illustrates the minimal distortion of the early portion and marked distortion of the late portion of the QRS complex (in lead V_1) that typically occurs with RBBB. The activation sequence of the interventricular septum and the right- and left-ventricular free walls contribute to the appearance of the QRS complex in lead V_1 (see **Figure 5.5**). Normal intraventricular conduction requires only two sequential 0.04-second periods, whereas a third is required when RBBB is present. The minimal contribution of the normal right-ventricular myocardium is completely subtracted from the early portion of the QRS complex and then added later, when the right ventricle is activated after the spread of impulses from the left ventricle through the interventricular septum to the right ventricle. This delay in RBBB conduction produces a late prominent positive wave in lead V_1 termed *R′* because it follows the earlier positive R wave produced by the normal left-to-right spread of activation through the interventricular septum (see **Figure 5.5**; **Table 5.1**).

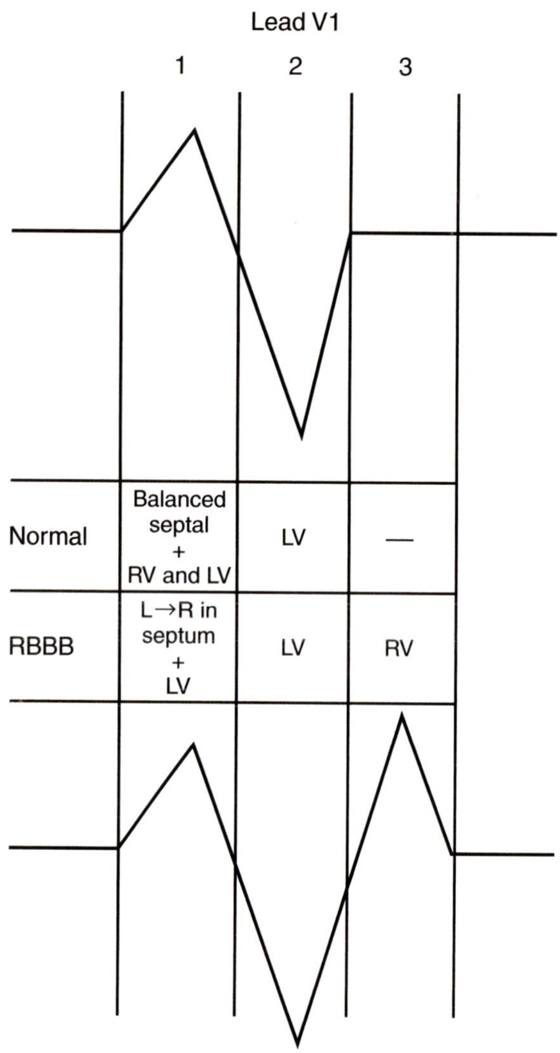

FIGURE 5.5. The contributions from activation of the interventricular septum and the right- and left-ventricular free walls to the appearance of the QRS complex in lead V_1, with normal intraventricular conduction (top) and with right-bundle-branch block (RBBB) (bottom). The numbers refer to the first, second, and third sequential 0.04-second periods of time. Only two 0.04-second periods are required for normal conduction, but a third is required when RBBB is present. LV, left ventricle; RV, right ventricle.

Table 5.1.

Criteria for Right-Bundle-Branch Block

QRS Duration ≥0.12 s	
Lead V_1	Late intrinsicoid (R′ peak or late R peak), M-shaped QRS (RSR′); sometimes wide R or qR
Lead V_6	Early intrinsicoid (R peak), wide S wave
Lead I	Wide S wave

The RBBB has many variations in its ECG appearance (**Figure 5.6A-C**). In **Figure 5.6A**, the RBBB is considered "incomplete" because the duration of the QRS complex is only 0.10 second, but in **Figure 5.6B,C**, the RBBB is considered "complete" because the duration of the QRS complex is ≥0.12 second.

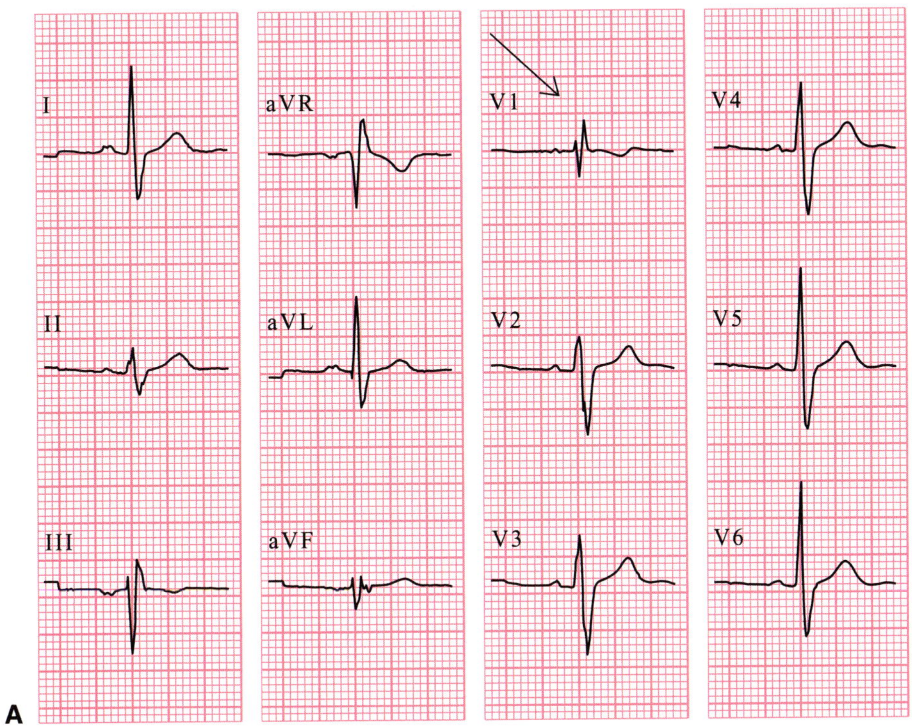

FIGURE 5.6. Twelve-lead electrocardiograms from a 17-year-old girl with an ostium secundum atrial septal defect (**A**), an 81-year-old woman with fibrosis of the right bundle branch (**B**), and an 82-year-old man with fibrosis of both the right bundle branch and the anterior fascicle of the left bundle branch (**C**). Arrows in **A**, **B**, and **C** indicate the prominent terminal R′ wave in V_1. *(continued)*

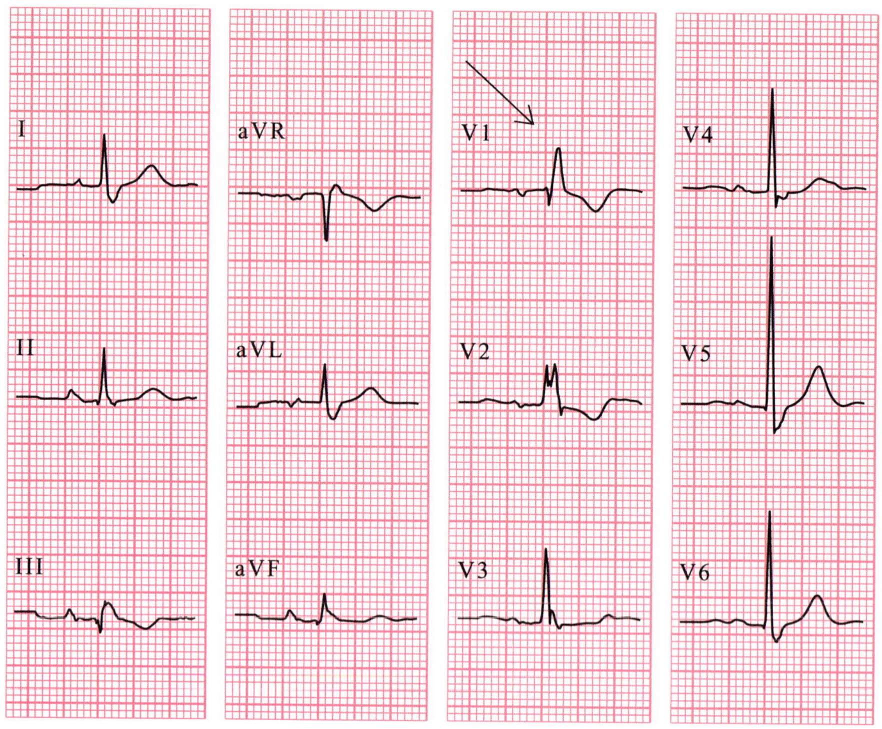

B

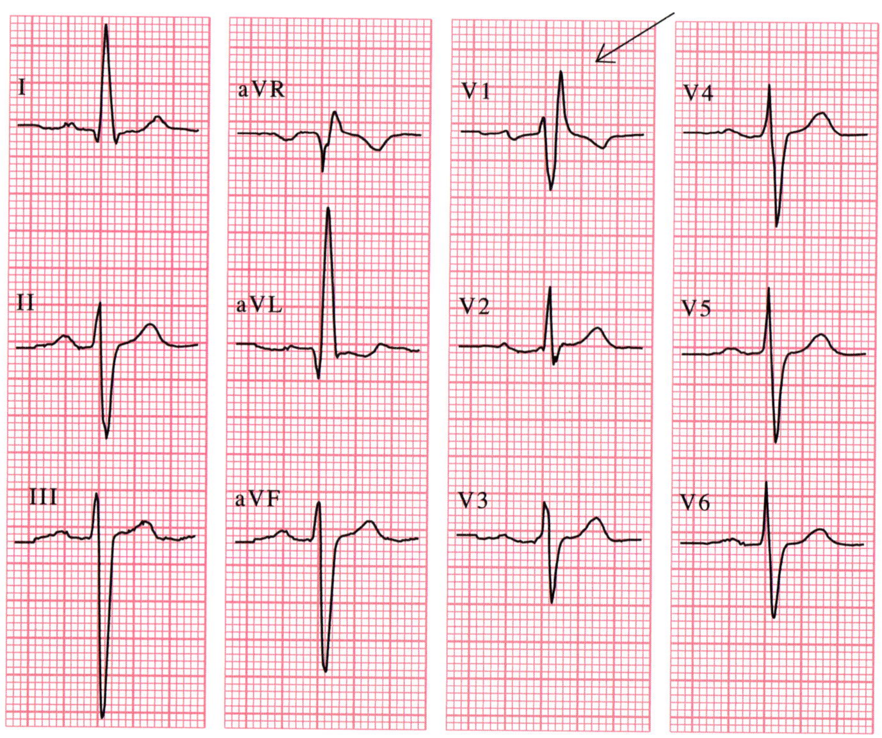

C

FIGURE 5.6. *(continued)*

Left Fascicular Blocks

Normal activation of the left-ventricular free wall spreads simultaneously from two sites (near the insertions of the papillary muscles of the mitral valve). Wavefronts of activation spread from these endocardial sites to the overlying epicardium. Because the wavefronts travel in opposite directions, they neutralize each other's influence on the ECG in a phenomenon called *cancellation*. When a block in either the LAF or LPF is present, activation of the free wall proceeds from one site instead of two. Because the cancellation is removed, the waveforms of the QRS complex change, as described in the following text (**Tables 5.2** and **5.3**). A schematic diagram of the left ventricle viewed from its apex upward toward its base is illustrated in **Figure 5.7**.

Table 5.2.

Criteria for Left Anterior Fascicular Block

1. Left-axis deviation (usually ≥−60 degrees)
2. Small Q in leads I and aVL; small R in II, III, and aVF
3. Minimal QRS prolongation (0.020 s) from baseline
4. Late intrinsicoid (R wave peak) deflection in aVL (>0.045 s)
5. Increased QRS voltage in limb leads

Table 5.3.

Criteria for Left Posterior Fascicular Block

1. Right-axis deviation (usually ≥+120 degrees)
2. Small R in leads I and aVL; small Q in II, III, and aVF
3. Usually normal QRS duration
4. Late intrinsicoid deflection in aVF (>0.045 s)
5. Increased QRS voltage in limb leads
6. No evidence of RVH

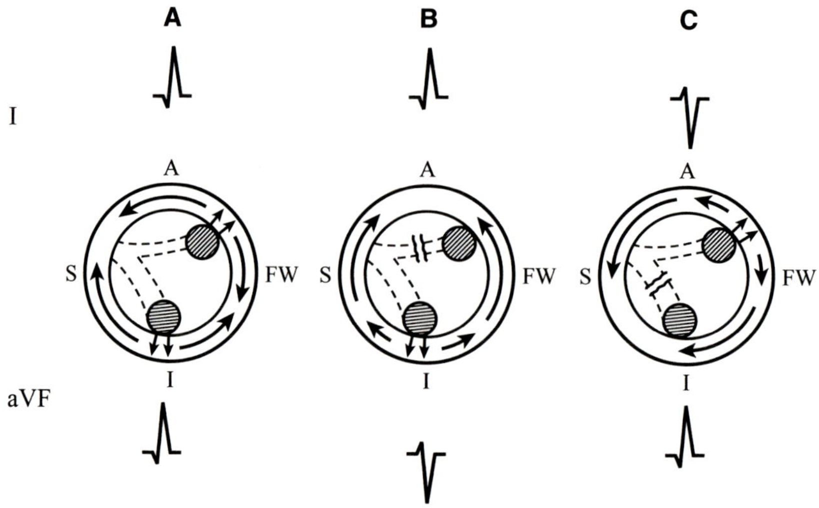

FIGURE 5.7. Schematic left ventricle viewed from its apex upward toward its base. The interventricular septum (S), left-ventricular free wall (FW; also known as lateral wall), and anterior (A) and inferior (I) regions of the left ventricle are indicated. The typical appearances of the QRS complexes in leads I (top) and aVF (bottom) are presented for normal (**A**), left anterior fascicular block (**B**), and left posterior fascicular block left-ventricular activation (**C**). Dashed lines, fascicles; wavy lines, sites of fascicular block; small crosshatched circles, papillary muscles; outer rings, endocardial and epicardial surface of the left-ventricular myocardium; arrows, directions of activation wavefronts.

Left Anterior Fascicular Block

If the LAF of the LBB is blocked (see **Figure 5.7B**), the initial activation of the left-ventricular free wall occurs via the LPF. Activation spreading from endocardium to the epicardium in this region is directed inferiorly and rightward. Because the block in the LAF has removed the initial superior and leftward activation, a Q wave appears in leads that have their positive electrodes in a superior-leftward position (ie, lead I), and an R wave appears in leads that have their positive electrodes in an inferior-rightward position (ie, lead aVF) (**Figure 5.8**). Following this initial period, the activation wave spreads over the remainder of the left-ventricular free wall in a superior-leftward direction, producing a prominent R wave in lead I and a prominent S wave in lead aVF. This change in the left-ventricular activation sequence produces a leftward shift of the axis of the QRS complex to at least −45 degrees. The overall duration of the QRS complex may be within the normal range but is usually prolonged by 0.02 second from the patient's baseline.[4]

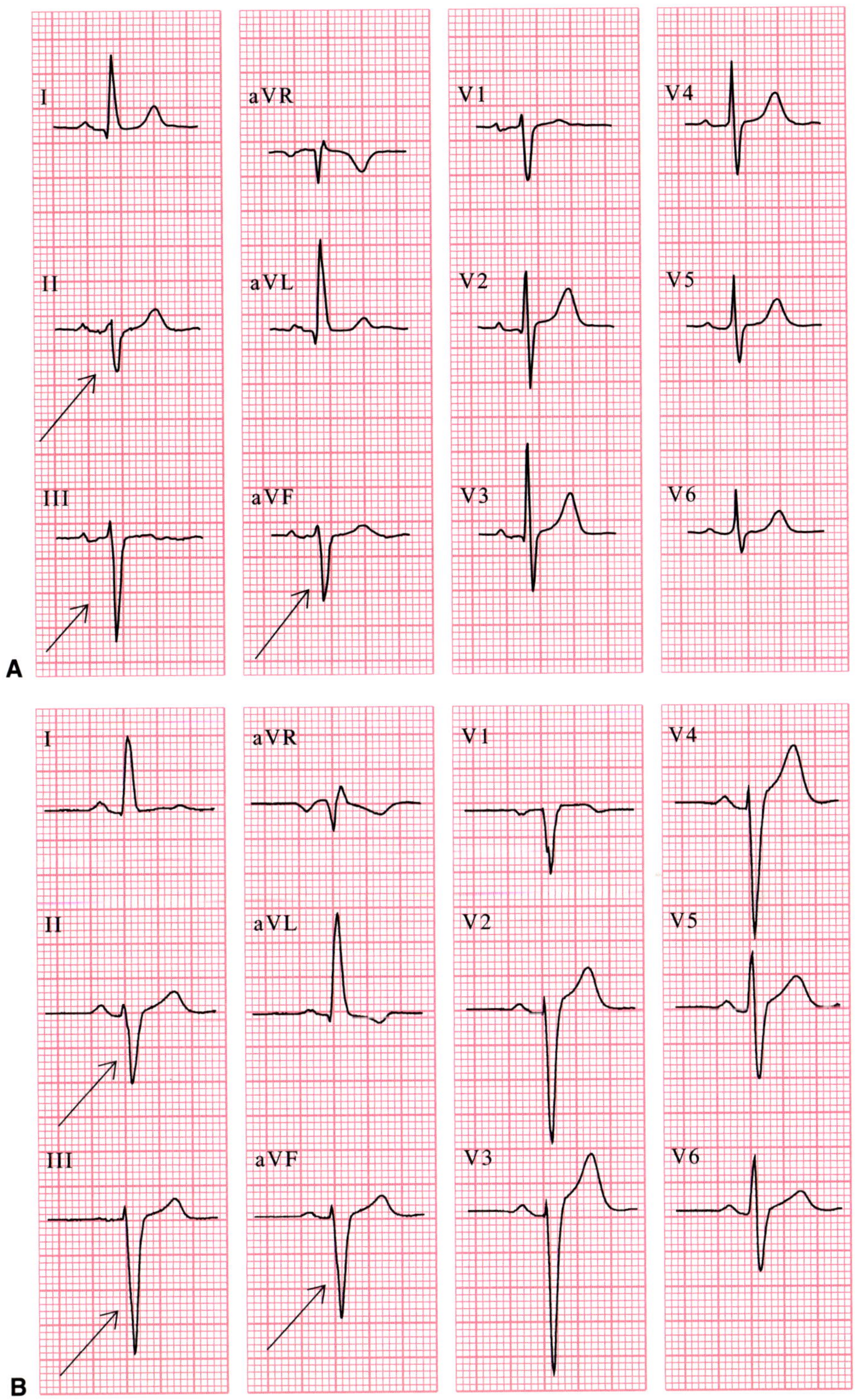

FIGURE 5.8. Twelve-lead electrocardiograms from a 53-year-old woman with no medical problems (**A**) and a 75-year-old man with a long history of poorly treated hypertension (**B**). Arrows indicate the deep S waves in leads II, III, and aVF that reflect extreme left-axis deviation.

Left Posterior Fascicular Block

If the LPF of the LBB is blocked (see **Figure 5.7C**), the situation is reversed from that in LAF block, and the initial activation of the left-ventricular free wall occurs via the LAF. Activation spreading from the endocardium to the epicardium in this region is directed superiorly and leftward. Because the block in the LPF has removed the initial inferior and rightward activation, a Q wave appears in leads with their positive electrodes in an inferior-rightward position (ie, lead aVF), and an R wave appears in leads with their positive electrodes in a superior-leftward direction (ie, lead I). Following this initial period, the activation spreads over the remainder of the left-ventricular free wall in an inferior/rightward direction, producing a prominent R wave in lead aVF and a prominent S wave in lead I. This change in the left-ventricular activation sequence produces a rightward shift of the axis of the QRS complex to ≥+90 degrees.[5] The duration of the QRS complex may be normal or slightly prolonged (**Figure 5.9**).

The consideration that LPFB may be present requires that there be no evidence of right-ventricular hypertrophy (RVH) from either the precordial leads (see **Figure 5.9**) or from other clinical data. Even the absence of RVH, however, does not allow diagnosis of LPFB because RVH can produce the same pattern as LPFB in the limb leads and RVH is much more common than LPFB.

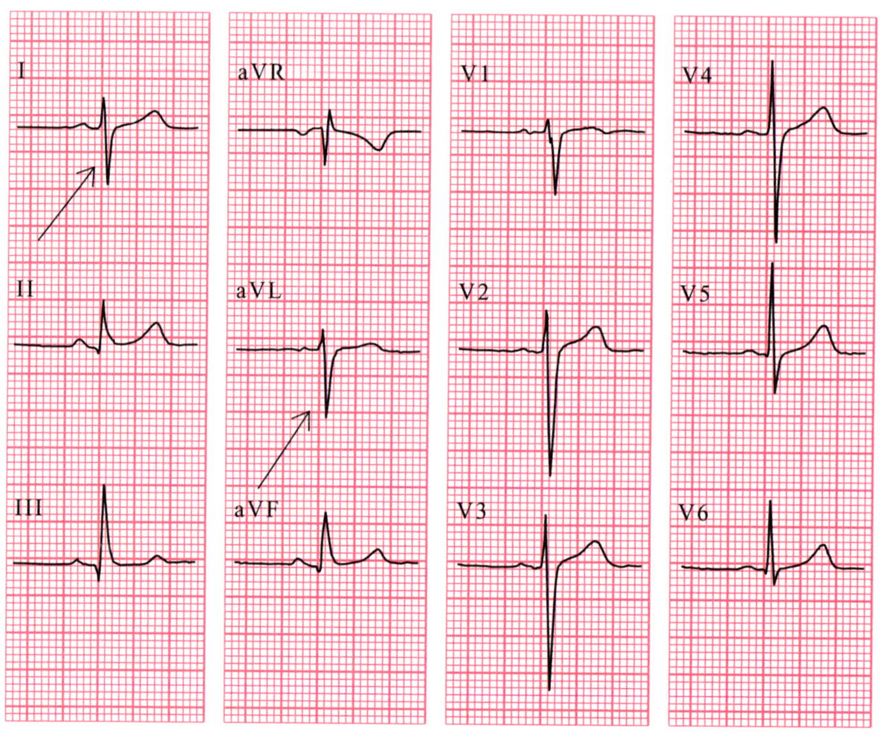

FIGURE 5.9. Electrocardiogram of an asymptomatic individual shows deep S waves in leads I and aVL, typical of both left posterior fascicular block and right-ventricular hypertrophy (arrows). Consideration that left posterior fascicular block may be present requires that there be no evidence of right-ventricular hypertrophy from either the precordial leads or from clinical data.

Bifascicular Blocks

The term *bifascicular block* is used when there is ECG evidence of involvement of any two of the RBBB, LAF, or LPF. Such evidence may appear at different times or may coexist on the same ECG. Bifascicular block is sometimes applied to complete LBBB and is commonly applied to the combination of RBBB with either LAFB or LPFB. The combination of RBBB with LAFB can be caused by a large anteroseptal infarct. The term *bilateral bundle-branch block* is also appropriate when RBBB and either LAFB or LPFB are present.[6] When there is bifascicular block, the duration of the QRS complex is prolonged to ≥0.12 second.

Left-Bundle-Branch Block

Figure 5.10 illustrates the QRS complex distortion produced by LBBB in lead V_1. It also identifies the various contributions from ventricular myocardium to the appearances of the QRS complex. Complete LBBB may be caused by disease in either the main LBB (*predivisional*) or in both of its fascicles (*postdivisional*). Complete LBBB can also be caused by disease in the His bundle. Light and electron microscopy studies conducted by James and Sherf[A] showed that fibers within the His bundle are predestined to form LBB and RBB,

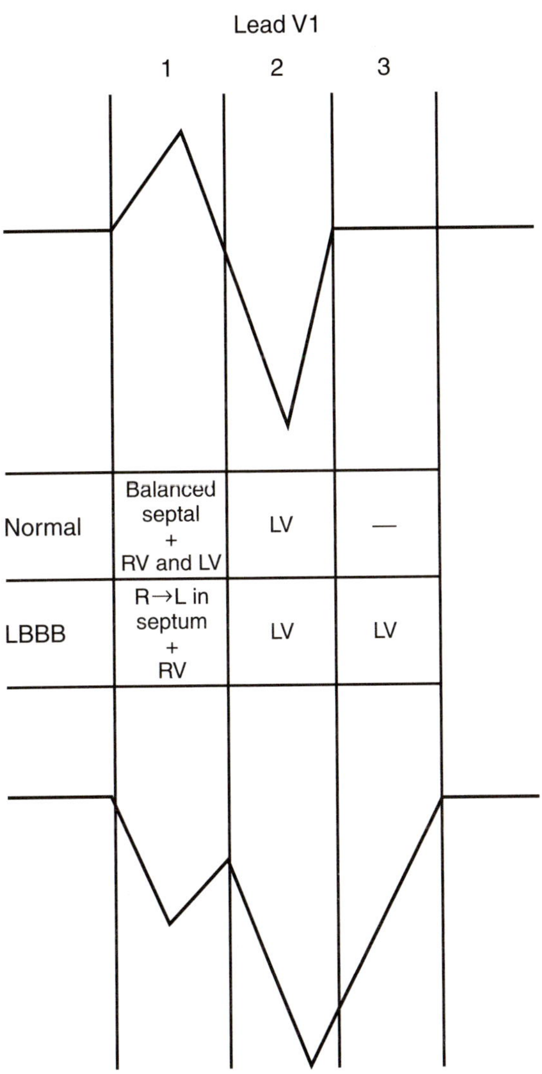

FIGURE 5.10. Contributors to the QRS complex in lead V_1. Top. Normal intraventricular conduction. Bottom. Left-bundle-branch block (LBBB). The numbers refer to the first, second, and third sequential 0.04-second periods of time. LV, left ventricle; RV, right ventricle.

a concept known as longitudinal dissociation of conduction fibers. This concept is validated by the recent development of His bundle pacing to correct LBBB. When the impulse cannot progress along the LBB, electrical activation must first occur in the right ventricle and then travel through the interventricular septum to the left ventricle.

Figure 5.11 shows the electrical activation in normal activation (**Figure 5.11A**) and in the presence of LBBB (**Figure 5.11B**). In normal activation, the interventricular septum is activated from left to right (see **Figure 5.11A** and **Figure 5.12A**), producing an initial R wave in the right precordial leads and a Q wave in leads I, aVL, and the left precordial leads. When complete LBBB is present, however, the septum is activated from right to left (see **Figure 5.11B** and **Figure 5.12C**). This right to left septal depolarization produces a small R wave followed by a large S wave or a large Q wave with no R wave in the right precordial leads (V_1 and V_2) and eliminates the normal *septal Q waves* in the leftward-oriented leads (leads V_5 through V_6, I, aVL). It should be noted, however, that patients with LBBB and an anterior myocardial infarction (MI) can have Q waves in leftward-oriented leads even with LBBB (see Chapter 9 Online Supplement, **eFigure 9.5B**). The activation of the left ventricle then proceeds sequentially from the interventricular septum to the adjacent anterior and inferior walls and then to the lateral free wall (see **Figure 5.11B** and **Figure 5.12C**).

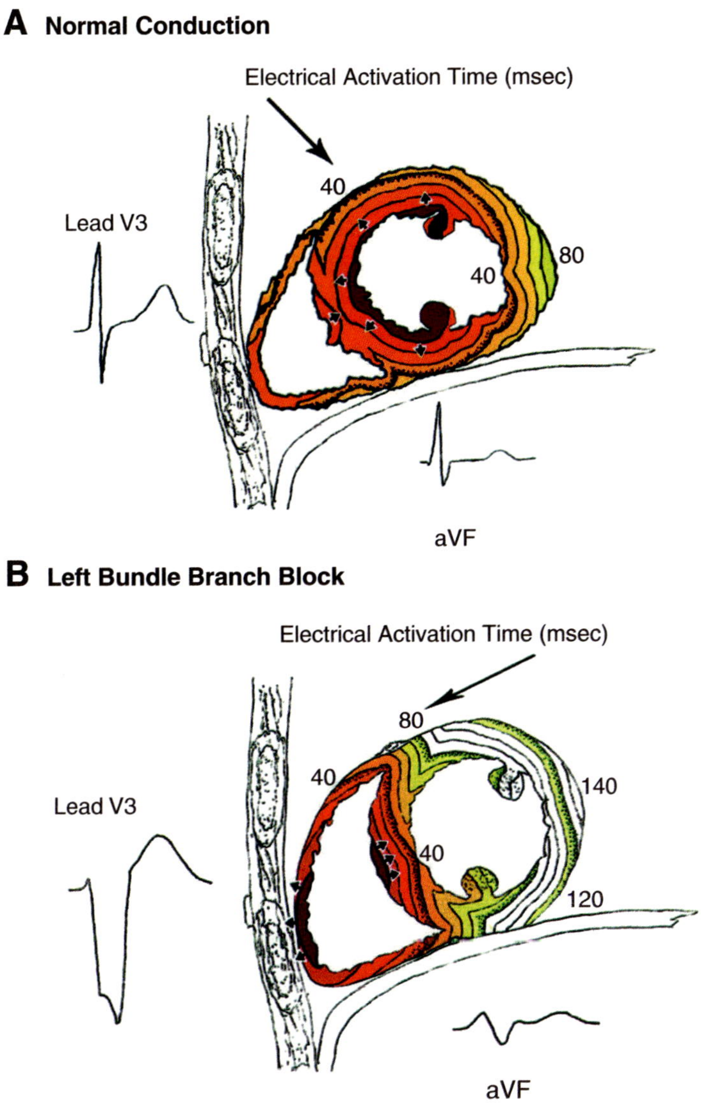

FIGURE 5.11. Ventricular activation in normal (**A**) and complete left-bundle-branch block (LBBB) (**B**) activation. For reference, two QRS-T waveforms are shown in their anatomic locations in each image. Electrical activation starts at the small arrows and spreads in a wavefront, with each colored line representing successive 0.01 second. Comparing **A** and **B** reveals the difference between normal and complete LBBB activation. In normal activation (**A**), activation begins within the left- and right-ventricular endocardium. In complete LBBB (**B**), activation only begins in the right ventricle and must proceed through the septum for 0.04 to 0.05 second before reaching the left ventricle endocardium. It then requires another 0.05 second for reentry into the left-ventricular Purkinje network and to propagate to the endocardium of the lateral wall. It then requires another 0.05 second to activate the lateral wall, producing a total QRS duration of 0.14 to 0.15 second. Any increase in septal or lateral wall thickness or left-ventricular endocardial surface area further increases QRS duration. Because the propagation velocity in human myocardium is 3 to 4 mm per 0.1 second, a circumferential increase in left-ventricular wall thickness by 3 mm will increase total QRS duration by 0.02 second in LBBB (0.1 s for the septum and 0.1 s for the lateral wall). (Reprinted with permission from Strauss DG, Selvester RH, Lima JA, et al. ECG quantification of myocardial scar in cardiomyopathy patients with or without conduction defects: correlation with cardiac magnetic resonance and arrhythmogenesis. *Circ Arrhythm Electrophysiol.* 2008;1:327-336.)

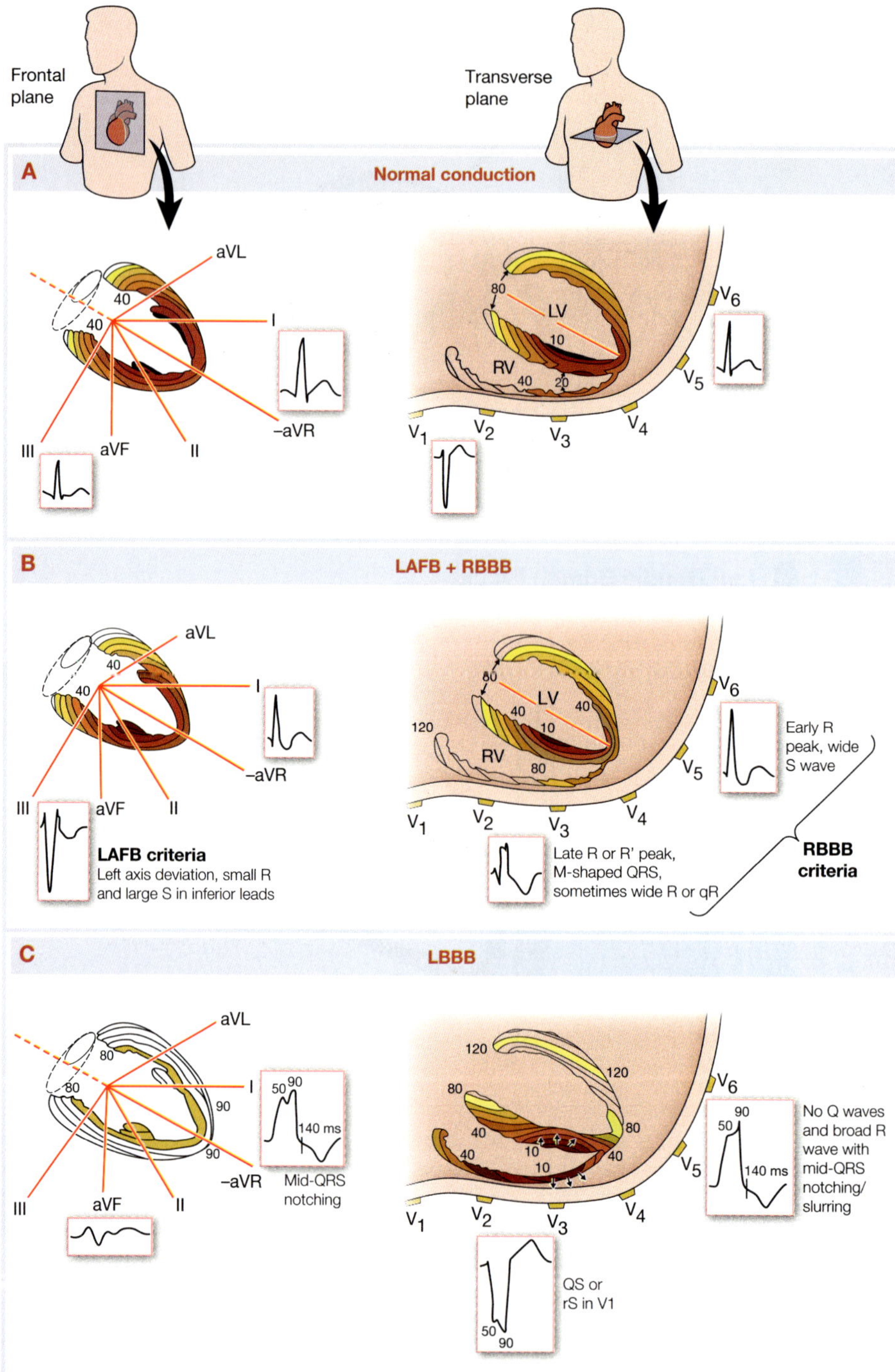

FIGURE 5.12. Ventricular activation sequence and ECG waveforms in the frontal and transverse planes. The frontal and transverse planes are shown in normal conduction (**A**), left anterior fascicular block and right-bundle-branch block (**B**), and left-bundle-branch block (**C**). Colored lines represent areas of myocardium activated within the same 10-millisecond period (*isochrones*). Numbers represent milliseconds since beginning of activation. (Modified from Strauss DG, Selvester RH. The QRS complex—a biomarker that "images" the heart: QRS scores to quantify myocardial scar in the presence of normal and abnormal ventricular conduction. *J Electrocardiol*. 2009;42:85-96. Copyright © 2009 Elsevier. With permission.)

A critical component of diagnosing LBBB on the ECG is the presence of mid-QRS notching/slurring in frontward-backward leads (V_1 and V_2) or leftward-rightward leads (V_5, V_6, I, and aVL) as shown in activation sequence (see **Figure 5.11B** and **Figure 5.12C**). **Figure 5.12** shows ECGs from an 82-year-old woman before (**Figure 5.13A**) and after (**Figure 5.13B**) the development of LBBB. Notice that QRS duration increases from 0.76 to 0.148 second with the development of LBBB. In addition to the marked increase in QRS duration, notice the change in QRS morphology that now includes distinctive mid-QRS notching in leads I and aVL, along with mid-QRS slurring in leads V_5 and V_6. **Figure 5.14** shows another example of a patient who has a sudden QRS prolongation due to LBBB with the appearance of prominent mid-QRS notching/slurring.

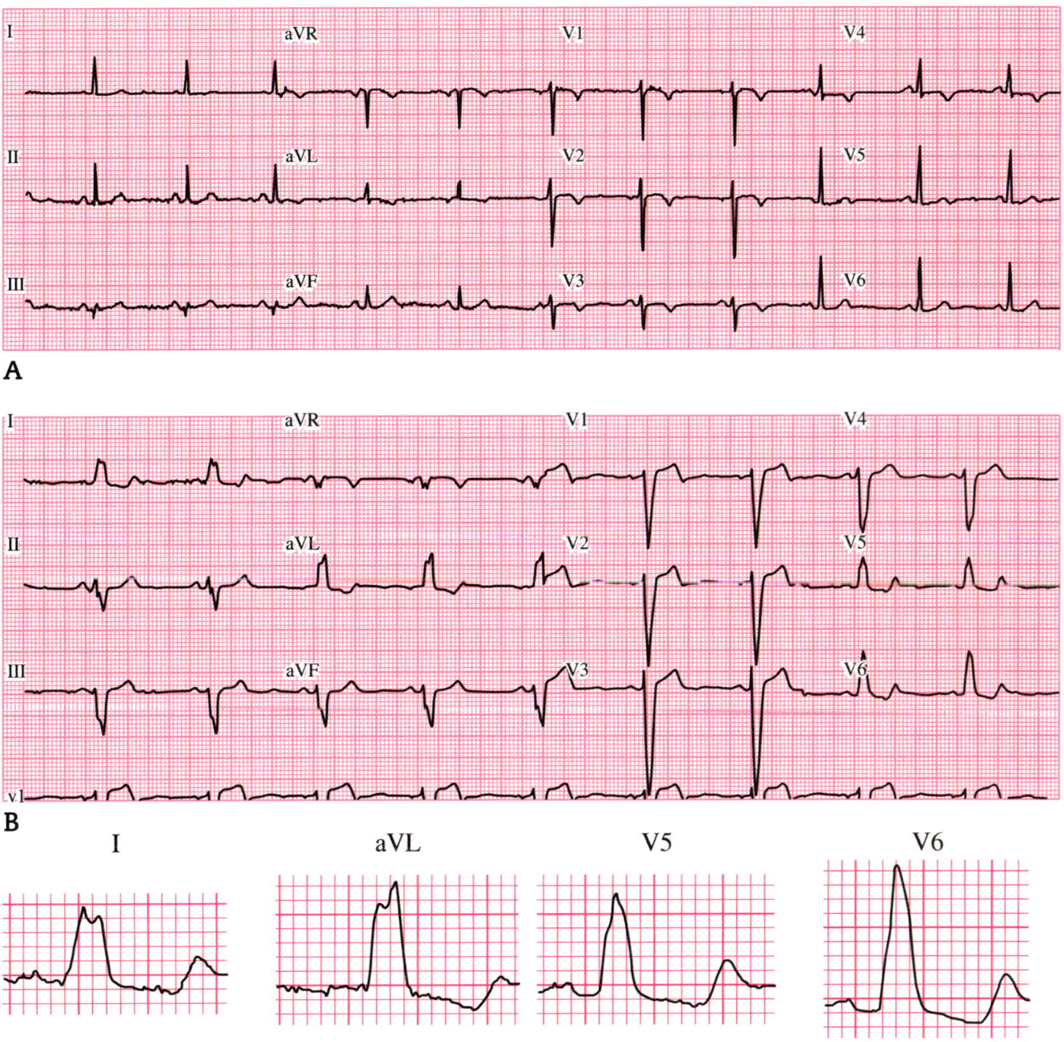

FIGURE 5.13. Electrocardiograms from an 82-year-old woman with a sudden increase in QRS duration from 0.076 (**A**) to 0.148 second (**B**) 1 year later (a 95% increase) with the development of complete left-bundle-branch block. In addition to the increase in QRS duration, notice the change in QRS morphology that includes distinctive mid-QRS notching in leads I and aVL, along with mid-QRS slurring in leads V_5 and V_6. (Reproduced from Strauss DG, Selvester RH, Wagner GS. Defining left bundle branch block in the era of cardiac resynchronization therapy. *Am J Cardiol.* 2011;107[6]:927-934. Copyright © 2011 Elsevier. With permission.)

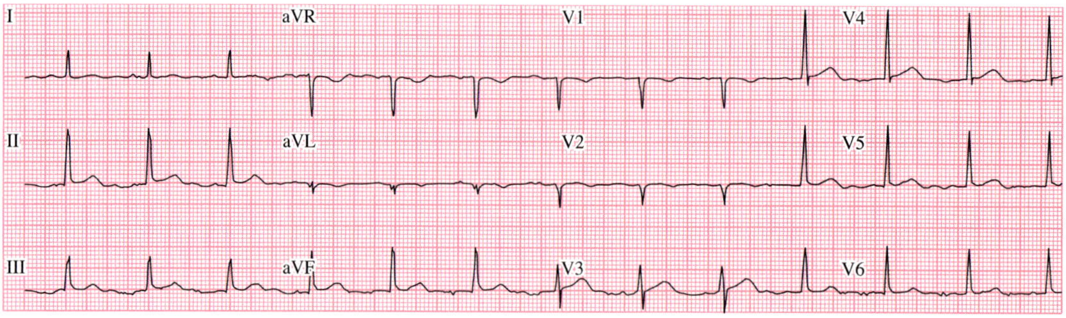

A

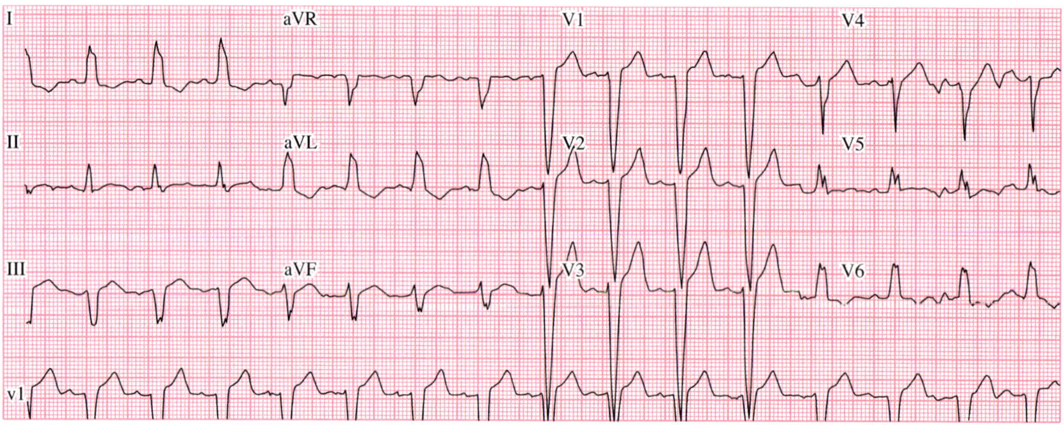

B

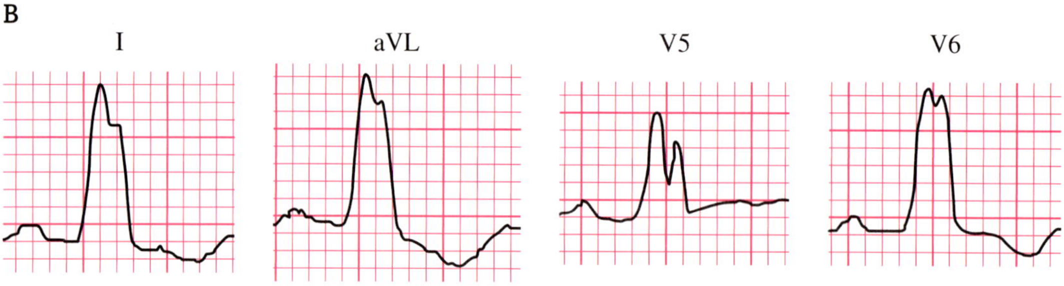

FIGURE 5.14. Electrocardiograms from a 75-year-old woman with a sudden increase in QRS duration from 0.092 (**A**) to 0.156 second (**B**) in 6 months (a 70% increase) with the development of complete left-bundle-branch block. The patient developed distinctive mid-QRS notching in leads I, aVL, V_5, and V_6. (Reproduced from Strauss DG, Selvester RH, Wagner GS. Defining left bundle branch block in the era of cardiac resynchronization therapy. *Am J Cardiol*. 2011;107[6]:927-934. Copyright © 2011 Elsevier. With permission.)

Table 5.4 contains "conventional" criteria for LBBB that consists primarily of a QRS duration ≥0.12 second and a leftward conduction delay (QS or rS) in lead V_1. Simulation and endocardial mapping research has demonstrated, however, that approximately 1 of 3 patients diagnosed with LBBB by conventional criteria do not have activation consistent with LBBB.[7] **Table 5.5** contains "strict" (Strauss et al.[7]) criteria for LBBB that requires QRS duration ≥0.13 second in women and QRS duration ≥0.14 seconds in men; a QS or rS in V_1; and mid-QRS notching/slurring in two of the leads I, aVL, V_1, V_2, V_5, or V_6.[7]

Table 5.4.

Conventional Criteria for Left-Bundle-Branch Block

Lead V_1	QS or rS
Lead V_6	Late intrinsicoid (R or R′ peak), no Q waves, monophasic R
Lead I	Monophasic R wave, no Q

Table 5.5.

Strict Criteria for Left-Bundle-Branch Block

QRS duration	≥0.13 s in women or ≥0.14 s in men
Lead V_1	QS or rS
Mid-QRS notching/slurring in two of the leads I, aVL, V_1, V_2, V_5, or V_6	

Right-Bundle-Branch Block With Left Anterior Fascicular Block

Just as LAFB appears as a unifascicular block much more commonly than does LPFB, it more commonly accompanies RBBB as a bifascicular block. The combination of RBBB and LAFB is commonly a sign of a large anteroseptal infarct because the RBB and LAF are perfused by the same coronary artery (see Chapter 9).[8] **Figure 5.12B** shows the ventricular activation sequence and corresponding QRST waveforms in the presence of RBBB plus LAFB. The diagnosis of LAFB plus RBBB is made by observing the late prominent R or R′ wave in precordial lead V_1 of RBBB and the initial R waves and prominent S waves in limb leads II, III, and aVF of LAFB. The duration of the QRS complex should be ≥0.12 second and the frontal plane axis of the complex should be between −45 and −120 degrees (**Figure 5.15**). In a 12-lead ECG from a 1-year previous examination (**Figure 5.15A**), only LAFB (deep S waves in II, III, and aVF) is present. In a current ECG evaluation of the same patient (**Figure 5.15B**), the presence of RBBB (prominent R′ wave in V_1) indicates that a second fascicle has been blocked.

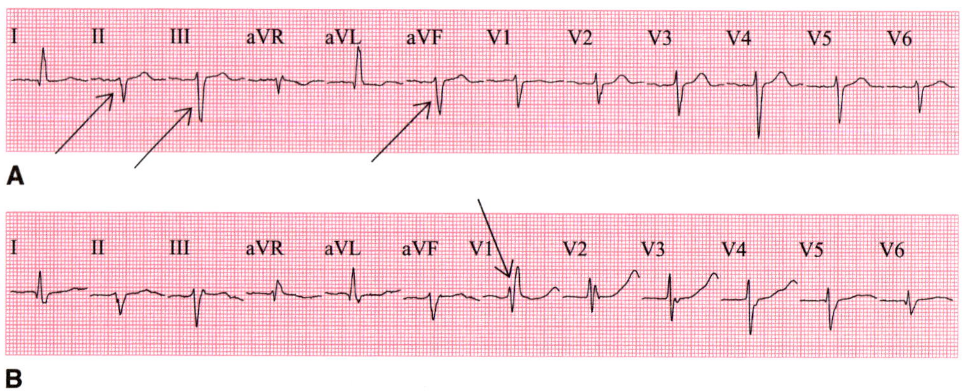

FIGURE 5.15. **A.** Deep S waves characteristic of left anterior fascicular block (arrows). **B.** Prominent R′ wave characteristic of right-bundle-branch block (arrow).

Right-Bundle-Branch Block With Left Posterior Fascicular Block

The example of bifascicular block consisting of RBBB with LPFB rarely occurs. Even when changes in the ECG are entirely typical of this combination, the diagnosis should be considered only if there is no clinical evidence of RVH. The diagnosis of RBBB with LPFB should be considered when precordial lead V_1 shows changes typical of RBBB, and limb leads I and aVL show the initial R waves and prominent S waves typical of LPFB. The duration of the QRS complex should be ≥0.12 second, and the frontal plane axis of the complex should be ≥+90 degrees (**Figure 5.16**).[9]

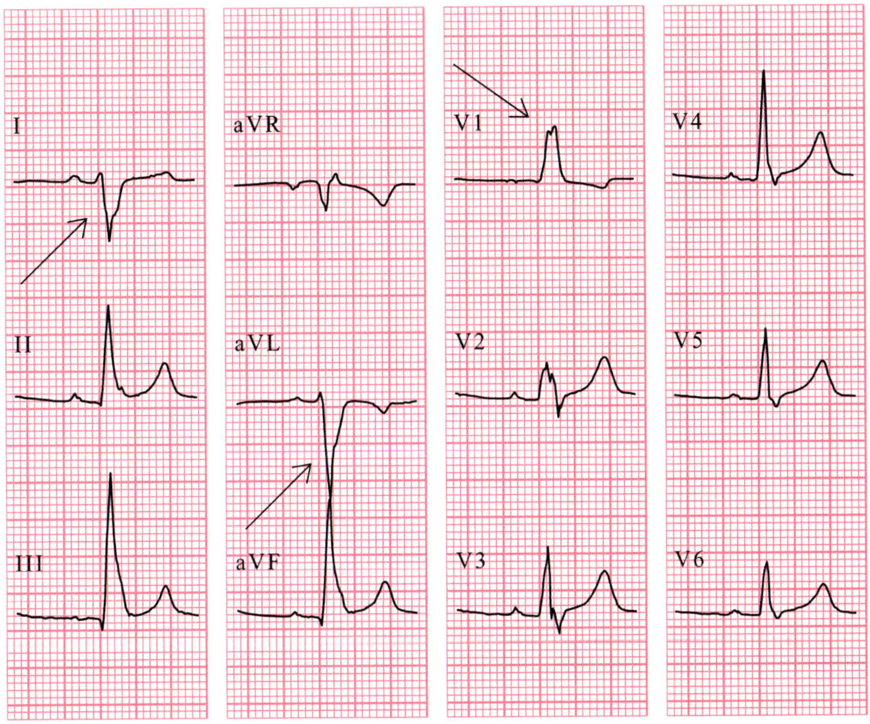

FIGURE 5.16. Right-bundle-branch block with left posterior fascicular block. Arrows, prominent S waves (I and aVL) and RR′ complex (V_1).

Systematic Approach to the Analysis of Bundle-Branch and Fascicular Blocks

The systematic approach to waveform analysis used in Chapter 3 should be applied in analyzing bundle-branch and fascicular blocks.

General Contour of the QRS Complex

The RBBB and LBBB have opposite effects on the contour of the QRS complex. The RBBB adds a new waveform directed toward the right ventricle following the completion of slightly altered waveforms directed toward the left ventricle (see **Figure 5.5**). Therefore, the QRS complex in RBBB tends to have a triphasic appearance. In lead V_1, which is optimal for visualizing right- versus left-sided conduction delay, the QRS in RBBB has the appearance of rabbit ears (see **Figure 5.6**). Typically, the "first ear" (R wave) is shorter than the "second ear" (R′ wave). (Although the term "rabbit ears" in this context refers to a triphasic QRS, it can also refer to two peaks found in monophasic QRS complexes.) When RBBB is accompanied by block in one of the LBB fascicles, the positive deflection in lead V_1 is often monophasic (see **Figure 5.15**).

In LBBB, a sequential spread of activation through the interventricular septum and left-ventricular free wall replaces the normal, competing, and simultaneous spread of activation through these areas. As a result, the QRS complex tends to have a monophasic appearance with mid-QRS notching in leads V_1, V_2, V_5, V_6, I, and/or aVL.

Although LBBB and left-ventricular hypertrophy (LVH) have many ECG similarities, they also show marked differences. Although the normal Q waves over the left ventricle may be present or even exaggerated in LVH, they are absent in LBBB (when there is no accompanying anteroapical infarction). In addition, clear mid-QRS notching is present in LBBB, but not LVH, although LVH and apical MI could cause mid-QRS notching, mimicking LBBB.

QRS Complex Duration

Complete RBBB usually increases the duration of the QRS complex by $\geq$0.04 second, and complete LBBB increases the duration of the complex by $\geq$0.06 second. Block within the LAF or LPF of the LBB usually prolongs the duration of the QRS complex by approximately 0.02 second (see **Figures 5.8B** and **5.9**).[4]

Positive and Negative Amplitudes

The BBB produces QRS waveforms with lower voltage and more definite notching than those that occur with ventricular hypertrophy. The amplitude of the QRS complex, however, does increase in LBBB because of the relatively unopposed spread of activation over the left ventricle.

One general rule for differentiating between LBBB and LVH is that the greater the amplitude of the QRS complex, the more likely is LVH to be the cause of this. Similarly, the more prolonged is the duration of the QRS complex, the more likely is LBBB to be the cause of this effect. Klein and colleagues[10] have suggested that in the presence of LBBB, either of the following criteria are associated with LVH:

Diagnosing LVH in the Presence of LBBB

1. S wave in V_2 + R wave in V_6 >45 mm
2. Evidence of left-atrial enlargement with a QRS complex duration >0.16 second

QRS Axis in the Frontal and Transverse Planes

Because complete RBBB and complete LBBB alter conduction to entire ventricles, they might not be expected to produce much net alteration of the frontal plane QRS axis. Rosenbaum et al[3] studied patients with intermittent LBBB in which blocked and unblocked complexes could be examined side by side. The LBBB was often observed to produce a significant left-axis shift and sometimes even a right-axis shift. The axis was unchanged in only a minority of patients.

Block in either the LAF or LPF of the LBB alone produces marked axis deviation. The initial 0.020 second of the QRS complex is directed away from the blocked fascicles, and the middle and late portions are directed toward the blocked fascicles, causing the overall direction of the QRS complex to be shifted toward the site of the block (see **Figures 5.8** and **5.9**).[2] When block in either of these LBB fascicles is accompanied by RBBB, an even later waveform is added to the QRS complex, thereby further prolonging its duration. The direction of this final waveform in the frontal plane is in the vicinity of 180 degrees, as a result of the RBBB (see **Figure 5.6C**).[2]

In BBB, the T wave is usually directed opposite to the latter portion of the QRS complex (eg, in **Figure 5.17A**, the T wave in lead I is inverted and the latter part of the QRS complex is upright; in **Figure 5.17B**, the T wave is upright and the latter part of the QRS complex is negative). This opposite polarity is the natural result of the depolarization-repolarization disturbance produced by the BBB and is therefore termed *secondary*. Indeed, if the direction of the T wave is similar to that of the terminal part of the QRS complex (**Figure 5.17C**), it should be considered abnormal. Such T-wave changes are *primary* and imply myocardial disease. The diagnosis of MI in the presence of BBB is considered in Chapter 9.

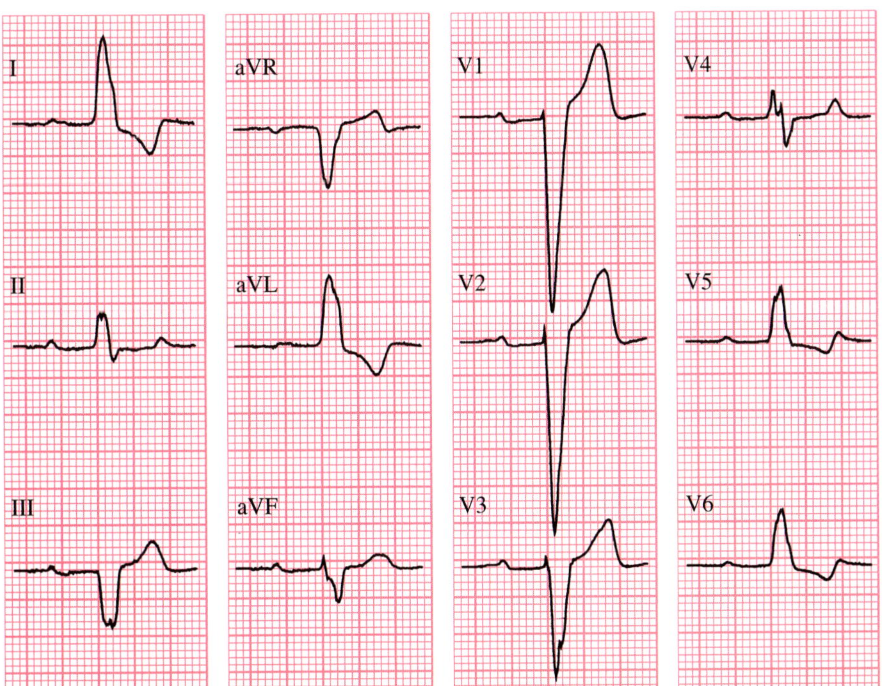

A

FIGURE 5.17. **A.** An 89-year-old woman during a routine health evaluation. *(continued)*

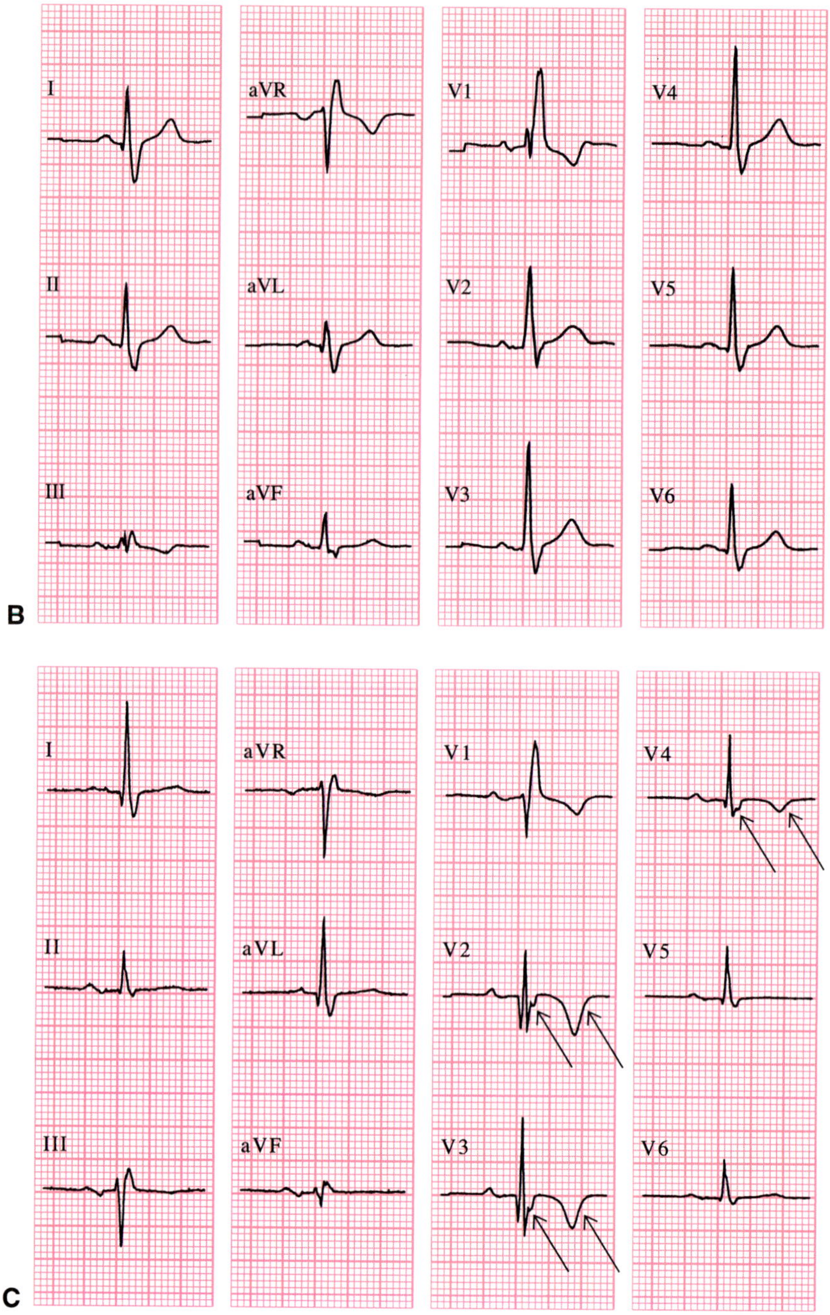

FIGURE 5.17. *(continued)* **B.** A 45-year-old pilot during an annual health evaluation. **C.** A 64-year-old woman on the first day after coronary bypass surgery. Arrows, concordant directions of the terminal QRS complex and T wave in leads V_2 to V_4.

One method of determining the clinical significance of T-wave changes in BBB is to measure the angle between the axis of the T wave and that of the terminal part of the QRS complex. Obviously, if the two are oppositely directed (as they are with secondary T-wave changes), the angle between them is wide and may approach 180 degrees. It has been proposed that if this angle is <110 degrees, myocardial disease is present. In **Figure 5.17B**, the angle is about 150 degrees, whereas in **Figure 5.17C**, it is only a few degrees.

Clinical Perspective on Intraventricular-Conduction Disturbances

Both RBBB and LBBB are often seen in apparently normal individuals.[11] The cause of this diffuse conduction delay is *fibrosis* of the Purkinje fibers. This fibrosis has been described as *Lenègre disease*[12] or *Lev disease*.[13] The process of Purkinje fibrosis progresses slowly: A 10-year follow-up study of healthy aviators with BBB revealed no incidence of complete *AV block*, *syncope*, or sudden death.[14] The pathologic process may be accelerated by systemic hypertension; it preceded the appearance of BBB in 60% of the individuals in the Framingham study. The mean age of onset of the BBB was 61 years.[15]

Insight into the long-term prognosis for individuals with chronic BBB but no other evidence of cardiac disease comes from studies of the ECG changes preceding the development of transient or permanent complete AV block. Lasser and associates[16] documented the common presence of some combination of bundle-branch or fascicular block immediately before onset of the AV block. The most common combination was RBBB with LAFB.

The combined results of these studies suggest that Lenègre or Lev disease is a slowly developing process of fibrosis of the Purkinje fibers that has the ultimate potential of causing complete AV block because of bilateral bundle branch involvement. Because the Purkinje cells lack the physiologic capacity of the AV nodal cells to conduct at varying speeds, a sudden progression from no AV block to complete AV block may occur.[17] When this rapid progression of block does occur, ventricular activation can result only from impulse formation within a Purkinje cell beyond the site of the block. Several clinical conditions may result, including syncope and sudden death.

Bundle-branch or fascicular block may also be the result of other serious cardiac diseases. In Central and South America, *Chagas disease*, produced by infection with *Trypanosoma cruzi*, is almost endemic and is a common cause of RBBB with LAFB.[18] As indicated in Chapter 4, RBBB is commonly produced by the distention of the right ventricle that occurs with volume overloading. Transient RBBB may be produced during right heart catheterization as a result of catheter tip–induced trauma (**Figure 5.18**). The resultant RBBB is displayed in the third and fourth beats of the schematic lead V_1 recording.

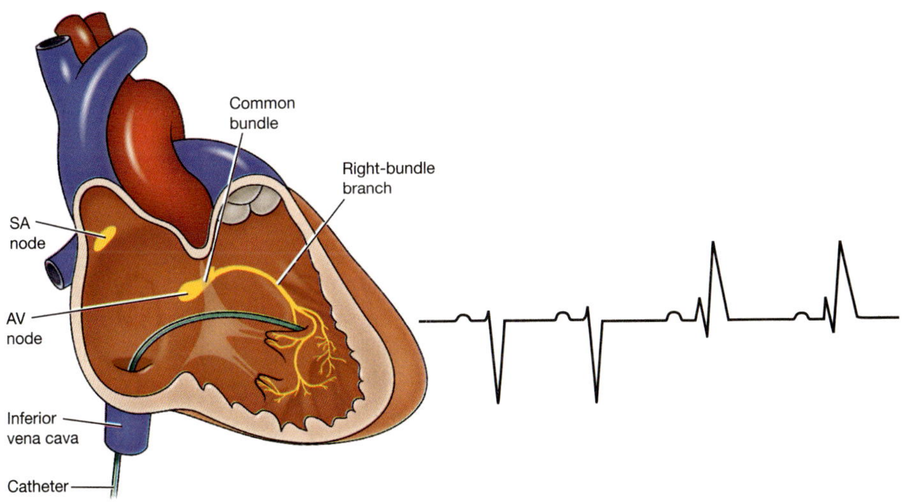

FIGURE 5.18. Right-bundle-branch block is induced by trauma to the right bundle branch. A catheter has been advanced from the leg via the inferior vena cava, and its tip lies against the right-ventricular endocardium in the vicinity of the right bundle branch. The resultant right-bundle-branch block is illustrated in the third and fourth beats of the schematic lead V_1 electrocardiogram recording. AV, atrioventricular; SA, sinoatrial. (From Netter FH, ed. *The CIBA Collection of Medical Illustrations*. Summit, NJ: CIBA-Geigy; 1978:13. *Heart*; vol 5, with permission.)

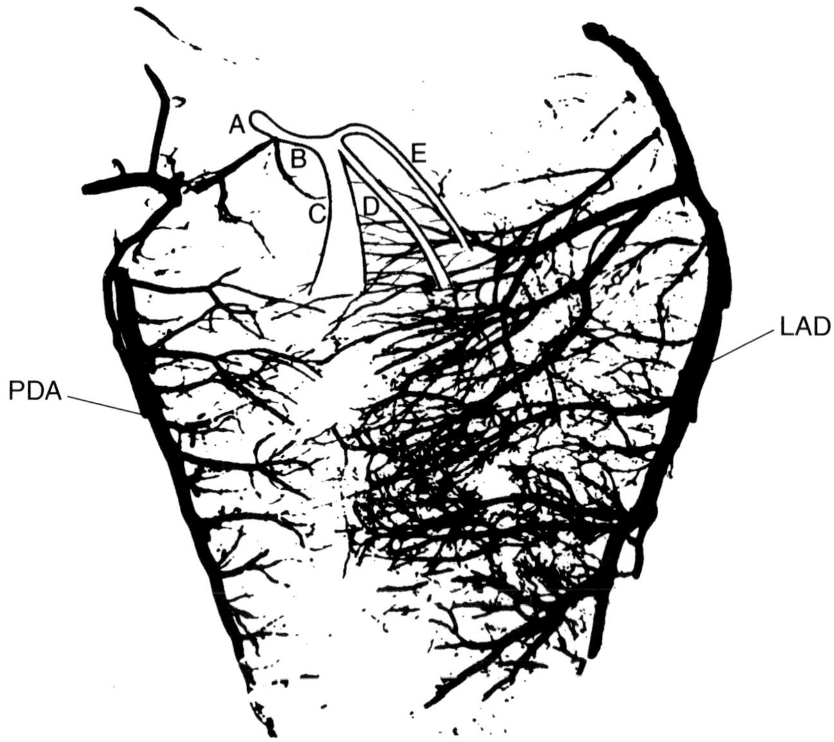

FIGURE 5.19. The proximal portion of specialized conduction system is shown in relation to its blood supply from a right anterior oblique view: A, atrioventricular node; B, common bundle; C, left posterior fascicle; D, left anterior fascicle; E, right bundle branch; LAD, left anterior descending artery; PDA, posterior descending artery. (Reprinted with permission from Rotman M, Wagner GS, Wallace AG. Bradyarrhythmias in acute myocardial infarction. *Circulation*. 1972;45:703-722, with permission. Copyright 1972, American Heart Association.)

Conventional teaching prescribes that new-onset LBBB or RBBB that occurs with acute MI is associated with massive MIs.[19] Pathology studies have demonstrated that the proximal left anterior descending coronary artery septal perforators perfuse the RBB and LAF of the LBB in 90% of cases, whereas the right coronary artery (via the AV nodal artery) perfuses the posterior fascicle of the LBB in 90% of cases, and there is dual blood supply to each of these fascicles in 40% to 50% of cases.[8] Thus, proximal left anterior descending artery occlusions could cause RBBB and/or LAFB; however, both proximal left anterior descending artery and right coronary artery occlusions would be required for MIs to be the direct cause of LBBB in 90% of patients. See **Figure 5.19** for a schematic of the relationship between the fascicles and coronary arteries. Of note, histopathology studies have found that interruption of the LBB almost always occurs at its junction with the main bundle where the LBB can be compressed between connective tissue at the base of the ventricular septum.[20-22] This compression likely occurs more frequently when the ventricles are subjected to mechanical strain from hypertrophy or dilatation.

Intermittent BBB (prolonged QRS complexes present at some times but not at others) usually represents a transition stage before permanent block is established. **Figure 5.20** shows an example of sudden-onset LBBB from a 62-year-old woman during routine ECG monitoring after uncomplicated abdominal surgery (**Figure 5.20A**) and sudden-onset RBBB from a 54-year-old man during 24-hour ECG monitoring for a complaint of dizziness (**Figure 5.20B**).

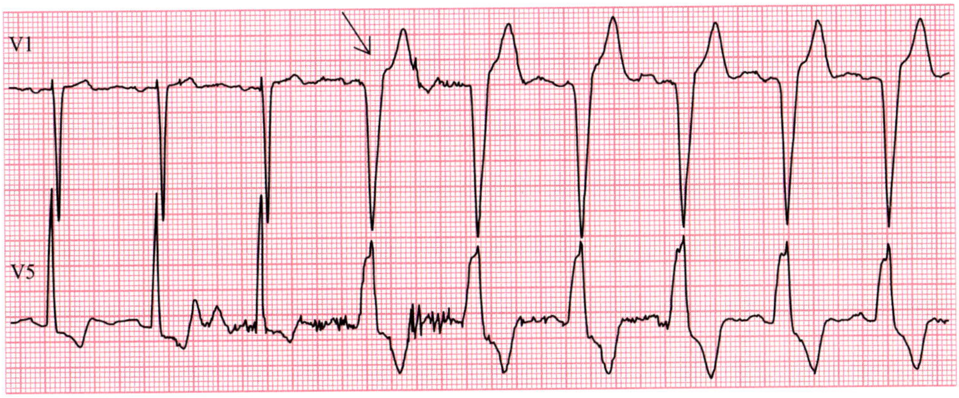

A

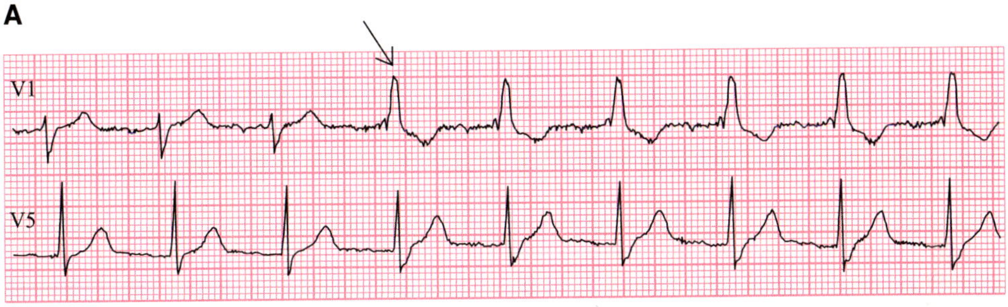

B

FIGURE 5.20. Precordial leads V_1 and V_5 are shown from a 62-year-old woman during routine electrocardiogram monitoring after uncomplicated abdominal surgery (**A**) and a 54-year-old man during 24-hour electrocardiogram monitoring for a complaint of dizziness (**B**). Arrows indicate the onsets in the V_1 leads of typically appearing left-bundle-branch block in **A** and right-bundle-branch block in **B**.

At times, intermittent BBB is determined by the heart rate. As the rate accelerates, the *R-R interval* shortens, and the descending impulse finds one of the bundle branches still in its *refractory period.* The appearance of incomplete RBBB following the shorter cycle intervals is illustrated in **Figure 5.21**. With this *tachycardia-dependent* BBB, slowing of the heart rate allows descending impulses to arrive after the refractory period of the entire conduction system, and normal conduction is resumed.

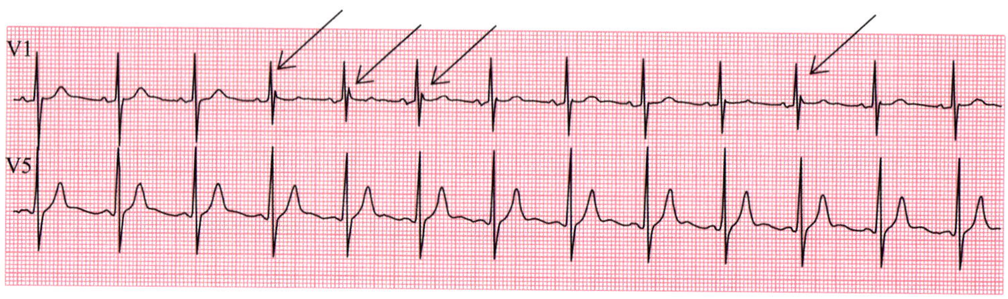

FIGURE 5.21. Appearance of tachycardia-dependent incomplete RBBB (arrows).

A rarer form of intermittent BBB, which develops only when the cardiac cycle lengthens rather than shortens, is termed *bradycardia-dependent BBB*. All beats are conducted sinus beats grouped in pairs. Those ending the shorter cycles are conducted normally, whereas those ending the longer cycles are conducted with LBBB (**Figure 5.22**). Intermittent BBB is a form of intermittent aberrant conduction of electrical impulses through the ventricular myocardium.

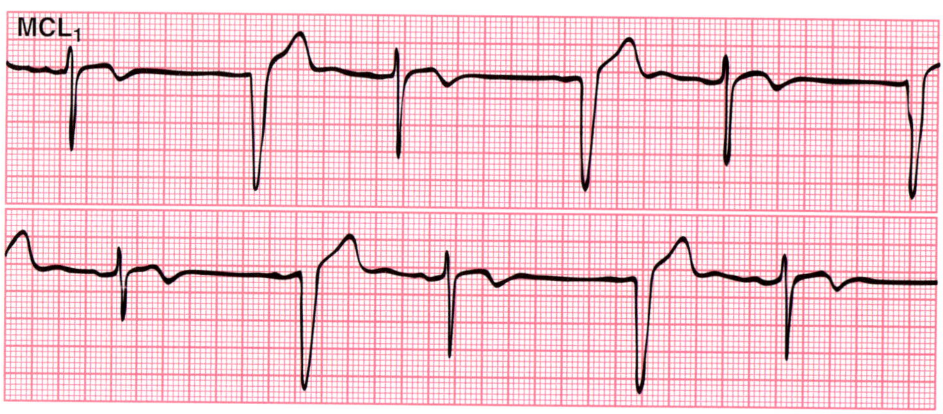

FIGURE 5.22. Bradycardia-dependent bundle-branch block.

CHAPTER 5 SUMMARY ILLUSTRATION

Right bundle branch block (RBBB)

Late intrinsicoid (R' peak or late R peak), M-shaped QRS (RSR'); sometimes wide R or qR

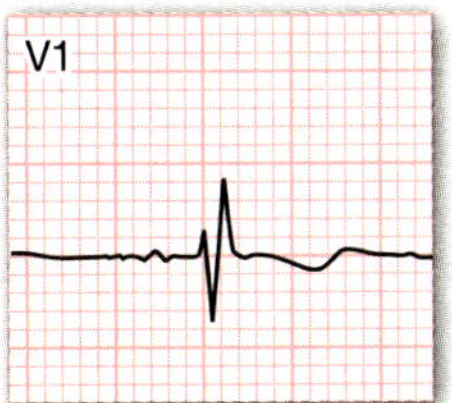

Early intrinsicoid (R peak), wide S wave

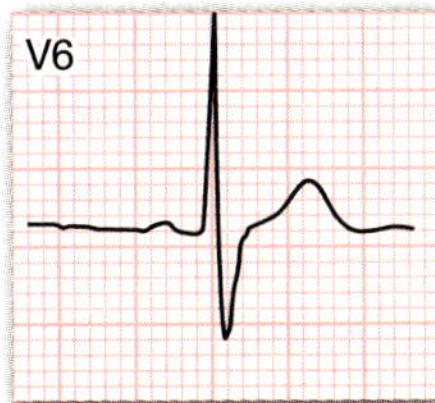

Wide S wave

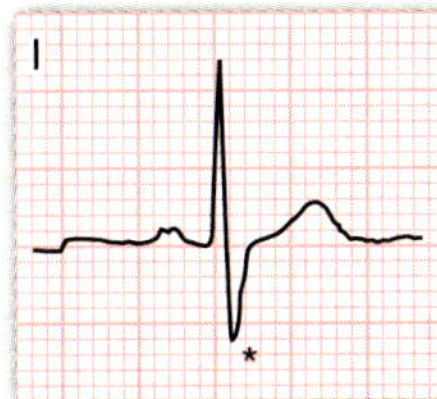

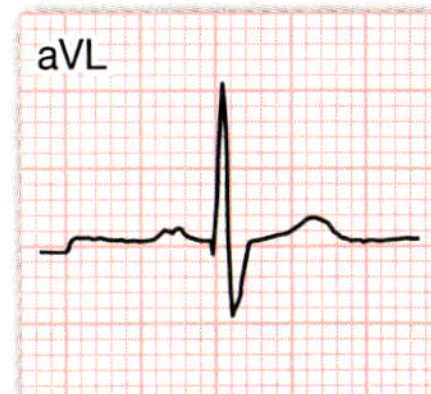

- QRS duration ≥120 ms

Left bundle branch block (LBBB)

QS or rS

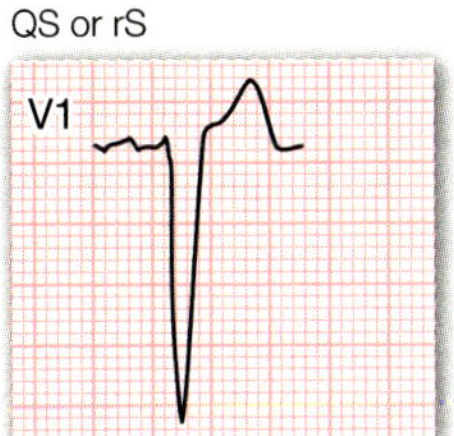

Mid-QRS notching/slurring in two of the leads

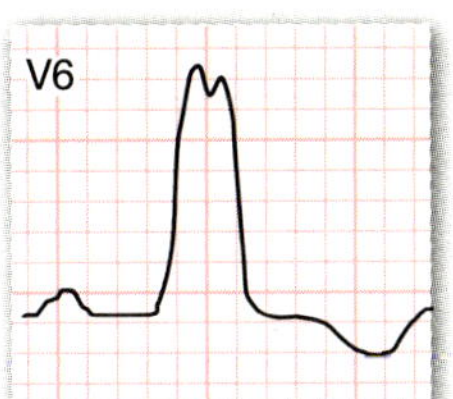

Mid-QRS notching/slurring in two of the leads

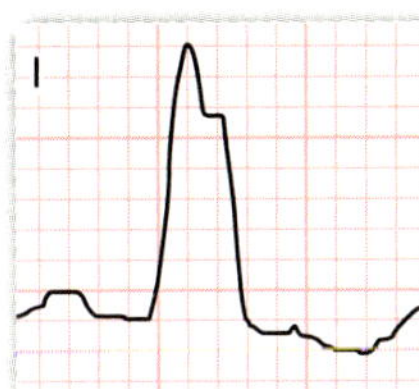

Mid-QRS notching/slurring in two of the leads

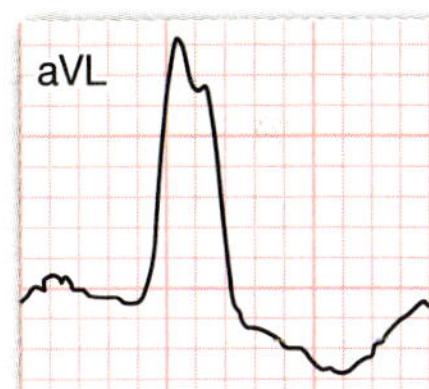

- Traditional criteria: QRS duration 120 ms
- Strict criteria: QRS duration 130 ms (women) or 140 ms (men) and the presence of mid-QRS notching in at least 2 of the leads I, aVL, V1, V2, V5 or V6.

Left Anterior Fascicular Block (LAFB)

Small Q, Large R

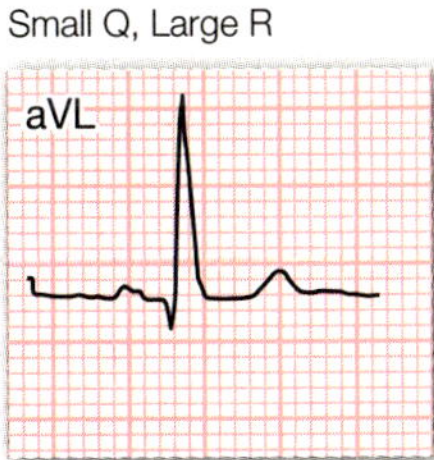

Small R, Large S

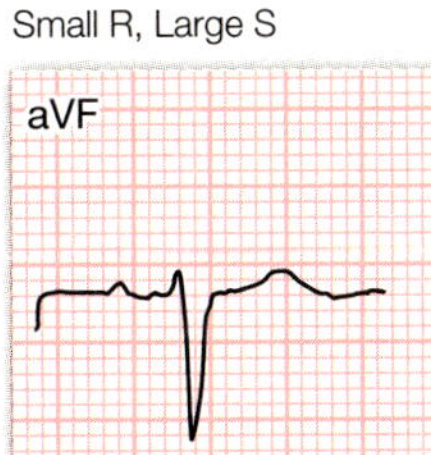

- LAFB – Left axis deviation, minimal QRS prolongation (20 ms)

Left Posterior Fascicular Block (LPFB)

Small R, Large S

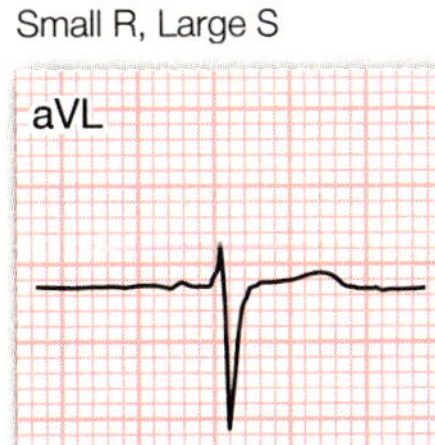

Small Q, Large R

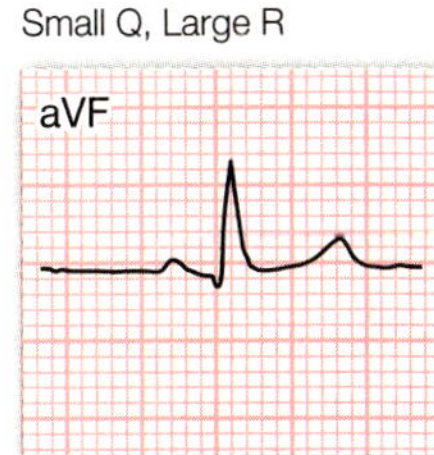

- LPFB – Right axis deviation, no evidence of RVH

RBBB+LAFB – Meets criteria for RBBB and LAFB

Late R or R' peak, M-shaped QRS-shaped QRS

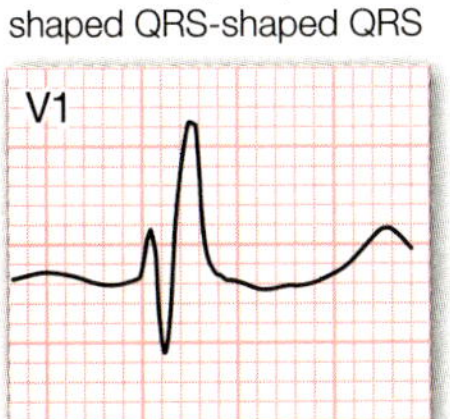

Early R peak, wide S wave

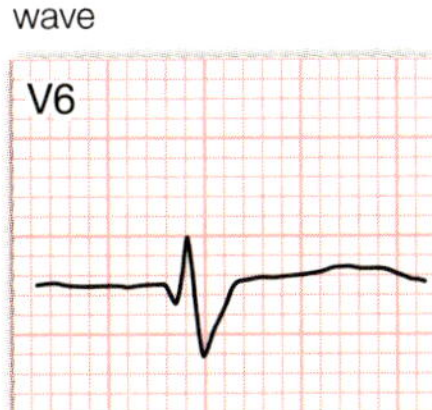

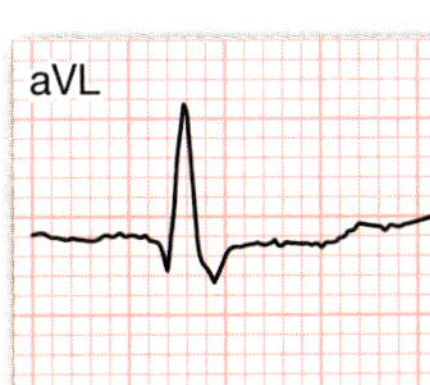

Small R & large S in inferior leads, left axis deviation

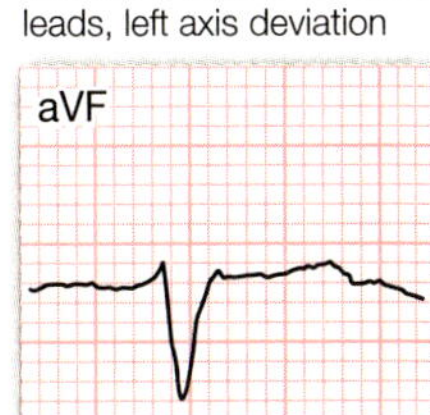

Abbreviations: LV, left ventricle; RV, right ventricle.

Glossary

AV block: a delay in the cardiac conduction system that causes a disruption of atrial-to-ventricular electrical conduction.

Bifascicular block: an intraventricular conduction abnormality involving any two of the following: RBB, the anterior division of the LBB, and the posterior division of the LBB.

Bilateral bundle-branch block: an intraventricular conduction abnormality involving both the right and left bundle branches, as indicated either by the presence of some conducted beats with RBBB and others with LBBB, or by AV block located distal to the common bundle.

Bradycardia-dependent BBB: RBBB or LBBB that is intermittent, appearing only with a slowing of the atrial rate.

Cancellation: elimination of an abnormality produced by a particular cardiac problem by a similar abnormality in another part of the heart or by a different abnormality in the same part of the heart because the ECG waveforms represent the summation of the wavefronts of activation and recovery within the heart.

Chagas disease: a tropical disease caused by the flagellate organism *T cruzi*, which is marked by prolonged high fever; edema; and enlargement of the spleen, liver, and lymph nodes and is complicated by cardiac involvement.

Fascicle: a group of Purkinje fibers too small to be called a "branch."

Fibrosis: a condition in which Purkinje fibers are replaced by nonconducting interstitial fibrous tissue.

Left anterior fascicular block: a conduction abnormality in the anterior fascicle of the LBB.

Left posterior fascicular block: a conduction abnormality in the posterior fascicle of the LBB.

Lenègre (Lev) disease: variations of fibrosis of the intraventricular Purkinje fibers in the absence of other significant cardiac disease, described by Lenegre[20] and Lev.[21]

Primary and secondary T-wave changes: in the presence of RBBB or LBBB, the term *primary T-wave changes* refers to abnormal T waves that are directed in the same direction as the latter portion of the QRS complex, and *secondary T-wave changes* refers to normal T waves that are directed opposite to the latter portion of the QRS complex.

Refractory period: the period following electrical activation during which a cardiac cell cannot be reactivated.

R-R interval: the period between successive QRS complexes.

Septal Q wave: a normal, initially negative small QRS waveform that appears in leftward-oriented ECG leads because the earliest activation of the interventricular septum via the septal fascicles of the LBB occurs in a left-to-right direction.

Syncope: a brief, sudden loss of consciousness associated with transient lack of cerebral blood flow.

Tachycardia-dependent BBB: RBBB or LBBB that is intermittent, appearing only with an acceleration of the atrial rate.

Trifascicular block: an intraventricular conduction abnormality involving the RBB and both the anterior and posterior fascicles of the LBB.

Unifascicular block: an intraventricular conduction abnormality involving only one of the three principal fascicles of the intraventricular Purkinje system.

Acknowledgment

We gratefully acknowledge the past contributions of the previous edition's author, Dr. Galen S. Wagner, as portions of that chapter were retained in this revision.

References

1. Wellens HJJ, Lie KI, Janse MJ, eds. *The Conduction System of the Heart: Structure, Function and Clinical Implications*. Hague, Netherlands: Martinus Nijhoff; 1978.
2. Demoulin JC, Kulbertus HE. Histopathological examination of concept of left hemiblock. *Br Heart J*. 1972;34:807-814.
3. Rosenbaum MB, Elizari MV, Lazzari JO. *The Hemiblocks*. Oldsmar, FL: Tampa Tracings; 1970.
4. Loring Z, Chelliah S, Selvester RH, Wagner G, Strauss DG. A detailed guide for quantification of myocardial scar with the Selvester QRS score in the presence of ECG confounders. *J Electrocardiol*. 2011;44:544-554.

5. Eriksson P, Hansson PO, Eriksson H, Dellborg M. Bundle-branch block in a general male population: the study of men born 1913. *Circulation.* 1998;98:2494-2500.
6. Hindman MC, Wagner GS, JaRo M, et al. The clinical significance of bundle branch block complicating acute myocardial infarction. 2. Indications for temporary and permanent pacemaker insertion. *Circulation.* 1978;58:689-699.
7. Strauss DG, Selvester RH, Wagner GS. Defining left bundle branch block in the era of cardiac resynchronization therapy. *Am J Cardiol.* 2011;107(6):927-934.
8. Frink RJ, James TN. Normal blood supply to the human His bundle and proximal bundle branches. *Circulation.* 1973;47:8-18.
9. Willems JL, Robles de Medina EO, Bernard R, et al. Criteria for intraventricular conduction disturbances and pre-excitation. *J Am Coll Cardiol.* 1985;5:1261-1275.
10. Klein RC, Vera Z, DeMaria AN, Mason DT. Electrocardiographic diagnosis of left ventricular hypertrophy in the presence of left bundle branch block. *Am Heart J.* 1984;108(3, pt 1):502-506.
11. Hiss RG, Lamb LE. Electrocardiographic findings in 122,043 individuals. *Circulation.* 1962;25:947-961.
12. Lenegre J. Etiology and pathology of bilateral bundle branch block in relation to complete heart block. *Prog Cardiovasc Dis.* 1964;6:409-444.
13. Lev M. Anatomic basis for atrioventricular block. *Am J Med.* 1964;37:742-748.
14. Rotman M, Triebwasser JH. A clinical and follow-up study of right and left bundle branch block. *Circulation.* 1975;51:477-484.
15. Schneider JF, Thomas HE Jr, McNamara PM, Kannel WB. Clinical-electrocardiographic correlates of newly acquired left bundle branch block: the Framingham Study. *Am J Cardiol.* 1985;55:1332-1338.
16. Lasser RP, Haft JI, Friedberg CK. Relationship of right bundle-branch block and marked left axis deviation (with left parietal or peri-infarction block) to complete heart block and syncope. *Circulation.* 1968;37:429-437.
17. Pick A, Langendorf R. *Interpretation of Complex Arrhythmias.* Philadelphia, PA: Lea & Febiger; 1979.
18. Acquatella H, Catalioti F, Gomez-Mancebo JR, Davalos V, Villalobos L. Long-term control of Chagas disease in Venezuela: effects on serologic findings, electrocardiographic abnormalities, and clinical outcome. *Circulation.* 1987;76:556-562.
19. Neeland IJ, Kontos MC, de Lemos JA. Evolving considerations in the management of patients with left bundle branch block and suspected myocardial infarction. *J Am Coll Cardiol.* 2012;60:96-105.
20. Lenegre J. *Contribution à l'etude des blocs de branche.* Paris, France: JB Bailliere et Fils; 1958.
21. Lev M, Unger PN, Rosen KM, Bharati S. The anatomic substrate of complete left bundle branch block. *Circulation.* 1974;50:479-486.
22. Sugiura M, Okada R, Okawa S, Shimada H. Pathohistological studies on the conduction system in 8 cases of complete left bundle branch block. *Jpn Heart J.* 1970;11:5-16.

Reference to the South Asian Edition

A James TN, Sherf L. Fine structure of the His bundle. *Circulation.* 1971;44:928. doi: 10.1161/01.cir.44.1.9.

SECTION III

Ischemia and Infarction

6 Introduction to Myocardial Ischemia and Infarction

DAVID G. STRAUSS,
DOUGLAS D. SCHOCKEN,
TOBIN H. LIM, AND
ANANDARAJA SUBRAMANIAN

Introduction to Ischemia and Infarction

The energy required to maintain the cardiac cycle is generated by a process known as *aerobic metabolism*, in which oxygen is required for energy production. Oxygen and essential nutrients are supplied by the blood to the cells of the myocardium via the *coronary arteries* (*myocardial perfusion*). If the blood supply to the myocardium becomes insufficient, an energy deficit occurs. To compensate for this diminished aerobic metabolism, the myocardial cells initiate a different metabolic process, *anaerobic metabolism*, in which oxygen is not required. In this process, the cells use their reserve supply of glucose stored in glycogen molecules to generate energy. Anaerobic metabolism, however, is less efficient than aerobic metabolism. Anaerobic metabolism produces only enough energy to survive but not function. Lastly, anaerobic metabolism is temporary, operating only until this glycogen is depleted.

In the period during which perfusion is insufficient to meet the myocardial demand required for both survival and function, the myocardial cells are *ischemic*. To sustain themselves, myocardial cells with an energy deficiency must uncouple their electrical activation from mechanical contraction and remain in their resting state. This state of electromechanical uncoupling has been termed myocardial *stunning* during acute, sudden-onset ischemia and *hibernation* during chronic ischemia.[1] Thus, the area of the myocardium that is ischemic cannot participate in the pumping process of the heart.[2,3]

Various areas of the myocardium are more or less susceptible to ischemia. There are several determining factors.

Factors Determining Susceptibility to Ischemia

1. Proximity to the intracavitary blood supply
2. Distance from the major coronary arteries
3. Workload as determined by the pressure required to pump blood

Proximity to the Intracavitary Blood Supply

The internal layers of myocardial cells (endocardium) have a secondary source of nutrients, the intracavitary blood, which provides protection from ischemia.[4,5] The entire myocardium of the right and left atria has so few cell layers that it is almost all endocardium and *subendocardium* (**Figure 6.1**). In the ventricles, however, only the innermost cell layers are similarly protected. The Purkinje system is located in these layers and is therefore well protected against ischemia.[6]

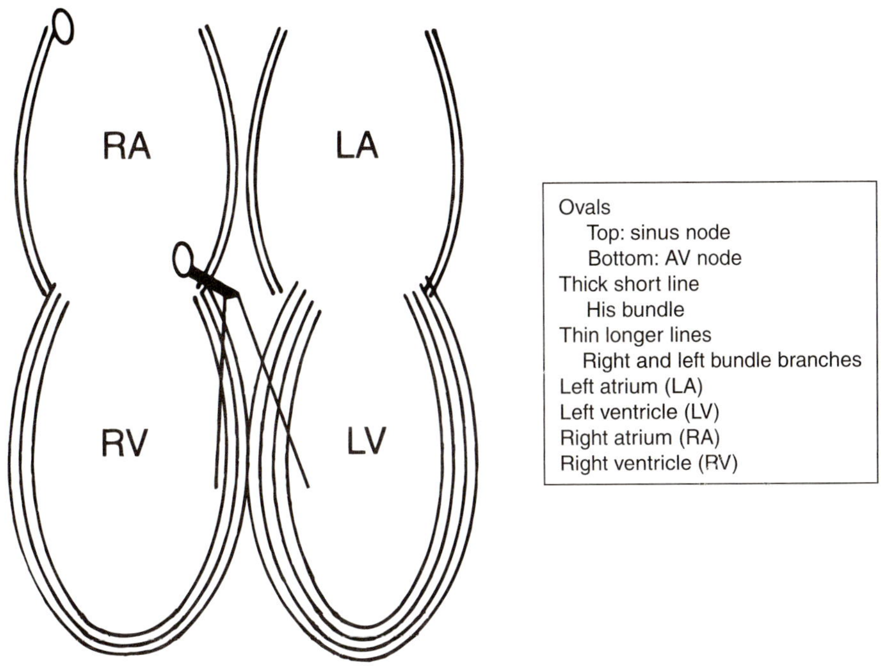

FIGURE 6.1. Schematic comparison of the relative thickness of the myocardium in the four cardiac chambers along with the sinoatrial node, atrioventricular node, His bundle, and right and left bundles. (Modified from Wagner GS, Waugh RA, Ramo BW. *Cardiac Arrhythmias*. New York, NY: Churchill Livingstone; 1983:2. Copyright © 1983 Elsevier. With permission.)

Distance From the Major Coronary Arteries

The ventricles consist of multiple myocardial layers that depend on the coronary arteries for their blood supply. These arteries arise from the aorta and course along the epicardial surfaces before penetrating the thickness of the myocardium. They then pass sequentially through the epicardial, middle, and subendocardial layers (**Figure 6.2**). The subendocardial layer is the most distant, innermost layer of the myocardium and is subjected to the highest myocardial wall tension, resulting in greater oxygen needs.[7] Therefore, the subendocardial layer is the most susceptible to ischemia.[8] The thicker walled left ventricle is much more susceptible to insufficient perfusion than is the thinner walled right ventricle because of both the wall thickness itself and the greater workload of the left ventricle.

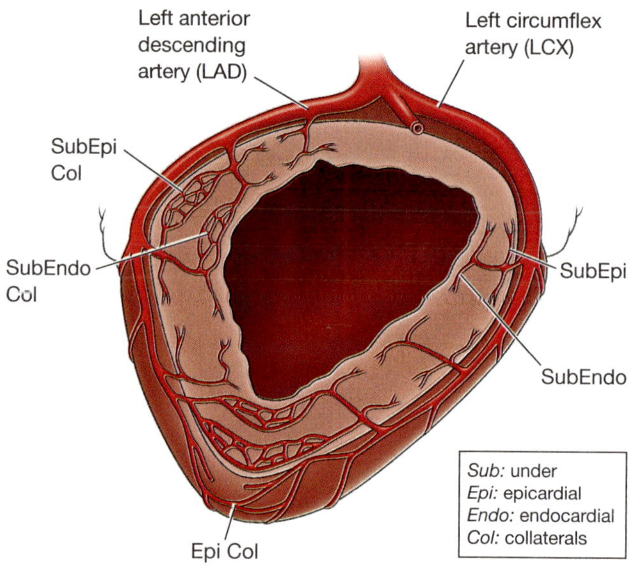

FIGURE 6.2. Cross-section of the left ventricle from the left anterior oblique view. The epicardial courses of the main branches of the main coronary arteries and their intramyocardial branches are shown. (Modified from Califf RM, Mark DB, Wagner GS, eds. *Acute Coronary Care*. 2nd ed. Chicago, IL: Mosby-Year Book; 1994. Copyright © 1994 Elsevier. With permission.)

Workload as Determined by the Pressure Required to Pump Blood

The greater the pressure required by a cardiac chamber to pump blood, the greater its workload and the greater its metabolic demand for oxygen. The myocardial workload is smallest in the atria, intermediate in the right ventricle, and greatest in the left ventricle. Therefore, the susceptibility to ischemia is also lowest in the atria, intermediate in the right ventricle, and greatest in the left ventricle.

Ischemia is a relative condition that depends on the balance among the coronary blood supply, the level of oxygenation of the blood, and the myocardial workload. Theoretically, an individual with normal coronary arteries and fully oxygenated blood could develop *myocardial ischemia* if the workload were increased either by an extremely elevated arterial blood pressure or an extremely high heart rate. Alternatively, an individual with normal coronary arteries and a normal myocardial workload could develop ischemia if the oxygenation of the blood became extremely diminished. Conversely, the myocardium of someone with severe narrowing (stenoses) in all coronary arteries might never become ischemic if the cardiac workload remained low and the blood was well oxygenated.

When ischemia is produced by an increased workload, this condition is normally reversed by returning to the resting state before the myocardial cells' reserve supply of glycogen is entirely depleted. However, a condition that produces myocardial ischemia by decreasing the coronary blood supply may not be reversed so easily.

Coronary arteries may gradually become partly obstructed by plaques in the chronic process of atherosclerosis (**Figure 6.3**). This condition produces ischemia when, even though the myocardial blood supply is sufficient at a resting workload, it becomes insufficient when the workload is increased by either emotional or physical stress. The gradual progression of the atherosclerotic process is accompanied by growth of collateral arteries, which supply blood to the myocardium beyond the level of obstruction. Indeed, these collateral arteries may be sufficient to entirely replace the blood-supplying capacity of the native artery if it becomes completely obstructed by the atherosclerotic plaque.[9]

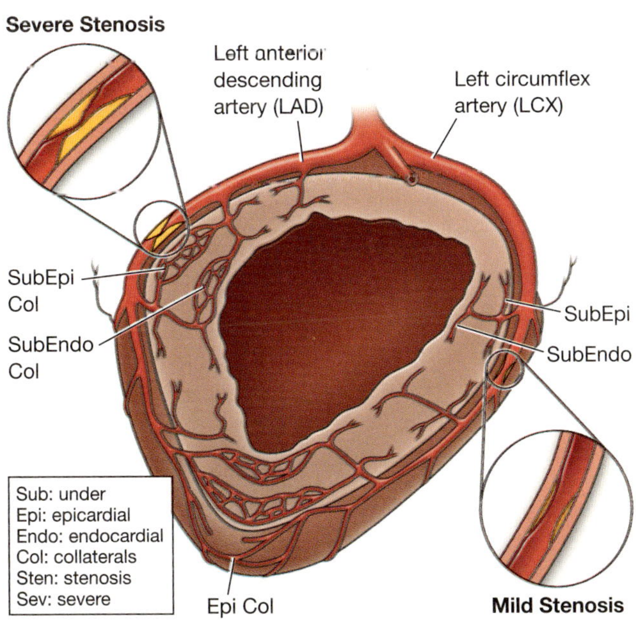

FIGURE 6.3. Stenosis of coronary arteries. (Reprinted from Califf RM, Mark DB, Wagner GS, eds. *Acute Coronary Care*. 2nd ed. Chicago, IL: Mosby-Year Book; 1994. Copyright © 1994 Elsevier. With permission.)

Partially obstructed atherosclerotic coronary arteries may suddenly become completely obstructed by the acute processes of spasm of their smooth-muscle layer or *thrombosis* within the remaining arterial lumen.[10,11] In either of these conditions, ischemia develops immediately unless the resting metabolic demands of the affected myocardial cells can be satisfied by the collateral blood flow. If the spasm is relaxed or the thrombus is resolved (thrombolysis) before the glycogen reserve of the affected cells is severely depleted, the cells promptly resume their contraction. If, however, the acute, complete obstruction continues until the myocardial cells' glycogen is severely depleted, they become *stunned.*[12] Even after blood flow is restored, these cells are unable to resume contraction until they have repleted their glycogen reserves. If the complete obstruction further persists until the myocardial cells' glycogen is entirely depleted, the cells are unable to sustain themselves, are irreversibly damaged, and die. This clinical process is termed a heart attack or *myocardial infarction*.

Electrocardiographic Changes

Electrophysiologic Changes During Ischemia

Knowing the action potential changes that occur during ischemia and the location of ischemia helps to understand what electrocardiogram (ECG) changes occur during ischemia. This process is illustrated with the use of the interactive ECG simulation program, ECGSIM.[13] With the onset of ischemia, there are three principle changes that occur to the action potential.

Changes in the Action Potential During Ischemia

1. Action potential duration shortens.
2. Action potential amplitude decreases.
3. Depolarization phase of the action potential is delayed (slowed conduction velocity).

Experimental and simulation studies have shown that changes in extracellular potassium and pH, along with opening of ATP-dependent potassium channels can account for the action potential (AP) changes that occur in acute ischemia.

Electrocardiographic Changes During Supply Ischemia (Insufficient Blood Supply)

Figure 6.4 and **Video 6.1** demonstrate the individual and the combined effect of these three action potential changes during supply ischemia (insufficient blood supply) due to sudden occlusion of the distal left anterior descending coronary artery. The principal ECG changes that occur are seen in the ECG leads that are directly above the ischemic area. In this case, they are leads V_3 and V_4.

ECG Changes in Leads with a Positive Pole above the Ischemic Region

1. Action potential duration shortening causes increased T-wave amplitude.
2. Decreased action potential amplitude causes increased ST-segment elevation.
3. Delayed depolarization causes the QRS complex to become more positive (increased R wave and decreased S wave).

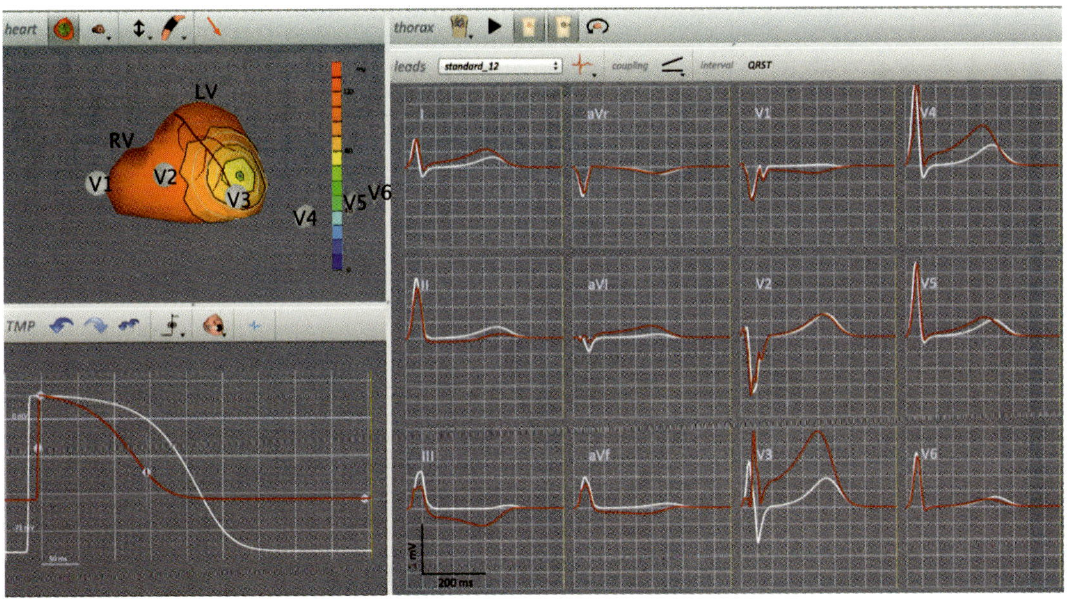

FIGURE 6.4. Screenshot from **Video 6.1** available with the online version of the book using ECG simulation software to study transmural myocardial ischemia from insufficient blood supply. The image shows the ischemic region on the heart (upper left), ischemic action potential (lower left; ischemia in red) and 12-lead ECG (right, ischemia in red) resulting from transmural ischemia due to an occluded left anterior descending artery. **Video 6.1** demonstrates how to use the software and shows how individual and combined ischemic action potential changes cause body surface ECG changes. After watching **Video 6.1**, the software can be downloaded for free at www.ecgsim.org for further exploration of the relationship between ischemia in different regions of the heart and the associated 12-lead ECG changes. LV, left ventricle; RV, right ventricle; TMP, transmembrane potential (also known as action potential).

To view the animation(s) and video(s) associated with this chapter please access lww.co.in. Instructions are located on the inside front cover.

Video 6.1 shows the combined effect of all three action potential changes during ischemia. When the location of ischemia occurs in a different part of the left ventricle, the same changes to the ECG occur in the leads that are above the ischemic area. This observation will be discussed in more detail in Chapter 8.

Based on clinical observations, Sclarovsky and Birnbaum developed a method for classifying the gradation of changes observed in decreased supply and have shown that patient prognosis worsens as the ischemia grade increases.[14]

Sclarovsky-Birnbaum Ischemia Grading[14]

- Grade 1: increase in T-wave amplitude only (**Figure 6.5A**)
- Grade 2: increase in T waves + ST segments (**Figure 6.5B**)
- Grade 3: increase in T waves + ST segments + QRS complexes; "tombstoning" (**Figure 6.5C**)

Going back to the lessons learned from **Video 6.1**, the least severe grade 1 ischemia (only increase in T-wave amplitude) means that the only ischemic change is a shortening of action potential duration. With grade 2 ischemia, there is also an increase in ST-segment elevation, indicating the presence of decreased action potential amplitude. With grade 3 ischemia, changes to the QRS complex are now present, indicating the presence of delayed depolarization. *Tombstoning* is a descriptive term for this most extreme severity of decreased supply. These changes illustrated by often remarkable ST elevations suggest the appearance of an old-fashioned tombstone and foretell the poor prognostic outcome in patients with such findings who do not receive prompt restoration of blood flow to the region of ischemia.

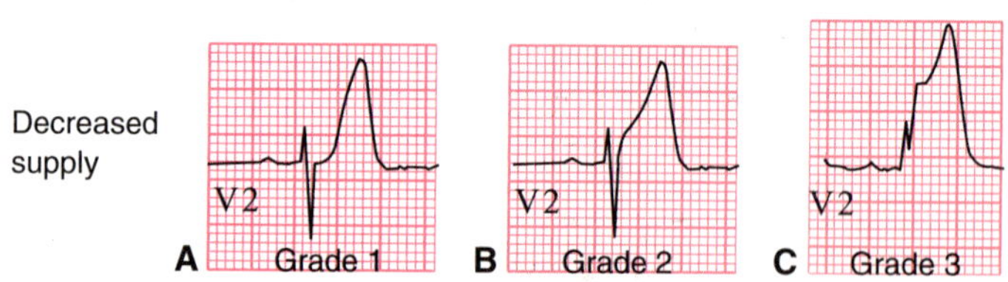

FIGURE 6.5. Lead V_2 waveforms in a patient with Sclarovsky-Birnbaum grade 1 ischemia (increase in T-wave amplitude only) (**A**), grade 2 ischemia (increase in ST segment and T wave) (**B**), and grade 3 (increase in QRS complex, ST segment, and T wave; "tombstoning") (**C**).

Electrocardiographic Changes During Demand Ischemia

An increase in demand is most commonly recognized on the ECG by changes in the ST segments; however, demand ischemia can also result in changes in the QRS complex and T wave.[15] Because increased demand is limited to the subendocardial layer of the left ventricle, it is termed *subendocardial ischemia*. In addition, demand ischemia usually occurs globally throughout the entire subendocardium of the left ventricle, and thus, it is not possible to localize demand ischemia to an individual coronary artery territory. Instead of the ST and T waves shifting toward the ischemic area as they do in supply ischemia, with demand ischemia, the ST and T waves shift away from the ischemic area (**Figure 6.6**). This subendocardial ischemia results in ST depression and T-wave inversion in most leads on the 12-lead ECG because the positive pole of the lead lies above the epicardium of the left ventricle. In aVR, which has a positive pole that points away from the endocardium of the left ventricle, demand ischemia results in ST elevation and an increase in T-wave amplitude.

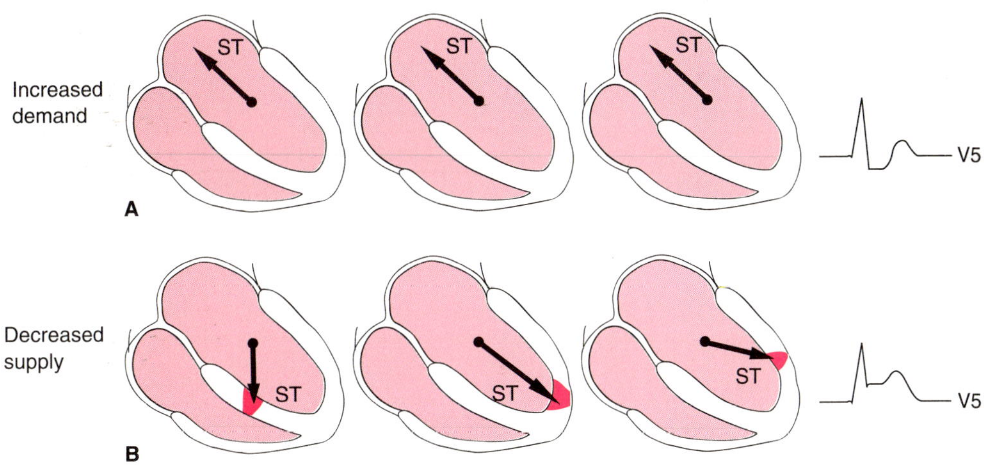

FIGURE 6.6. Electrocardiogram changes with abnormal perfusion. **A.** Global subendocardial ischemia from increased demand causes the ST-segment vector to point away from the entire left ventricle (appears as ST depression in lead V_5). **B.** Transmural ischemia from an occluded coronary artery (ie, decreased supply) causes the ST-segment vector to point toward the involved region resulting in ST elevation in the electrocardiogram leads above the ischemia zone. Arrows, ST-segment direction.

Figure 6.7 and **Video 6.2** demonstrate ischemic action potential changes throughout the left ventricular endocardium representative of global subendocardial ischemia.

Global Subendocardial Ischemia Action Potential Changes and the Corresponding ECG Changes

1. Action potential duration shortening causes T-wave flattening and then inverted T waves in all leads except aVR. In aVR, T waves flip from negative to positive.
2. Decreased action potential amplitude causes ST-segment depression in all leads except aVR, where ST elevation occurs.

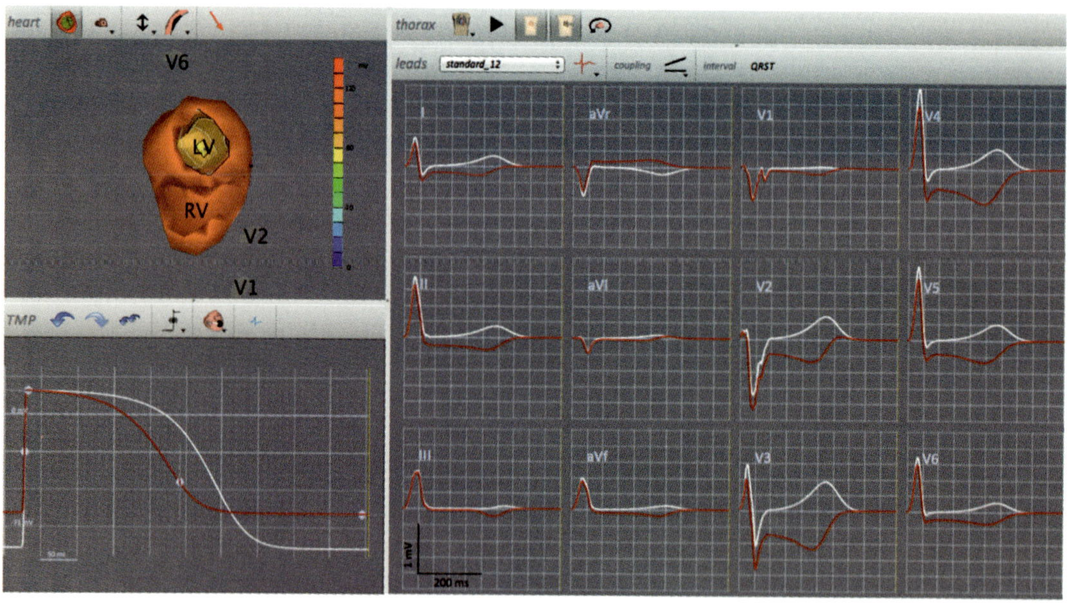

FIGURE 6.7. Screenshot from **Video 6.2** available with the online version of the book using ECG simulation software to study subendocardial ischemia from increased myocardial demand. The image shows the ischemic region in yellow throughout the inside of the left ventricle (upper left), ischemic action potential (lower left; ischemia in red) and 12-lead ECG (right, ischemia in red) resulting from global subendocardial ischemia. **Video 6.2** demonstrates how to use the software and shows why global subendocardial ischemia causes ST-segment depression in the precordial leads, but causes ST-segment elevation in lead aVR. After watching **Video 6.2**, the software can be downloaded for free at www.ecgsim.org for further exploration. LV, left ventricle; RV, right ventricle; TMP, transmembrane potential (also known as action potential).

Progression of Transmural Ischemia to Infarction

Insufficient myocardial perfusion of the left ventricle caused by complete coronary arterial occlusion results initially in *hyperacute T-wave* changes (see **Figure 6.8A**). Unless the occlusion is very brief or the myocardium is very well protected, the epicardial injury current is generated as represented by ST-segment deviation (see **Figure 6.8B**). Both the T wave and ST segments deviate toward the involved region. If delayed depolarization occurs, the terminal part of the QRS complex also deviates toward the involved region. If the complete occlusion persists, and myocardial reperfusion is not attained while the cells retain their viability, a myocardial infarction occurs (see **Figure 6.8C**; see Chapter 9). As this infarction process evolves, both the QRS complex and T wave are directed away from the involved region.[16,17]

The abnormal Q wave is the hallmark of an established infarction and the abnormal T wave is termed the *postischemic T wave*.[18] It is inverted in its relationship to the QRS complex in many of the ECG leads (see **Figure 6.8C**). The ECG changes associated with each of the three pathologic processes introduced in this chapter are presented in Chapters 7, 8, and 9.

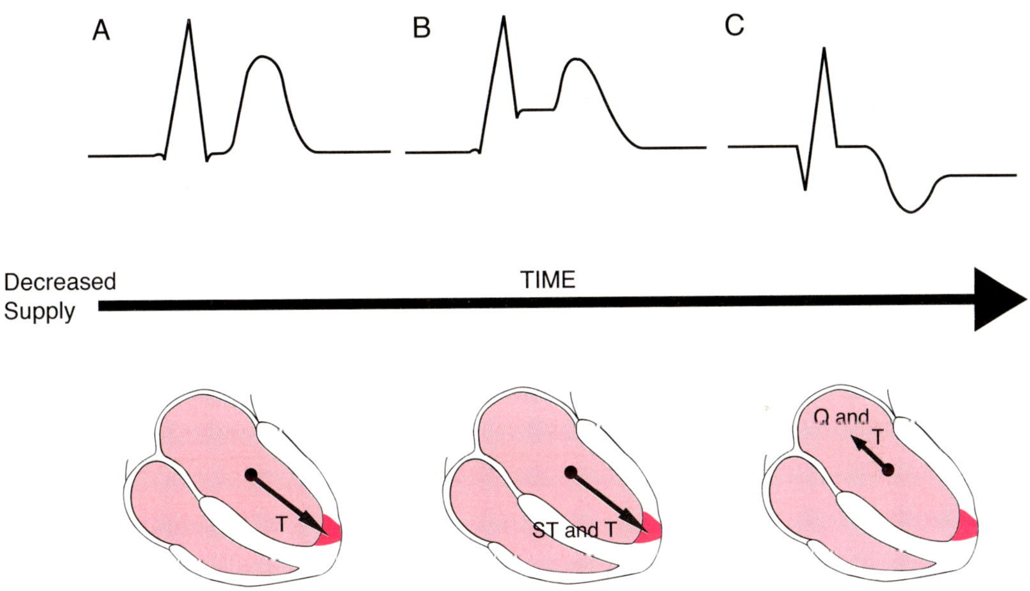

FIGURE 6.8. Results of myocardial ischemia over time. Early transmural myocardial ischemia produces increased T-wave amplitude (**A**), which is followed by ST-segment elevation (**B**). **C**, after infarction (cell death occurs), Q waves develop and T waves invert. The arrow on the heart indicates the direction of the T wave (**A**), ST segment and T wave (**B**) and Q and T waves (**C**).

CHAPTER 6 SUMMARY ILLUSTRATION

Myocardial Ischemia and Infarction

Increased demand

Global subendocardial ischemia from increased demand causes the ST-segment vector to point away from the entire left ventricle (appears as ST depression in lead V5).

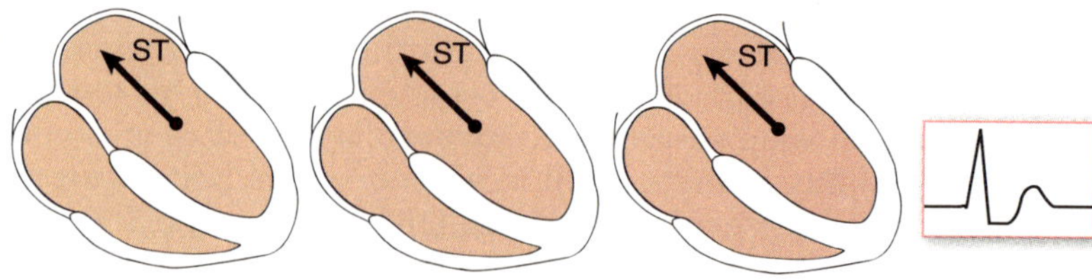

Decreased supply

Transmural ischemia from an occluded coronary artery (i.e., decreased supply) causes the ST-segment vector to point toward the involved region resulting in ST elevation in the ECG leads above the ischemia zone. Arrows, ST-segment direction.

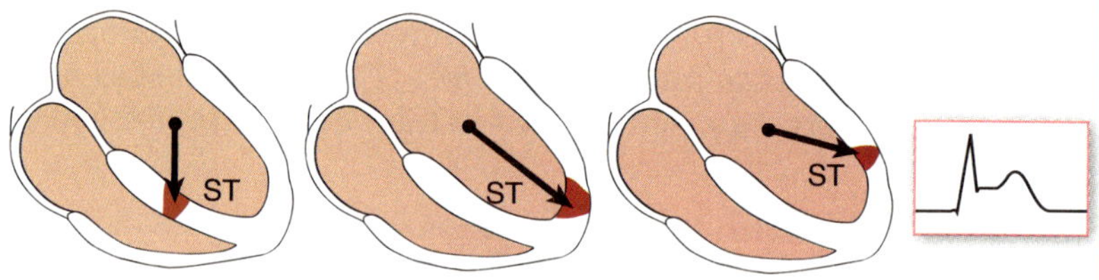

Results of myocardial ischemia over time

Early transmural myocardial ischemia produces increased T-wave amplitude (A), which is followed by ST-segment elevation (B). After infarction (cell death occurs), Q waves develop and T waves invert (C).

Decreased supply

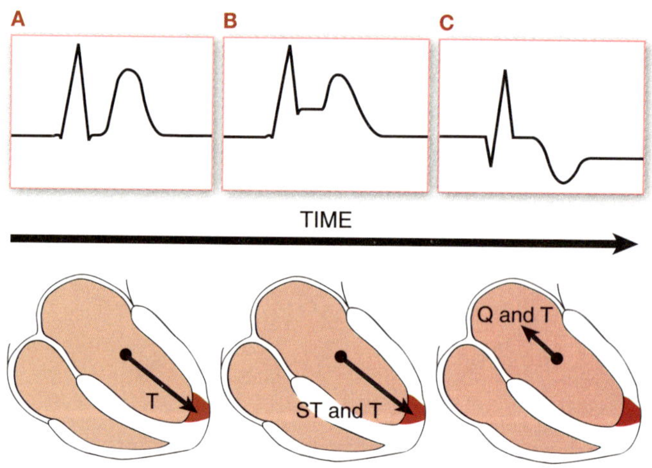

Glossary

Aerobic metabolism: the intracellular method for converting glucose into energy that requires the presence of oxygen and produces enough energy to nourish the myocardial cell and also to cause it to contract.

Anaerobic metabolism: the intracellular method for converting glucose into energy that does not require oxygen but produces only enough energy to nourish the cell.

Coronary arteries: either of the two arteries (right or left) that arise from the aorta immediately above the semilunar valves and supply the tissues of the heart itself.

Hyperacute T waves: T waves directed toward the ischemic area of the left-ventricular epicardium that can be identified in leads involved with the ischemic area by an increased positive amplitude.

Myocardial infarction: death of myocardial cells as a result of failure of the circulation to provide sufficient oxygen to restore metabolism after the intracellular stores of glycogen have been depleted.

Myocardial ischemia: a reduction in the supply of oxygen to less than the amount required by myocardial cells to maintain aerobic metabolism.

Myocardial perfusion: the flow of oxygen and nutrients into the cells of the heart muscle.

Postischemic T waves: T waves directed away from the ischemic area of the left-ventricular myocardium when the ischemic process is resolving either from infarction or to reperfusion.

Stunned myocardium: a region of myocardium consisting of cardiac cells that are using anaerobic metabolism and are therefore ischemic and incapable of contraction but which are not infarcted.

Subendocardium: the region of the myocardium just deep to the endocardium, most vulnerable to demand ischemia.

Thrombosis: the formation or presence of a blood clot within a blood vessel or cardiac chamber.

Tombstoning: severe supply ischemia that obscures the transition from QRS to ST segment to T wave.

Transmural: involving the full thickness of the myocardial wall.

Acknowledgment

We gratefully acknowledge the past contributions of the previous edition's author, Dr. Galen S. Wagner, as portions of that chapter were retained in this revision.

References

1. Kloner RA, Bolli R, Marban E, Reinlib L, Braunwald E. Medical and cellular implications of stunning, hibernation, and preconditioning: an NHLBI workshop. *Circulation*. 1998;97(18):1848-1867.
2. Reimer KA, Jennings RB, Tatum AH. Pathobiology of acute myocardial ischemia: metabolic, functional and ultrastructural studies. *Am J Cardiol*. 1983;52(2):72A-81A.
3. Lanza G, Coli S, Cianflone D, Maseri A. Coronary blood flow and myocardial ischemia. In: Fuster V, Alexander RW, O'Rourke RA, et al, eds. *Hurst's the Heart*. 11th ed. New York, NY: McGraw-Hill; 2004:1153-1172.
4. Reimer KA, Jennings RB. The "wavefront phenomenon" of myocardial ischemic cell death. II. Transmural progression of necrosis within the framework of ischemic bed size (myocardium at risk) and collateral flow. *Lab Invest*. 1979;40(6):633-644.
5. Reimer KA, Lowe JE, Rasmussen MM, Jennings RB. The wavefront phenomenon of ischemic cell death. 1. Myocardial infarct size vs duration of coronary occlusion in dogs. *Circulation*. 1977;56(5):786-794.
6. Hackel DB, Wagner G, Ratliff NB, Cies A, Estes EH Jr. Anatomic studies of the cardiac conducting system in acute myocardial infarction. *Am Heart J*. 1972;83(1):77-81.
7. Reimer KA, Jennings RB. Myocardial ischemia, hypoxia and infarction. In: Fozzard HA, ed. *The Heart and Cardiovascular System*. New York, NY: Raven Press Ltd; 1992:1875-1973.
8. Bauman R, Rembert J, Greenfield J. The role of the collateral circulation in maintaining cellular viability during coronary occlusion. In: Califf RM, Mark DB, Wagner GS, eds. *Acute Coronary Care*. 2nd ed. Chicago, IL: Mosby-Year Book; 1994.
9. Cohen M, Rentrop KP. Limitation of myocardial ischemia by collateral circulation during sudden controlled coronary artery occlusion in human subjects: a prospective study. *Circulation*. 1986;74(3):469-476.

10. Kolodgie FD, Virmani R, Burke AP, et al. Pathologic assessment of the vulnerable human coronary plaque. *Heart.* 2004;90(12): 1385-1391.
11. Davies MJ, Fulton WF, Robertson WB. The relation of coronary thrombosis to ischaemic myocardial necrosis. *J Pathol. 1979*;127(2):99-110.
12. Cooper HA, Braunwald E. Clinical importance of stunned and hibernating myocardium. *Coron Artery Dis.* 2001;12(5):387-392.
13. van Oosterom A, Oostendorp TF. ECGSIM: an interactive tool for studying the genesis of QRST waveforms. *Heart.* 2004;90(2): 165-168.
14. Billgren T, Birnbaum Y, Sgarbossa EB, et al. Refinement and interobserver agreement for the electrocardiographic Sclarovsky-Birnbaum Ischemia Grading System. *J Electrocardiol.* 2004;37(3):149-156.
15. Michaelides AP, Triposkiadis FK, Boudoulas H, et al. New coronary artery disease index based on exercise-induced QRS changes. *Am Heart J.* 1990;120(2):292-302.
16. Wagner N, Wagner G, White R. The twelve-lead ECG and the extent of myocardium at risk of acute infarction: cardiac anatomy and lead locations, and the phases of serial changes during acute occlusion. In: Califf RM, Mark DB, Wagner GS, eds. *Acute Coronary Care in the Thrombolytic Era.* Chicago, IL: Mosby-Year Book; 1988:31-45.
17. Sclarovsky S. *Electrocardiography of Acute Myocardial Ischemic Syndromes.* London, United Kingdom: Martin Duntz; 1999: 99-122.
18. Surawicz B. ST-T abnormalities. In: MacFarlane PW, Lawrie TDV, eds. *Comprehensive Electrocardiology.* New York, NY: Pergamon Press; 1988:511-563.

To view digital content associated with this chapter please access lww.co.in. Instructions are located on the inside front cover.

7

Subendocardial Ischemia from Increased Myocardial Demand

DAVID G. STRAUSS, TOBIN H. LIM, MURALIDHARAN T R, AND PREETAM KRISHNAMURTHY

Changes in the ST Segment

Normal Variants

The ST segment of the electrocardiogram (ECG) is normally at approximately the same baseline level as the PR and TP segments (see **Figure 1.12**). The stability of the position of the ST segment on the ECG during a graded exercise stress test provides clinical information about the presence or absence of myocardial ischemia.[1] If coronary blood flow is capable of increasing enough to satisfy the metabolic demands of the cells in the left-ventricular subendocardium, minimal alteration occurs in the appearance of the ST segment. Often, however, some changes appear in the ST segment that may be falsely considered "positive" for ischemia. A common normal variation in the 12-lead ECG before, during, and after exercise stress testing[2] is shown in **Figure 7.1A, B,** and **C**, respectively. Note the minor depression of the J point with the ST segment upsloping toward the upright T wave (arrows). The apparent ST-J point depression with upward sloping ST segment may occur because at faster heart rates, ventricular repolarization occurs sooner (note the shorter length of the ST segment and shorter overall QT interval in **Figure 7.1B** during exercise) and the QRS and T wave almost merge together.

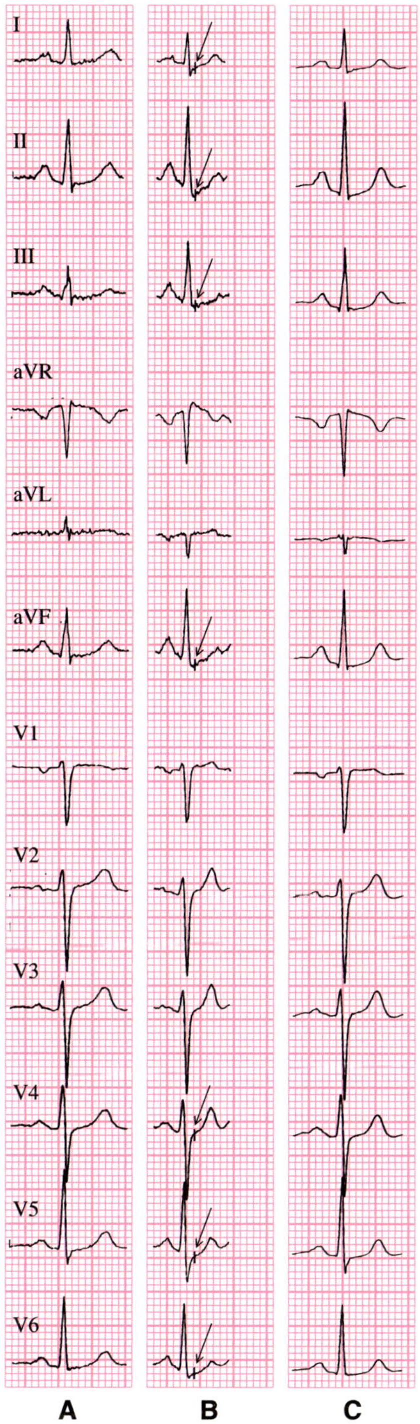

FIGURE 7.1. Twelve-lead electrocardiograms recorded from a 54-year-old man at rest (**A**), during an exercise stress test (**B**), and immediately after the test (**C**). Arrows indicate the depression of the ST-J point in many leads in **B**. This minor ST-J point depression with upward sloping ST segments is a benign common normal variation in the electrocardiogram during exercise. Enhanced Ta wave of atrial repolarization could also result in this appearance (see Chapter 3).

Typical Subendocardial Ischemia

Partial obstructions within the coronary arteries do not produce insufficient blood supply at rest and, therefore, cannot be detected on the resting ECG (**Figure 7.2A**). When such a partial obstruction, however, prevents myocardial blood flow from increasing enough to meet the increased metabolic demand during stress, the resulting ischemia (limited to the subendocardial layer of the left ventricle) is manifested by horizontal (**Figure 7.2B**) or downsloping ST-segment depression. The ST-segment depression typically disappears within several minutes after the demand on the myocardium is returned to baseline levels by stopping the exercise (**Figure 7.2C**) because the myocardial cells have been only reversibly ischemic. It cannot be emphasized enough that ECGs during and shortly after exercise are different from the standard resting ECGs and need to be interpreted carefully in their clinical context.

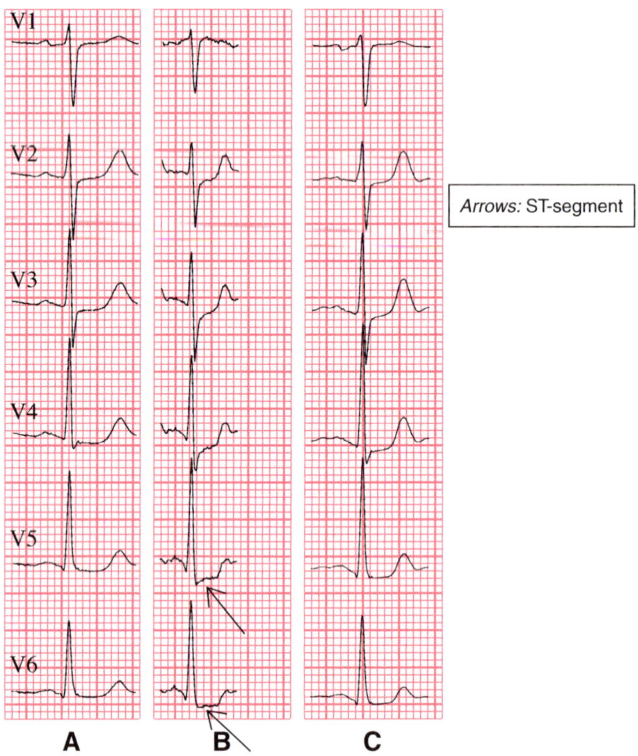

FIGURE 7.2. Serial recordings of the six precordial leads from a 60-year-old man with a history of exertional chest pain made at rest (**A**), during exercise at a heart rate of 167 beats per minute (**B**), and 5 minutes after exercise (**C**). Arrows indicate the horizontal ST-segment depression in leads V_5 and V_6 in **B**.

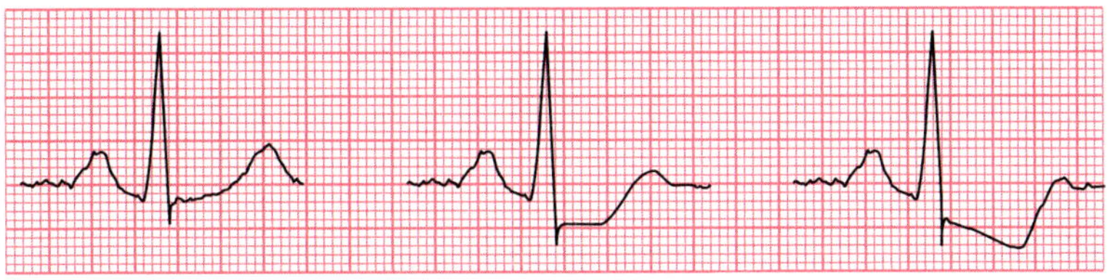

A B C

FIGURE 7.3. Single electrocardiogram waveforms at rest (**A**) and two variations of the abnormal condition of exercise-induced subendocardial ischemia (**B**,**C**).

A combination of two diagnostic criteria in at least one ECG lead is typically required for diagnosing left-ventricular subendocardial ischemia (**Figure 7.3**).

Diagnostic Criteria for Stress-Induced Left-Ventricular Subendocardial Ischemia

1. ST-segment depression of ≥1 mm (0.10 mV) at the J point
2. Either a horizontal or a downward slope toward the end of the ST segment at its junction with the T wave

The terminal part of the T wave typically remains positive (see **Figure 7.3A-C**) but with progressively diminished amplitude from **Figure 7.3B,C**.

As indicated in Chapter 2, the positive poles of most of the standard limb and precordial ECG leads are directed toward the left ventricle. Subendocardial ischemia causes the ST segment to move generally away from the left ventricle (see **Figure 6.6A**). The changes in the ST segment appear negative or depressed in the leftward (I, aVL, or V_2-V_6) and inferiorly oriented leads (II, III, and aVF), which have their positive poles directed toward the left ventricle (**Figure 7.4A,B**). As previously stated in Chapter 6, the location of the ECG leads showing ST-segment depression is not indicative of the involved region of left-ventricular subendocardial ischemia. In leads that have their positive poles directed away from the left ventricle (limb lead aVR and precordial leads V_1 and V_2), ST elevation is typically present (see **Figure 7.4A,B**).

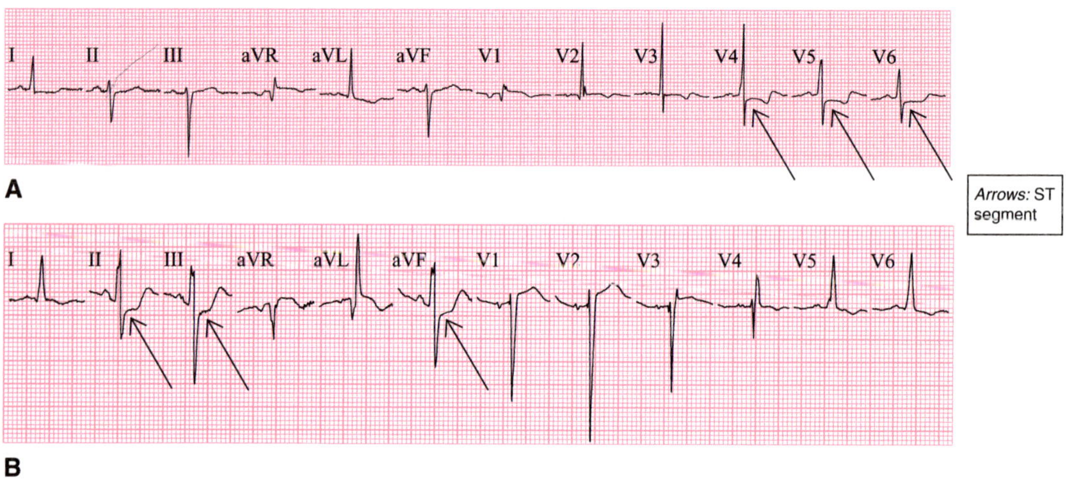

FIGURE 7.4. Twelve-lead electrocardiograms from two different patients with left-ventricular subendocardial ischemia. Patient **A** has most prominent ST-segment depression in leads V_4 to V_6 (arrows), with a negative beginning of the T wave in these leads. Patient **A** also has slightly depressed ST segments in I and aVL. Patient **B** has prominent ST-segment depression in leads II, III, and aVF. All of these leads have positive poles pointing away from the epicardium of the left ventricle, thus ST depression occurs with subendocardial ischemia.

By way of emphasis, the earlier concept is nicely shown in **Video 6.2**, which demonstrates how ischemic action potentials in the subendocardium create the ECG pattern of subendocardial ischemia.

The change in the ST segments that occurs with left-ventricular subendocardial ischemia (**Figure 7.5A**) is similar to that described in Chapter 4 for left-ventricular strain. Left-ventricular strain, however, also causes the T waves to be directed away from the left ventricle and is accompanied by the QRS changes of left-ventricular hypertrophy (**Figure 7.5B**). Therefore, a diagnostic dilemma exists when a patient with symptoms suggesting an acute coronary syndrome has a resting ECG not suggestive of left-ventricular hypertrophy but with ST depression and inverted T waves (**Figure 7.5C**). Resolution of this conundrum can be vexing, indeed.

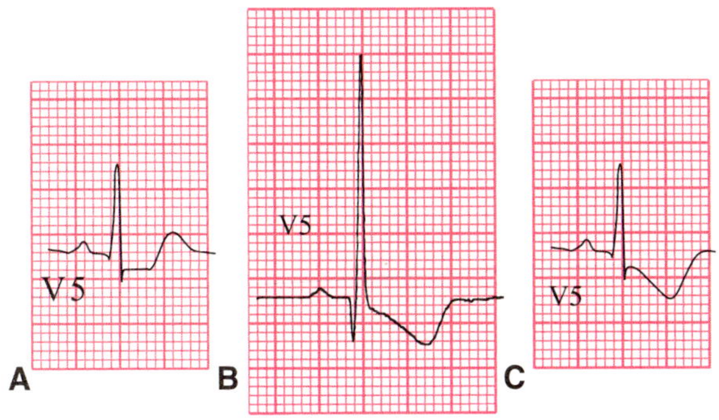

FIGURE 7.5. **A.** Horizontal ST-segment depression with upright T wave consistent with subendocardial ischemia. **B.** Left-ventricular strain causing ST-segment depression; however, it is accompanied by increased QRS voltage and an inverted T wave. **C.** Diagnostic dilemma (subendocardial ischemia versus left-ventricular strain) of depressed ST segment and inverted T wave but normal QRS voltage.

Atypical Subendocardial Ischemia

Deviation of the junction of the ST segment with the J point, followed by an upsloping ST segment, may also be indicative of subendocardial ischemia.[2] A 0.1- to 0.2-mV depression of the J point, followed by an upsloping ST segment that remains 0.1 mV depressed for 0.08 second[3] or by a 0.2-mV depression of the J point followed by an upsloping ST segment that remains 0.2 mV depressed for 0.08 second, may also be considered "diagnostic" of subendocardial ischemia.[4] A short-hand rule based on this observation is the "two-by-two" criteria of two small blocks below the baseline and two small blocks after the J point (80 ms), which is indicative of subendocardial ischemia even if upsloping at that point, also sometimes referred to as the "slowly upsloping rule" (**Figure 7.6**; **Table 7.1**).[3-5]

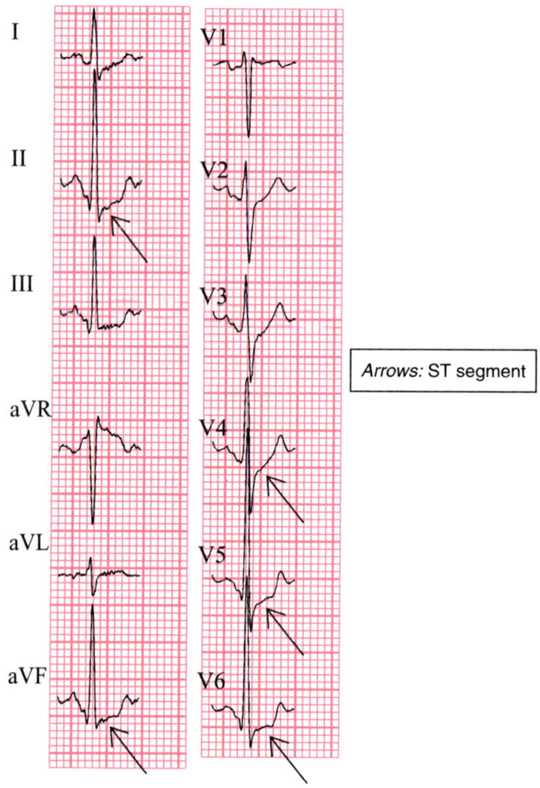

FIGURE 7.6. ST-J point depression with an upsloping ST segment (arrows) that may be indicative of subendocardial ischemia. See **Table 7.1** for proposed criteria for subendocardial ischemia.

Table 7.1.

Varying Electrocardiographic Criteria for Subendocardial Ischemia

J Point Depression (mV)	Slope	J + 0.08-s Depression
≥0.1	Flat, down	≥ same level
0.1–0.2	Up	≥0.1 mV
≥0.2	Up	≥0.2 mV

Normal Variant or Subendocardial Ischemia?

Lesser deviations of the ST segments (**Figure 7.7**) could be caused by subendocardial ischemia or could be a variation of normal. Even the ST-segment changes "diagnostic" of left-ventricular subendocardial ischemia could be an extreme variation of normal. When these lesser ECG changes appear, they should be considered in the context of other manifestations of coronary insufficiency, such as precordial pain, dyspnea, abnormal blood pressure, or cardiac arrhythmias.[1] Additional testing using cardiac imaging is typically required for definitive diagnosis or exclusion of myocardial ischemia, especially for women, a source of false-positive ECG changes otherwise indicative of subendocardial ischemia on stress testing.[6-8]

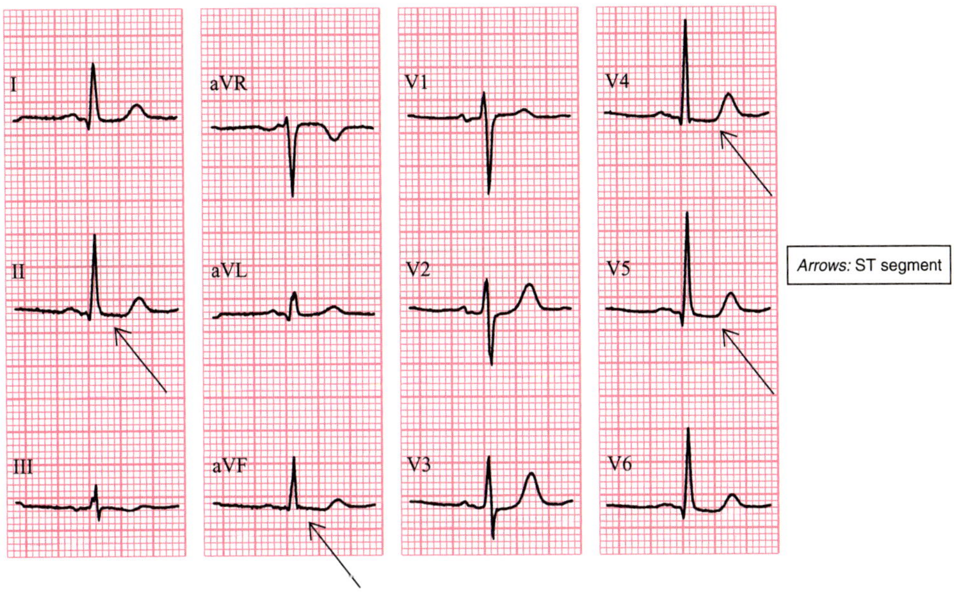

FIGURE 7.7. Twelve-lead electrocardiogram from a 69-year-old woman with severe substernal pain at rest and who was transported by ambulance to the emergency department of a hospital. Arrows indicate minimal ST-segment depression in many leads. This finding could be representative of subendocardial ischemia or could be a normal variant.

Abnormal Variants of Subendocardial Ischemia

The maximal ST-segment depression during stress tests is almost never seen in leads V_1 to V_3.[9] When these leads do exhibit the maximal ST depression in the ECG, the cause is either right-ventricular subendocardial ischemia (**Figure 7.8A**) or transmural ischemia in the lateral wall of the left ventricle due to occlusion of the left circumflex coronary artery (**Figure 7.8B**). The ST-segment depression of left-ventricular subendocardial ischemia usually resolves after several minutes following removal of the excessive cardiovascular stress. Occasionally, ST-segment depression is observed in the absence of an obvious increase in left-ventricular workload. In this case, the possibility of subendocardial infarction should be investigated.

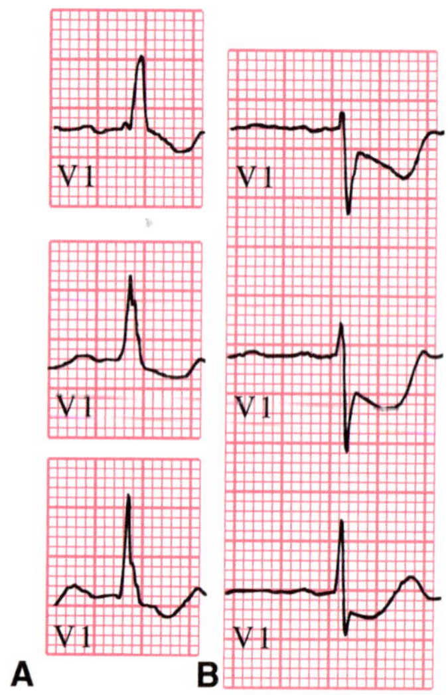

FIGURE 7.8. **A.** Electrocardiogram lead V_1 from three patients with right-ventricular subendocardial ischemia. **B.** Electrocardiogram lead V_1 from three patients with transmural ischemia in the lateral wall of the left ventricular due to occlusion of the left circumflex coronary artery.

Ischemia Monitoring

Another clinical test used in the diagnosis of subendocardial ischemia is continuous ischemia monitoring. This testing may be performed either during the activities of daily living (ambulatory monitoring) or during hospitalization (bedside monitoring). This method of continuous ischemia monitoring has been termed *Holter monitoring* after its developer and is discussed in Chapter 2. Originally, only a single ECG lead was used, but current methods provide 3 leads or even all 12 leads. The limb leads must be moved to the torso positions to avoid excessive skeletal muscle artifact (see Chapter 2).

Figure 7.9 illustrates an episode of ST-segment depression during walking, accompanied by nonsustained ventricular tachycardia (see Chapter 17). An entry to the diary kept to accompany Holter monitoring relates the cardiac event to the precipitating activity (walking) and to the symptoms perceived (slight breathlessness). Although ischemia is typically accompanied by chest pain called angina, other symptoms may be present as in this case, and these are called angina equivalents. Sometimes, ischemia may occur without any symptoms, in which case it is termed *silent ischemia*.[10,11]

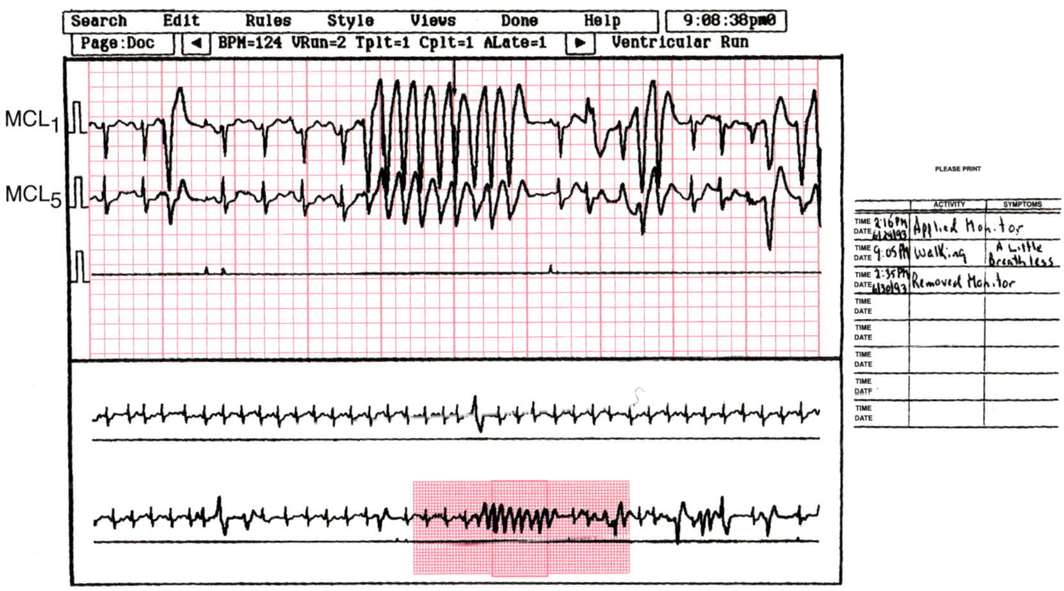

FIGURE 7.9. Modified chest lead. See text for patient's history.

CHAPTER 7 SUMMARY ILLUSTRATION

Rest | **Subendocardial Ischemia**

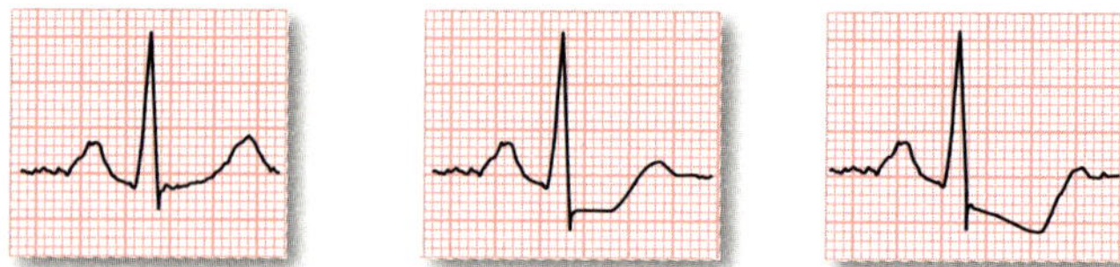

1. ST-segment depression of ≥1 mm (0.10 mV) at the J point.
2. Either a horizontal or a downward slope toward the end of the ST segment at its junction with the T wave.

Rest | **Exercise** | **Post-exercise**

Arrows: ST segment

ST-J point depression with upward sloping ST segments is a benign normal variation during exercise

Typical subendocardial ischemia: Horizontal ST-segment depression in leads V5 and V6

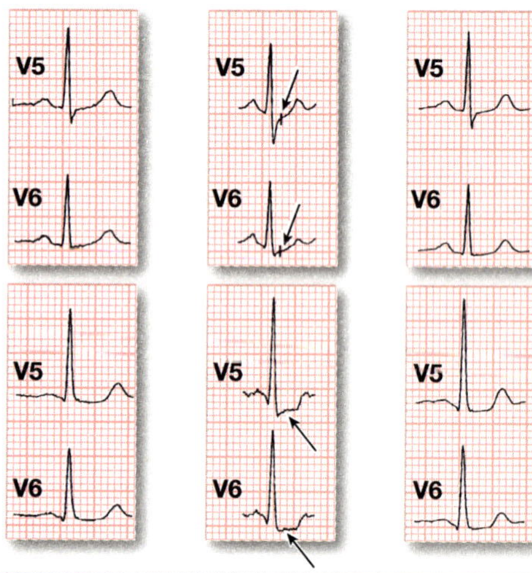

Patient A | **Patient B**

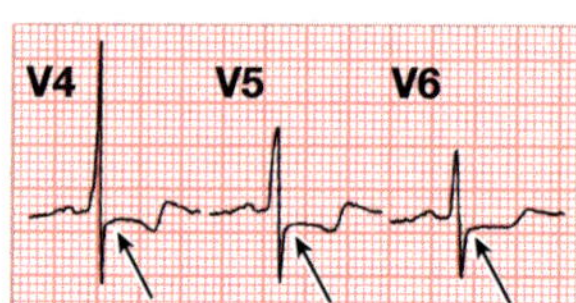

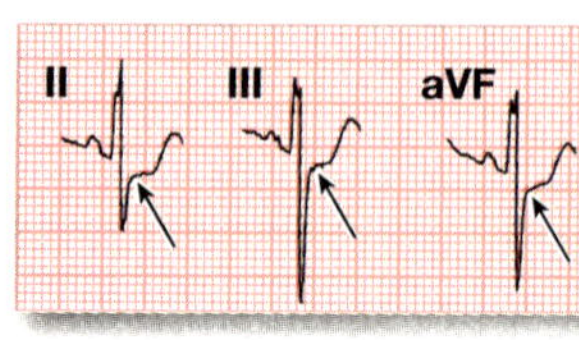

Subendocardial ischemia presents as ST-segment depression, typically in V4-V6 or in II, III, aVF

Arrows: ST segment

Subendocardial Ischemia vs. Left Ventricular Hypertrophy

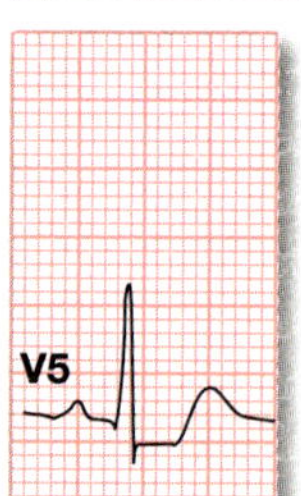

Typical subendocardial ischemia: horizontal ST-segment depression

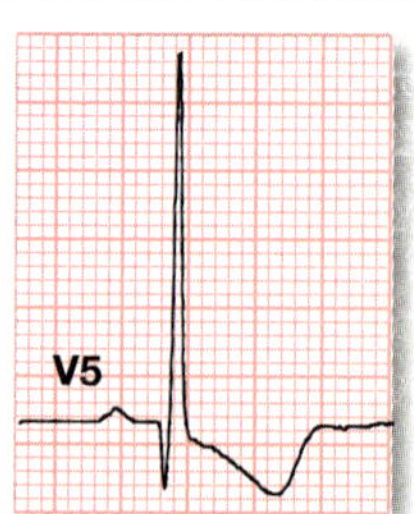

Typical Left ventricular hypertrophy with strain: increased QRS voltage, downward sloping ST segment and inverted T wave

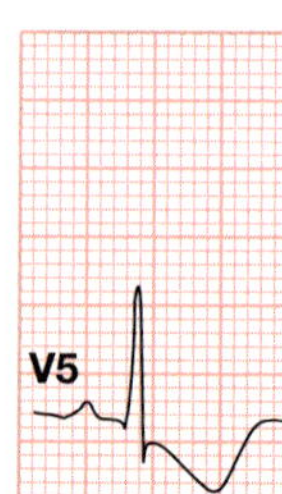

Diagnostic dilemma: subendocardial ischemia versus left ventricular strain

Glossary

Holter monitoring: continuous ECG recording of one or more leads, either for the detection of abnormalities of morphology suggestive of ischemia or abnormalities of rhythm.

Silent ischemia: evidence of myocardial ischemia appearing on an ECG recording in the absence of any awareness of symptoms of ischemia.

Stress testing: cardiovascular testing under conditions other than the resting state using exercise, mental stress, drugs to mimic exercise, drugs that alter coronary vasodilation, or even artificial cardiac pacemakers to simulate one aspect of the stress of exercise by increasing heart rate. Before, during, and after the stress, multiple variables are observed including symptoms, vital signs, rhythm, ECG waveforms, and intervals, especially ST segments and T waves. The utility of stress testing can be expanded greatly by addition of imaging to the variables under examination. Imaging can take on many forms, including echocardiography, nuclear imaging, positron emission tomography scanning, and cardiac magnetic resonance imaging.

Subendocardial ischemia: a condition marked by deviation of the ST segments of an ECG away from the ventricle (always the left ventricle) and in which only the inner part of the myocardium is ischemic.

Ventricular strain: deviation of the ST segments and T waves of an ECG away from the ventricle in which there is either a severe systolic overload or marked hypertrophy.

Acknowledgment

We gratefully acknowledge the past contributions of the previous edition's author, Dr. Galen S. Wagner, as portions of that chapter were retained in this revision.

References

1. Thomas GS, Wann LS, Ellestad MH. *Ellestad's Stress Testing: Principles and Practice*. 6th ed. New York, NY: Oxford University Press; 2018.
2. Ryik TM, O'Connor FC, Gittings NS, Wright JG, Khan AA, Fleg JL. Role of nondiagnostic exercise-induced ST-segment abnormalities in predicting future coronary events in asymptomatic volunteers. *Circulation*. 2002;106:2787-2792.
3. Sansoy V, Watson DD, Beller GA. Significance of slow upsloping ST-segment depression on exercise stress testing. *Am J Cardiol*. 1997;79:709-712.
4. Rijneke RD, Ascoop CA, Talmon JL. Clinical significance of upsloping ST segments in exercise electrocardiography. *Circulation*. 1980;61:671-678.
5. Kurita A, Chaitman BR, Bourassa MG. Significance of exercise-induced junctional S-T depression in evaluation of coronary artery disease. *Am J Cardiol*. 1977;40:492-497.
6. Ellestad MH, Savitz S, Bergdall D, Teske J. The false positive stress test. Multivariate analysis of 215 subjects with hemodynamic, angiographic and clinical data. *Am J Cardiol*. 1977;40:681-685.
7. Kohli P, Gulati M. Exercise stress testing in women: going back to the basics. *Circulation*. 2010;122:2570-2580.
8. Fitzgerald BT, Scalia WM, Scalia GM. Female false positive exercise stress ECG testing—fact versus fiction. *Heart Lung Circ*. 2019;28:735-741.
9. Shah A, Wagner GS, Green CL, et al. Electrocardiographic differentiation of the ST-segment depression of acute myocardial injury due to the left circumflex artery occlusion from that of myocardial ischemia of nonocclusive etiologies. *Am J Cardiol*. 1997;80:512-513.
10. Cohn PF, Fox KM, Daly C. Silent myocardial ischemia. *Circulation*. 2003;108:1263-1277.
11. Krucoff MW, Pope JE, Bottner RK, et al. Dedicated ST-segment monitoring in the CCU after successful coronary angioplasty: incidence and prognosis of silent and symptomatic ischemia. In: van Armin T, Maseri A, eds. *Silent Ischemia: Current Concepts and Management*. Darmstadt, Germany: Steinkopff Verlag; 1987:140-146.

8 Transmural Myocardial Ischemia From Insufficient Blood Supply

DAVID G. STRAUSS, TOBIN H. LIM,
MURALIDHARAN T R, AND
PREETAM KRISHNAMURTHY

Changes in the ST Segment

Just as changes in the ST segment of the electrocardiogram (ECG) are reliable indicators of subendocardial ischemia (caused by increased myocardial demand), they are also reliable indicators of transmural myocardial ischemia from insufficient coronary blood flow. Observation of the position of the ST segments (relative to the PR and TP segments) in a patient experiencing acute precordial pain provides clinical evidence of the presence or absence of severe transmural myocardial ischemia that typically progresses to myocardial infarction. However, many normal individuals show ST-segment elevation on their routine standard ECGs in the absence of ischemia (**Figure 8.1**).[1-3]

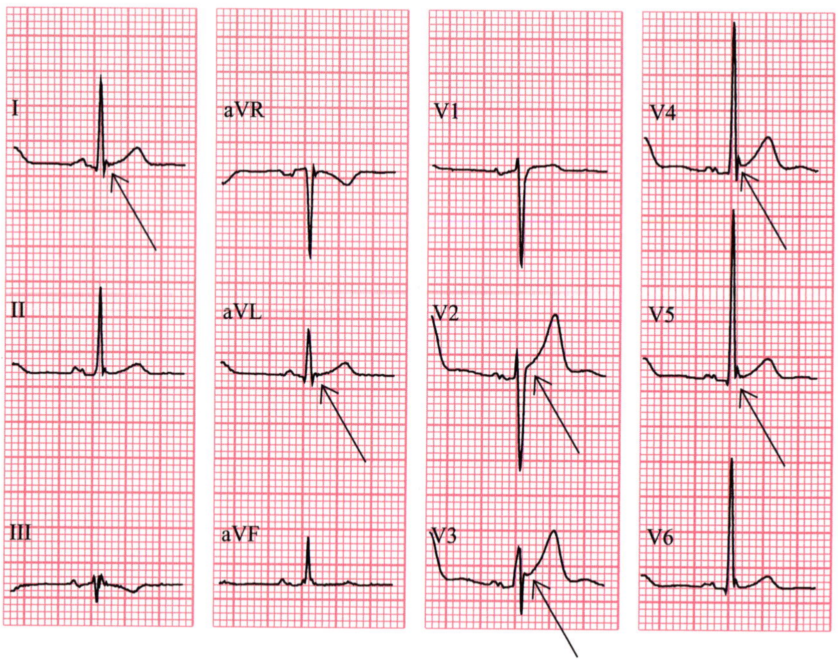

FIGURE 8.1. A 12-lead electrocardiogram (ECG) from a 34-year-old man presenting for the fourth time within a year to an emergency room with severe chest pain. The patient had no other signs of ischemia, and his ECG did not change from visit to visit. Individuals without ischemia can have ST elevation on routine standard ECGs. Arrows indicate ST-segment elevation in many leads.

When a sudden, complete occlusion of a coronary artery prevents blood flow from reaching an area of myocardium, the resulting transmural myocardial ischemia[4-6] is manifested by deviation of the ST segment toward the involved region. This ST-segment elevation is shown in the ECG of a patient before, during, and after receiving brief therapeutic balloon occlusion with percutaneous transluminal coronary angioplasty (**Figure 8.2A-C**). The ST-segment changes typically disappear abruptly when coronary blood flow is restored by deflating the angioplasty balloon after a brief period. This return to baseline after occlusion is relieved indicates that the myocardial cells have been reversibly ischemic and have not actually become infarcted.

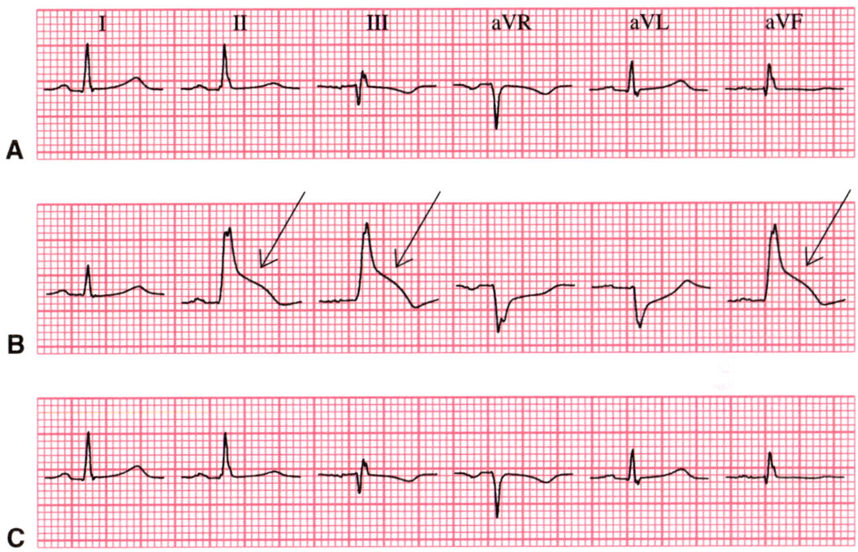

FIGURE 8.2. The six limb leads of the electrocardiogram recorded serially from a 58-year-old man with chest pain on exertion caused by a 90% obstruction of the right coronary artery. Electrocardiograms before (**A**), during (**B**), and after (**C**) 2 minutes of angioplasty balloon occlusion. Arrows, ST-segment elevation in leads II, III, and aVF that move toward the involved myocardial region during transmural myocardial ischemia.

It may be difficult to differentiate the abnormal changes in the ST segment produced by transmural myocardial ischemia from variations of normal, particularly when the deviation of the ST segment is minimal. Presence of one of the following criteria is typically required for the diagnosis of transmural myocardial ischemia[7]:

Electrocardiogram Criteria for Diagnosis of Transmural Myocardial Ischemia

1. Elevation of the origin of the ST segment at its junction (J point) with the QRS complex in two or more leads of
   - 0.1 mV (1 mm) in any lead except for leads V_2 and V_3
   - In leads V_2 and V_3, ST-J elevation should be
     a. 0.25 mV (2.5 mm) in men less than 40 years of age
     b. 0.20 mV (2.0 mm) in men 40 years of age or older
     c. 0.15 mV (1.5 mm) in women of any age
2. Depression of the origin of the ST segment at the J point of 0.10 mV (1 mm) in two or more of leads V_1 to V_3

A greater threshold is required for ST-segment elevation in leads V_2 to V_3 because a normal, slight elevation of the ST segment is often present (see **Figure 3.12**). In addition, younger men are most likely to have "normal" ST elevation in leads V_2 to V_3, which is the reason for different thresholds by age and gender.

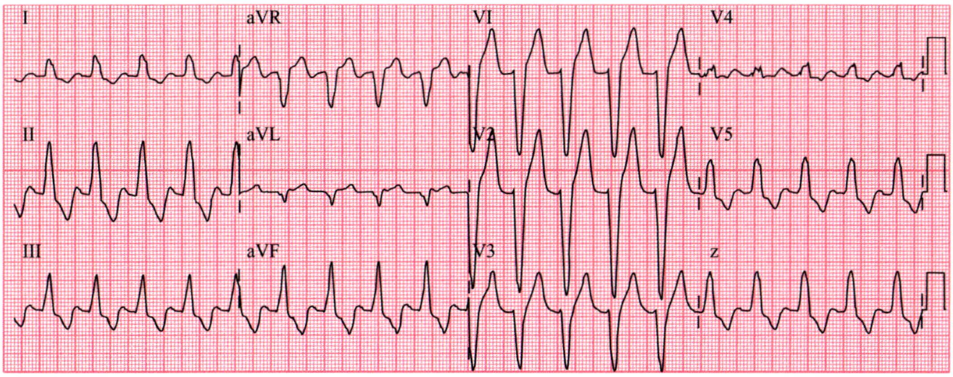

FIGURE 8.3. A 12-lead electrocardiogram of a patient with left-bundle-branch block. ST-segment elevation in leads V_1 to V_3 is normal in LBBB and should exceed 5 mm (0.5 mV) in order to be diagnostic of acute transmural myocardial ischemia. See **Table 8.1** for a complete description of criteria to diagnose acute transmural myocardial ischemia in the presence of left-bundle-branch block. From Sgarbossa et al.[8]

When the amplitude and duration of the terminal S wave is further increased in leads V_1 to V_3 as a result of left-ventricular dilation (see **Figure 4.6**) or left-bundle-branch block (**Figure 8.3**), an even greater "normal" elevation of the ST segment is typically present. A study has shown that elevation of the ST segment to ≥0.5 mV is required in leads V_1 to V_3 to diagnose acute anterior transmural myocardial ischemia in the presence of left-bundle-branch block.[8] This and other electrocardiographic criteria are presented in **Table 8.1**. However, the 0.1-mV threshold remains applicable for diagnosis of acute transmural ischemia when the deviation of the ST segment is in the same direction (concordant with) as that of the terminal QRS waveform.

Table 8.1.

Electrocardiographic Criteria of Acute Myocardial Infarction in the Presence of Left-Bundle-Branch Block[a]

Criteria
• ST-segment elevation ≥1 mm and concordant with a predominantly negative QRS complex
• ST-segment depression ≥1 mm in leads V_1, V_2, or V_3
• ST-segment elevation ≥5 mm and discordant with a predominantly negative QRS complex

[a]From Sgarbossa et al.[8]

Various positions along the ST segment are sometimes selected for measuring the amount of deviation from the horizontal PR-TP baseline. Measurement of ST-segment deviation is useful for establishing the diagnosis of transmural myocardial ischemia or for estimating its extent. "J" and "J + 0.08 second" have been used in some clinical situations (**Figure 8.4**). The deviated ST segment may be horizontal (**Figure 8.4A**), downsloping (**Figure 8.4B**), or upsloping (**Figure 8.4C**). The sloping produces different amounts of deviation of the ST segment as it moves from the J point toward the T wave. Note that the J point is more elevated than the J + 0.08-second point in **Figure 8.4B**, equally elevated in **Figure 8.4A**, and less elevated in **Figure 8.4C**. The ECG criteria for ST-elevation myocardial infarction may be

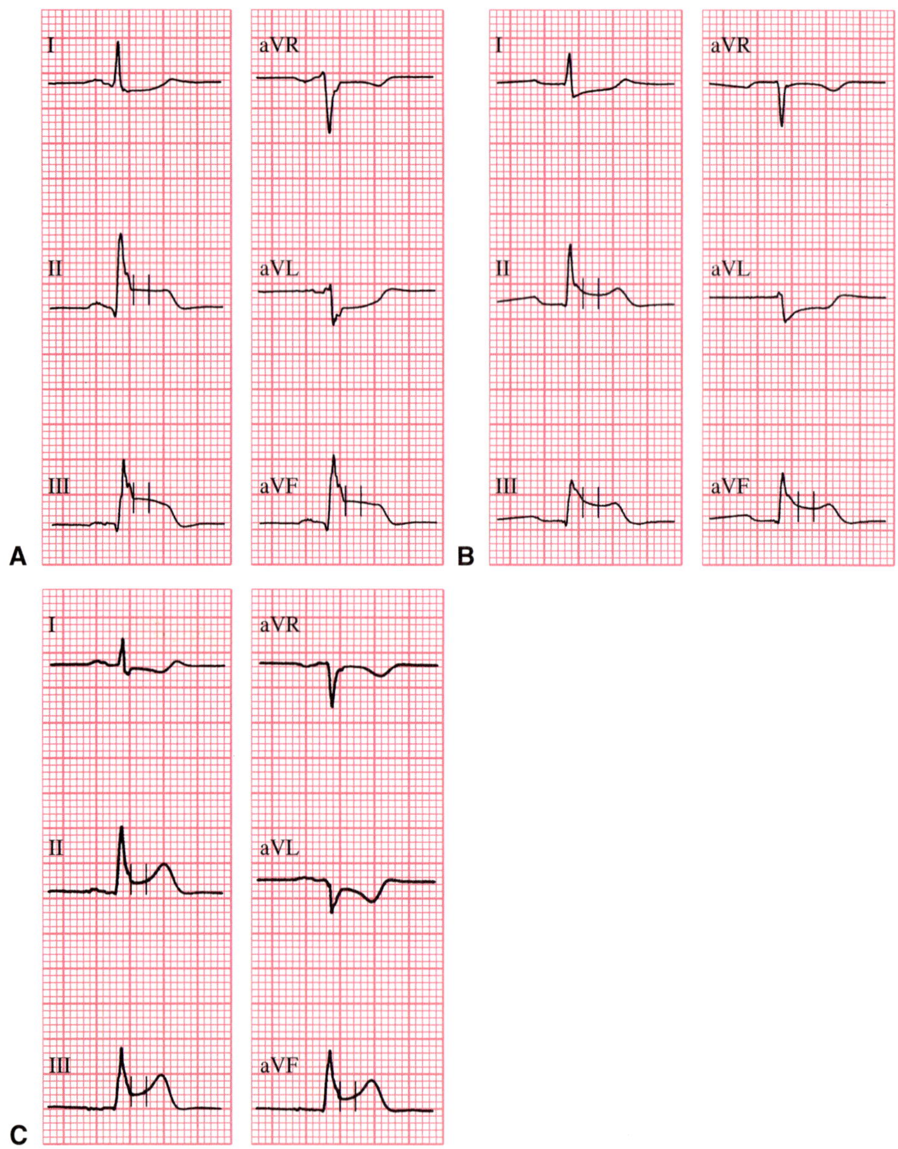

FIGURE 8.4. Variations in the appearances of the ST-segment elevation (**A**, horizontal; **B**, downsloping; and **C**, upsloping) indicative of transmural myocardial ischemia in three patients during occlusion of the right coronary artery. Vertical lines, locations of J and J + 0.08-second time points for measuring the amount of ST-segment deviation from the horizontal PR-TP baseline.

accompanied by other manifestations of insufficient myocardial perfusion, such as typical or atypical precordial pain, decreased blood pressure, cardiac arrhythmias, or other symptoms of autonomic nervous system activation such as nausea or diaphoresis.

> "The key element in confirming that inferior ischemia is present and not some other misleading reason for ST elevation [in the inferior leads] is depression of the ST segment in aVL. That is the clincher."
>
> HJL Marriott

Because the ST-segment axis in transmural myocardial ischemia deviates toward the involved area of myocardium, the changes described appear positive or elevated in leads with their positive poles pointing toward ischemic inferior (**Figure 8.5A**) or anterior (**Figure 8.5B**) aspects of the left ventricle (LV). Often, both ST-segment elevation and depression appear in different leads of a standard 12-lead ECG. Usually, the direction of greater deviation should be considered primary and the direction of lesser deviation should be considered secondary or reciprocal. When transmural myocardial ischemia involves both inferior and lateral aspects of the LV, the ST-segment depression of lateral involvement in leads V_1 to V_3 may equal or exceed the elevation produced by inferior involvement in leads II, III, and aVF.

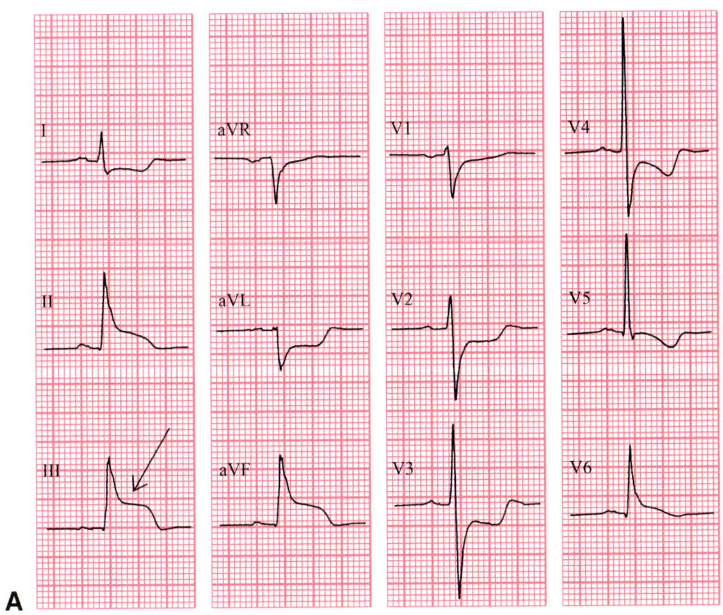

FIGURE 8.5. Twelve-lead electrocardiograms illustrating acute transmural myocardial ischemia after 1 minute of balloon occlusion in the mid–right coronary artery of a 47-year-old man with symptoms of unstable angina (**A**) and the proximal left anterior descending of a 73-year-old woman with a recent acute anterior infarction (**B**). Arrows, maximal ST-segment deviation directed toward the involved regions. *(continued)*

B

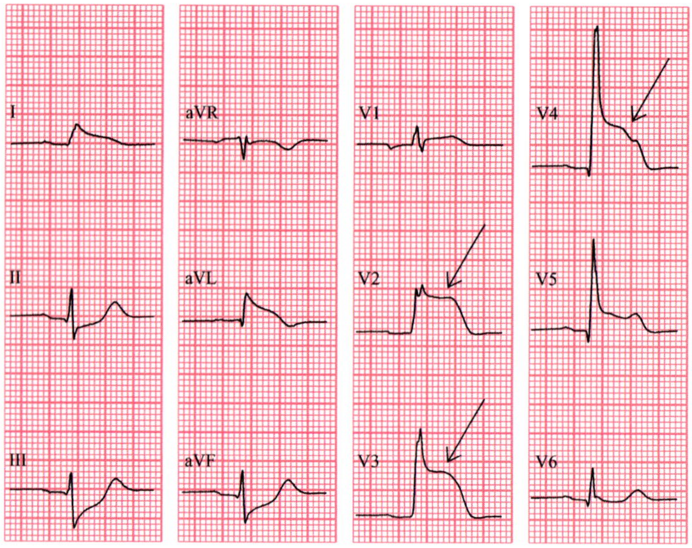

FIGURE 8.5. *(continued)*

As when considering a map of the earth, these pseudocylindrical modifications of "Mercator" views provide a planar perspective of the spatial relationships of the anatomy and pathology to the basal, middle, and apical segments of the four quadrants or "walls" of the LV in **Figure 8.6**.[9] The LV is typically divided into septal, anterior, lateral, and inferior quadrants. Distributions of the major coronary arteries (left coronary artery, left anterior descending [LAD] coronary artery, left circumflex artery [LCX], right coronary artery [RCA], and the posterior descending artery [PDA]; see **Figure 8.6**, top) are related to the distributions of insufficient blood supply resulting from occlusions of the respective arteries (see **Figure 8.6**, bottom).

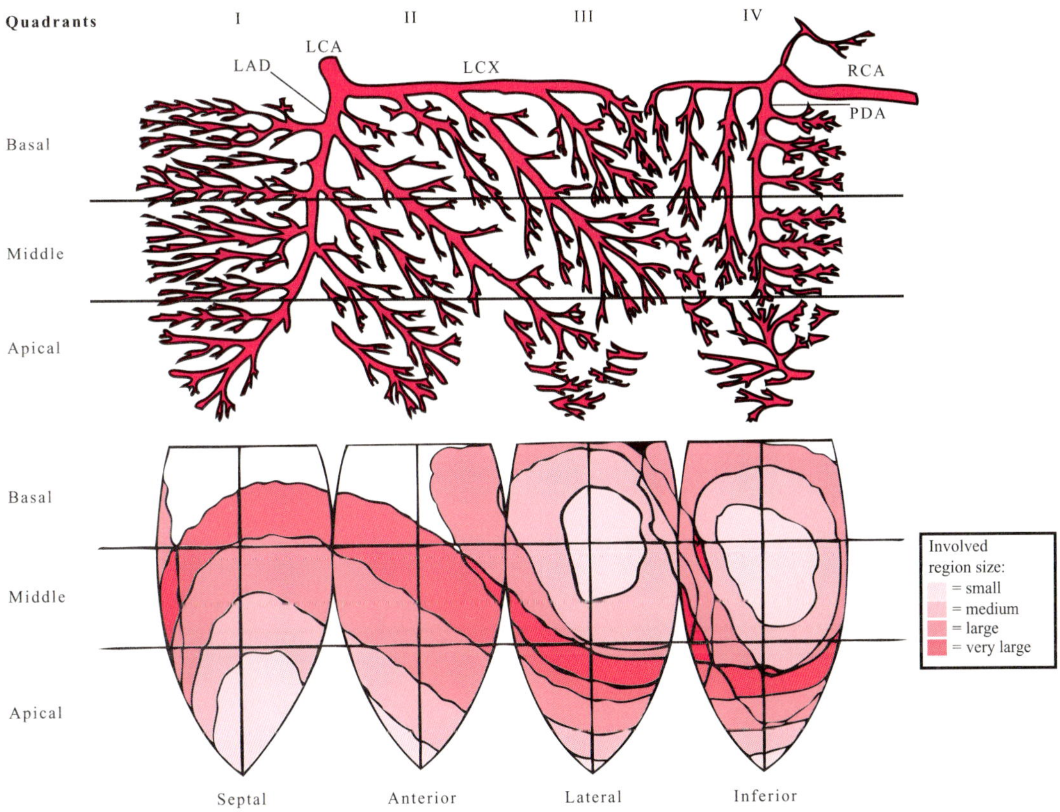

FIGURE 8.6. The 12 sections of the left ventricle myocardium defined by the four quadrants and the three levels. The distributions of the coronary arteries (left coronary artery [LCA], left anterior descending [LAD] coronary artery, left circumflex artery [LCX], right coronary artery [RCA], and posterior descending [PDA]) (top) are related to the distributions of insufficient blood supply resulting from occlusion of the respective arteries (bottom). The four grades of shading from light to dark indicate the size of the involved region as small, medium, large, and very large, respectively. (Adapted from Califf RM, Mark DB, Wagner GS. *Acute Coronary Care in the Thrombolytic Era*. Chicago, IL: Year Book; 1988:20–21. Copyright © 1988 Elsevier. With permission.)

Transmural myocardial ischemia most commonly occurs in the distal aspect of the area of the left-ventricular myocardium supplied by one of the three major coronary arteries. Note that involvement of basal and middle segments of the lateral quadrant may be due to occlusion of the proximal LCX or a large (marginal) branch. The relationship between seven culprit areas in the three coronary arteries and the leads commonly with ST elevation or depression are shown in **Table 8.2**.

In about 90% of individuals, the PDA originates from the RCA, and the LCX supplies only part of a single left-ventricular quadrant. This anatomic arrangement has been termed *right coronary dominance*. In most of the other 10% of individuals with left coronary dominance, the PDA originates from the LCX, and the RCA supplies only the right ventricle.

Table 8.2.

Seven Culprit Risk Areas in the Three Coronary Arteries[a]

1. Proximal LAD
   ST elevation: V_1, $\mathbf{V_2}$, $\mathbf{V_3}$, V_4, I, aVL
   ST depression: ***aVF***, ***III***
2. Main diagonal LAD
   ST elevation: I, aVL (minimal-to-no ST elevation in V_1, V_2, V_3)
   ST depression: ***III***, ***aVF***
3. Mid-to-distal LAD
   ST elevation: V_3, $\mathbf{V_4}$, $\mathbf{V_5}$, V_6, I, ***II***, aVF
   ST depression: aVR
4. Nondominant LCX
   ST elevation: (minimal-to-no ST elevation in II, III, aVF)
   ST depression: V_1, $\mathbf{V_2}$, $\mathbf{V_3}$, V_4
5. Dominant LCX
   ST elevation: II, ***III***, ***aVF***
   ST depression: V_1, $\mathbf{V_2}$, $\mathbf{V_3}$, V_4
6. Proximal RCA
   ST elevation: II, ***III***, ***aVF***, V_4R
   ST depression: V_1, V_2, V_3
7. Distal RCA
   ST elevation: II, ***III***, ***aVF***
   ST depression: (minimal-to-no ST depression in V_1, V_2, V_3)

Abbreviations: LAD, left anterior descending; LCX, left circumflex artery; RCA, right coronary artery.

[a]Bold/italics indicate usual leads with maximal deviation.

The basal and middle sectors of the lateral quadrant of the LV are typically supplied by the LCX. The LCX branches are located distant from the positive poles of all 12 of the standard ECG leads. Therefore, occlusion of the LCX is typically indicated by anterior ST-segment depression rather than elevation (**Figure 8.7**). Note that no ST-segment elevation is present in any standard lead. Consideration of the mirror-lake image obtained by viewing the recording upside down and backward, or placement of additional leads on the posterior-lateral thorax would be required to visualize ST-segment elevation due to transmural myocardial ischemia in this area.[10]

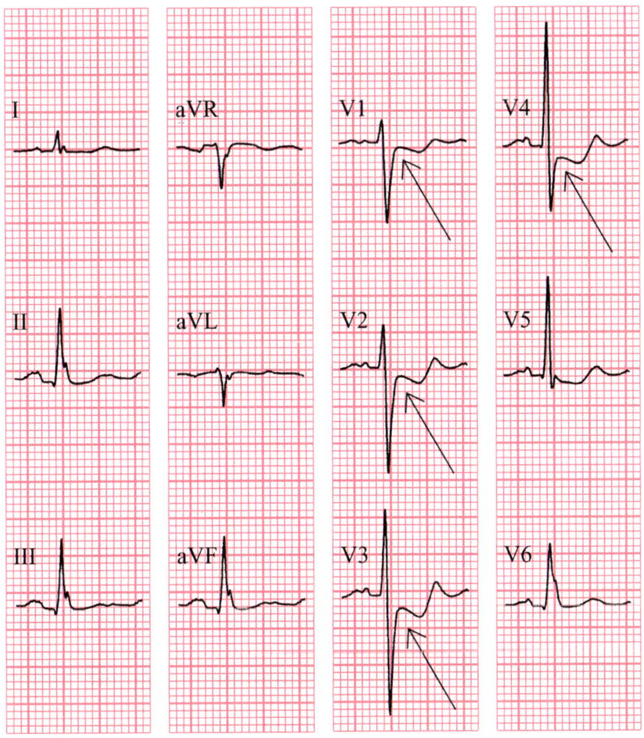

FIGURE 8.7. A 12-lead electrocardiogram recorded after 1 minute of balloon occlusion in the mid–left circumflex artery of a 54-year-old man with symptoms of acute unstable angina. Arrows indicate ST-segment depression in leads V_1 to V_4 from transmural myocardial ischemia in the lateral wall of the left ventricle.

Transmural myocardial ischemia may also involve the thinner walled right-ventricular myocardium when its blood supply via the RCA becomes insufficient. Right-ventricular transmural myocardial ischemia is represented on the standard ECG as ST-segment elevation in lead V_1 greater than V_2 (**Figure 8.8**). There would be even greater ST elevation present in the more rightward additional leads V_3R and V_4R than in lead V_1, which can also be considered lead V_2R.

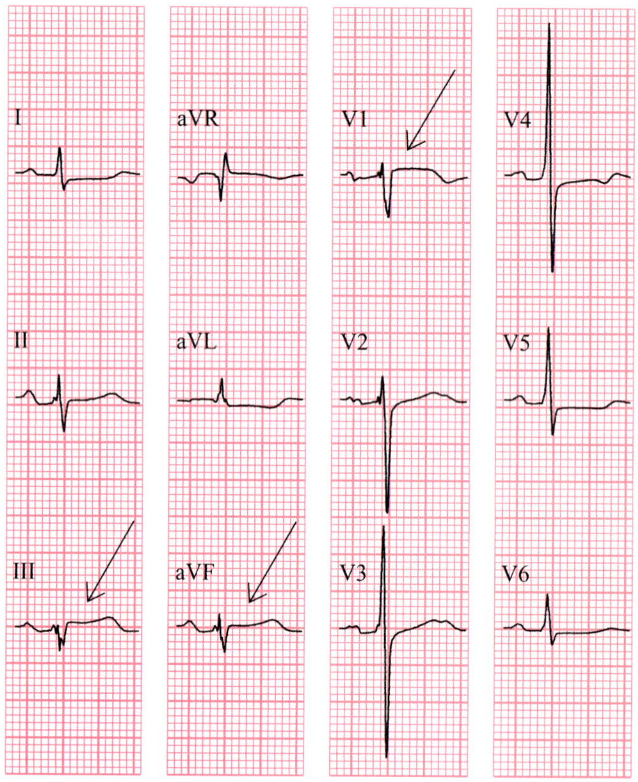

FIGURE 8.8. A 12-lead electrocardiogram after 1 minute of balloon occlusion in the proximal right coronary artery in a 65-year-old woman presenting with acute precordial pain of sudden onset. Arrows indicate the transmural myocardial ischemia appearing as ST-segment elevation in leads III and aVF and transmural myocardial ischemia in the right ventricle appearing as ST-segment elevation in lead V_1.

When ST elevation is confined to the lead aVR and is accompanied by diffuse ST depression in the other leads, it indicates subendocardial ischemia involving a large area of the heart. This is typically seen in critical narrowing of the left main coronary artery, though it may also be seen in narrowing of the proximal left anterior descending artery.

Changes in the T Wave

Although T waves are not typically recognized as indicators of ischemia caused by increased myocardial demand, they are reliable indicators of ischemia from insufficient coronary blood supply (see Chapter 6). **Figure 8.9** presents the changes in ST segments and T waves immediately after acute balloon occlusion of the LAD of two patients. In both examples, the ST segments and T waves deviate toward the involved anterior aspect of the LV. In some patients, the degree of deviation of the T wave is similar to that of the ST segment (**Figure 8.9A**). In other patients, there is the markedly greater deviation of the T-wave axis that is characteristic of "hyperacute" T waves (**Figure 8.9B**). These T-wave elevations typically persist only transiently after acute coronary thrombosis.[11] Hyperacute T waves may therefore be useful in timing the duration of the ischemia/infarction process when a patient presents with acute precordial pain.

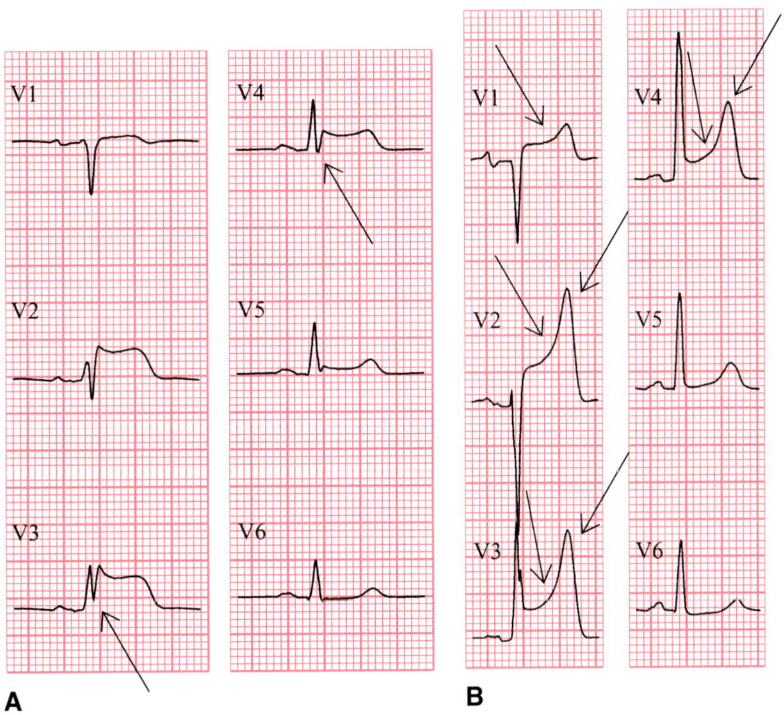

FIGURE 8.9. The six precordial leads of the electrocardiogram after 1 minute of balloon occlusion of the left anterior descending in a 74-year-old woman with a 5-year history of exertional angina (**A**) and a 51-year-old man with an initial episode of precordial pain (**B**). Arrows in **A**, disappearance of the S wave from below the TP-PR segment baseline; arrows in **B**, ST-segment elevation and hyperacute T waves.

Changes in the QRS Complex

The changes in the ST segment are the most prominent ECG manifestation of transmural myocardial ischemia, like that of subendocardial ischemia described in Chapter 7. These changes occurring due to transmural myocardial ischemia may be accompanied by deviation of the adjacent waveforms (QRS complex and T wave) in the same direction of the ST segments, as illustrated in LAD balloon inflation 2 (**Figure 8.10**). This deviation affects the amplitudes of the later QRS waveforms to a greater extent than those of the earlier QRS waveforms. This concept can be appreciated by comparing the inflation 2 and control recordings.[12] During inflation 1, the distortion of the QRS complex is much greater, indicating that there is a delayed depolarization of the ischemic zone. During the second inflation, however, there is minimal change in the QRS complex but significantly greater increase in T-wave amplitude. This phenomenon may be due to "preconditioning," where an initial sublethal ischemic episode protects the myocardium from future ischemic episodes.[13]

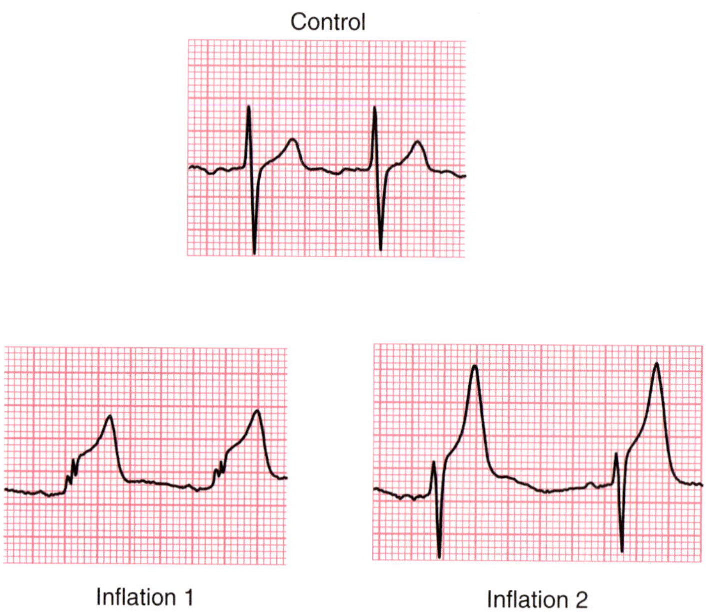

FIGURE 8.10. Recordings of two cardiac cycles in lead V_2 from baseline (control) and after 2 minutes each of two different periods of balloon occlusion of the left anterior descending. Reprinted with permission from Murry et al.[13]

The primary changes in the QRS complexes representing "tombstoning" may occur after the onset of transmural myocardial ischemia, as seen in inflation 1 of **Figures 8.10** and **8.11B**. The deviation of the QRS complex toward the area of transmural ischemia occurs because of slowed conduction (delayed depolarization) in the ischemic zone (lead V_2 of **Figure 8.11B**). The duration of the QRS complex may also be prolonged, as in the patient whose ECG is shown in the figure. Typically, acute ischemia of a higher grade of severity (grade 3) occurs during initial balloon occlusion when either collateral arteries or preconditioning provide the least protection. The ischemic zone is activated late, thereby producing an unopposed positive QRS complex waveform. With transmural myocardial ischemia in the lateral wall of the LV (typically from LCX occlusion), the QRS complex would deviate in the negative direction in leads V_1 to V_3.[14]

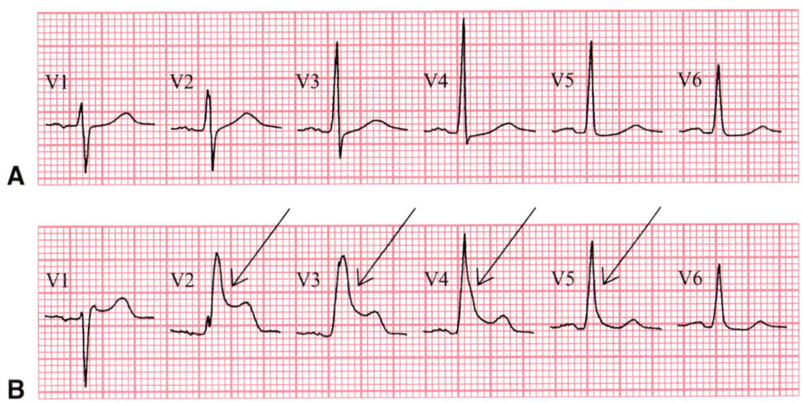

FIGURE 8.11. The six precordial leads of the electrocardiogram are presented from serial recordings from a 64-year-old man with acute unstable angina. **A.** Baseline recording prior to angiography after pain had resolved. **B.** After 2 minutes of the initial balloon occlusion of the left anterior descending. Arrows indicate the increased QRS complex duration in **B** that is apparent in leads V_2 to V_5.

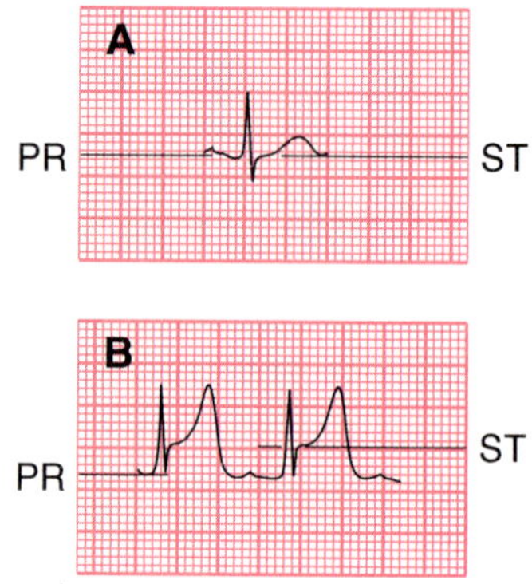

FIGURE 8.12. **A.** An electrocardiogram recording made before balloon inflation, in which the PR and ST baselines are at the same level and a 0.03-mV S wave is present. PR and ST baselines. **B.** During balloon occlusion, the ST segment is elevated by 0.03 mV by the epicardial injury current, and the S wave also deviates upward so that it just reaches the PR-segment baseline.

The deviation of the ST segments in transmural myocardial ischemia confounds measurement of the amplitudes of the QRS complex waveforms of the ECG because there are no longer isoelectric PR-ST-TP segments. As illustrated in **Figure 8.12**, the baseline of the PR segment remains as the reference for the initial waveform of the QRS complex, but with deviation of the QRS complex (**Figure 8.12B**), the terminal waveform maintains its relationship with the ST-segment baseline. The S-wave amplitude of 0.03 mV measured from the ST-segment baseline is the same in **Figure 8.12A** and **B**.

Having now learned more about the ST-segment, T-wave, and QRS-complex changes during transmural ischemia, it is recommended to return to **Video 6.1**. Video 6.1 uses the simulation program ECGSIM to make the connection between ischemic action potential changes and the characteristic ECG patterns of transmural ischemia.

Estimating Extent, Acuteness, and Severity of Ischemia

Visit lww.co.in to learn more about how to estimate the extent, acuteness, and severity of ischemia with ECG scoring systems. Instructions are noted on the inside front cover.

CHAPTER 8 SUMMARY ILLUSTRATION

Diagnosing Transmural Myocardial Ischemia

1. Elevation of the origin of the ST segment at its junction (J point) with the QRS complex in two or more leads of:
   - 0.1 mV (1 mm) in any lead except for leads V2 and V3
   - in leads V2 and V3 ST-J elevation should be:
     a. 0.25 mV (2.5 mm) in men less than 40 years of age
     b. 0.20 mV (2.0 mm) in men 40 years of age or older
     c. 0.15 mV (1.5 mm) in women of any age.
2. Depression of the origin of the ST segment at the J point of 0.10 mV (1 mm) in two or more of leads V1-V3.

Seven Culprit Risk Areas in the Three Coronary Arteries (Bold/Italics indicates usual leads with maximal deviation)

1. Proximal LAD
ST elevation: V1, ***V2***, ***V3***, V4, I, aVL
ST depression: ***aVF***, ***III***

2. Main diagonal LAD
ST elevation: I, aVL (minimal-to-no ST elevation in V1, V2, V3)
ST depression: ***III***, ***aVF***

3. Mid-to-distal LAD
ST elevation: V3, ***V4***, ***V5***, V6, I, ***II***, aVF
ST depression: aVR

Proximal LAD

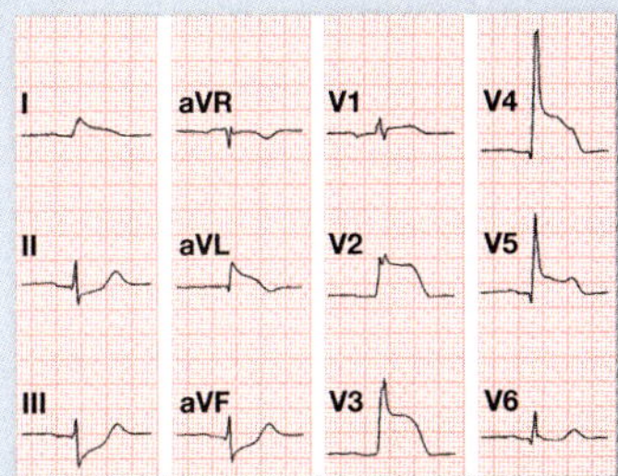

4. Nondominant LCX
ST elevation: (minimal-to-no ST elevation in II, III, aVF)
ST depression: V1, ***V2***, ***V3***, V4

5. Dominant LCX
ST elevation: II, ***III***, ***aVF***
ST depression: V1, ***V2***, ***V3***, V4

Dominant LCX

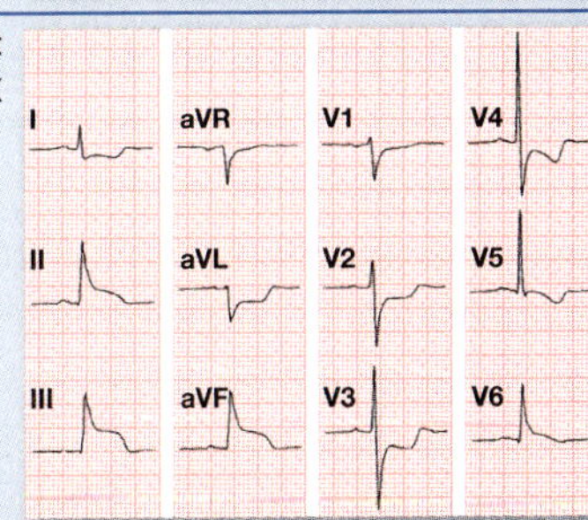

6. Proximal RCA
ST elevation: II, ***III***, ***aVF***, V4R
ST depression: V1, V2, V3

7. Distal RCA
ST elevation: II, ***III***, ***aVF***
ST depression: (minimal-to-no ST depression in V1, V2, V3)

Proximal RCA

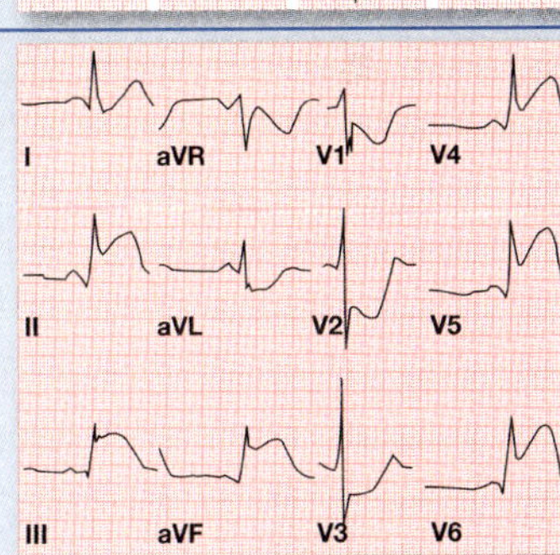

Electrocardiographic Criteria of Acute Myocardial Infarction in the Presence of Left-Bundle-Branch Block

Criteria

- ST-segment elevation ≥1 mm and concordant
- with a predominantly negative QRS complex.
- ST-segment depression ≥1 mm in
- leads V1, V2, or V3.
- ST-segment elevation ≥5 mm and discordant
- with a predominantly negative QRS complex.

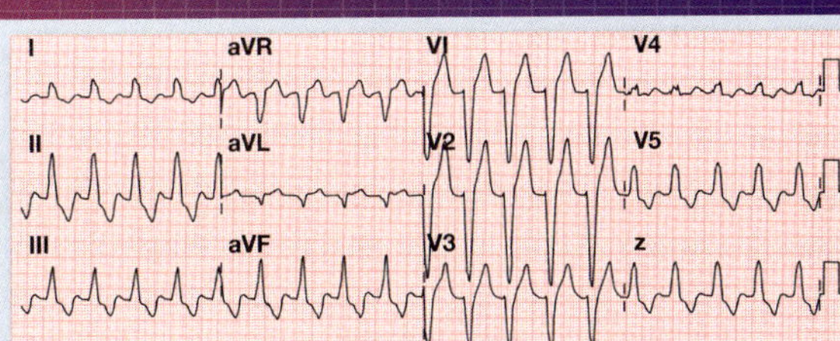

Abbreviations: LAD, left anterior descending; LCX, left circumflex artery; RCA, right coronary artery.

Glossary

Left coronary dominance: less common coronary artery anatomy (10%) in which the PDA is a branch of the LCX.

Reciprocal: a term referring to deviation of the ST segments in the opposite direction from that of their maximal deviation.

Right coronary dominance: the usual coronary artery anatomy in which the PDA is a branch of the RCA.

Acknowledgment

We gratefully acknowledge the past contributions of the previous edition's author, Dr. Galen S. Wagner, as portions of that chapter were retained in this revision.

References

1. Prinzmetal M, Goldman A, Massumi RA, et al. Clinical implications of errors in electrocardiographic interpretation; heart disease of electrocardiographic origin. *J Am Med Assoc*. 1956;161:138-143.
2. Levine HD. Non-specificity of the electrocardiogram associated with coronary artery disease. *Am J Med*. 1953;15:344-355.
3. Marriott HJ. Coronary mimicry: normal variants, and physiologic, pharmacologic and pathologic influences that simulate coronary patterns in the electrocardiogram. *Ann Intern Med*. 1960;52:413-427.
4. Vincent GM, Abildskov JA, Burgess MJ. Mechanisms of ischemic ST-segment displacement. Evaluation by direct current recordings. *Circulation*. 1977;56(4 pt 1):559-566.
5. Kléber AG, Janse MJ, van Capelle FJ, Durrer D. Mechanism and time course of S-T and T-Q segment changes during acute regional myocardial ischemia in the pig heart determined by extracellular and intracellular recordings. *Circ Res*. 1978;42:603-613.
6. Janse MJ, Cinca J, Moréna H, et al. The "border zone" in myocardial ischemia. An electrophysiological, metabolic, and histochemical correlation in the pig heart. *Circ Res*. 1979;44:576-588.
7. Wagner GS, Macfarlane P, Wellens H, et al. AHA/ACCF/HRS recommendations for the standardization and interpretation of the electrocardiogram: part VI: acute ischemia/infarction: a scientific statement from the American Heart Association Electrocardiography and Arrhythmias Committee, Council on Clinical Cardiology; the American College of Cardiology Foundation; and the Heart Rhythm Society. Endorsed by the International Society for Computerized Electrocardiology. *J Am Coll Cardiol*. 2009;53:1003-1011.
8. Sgarbossa EB, Pinski SL, Barbagelata A, et al. Electrocardiographic diagnosis of evolving acute myocardial infarction in the presence of left bundle-branch block. GUSTO-1 (Global Utilization of Streptokinase and Tissue Plasminogen Activator for Occluded Coronary Arteries) Investigators. *N Engl J Med*. 1996;334:481-487.
9. Wagner N, Wagner G, White R. The twelve-lead ECG and the extent of myocardium at risk of acute infarction: cardiac anatomy and lead locations, and the phases of serial changes during acute occlusion. In: Califf RM, Mark DB, Wagner GS, eds. *Acute Coronary Care in the Thrombolytic Era*. Chicago, IL: Year Book; 1988:31-45.
10. Seatre H, Selvester R, Solomon J, Baron KA, Ahmad J, Ellestad ME. 16-lead ECG changes with coronary angioplasty. Location of ST-T changes with balloon occlusion of five arterial perfusion beds. *J Electrocardiol*. 1992;24(suppl):153-162.
11. Dressler W, Roesler H. High T waves in the earliest stage of myocardial infarction. *Am Heart J*. 1947;34:627-645.
12. Wagner NB, Sevilla DC, Krucoff MW, et al. Transient alterations of the QRS complex and ST segment during percutaneous transluminal balloon angioplasty of the left anterior descending coronary artery. *Am J Cardiol*. 1988;62:1038-1042.
13. Murry CE, Jennings RB, Reimer KA. Preconditioning with ischemia: a delay of lethal cell injury in ischemic myocardium. *Circulation*. 1986;74:1124-1136.
14. Selvester RH, Wagner NB, Wagner GS. Ventricular excitation during percutaneous transluminal angioplasty of the left anterior descending coronary artery. *Am J Cardiol*. 1988;62:1116-1121.

To view digital content associated with this chapter please access lww.co.in. Instructions are located on the inside front cover.

9

Myocardial Infarction

DAVID G. STRAUSS, TOBIN H. LIM,
AND ANANDARAJA SUBRAMANIAN

Infarcting Phase

Transition From Ischemia to Infarction

When insufficient coronary blood supply persists after myocardial energy reserves have been depleted, the myocardial cells become irreversibly ischemic and the process of *necrosis* termed myocardial infarction (MI) occurs. The QRS complex is the most useful aspect of the electrocardiogram (ECG) for evaluating the presence, location, and extent of MI, which is discussed in detail in this chapter.

The online supplement to Chapter 8 discusses the transition from acute myocardial ischemia to cellular necrosis (infarction) and how ECG scores can be used to estimate the extent,[1] severity,[2] and acuteness[3] of ischemia. The Anderson-Wilkins acuteness score (see also Chapter 8 Online Supplement, **eTable 8.1**, **eFigure 8.2**) can estimate where in the process from acute ischemia to completed infarction a particular patient is. A key message is that during acute transmural ischemia, the electrical vector (axis) of the QRS complex, ST segment, and T wave all point toward the ischemic region. In other words, in ECG leads above the ischemic region, S waves disappear and/or R waves increase; ST-segment elevation develops (Pardee's sign); and T waves increase in amplitude. As the process of ischemia transitions to infarction, T waves decrease in amplitude (later becoming negative); Q waves develop; and ST segments decrease in amplitude.

In the world of cardiology, much has been made of the distinction between ST-segment elevation MI and MI without ST elevation. These distinctions are important for the urgency of evaluation and kinds of intervention used in most cases. ST elevation continues to serve as a major indicator of the need for prompt restoration of coronary blood flow to the ischemic area. Therefore, much of the material in this book addressing MI will concern ST segments and their appearance. All of this having been said, providers treat patients, and ECGs must always be interpreted in their clinical context.

Resolving ST-Segment Deviation: Toward the Infarct

The changes in the ST segment that are prominent during transmural myocardial ischemia typically disappear when the jeopardized myocardium either infarcts or is salvaged. The time course of resolution of the injury current is accelerated by therapeutic reperfusion via the culprit artery (see Chapter 8).[4] Schröder and coworkers[5] identified the threshold of ≥70% reduction in ST-segment elevation in the maximally involved lead as indicative of successful reperfusion.

When reelevation of the ST segments is observed, further myocardial ischemia is suggested (**Figure 9.1**). The reperfusing phase may be complicated by infarction of the myocardium in the periphery of the initially ischemic area. The initially occluding thrombus may embolize downstream to interfere with salvage that would have been attained via *collateral blood supply*.

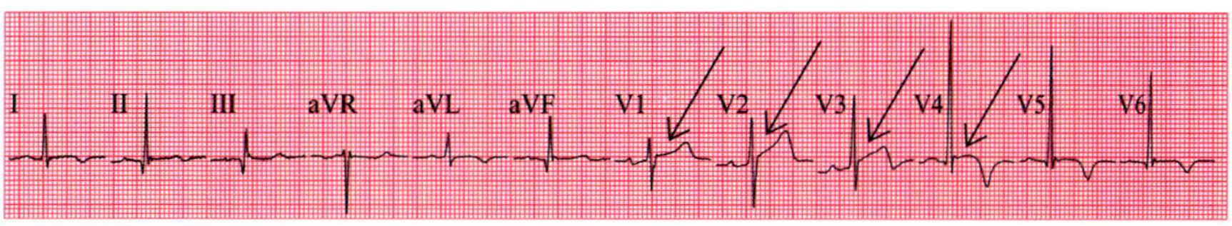

FIGURE 9.1. A 12-lead electrocardiogram from a 68-year-old man 4 days after thrombolytic therapy for an acute infarction. Acute chest pain has returned and new ST-segment elevation is apparent. Arrows, ST-segment elevation in multiple leads.

In some patients, the ST-segment elevation does not completely resolve and T-wave inversion fails to occur during the reperfusing phase of an MI (**Figure 9.2**). This condition more commonly occurs with anterior infarcts than with those in the other locations in the left ventricle (LV).[6] The lack of ST-segment resolution has been associated acutely with failure to reperfuse and chronically with thinning of the left-ventricular wall caused by *infarct expansion*.[7,8] The most extreme manifestation of infarct expansion is the development of a *ventricular aneurysm*, but ventricular aneurysm formation is very often prevented by successful reperfusion therapy.

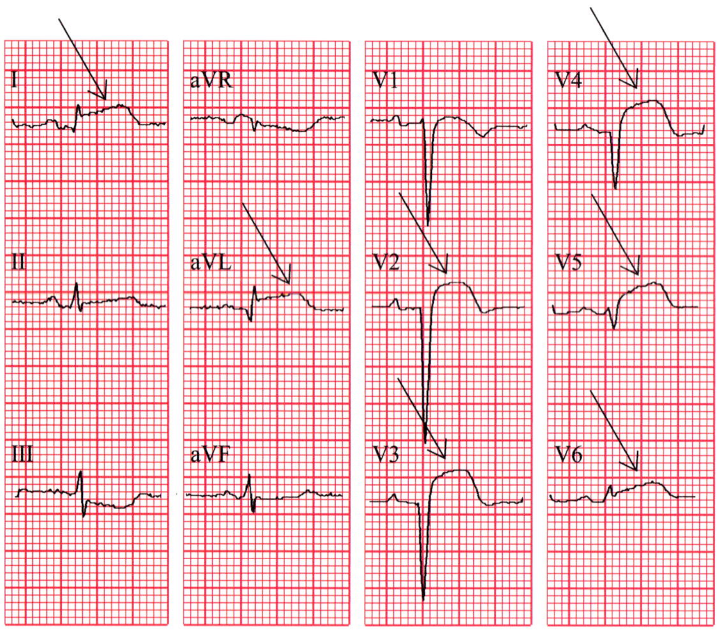

FIGURE 9.2. A 12-lead electrocardiogram obtained 2 weeks after an acute left anterior descending occlusion leading to an extensive anteroseptal infarction. Arrows, indicate persistent ST-segment elevation without evolution of T-wave inversion.

T-wave Migration: Toward to Away From the Infarct

The movement of the T waves toward the involved region of the LV also resolves as the jeopardized myocardium either recovers or infarcts. Unlike the ST segment, however, T waves do not typically return only to their original positions. The T waves typically migrate past the isoelectric baseline until they are directed away from the involved region.[9] They assume an appearance identical to that described in Chapter 6 as postischemic T waves, indicating that there is no ongoing myocardial ischemia. This evolution of the T wave is illustrated in serial ECGs at 3 and 7 days after *anterior infarction* (**Figure 9.3A,B**). Typically, the terminal portion of the T wave is the first to become inverted, followed by the middle and initial portions.

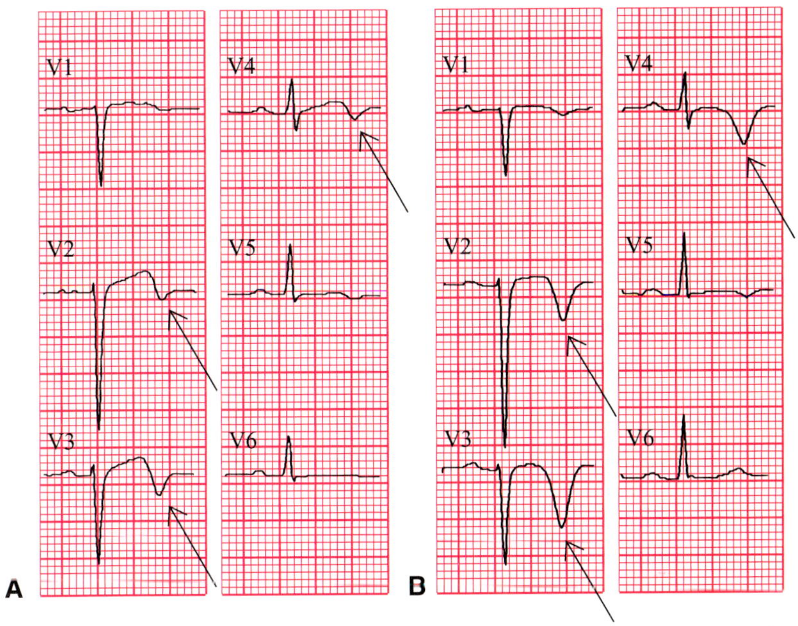

FIGURE 9.3. Serial 12-lead electrocardiograms from a 64-year-old woman at 3 days (**A**) and 7 days (**B**) after an uncomplicated acute anteroseptal infarction. Arrows indicate the terminal T-wave negativity (**A**) and total T-wave negativity (**B**).

Similarly, when the lateral wall of the LV is involved, the T waves eventually become markedly positive in the leads in which the injury current was represented by ST depression. **Figure 9.4** illustrates the prominent positive T waves (arrows) with abnormal R waves in leads V_1 and V_2 that accompany the negative T waves (arrows) with abnormal Q waves in other leads (II, III, aVF, V_5, and V_6) during the healing phase of an extensive inferolateral infarction (formerly termed infero-postero-lateral infarction).

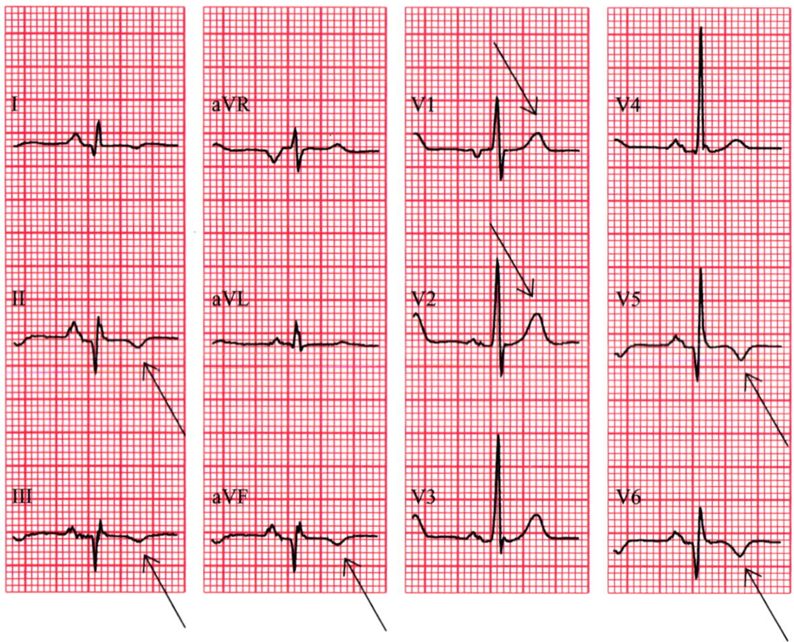

FIGURE 9.4. A 12-lead electrocardiogram from a 53-year-old man 5 days after an infarction involving the inferior and lateral walls extending to the apex. Arrows indicate negative T waves in leads with abnormal Q waves but positive T waves in leads with abnormal R waves.

Evolving QRS Complex Away From the Infarct

The QRS complex is the key waveform for evaluating the presence, location, and extent of a healing or chronic MI. As indicated in Chapter 8, almost immediately after a complete coronary artery occlusion, the QRS complex deviates toward the involved myocardial region, primarily because of delay in myocardial activation and secondarily because of the ischemia current of injury. Because the process of infarction begins in the most poorly perfused subendocardial layer of the myocardium, the deviation of the terminal QRS waveforms toward the ischemic region is replaced by deviation of the initial QRS waveforms away from the infarcted region (**Figure 9.5**).[10] Absence of any electrical activation of the infarcted myocardium has replaced the delayed activation of the severely ischemic myocardium, as illustrated in **Figure 9.5**.

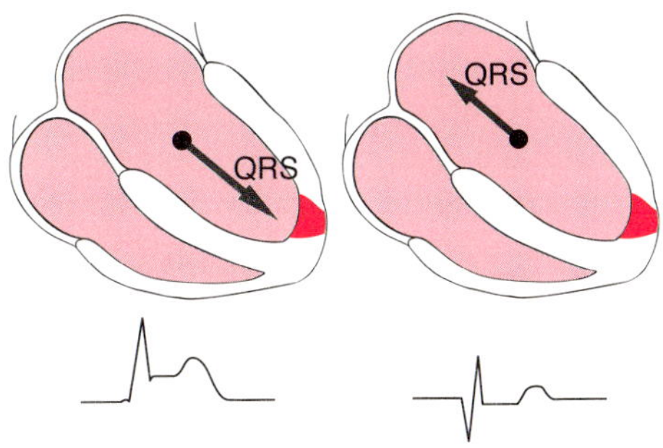

FIGURE 9.5. Schematic cross-sections.

The evolving appearance of the abnormalities of the QRS complex produced by an anterior infarction during the first few minutes of intravenous thrombolytic therapy with continuous monitoring for ischemia is shown in **Figure 9.6**. Secondary changes in the morphology of the QRS complex during transmural myocardial ischemia have shifted the axis of the complex toward the anterior left-ventricular wall. Myocardial reperfusion is accompanied by rapid resolution of the transmural myocardial ischemia and a shift of the QRS complex away from the anterior left-ventricular wall. Although it may appear that the reperfusion itself has caused the infarction, it is much more likely that the infarction occurred before initiation of the therapy that led to reperfusion and that its detection on the ECG was obscured by the secondary changes of the QRS complex caused by the ischemic injury currents.

Transmural myocardial ischemia involving the thin right-ventricular free wall may be manifested on the ECG by deviation of the ST segment (see Chapter 8), but right-ventricular infarction is not manifested by significant alteration of the QRS complex. This lack of QRS alteration is because activation of the right-ventricular free wall is insignificant in comparison with activation of the thicker interventricular septum and left-ventricular free wall. The MI evolves from transmural myocardial ischemia in the distal aspects of the left-ventricular myocardium supplied by one of the three major coronary arteries (see **Figure 8.6**).[11]

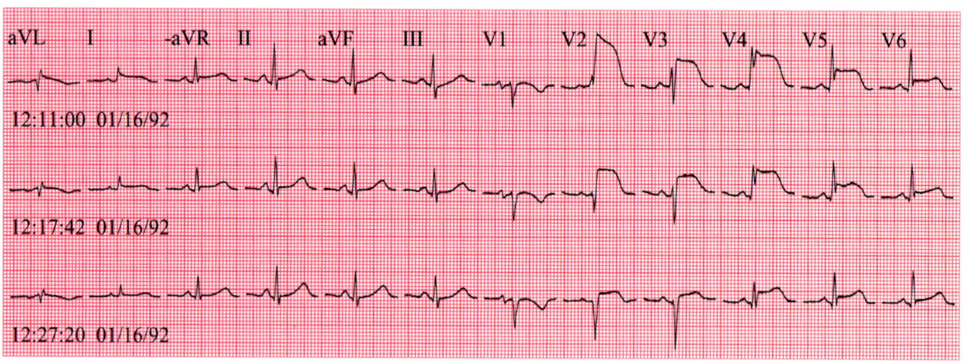

FIGURE 9.6. Continuous electrocardiogram monitoring during the first 27 minutes of intravenous thrombolytic therapy (begun at 12:00:00) in a 69-year-old man with acute thrombotic occlusion of the left anterior descending. The 12 standard leads of the electrocardiogram are presented in panoramic format after 11, 17, and 27 minutes of therapy.

Chronic Phase

QRS Complex for Diagnosing

The initial portion of the axis of the QRS complex deviates most prominently away from the area of infarction and is represented on the ECG by a prolonged Q-wave duration. As presented in **Figure 3.6**, the initial QRS waveform may normally be negative in all leads except V_1 to V_3. The presence of any Q wave is considered abnormal only in these 3 of the 12 standard ECG leads. **Table 9.1** indicates the upper limits of normal Q-wave duration in the various ECG leads.[12] The duration of the Q wave should be the primary measurement used in the definition of abnormality because the amplitudes of the individual QRS waveforms vary with the overall amplitude of the QRS complex. As discussed in the next section, Q-wave amplitude should be considered abnormal only in relation to the amplitude of the following R wave.

Table 9.1.

Abnormal Q Waves Suggesting Myocardial Infarction[a]

Limb Leads		Precordial Leads	
Lead	Criteria for Abnormal	Lead	Criteria for Abnormal
I	≥0.03 s	V_1	Any Q
II	≥0.03 s	V_2	Any Q
III	None	V_3	Any Q
aVR	None	V_4	≥0.02 s
aVL	≥0.03 s	V_5	≥0.03 s
aVF	≥0.03 s	V_6	≥0.03 s

[a]Modified with permission from Wagner et al.[12]

Many cardiac conditions other than MI are capable of producing abnormal initial QRS waveforms. As indicated in Chapters 4, 5, and 19, abnormalities that commonly prolong the duration of the Q wave are the following:

Abnormalities That Commonly Prolong the Duration of the Q Wave

1. Ventricular hypertrophy
2. Intraventricular conduction abnormalities (such as bundle branch block)
3. Ventricular preexcitation

The term Q wave as used here also refers to the Q-wave equivalent of abnormal R waves in leads V_1 and V_2. Therefore, the following steps should be considered in the evaluation of Q waves for the presence of MI:

Steps in the Evaluation of Q Waves for the Presence of Myocardial Infarction

1. Are abnormal Q waves present in any lead?
2. Are criteria present for other cardiac conditions that can produce abnormal Q waves?
3. Does the extent of Q-wave abnormality exceed that which could have been produced by some other cardiac condition?

Table 9.2.

Abnormally Small R Waves Suggesting Myocardial Infarction

Limb Leads		Precordial Leads	
Lead	Criteria for Abnormal	Lead	Criteria for Abnormal
I	R amp ≤0.20 mV	V_1	None
II	None	V_2	R dur ≤0.01 s or amp ≤0.10 mV
III	None	V_3	R dur ≤0.02 s or amp ≤0.20 mV
aVR	None	V_4	R amp ≤0.70 mV or ≤Q amp
aVL	R amp ≤Q amp	V_5	R amp ≤0.70 mV or ≤2 × Q amp
aVF	R amp ≤2 × Q amp	V_6	R amp ≤0.60 mV or ≤3 × Q amp

Abbreviations: amp, amplitude; dur, duration.

The deviation of the QRS axis away from the area of an MI may, in the absence of abnormal Q waves, be represented by diminished R waves. **Table 9.2** indicates the leads in which R waves of less than a certain amplitude or duration may be indicative of MI.[12]

Infarction in the lateral wall (old terminology posterior wall) of the LV is represented by a positive rather than a negative deviation of the QRS complex. This infarction results in an increased rather than a decreased R-wave duration and amplitude in precordial leads V_1 and V_2 (**Table 9.3**).[13]

Table 9.3.

Abnormally Large R Waves Suggesting Myocardial Infarction

Lead	Criteria for Abnormal
V_1	R dur ≥0.04 s, R amp ≥0.60 mV, R amp ≥S amp
V_2	R dur ≥0.05 s, R amp ≥1.50 mV, R amp ≥1.5 × S amp

Abbreviations: amp, amplitude; dur, duration.

QRS Complex for Localizing

Table 9.4 indicates the relationships among the coronary arteries, left-ventricular walls, and ECG leads that provide a basis for localizing MIs.[14] It may also be helpful to refer to **Figure 8.6**.

Table 9.4.

Infarction Terminology Relationships

Septal Wall - LAD occlusion **Q waves or diminished R waves: V_1-V_3** (V_4-V_5 if extends toward apex)
Anterior Wall - LAD occlusion **Q waves or diminished R waves: I, aVL** (V_3-V_5 if extends toward septum and apex)
Inferior Wall Infarct - RCA occlusion **Q waves or diminished R waves: II, III, aVF** (V_6 if extends toward apex)
Lateral Wall Infarct - LCX occlusion **Large R waves: V_1, V_2** (Q waves or diminished R waves in V_6 if extends toward apex)

Abbreviations: LAD, left anterior descending; LCX, left circumflex artery; RCA, right coronary artery.

An infarct produced by insufficient blood flow via the left anterior descending (LAD) coronary artery and limited to the septal quadrant (**Figure 9.7A**) is termed an anteroseptal infarct. When the infarct extends into the anterior quadrant (**Figure 9.7B**) and/or into the apical segments of other quadrants (**Figure 9.7C**), it is commonly referred to as an "extensive anterior" infarct. Although these two additional myocardial regions that may be infarcted by occlusion of the LAD are anatomically separate, they commonly share the same "apical" designation. One useful tip for localizing *apical infarction* is to look for findings that suggest simultaneous inferior and anterior infarctions. These findings are consistent with an anatomically large region supplied by an LAD that "wraps around" the apex and extends on to the distal or apical segment of the inferior wall.

A

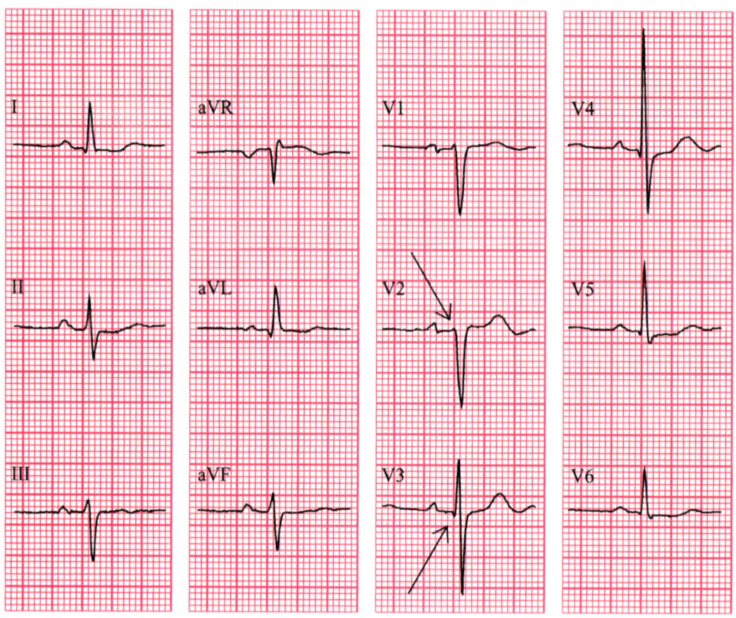

FIGURE 9.7. Twelve-lead electrocardiograms from a 75-year-old man with a previous infarct limited to the septum (**A**), a 61-year-old man with a previous infarct involving the anterior wall (**B**), and a 55-year-old man with a previous anterior infarct involving multiple apical sectors (**C**). Arrows, Q waves or diminished R waves. *(continued)*

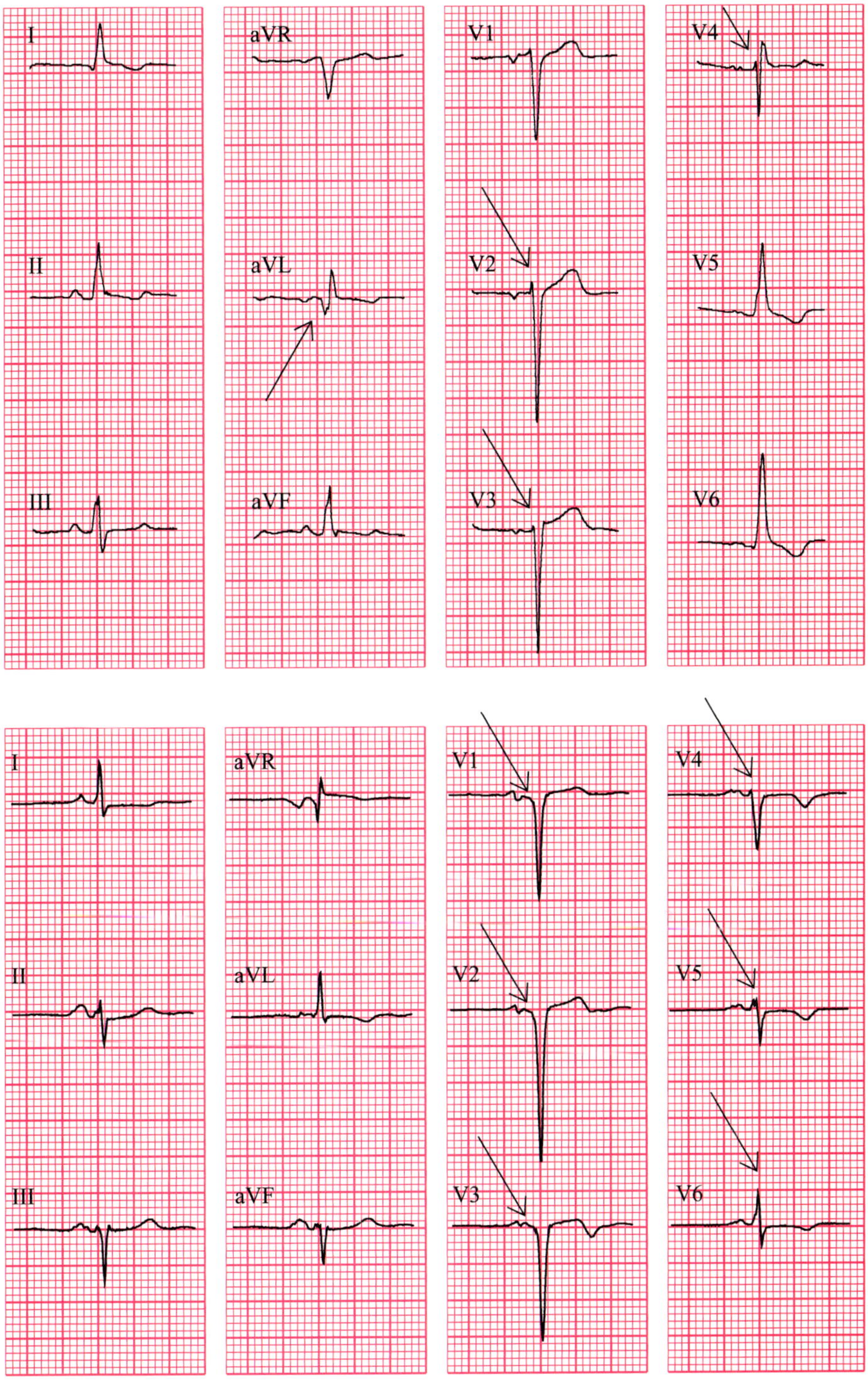

B

C

FIGURE 9.7. *(continued)*

In most individuals, the right coronary artery (RCA) is "dominant" (supplying the posterior descending artery). Its complete obstruction typically produces an *inferior infarction* involving the basal and middle segments of the inferior quadrant resulting in abnormal Q waves. **Figure 9.8** was recorded 3 days after an acute inferior MI. Abnormal Q waves appear only in the three limb leads with inferiorly oriented positive poles (leads II, III, and aVF).

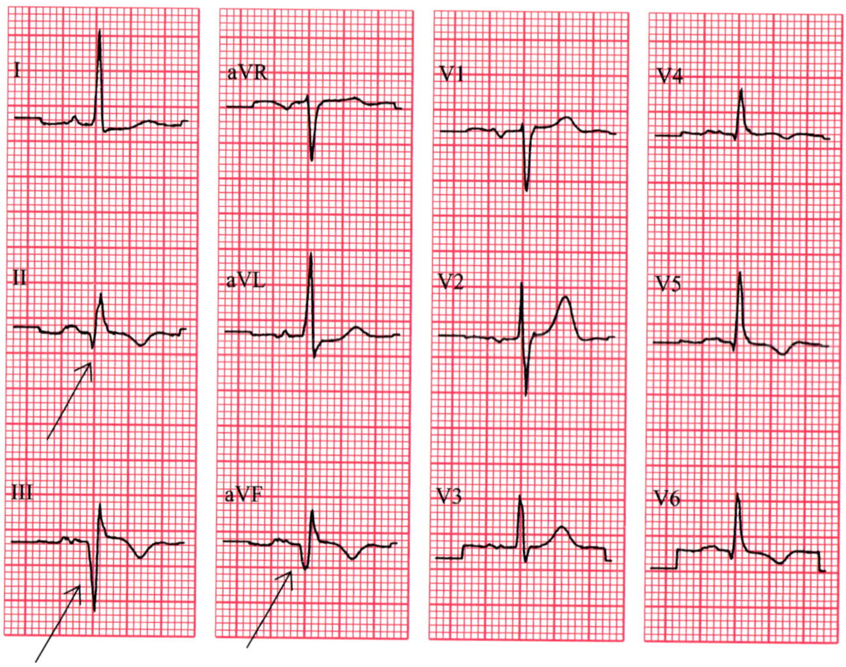

FIGURE 9.8. A 12-lead electrocardiogram from a 72-year-old woman 3 days after an acute inferior myocardial infarction from occlusion of the right coronary artery. Arrows, abnormal Q.

Also, when the RCA is dominant, the typical distribution of the left circumflex artery (LCX) supplies only the left-ventricular free wall between the distributions of the LAD and posterior descending artery. The basal and middle segments of the lateral wall of the LV are located away from the positive poles of all 12 of the standard ECG leads. Therefore, complete occlusion of a nondominant LCX is indicated by a positive (in leads V_1 and V_2) rather than a negative deviation of the QRS complex (**Figure 9.9**) and termed *lateral infarction* (formerly termed posterior or posterolateral). Additional leads on the posterior thorax are required to record the elevation of the ST segment caused by transmural myocardial ischemia and the negative deviation of the QRS complex caused by MI in this region.[13]

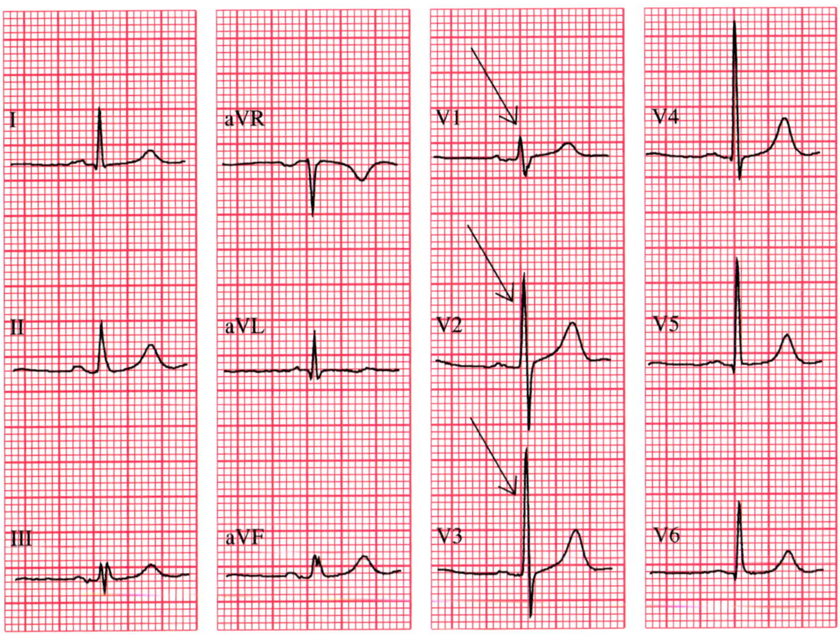

FIGURE 9.9. A 12-lead electrocardiogram from a 70-year-old man 1 year after an acute lateral-wall myocardial infarction. Coronary angiography showed complete occlusion of a nondominant left circumflex artery (the right coronary artery supplied the posterior descending artery). Arrows, abnormally prominent R waves.

Figure 9.10 presents an example of the almost complete QRS-axis deviation away from the left-ventricular free wall expected from a more extensive infarction of the LV lateral wall. Note the almost completely positive QRS forces in leads V_1 to V_3 and the abnormal Q wave in lead V_6.

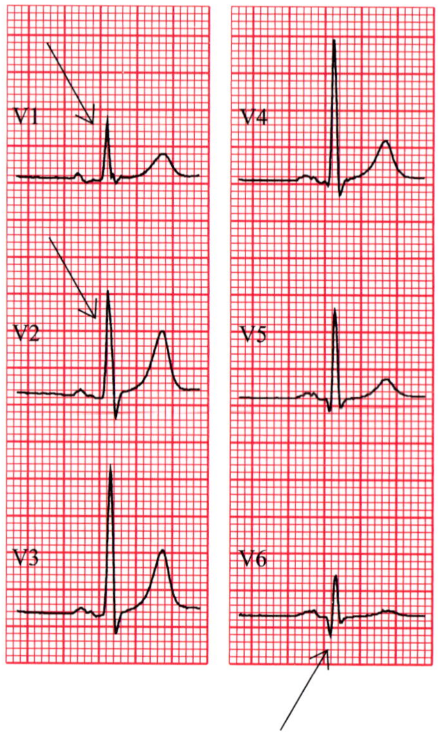

FIGURE 9.10. The six precordial leads of the electrocardiogram from a 63-year-old man 1 week after an acute infarction of the lateral wall of the left ventricle from an left circumflex artery occlusion. Arrows, abnormally large R waves in V_1 and V_2 and presence of a Q wave in aVF.

When the left coronary artery is dominant (supplying the posterior descending artery), a sudden complete obstruction of the RCA can produce infarction only in the right ventricle, which is not likely to produce changes in the QRS complex. The LCX supplies the middle and basal segments of both the lateral and inferior LV walls, and its obstruction can produce an inferolateral infarction (**Figure 9.11**). This same combination of left-ventricular locations can be involved when there is dominance of the RCA and one of its branches extends into the typical distribution of the LCX. The ECG in this instance indicates the region infarcted but not whether the RCA or the LCX is the "culprit artery."

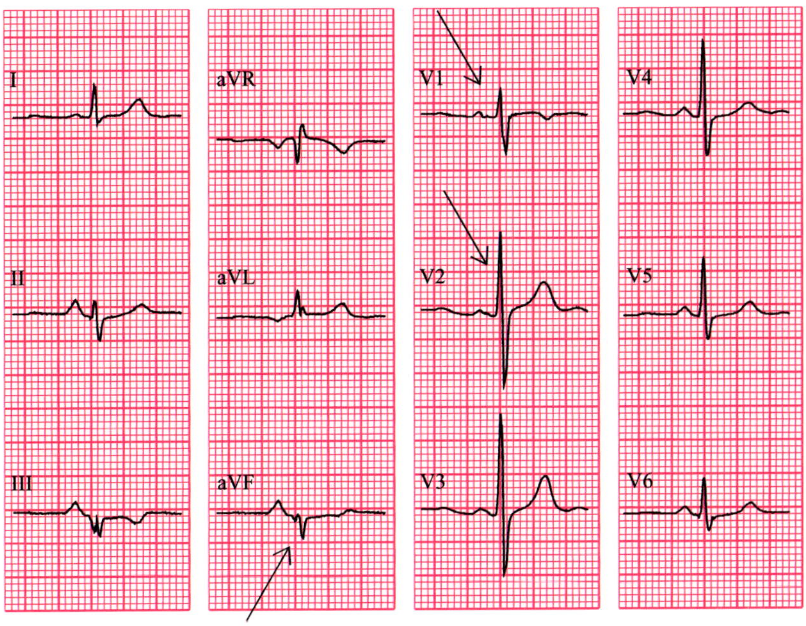

FIGURE 9.11. A 12-lead electrocardiogram from a 70-year-old woman with a healed inferolateral infarction. Arrows, abnormal Q wave in aVF and abnormally prominent R waves in V_1 to V_2.

The lateral wall of the apex of the heart may be involved when either a dominant RCA or LCX is acutely obstructed and inferior, lateral, and apical locations of infarctions are apparent on the serial 12-lead ECGs (**Figure 9.12**). A patient's baseline ECG is shown in **Figure 9.12A** without abnormal QRS forces. The ECG at the time of hospital admission (**Figure 9.12B**) already shows abnormal Q waves, and the recording at hospital discharge (**Figure 9.12C**) shows that an abnormally prominent R wave has appeared in leads V_1 and V_2.

A

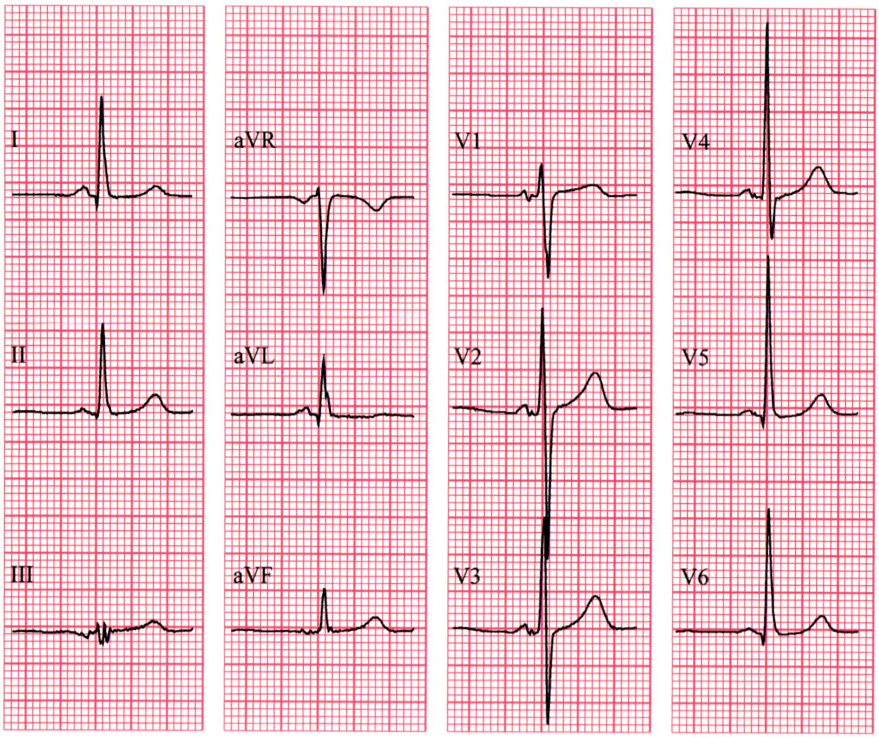

FIGURE 9.12. Serial 12-lead electrocardiograms from a previous routine examination (**A**), the time of hospital admission (**B**), and the time of hospital discharge (**C**) of an 81-year-old man. *(continued)*

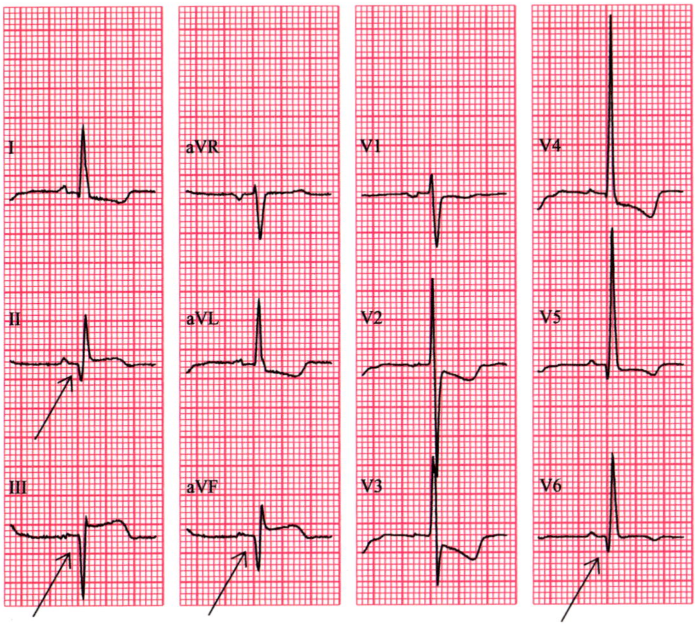

B

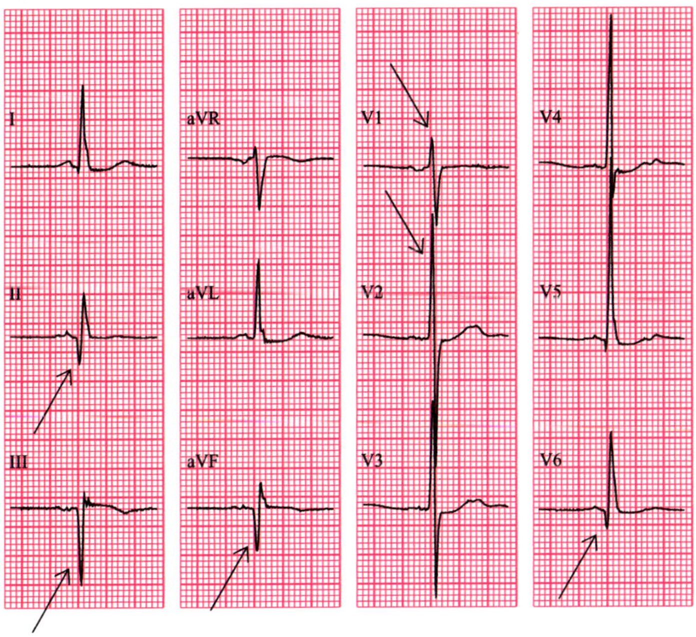

C

FIGURE 9.12. *(continued)*

Fragmented QRS (fQRS)

The term fragmented QRS is used to indicate the presence of a second R wave or a notch in the nadir of the R or S wave in two contiguous leads corresponding to a coronary artery territory. When the QRS is wide, two or more notches are required to called it fQRS. fQRS has been identified in many abnormalities, but it is a typical finding in coronary artery disease. The presence of fQRS is a better marker of prior MI compared to q wave.[A] The presence of fQRS also has prognostic importance, identifying patients with a poorer long-term outcome.

CHAPTER 9 SUMMARY ILLUSTRATION

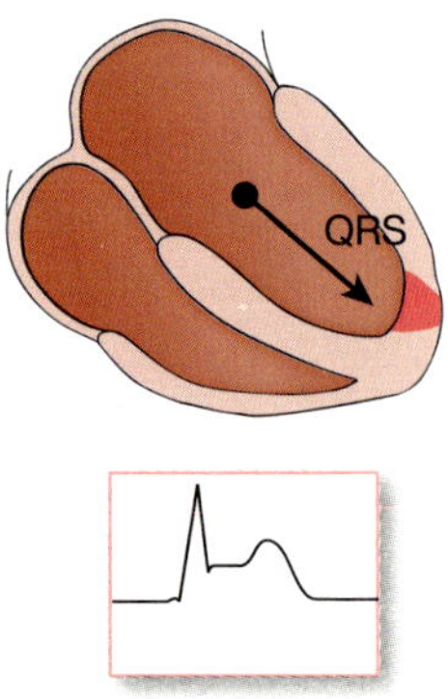

Initial transmural myocardial ischemia causes the ST-segment to increase above the ischemic area

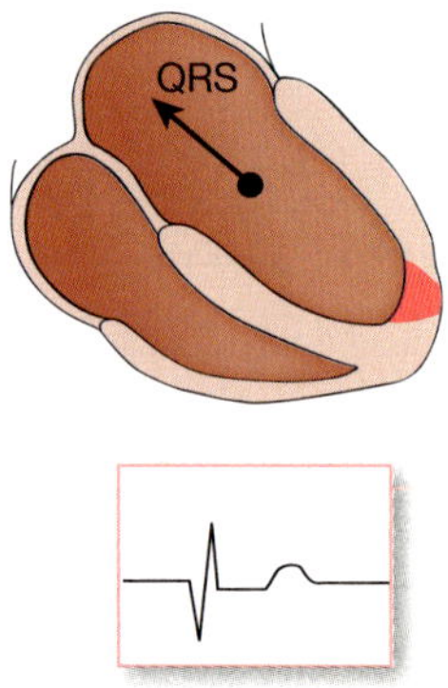

With chronic myocardial infarction the ST segment returns to baseline and Q waves form

Abnormal Q Waves Suggesting MI

Limb Leads		Precordial Leads	
Lead	**Criteria for Abnormal**	**Lead**	**Criteria for Abnormal**
I	≥0.03 s	V1	Any Q
II	≥0.03 s	V2	Any Q
III	None	V3	Any Q
aV	None	V4	≥0.02 s
aVL	≥0.03 s	V5	≥0.03 s
aVF	≥0.03 s	V6	≥0.03 s

Modified from Wagner GS, Freye CJ, Palmeri ST, et al. Evaluation of a QRS scoring system for estimating myocardial infarct size. I. Specificity and observer agreement. Circulation. 1982;65:345, with permission.

Infarction Terminology Relationships

Septal Wall - LAD occlusion
Q waves or diminished R waves: V1-V3 (V4-V5 if extends toward apex)

Anterior Wall - LAD occlusion
Q waves or diminished R waves: I, aVL (V3-V5 if extends toward septum and apex)

Inferior Wall Infarct - RCA occlusion
Q waves or diminished R waves: II, III, aVF (V6 if extends toward apex)

Lateral Wall Infarct - LCX occlusion
Large R Waves: V1, V2 (Q Waves or diminished R waves in V6 if extends toward apex)

LAD, left anterior descending; LCX, left circumflex artery; LV, left ventricle; RCA, right coronary artery; RV, right ventricle.

LAD occlusion with septal wall infarct extending to the apex

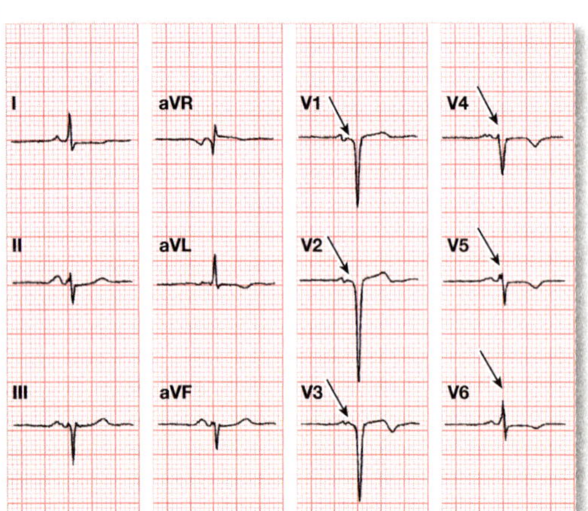

Dominant RCA or LCX with large inferior (Q wave in II, III, aVF) and lateral (large R wave in V1, V2) infarct extending toward the apex (Q wave in V6)

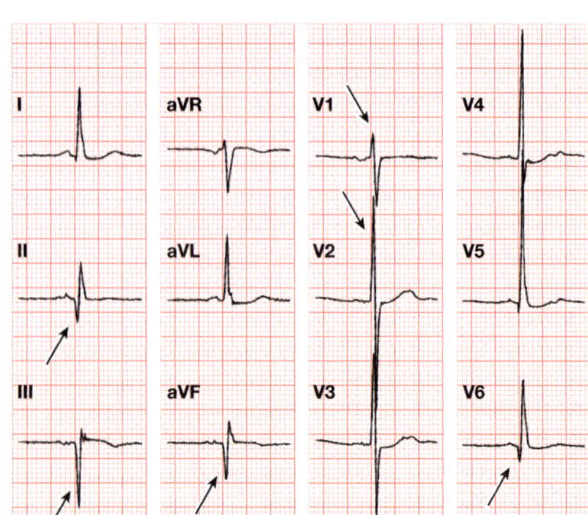

Glossary

Anterior infarction: an infarction in the distribution of the LAD, involving primarily the middle and apical sectors of the anterior septal quadrant of the LV.

Apical infarction: an infarction in the distribution of any of the major coronary arteries, involving primarily the apical sectors of the posterior-lateral and inferior quadrants of the LV.

Collateral blood supply: the perfusion of an area of myocardium via arteries that have developed to compensate for an obstruction of one of the principal coronary arteries.

Infarct expansion: partial disruption of the myocardial wall in the area of a recent infarction that results in thinning of the wall and dilation of the involved chamber.

Inferior infarction: an infarction in the distribution of the posterior descending coronary artery, involving primarily the basal and middle sectors of the inferior quadrant of the LV but often extending into the posterior aspect of the right ventricle.

Lateral infarction: infarction in the distribution of the LCX, involving primarily the basal and middle sectors of the lateral quadrant of the LV (see **Figure 8.6**). Note that this lateral quadrant has previously been called "posterior" or "posterior-lateral."

Necrosis: death of a living tissue; termed an *infarction* when it is caused by insufficient supply of oxygen via the circulation.

Ventricular aneurysm: the extreme of infarct expansion in which the ventricular wall becomes so thin that it bulges outward (dyskinesia) during systole.

Acknowledgment

We gratefully acknowledge the past contributions of the previous edition's author, Dr. Galen S. Wagner, as portions of that chapter were retained in this revision.

References

1. Aldrich HR, Wagner NB, Boswick J, et al. Use of initial ST-segment deviation for prediction of final electrocardiographic size of acute myocardial infarcts. *Am J Cardiol.* 1988;61:749-753.
2. Billgren T, Birnbaum Y, Sgarbossa EB, et al. Refinement and interobserver agreement for the electrocardiographic Sclarovsky-Birnbaum Ischemia Grading System. *J Electrocardiol.* 2004;37:149-156.
3. Corey KE, Maynard C, Pahlm O, et al. Combined historical and electrocardiographic timing of acute anterior and inferior myocardial infarcts for prediction of reperfusion achievable size limitation. *Am J Cardiol.* 1999;83:826-831.
4. de Lemos JA, Antman EM, Giugliano RP, et al. ST-segment resolution and infarct-related artery patency and flow after thrombolytic therapy. Thrombolysis in Myocardial Infarction (TIMI) 14 investigators. *Am J Cardiol.* 2000;85:299-304.
5. Schröder R, Dissmann R, Brüggemann T, et al. Extent of early ST segment elevation resolution: a simple but strong predictor of outcome in patients with acute myocardial infarction. *J Am Coll Cardiol.* 1994;24:384-391.
6. Arvan S, Varat MA. Persistent ST-segment elevation and left ventricular wall abnormalities: a 2-dimensional echocardiographic study. *Am J Cardiol.* 1984;53:1542-1546.
7. Lindsay J Jr, Dewey RC, Talesnick BS, Nolan NG. Relation of ST-segment elevation after healing of acute myocardial infarction to the presence of left ventricular aneurysm. *Am J Cardiol.* 1984;54:84-86.
8. Oliva PB, Hammill SC, Edwards WD. Electrocardiographic diagnosis of postinfarction regional pericarditis. Ancillary observations regarding the effect of reperfusion on the rapidity and amplitude of T wave inversion after acute myocardial infarction. *Circulation.* 1993;88:896-904.
9. Mandel WJ, Burgess MJ, Neville J Jr, Abildskov JA. Analysis of T-wave abnormalities associated with myocardial infarction using a theoretic model. *Circulation.* 1968;38:178-188.
10. Wagner NB, White RD, Wagner GS. The 12-lead ECG and the extent of myocardium at risk of acute infarction: cardiac anatomy and lead locations, and the phases of serial changes during acute occlusion. In: Califf RM, Mark DB, Wagner GS, eds. *Acute Coronary*

Care in the Thrombolytic Era. Chicago, IL: Year Book; 1988:36-41.

11. Wagner GS, Wagner NB. The 12-lead ECG and the extent of myocardium at risk of acute infarction: anatomic relationships among coronary, Purkinje, and myocardial anatomy. In: Califf RM, Mark DB, Wagner GS, eds. *Acute Coronary Care in the Thrombolytic Era*. Chicago, IL: Year Book; 1988:16-30.
12. Wagner GS, Freye CJ, Palmeri ST, et al. Evaluation of a QRS scoring system for estimating myocardial infarct size. I. Specificity and observer agreement. *Circulation*. 1982;65:342-347.
13. Flowers NC, Horan LG, Sohi GS, Hand RC, Johnson JC. New evidence for inferoposterior myocardial infarction on surface potential maps. *Am J Cardiol*. 1976;38:576-581.
14. Bayés de Luna A, Wagner G, Birnbaum Y, et al. A new terminology for left ventricular walls and location of myocardial infarcts that present Q wave based on the standard of cardiac magnetic resonance imaging: a statement for healthcare professionals from a committee appointed by the International Society for Holter and Noninvasive Electrocardiography. *Circulation*. 2006;114:1755-1760.

Reference to the South Asian Edition

A. Das MK, Khan B, Jacob S, Kumar A, Mahenthiran J. Significance of a fragmented QRS complex versus a Q wave in patients with coronary artery disease. *Circulation*. 2006;113:2495-2501.

SECTION IV

Drugs, Electrolytes, and Miscellaneous Conditions

10 Electrolytes and Drugs

ROBBERT ZUSTERZEEL,
JOSE VICENTE RUIZ,
DAVID G. STRAUSS, AND
MUKUND ARAVIND PRABHU

This chapter provides an overview of the cardiac action potential and explains how abnormalities in the body's electrolytes as well as certain drugs can cause changes in the action potential that can be seen on the body surface electrocardiogram (ECG). This chapter begins with a more detailed description of the cardiac action potential and which electrolytes (or more specifically, ions) and ion channels play a role in depolarization and repolarization. Subsequent sections cover which ECG waveform changes can be expected in the presence of electrolyte abnormalities or the presence of certain commonly used antiarrhythmic drugs.

Cardiac Action Potential

The cardiac action potential was already discussed in Chapter 1. The action potential's shape varies at different locations in the heart (ie, endocardial action potentials are longer than epicardial action potentials). This chapter focuses on the different phases of the action potential in more detail. The following paragraphs explain which ions cause the depolarization and repolarization of each cardiac cell in order to describe the effects of electrolyte abnormalities and drugs on the ECG.

The cardiac action potential has five phases as shown in **Figure 10.1**. Each phase is characterized by the movement of different ions across the myocardial cell membrane. The most important ions are sodium, potassium, and calcium. The action potential "starts" with phase 4 (black), the resting phase. During this phase, the action potential remains more or less constant around −90 mV (see black in **Figure 10.1**). During phase 0, depolarization, there is rapid influx of sodium ions into the cells, making the inside of the cell more positive compared to the outside, and causing a spike in the action potential (purple). In phase 1, the repolarization starts by a decrease in the rapid sodium influx forcing the action potential back down but not completely back to baseline. This decrease in sodium influx occurs because during phase 2, the permeability of the membrane for other depolarizing currents increases. There is a slow influx of both calcium and sodium (green) into the cells counteracting the initial repolarization from phase 1. This influx during phase 2 is, however, opposed by another repolarizing current, the major efflux of potassium ions (red). The result of these opposing currents during phase 2 (influx of calcium and sodium and efflux of potassium) leads to a plateau in the cardiac action potential ("plateau" phase). During the rapid repolarization in phase 3, the permeability of the cell membrane for entry of sodium and calcium ions stops while potassium ions continue to exit the cell (red) and return the action potential completely back to baseline after which the resting state, phase 4, is achieved (black).

Although action potential waveforms and ion channel currents are largely similar in the atria and the ventricles, they are very different in both the sinoatrial (SA) and atrioventricular (AV) nodes. The SA and AV nodes do not have a rapid upstroke in phase 0, and phases 1 and 2 are nonexistent due to a lack of rapid inward sodium channels (see **Figure 10.1**). Their action potential depolarizations therefore heavily rely on slow-acting calcium influx (blue) causing a much smoother action potential waveform.

Figure 10.1 also shows the body surface ECG beneath the cardiac action potential. Parts of the action potential are color coded to indicate their temporal alignment with the ECG. In general, phases 0 and 1 account for the QRS complex (rapid depolarization and earliest phase of repolarization). Phase 2 aligns with the flat ST segment (plateau phase—almost no net current across the membrane) and upstroke of the T wave (i.e. J-Tpeak interval). Phase 3 accounts for the descending part of the T wave (i.e. Tpeak–Tend interval). Finally, the ECG baseline is reflected by phase 4 of the cardiac action potential (resting phase).

Overview of Cardiac Action Potential and Ion Channel Currents

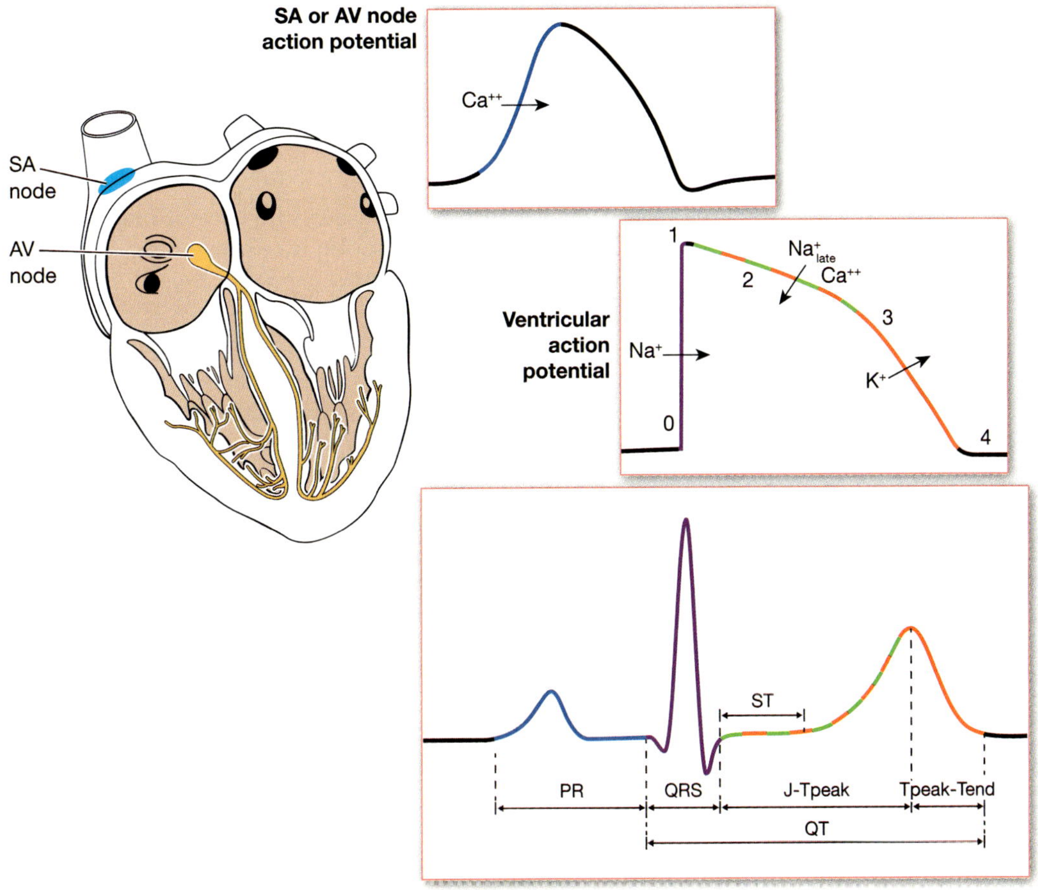

FIGURE 10.1. The arrows depict flow of ions across the cell membrane (eg, Na^+, Ca^{2+} influx, K^+ efflux) and colors on the action potentials correlate with colors on the ECG. SA, sino-atrial; AV, atrio-ventricular.

Electrolyte Abnormalities

Either abnormally low (hypo-) or high (hyper-) serum levels of the electrolytes potassium or calcium may produce marked abnormalities of the ECG waveforms. Indeed, typical ECG changes may provide the first clinical evidence of the presence of these conditions. Changes in sodium levels, however, do not have any effect on the ECG.

Potassium

The terms *hypokalemia* and *hyperkalemia* are commonly used for alterations in serum levels of potassium. Because either of these conditions may be life-threatening, an understanding of the ECG changes they produce is very important.

Hypokalemia

Hypokalemia may have many causes[1] and often occurs with other electrolyte disturbances (eg, reduced serum magnesium levels, thiazide, or loop diuretics) and is particularly dangerous in the presence of cardiac glycoside therapy (eg, *digitalis* or digoxin). The typical ECG signs of hypokalemia may appear when the serum potassium concentration is within normal limits, and conversely, the ECG may be normal when serum levels of potassium are elevated. The ECG changes in hypokalemia are the following[2]:

Electrocardiogram Features in Hypokalemia

1. Flattening or inversion of the T wave
2. Increased prominence of the U wave
3. Slight depression of the ST segment
4. Increased amplitude and width of the P wave
5. Prolongation of the PR interval
6. Premature beats and sustained tachyarrhythmias
7. Prolongation of the heart-rate corrected QT interval (QTc)

Figure 10.2 illustrates several characteristics from a patient with hypokalemia.

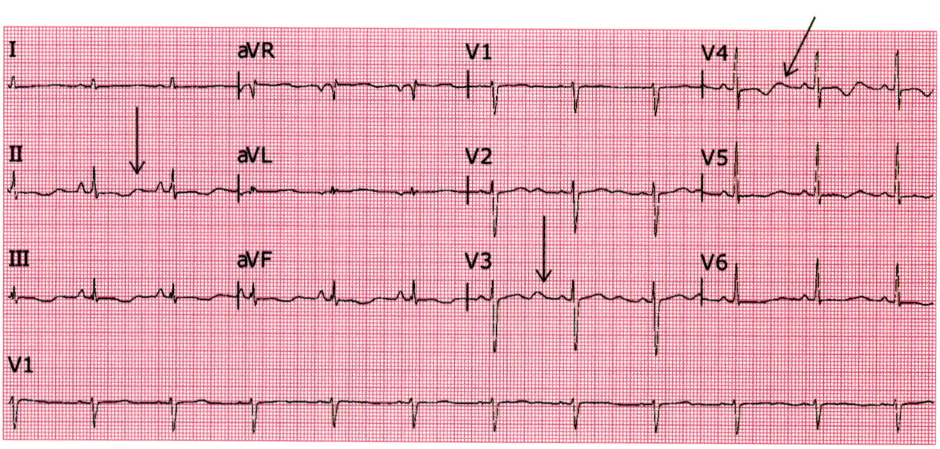

FIGURE 10.2. A multilead ECG recording from a 53-year-old man receiving diuretic therapy for chronic heart failure. The patient's serum potassium level was 1.7 mEq/L (normal 3.5–5.0 mEq/L). QT is prolonged and arrows indicate prominent U waves.

The reversal in the relative amplitudes of the T and U waves is the most characteristic change in waveform morphology in hypokalemia. The U-wave prominence is caused by prolongation of phase 3 of the cardiac action potential. This prolongation of the recovery phase can lead to the life-threatening *torsades de pointes*, a specific type of ventricular tachyarrhythmia (see Chapter 17).[3] Hypokalemia also potentiates the tachyarrhythmias produced by digitalis toxicity.

Hyperkalemia

As with hypokalemia, there may be a poor correlation between serum potassium levels and the typical ECG changes of hyperkalemia.[4] The earliest ECG evidence of hyperkalemia usually appears in the T waves (**Figure 10.3**).

Progressive Electrocardiogram Changes With Increasing Hyperkalemia

1. Increased amplitude and peaking of the T wave
2. Prolongation of the QRS interval
3. Prolongation of the PR interval
4. Flattening of the P wave
5. Loss of P wave
6. Sine wave appearance

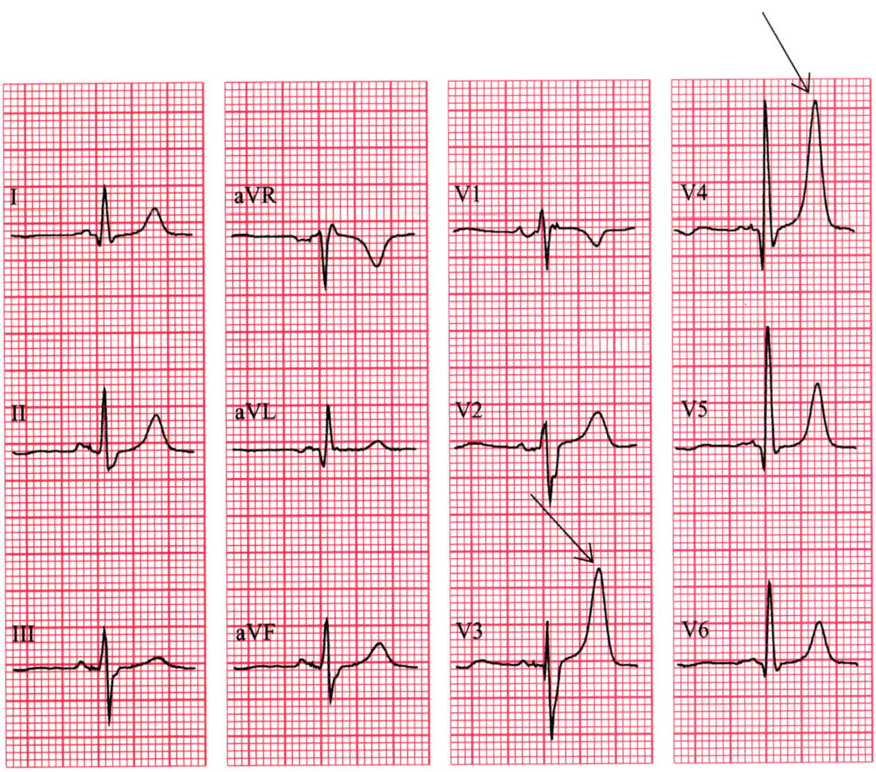

FIGURE 10.3. A 12-lead ECG recording from a 42-year-old man with acute renal failure. The patient's serum potassium level was 7.1 mEq/L. Arrows indicate unusually prominent and peaked positive T waves.

The AV conduction in hyperkalemia may become so delayed that advanced AV block appears (see Chapter 18).[5] Prolongation of the QRS complex and flattening of the P waves occur because the high potassium levels in hyperkalemia delay the spread of the cardiac activating impulse through the myocardium (prolongation of phases 1 through 3 of the cardiac action potential). This abnormally slow intraventricular conduction can lead to ventricular fibrillation and cardiac arrest (see Chapter 17).[6]

Figure 10.4A is from a patient with end-stage renal disease and an initial serum potassium level of 7.8 mEq/L. The tracing shows peaked T waves, QRS prolongation throughout, and an absence of P waves (*atrial fibrillation*). In **Figure 10.4B**, the T waves and the QRS complexes return to their normal duration, and the P waves reappear (normal sinus rhythm) when the serum potassium concentration returns to normal (corrected with dialysis to 4.5 mEq/L). Hyperkalemia may also reduce the myocardial response to artificial electronic pacemaker stimulation (failure to capture).[7]

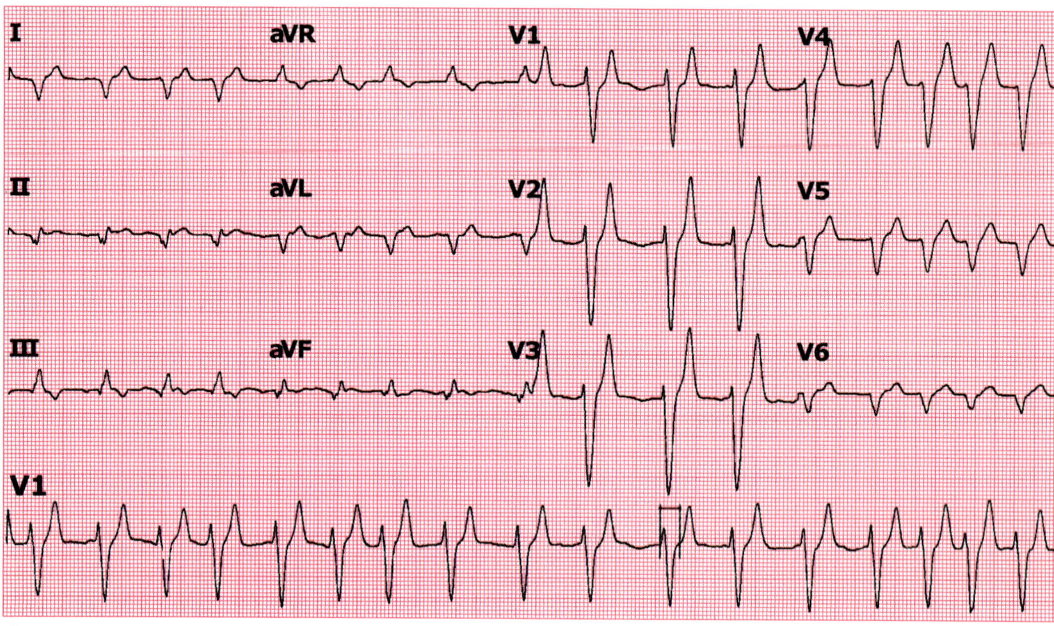

A

FIGURE 10.4. Twelve-lead ECG and V1 rhythm recordings from a 72-year-old woman with end-stage renal disease. The patient's serum potassium level was initially 7.8 mEq/L (**A**) and was then corrected to 4.5 mEq/L (**B**) after dialysis. Caliper indicates the markedly prolonged QRS complex in **A**, and asterisks indicate reappearing P waves in **B**. *(continued)*

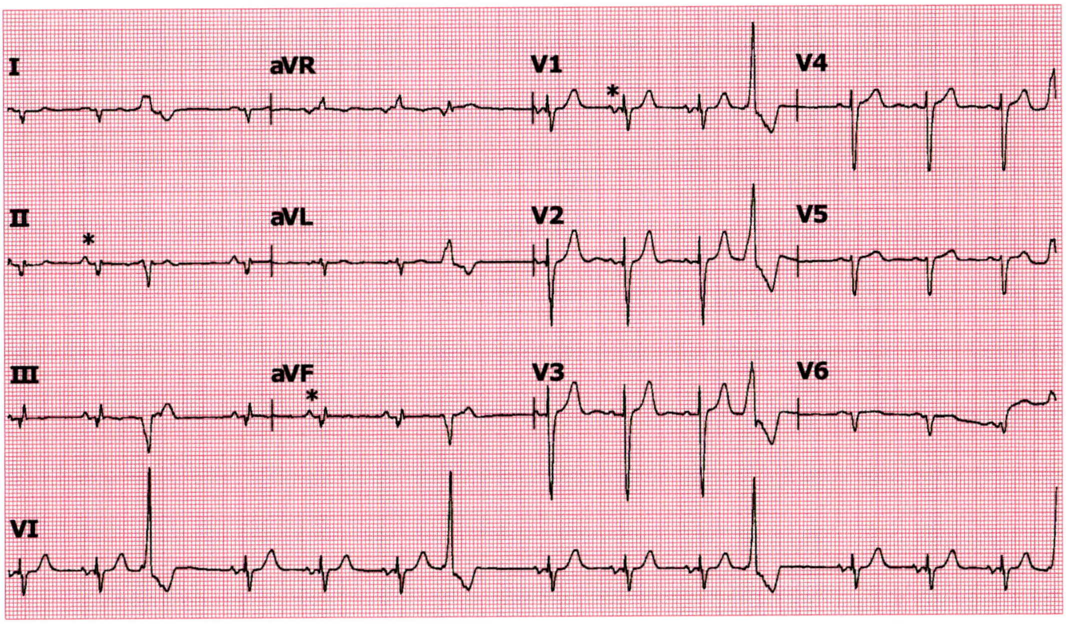

B

FIGURE 10.4. *(continued)*

Calcium

The ventricular recovery time, as represented on the ECG by the heart rate QTc interval (see Chapter 3), is altered by the extremes of serum calcium levels:

Electrocardiogram Effects of Extremes of Serum Calcium Levels

1. Deficiency = hypocalcemia → prolonged QTc interval
2. Excess = hypercalcemia → shortened QTc interval

These changes are predominantly driven by the ST-segment duration since changes in calcium levels affect the duration of phase 2 of the action potential.

Hypocalcemia

Figure 10.5 illustrates this change in the QTc interval from a patient with chronic renal failure. The serum calcium level was 7.2 mg/100 mL (normal range, 8.5-10.5 mg/100 mL). Because the ventricular rate is 88 beats/min, the QTc interval is 493 milliseconds ($434 / 0.681^{1/3}$), using Fridericia formula QTc = QT (ms) / (RR interval (s)$^{1/3}$); see Chapter 3. In *hypocalcemia*, the prolonged QT interval may be accompanied by terminal T-wave inversion in some leads. **Figure 10.6** illustrates the prolonged QT interval with some terminal T-wave changes in a patient with chronic renal failure. Low calcium prolongs phase 2, the plateau phase, of the cardiac action potential. The serum calcium level was 4.7 mEq/L. The ventricular rate is 100 beats/min; therefore, the QTc = 592 milliseconds ($500 / 0.6^{1/3}$), using Fridericia formula.

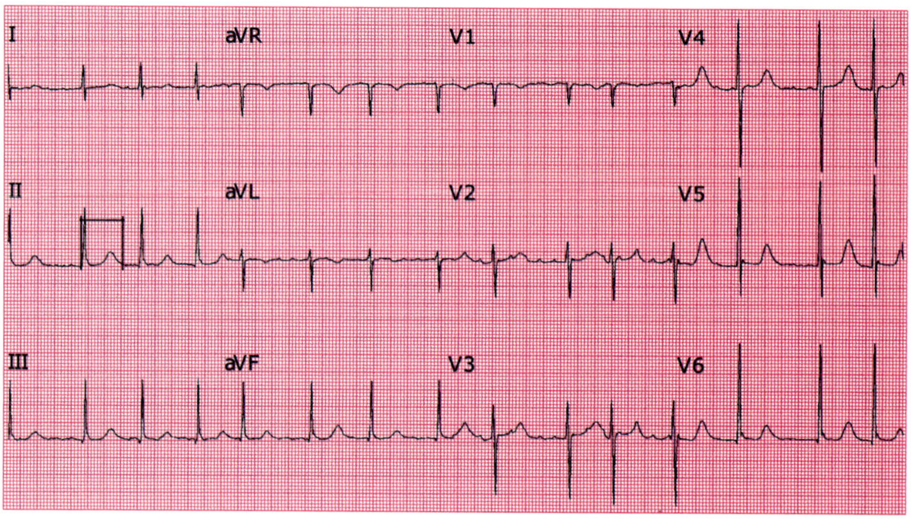

FIGURE 10.5. A 12-lead ECG from a 49-year-old man with chronic renal failure. The patient's serum calcium level was 7.2 mg/100 mL (normal range, 8.5–10.5 mg/100 mL). Caliper indicates the prolonged QT interval.

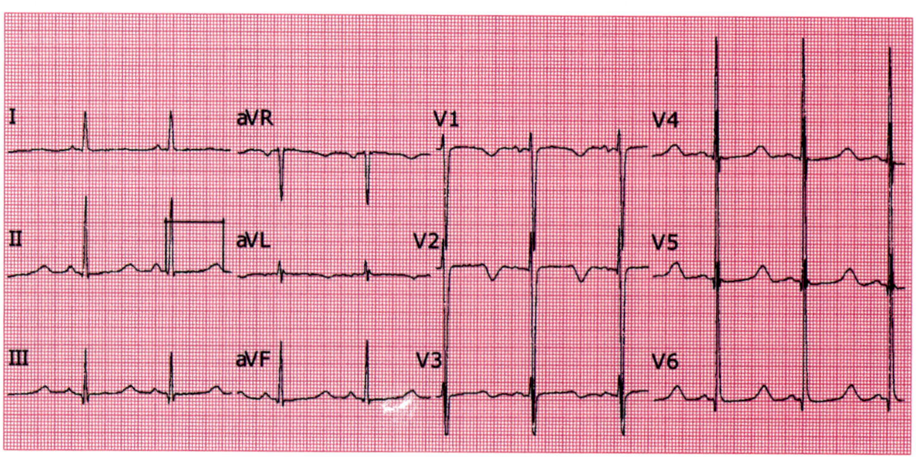

FIGURE 10.6. A 12-lead ECG from a 24-year-old woman with chronic renal failure and hypocalcemia (serum calcium 4.7 mEq/L). Caliper indicates the prolonged QT interval.

Hypercalcemia

In *hypercalcemia*, the proximal limb of the T wave acutely slopes to its peak, and the ST segment may not be apparent, as illustrated in leads V_2 and V_3 in **Figure 10.7**.[8] The short QT in this circumstance gives the impression that there is ST elevation when, in fact, the ST segment is so short that the T wave begins at the J point (termination of the QRS). This T wave appearing at the end of the QRS resembles transmural ischemia but appears throughout all the leads. Moreover, the QT interval is much less than one-third to one-half the R-R interval at rates less than 100 beats/min. In extreme hypercalcemia, an increase in amplitude of the QRS complex, biphasic T waves, and *Osborn waves* have been described.[9,10] The QTc interval shortens due to a more rapid phase 2 of the action potential. Because the heart rate is 56 beats/min, the QTc is 300 milliseconds ($307 / 1.071^{1/3}$).

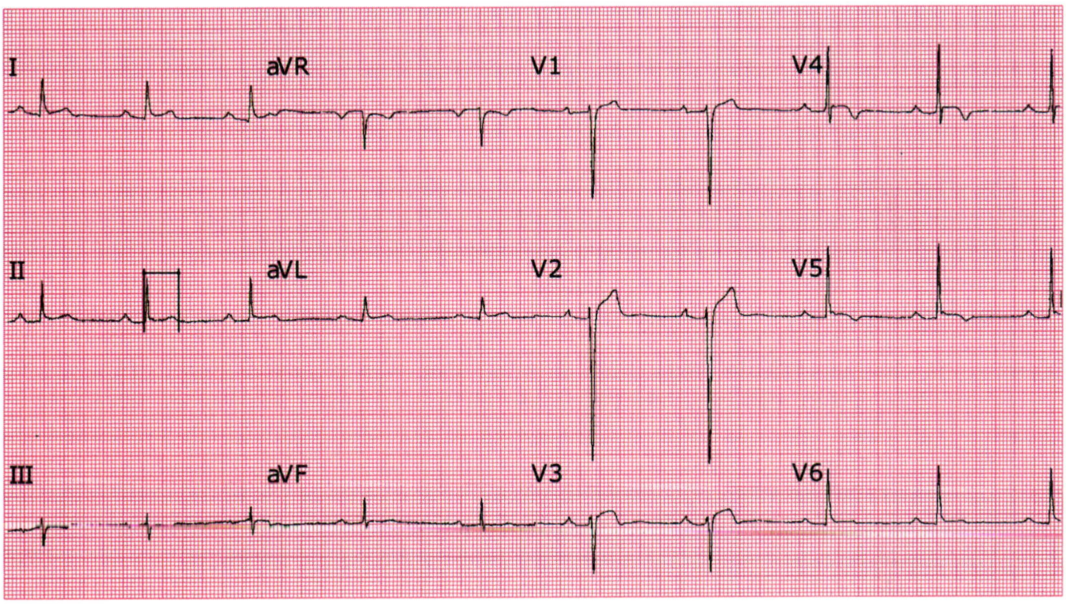

FIGURE 10.7. A 12-lead ECG from a 33-year-old man with hyperparathyroidism and a serum calcium level of 15 mg/100 mL. Caliper indicates the shortened QT interval.

Magnesium Imbalance

Magnesium imbalance is commonly accompanied by changes in calcium and potassium balance as well. In patients with isolated hypomagnesemia, the P wave duration and the QTc interval are increased, suggesting prolongation of repolarization of both atrial and ventricular tissues. Changes seen in severe hypermagnesemia are similar to that of hyperkalemia and include prolongation of the PR interval, higher degrees of atrioventricular conduction disturbances, increased duration of QRS complex, prolonged QT interval, delayed intraventricular conduction, and increased height of the T wave.

Drug Effects

Either therapeutic or toxic cardiac effects of various medications can sometimes be detected on the ECG. The term **drug effect** refers to the therapeutic cardiac manifestations of a drug on the ECG, and the term **drug toxicity** refers to the cardiac *arrhythmias* caused by various medications (see Chapters 17 and 18). The level of a drug in blood and tissue at which toxicity occurs can vary widely depending on several factors, including the underlying pathology for which the drug is being used, the patient's premedication ECG status, the variations in electrolytes such as potassium and calcium, and the presence of other drugs.

The ECG effects of drugs can most commonly be explained by the effects they have on cardiac ion channels and action potentials. These effects are potentially similar to certain electrolyte abnormalities discussed previously as they share similar interactions with these ion channels. This chapter addresses the ECG effects of antiarrhythmic drugs only. There are, however, other commonly prescribed drugs (eg, some antibiotics, antihistamines, antidepressants, and antipsychotics) that can also cause changes in the ECG by similar mechanisms.

Antiarrhythmic Drugs

The effect of an antiarrhythmic drug may be modified by the underlying cardiac disorder for which it is being used, by coexisting electrolyte imbalance, and by interaction of the drug with concomitant medications. An example of a drug interaction is the marked increase in blood levels of drug A (eg, digitalis) that occurs with the introduction of drug B (eg, *quinidine* or *amiodarone*). The commonly used antiarrhythmic drugs are classified according to Vaughan Williams and associates[11,12] and are grouped by their effects on specific cardiac ion channels (**Table 10.1**). Keep in mind that even though a drug is a member of a certain class, it can also have effects on ion channels similar to those of other classes. Examples of these characteristics are discussed in text that follows (eg, see sotalol and amiodarone). It should be noted that a newer version of the Vaughan Williams scheme that includes both established and potential antiarrhythmic agents has been recently published and includes other drugs like ivabradine and adenosine.[A]

Table 10.1.

Overview of Vaughan Williams Classification and Drug Examples

Class of Action	Drug Examples
Class I: Sodium channel blockers	
Ia: Moderate prolongation of conduction and repolarization	Quinidine Procainamide Disopyramide
Ib: Minimal effect on conduction and repolarization	Lidocaine Mexiletine Phenytoin
Ic: Marked prolongation of conduction but not repolarization	Flecainide Propafenone
Class II: β-adrenergic receptor blockers	Propranolol Metoprolol
Class III: potassium channel blockers	Amiodarone Sotalol Dofetilide Ibutilide
Class IV: calcium channel blockers	Verapamil Diltiazem
Others: mechanisms of action not fully elucidated	Adenosine Cardiac glycosides (digitalis, digoxin)

Class I Drugs

Drugs in class I of the Vaughan Williams classification have direct action on the sodium channels of the myocardial cell membrane and have been subdivided according to their effect on the different phases of the action potential. The more common drugs and their effects on the action potential are as follows:

Class Ia (Including Quinidine, Procainamide, and Disopyramide)

Class Ia drugs generally cause a moderate prolongation of conduction as well as repolarization. As an example, quinidine changes the ECG by a delay in the recovery or repolarization of myocardial cells. Even though quinidine is grouped into class Ia, most of its ECG effects are caused by blocking potassium channels and not as much by sodium channel blockade (ie, it has Vaughan Williams class III effects as well). This combination of effects results in prolongation of the QTc interval,[13] a decreased T-wave amplitude, and an increased U-wave amplitude, similar to hypokalemia, by prolonging phases 2 and 3 of the cardiac action potential. These changes are illustrated in **Figure 10.8** from a patient with recent acute anterior infarction complicated by ventricular tachycardia. The arrhythmia was controlled by quinidine, and a quinidine effect appeared on the ECG. In this example, the QT interval is 390 milliseconds, and because the ventricular rate is 100 beats/min, the QTc interval is prolonged to 462 milliseconds (Fridericia formula). Minimal prolongation of the QRS complex occurs rarely with quinidine effect; an increase in duration of the QRS complex of 25% to 50% is evidence of quinidine toxicity. Quinidine effect is also exaggerated by the presence of digitalis. The phenothiazine group of drugs, which are commonly used in treating psychiatric disorders, produce ECG changes similar to quinidine effect.

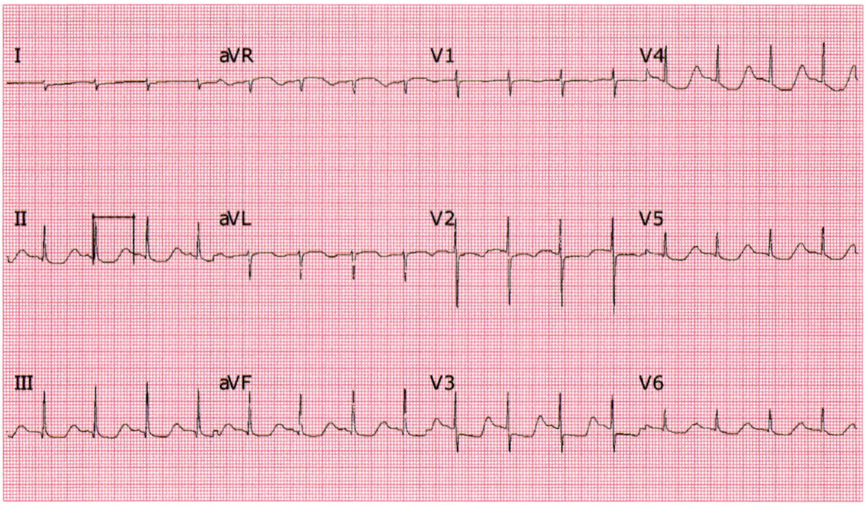

FIGURE 10.8. A 12-lead ECG from a 68-year-old woman with recent acute anterior infarction complicated by ventricular tachycardia. The arrhythmia has been controlled by quinidine, and a quinidine effect appears on the ECG. Caliper indicates markedly prolonged QT interval, extending from the QRS complex onset to the end of the T wave.

Class Ib (Lidocaine and Mexiletine)

Class Ib drugs are also sodium channel blockers, but usually, the surface ECG appears to be unaltered by lidocaine and mexiletine. They can, however, produce action potential and QT interval shortening due to them blocking the late sodium current. **Figure 10.9** shows the ECG of a healthy volunteer on lidocaine.

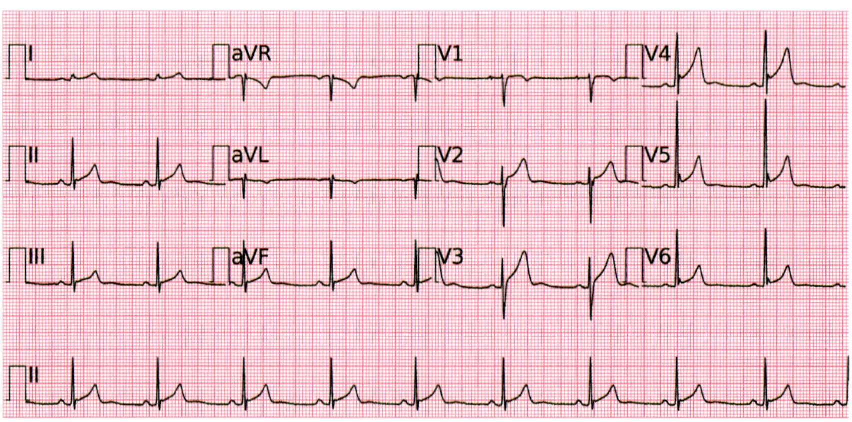

FIGURE 10.9. Electrocardiogram from normal volunteer on lidocaine. Diffuse ST elevation seen here is likely due to early repolarization and is not a lidocaine effect. From PhysioNet.[14]

Class Ic (Flecainide)

Class Ic sodium channel blockers cause a marked prolongation of conduction but not repolarization. Flecainide produces broadening of the QRS complex, with the interval between the J point and the end of the T wave remaining unaltered, thus slightly prolonging the QT interval.

Class II Drugs

The drugs in class II of the Vaughan Williams classification system are the β-adrenergic blocking agents. By decreasing sympathetic effects on the heart, there is a slowing of heart rate due to the decreased SA node impulse formation. Conduction through the AV node is also delayed, prolonging the PR interval of the ECG. If there is underlying SA or AV nodal dysfunction, these changes may be increased. Sotalol is a drug with both class II and III properties, which is discussed further in the Class III Drugs section.

Class III Drugs

The drugs in class III of the Vaughan Williams system are potassium channel blockers and prolong myocardial repolarization and may therefore markedly prolong the QTc interval on the ECG. Among the class III drugs are the following:

Dofetilide

Dofetilide predominantly blocks potassium channels and prolongs phases 2 and 3 of the cardiac action potential. **Figure 10.10** shows the ECGs of a healthy volunteer before dofetilide administration (**Figure 10.10A**) and after administration (**Figure 10.10B**). Compared to **Figure 10.10A**, **Figure 10.10B** demonstrates prolongation of the QTc interval and decreased T-wave amplitude (no clear U wave in this example), which are similar to the ECG effects of hypokalemia.

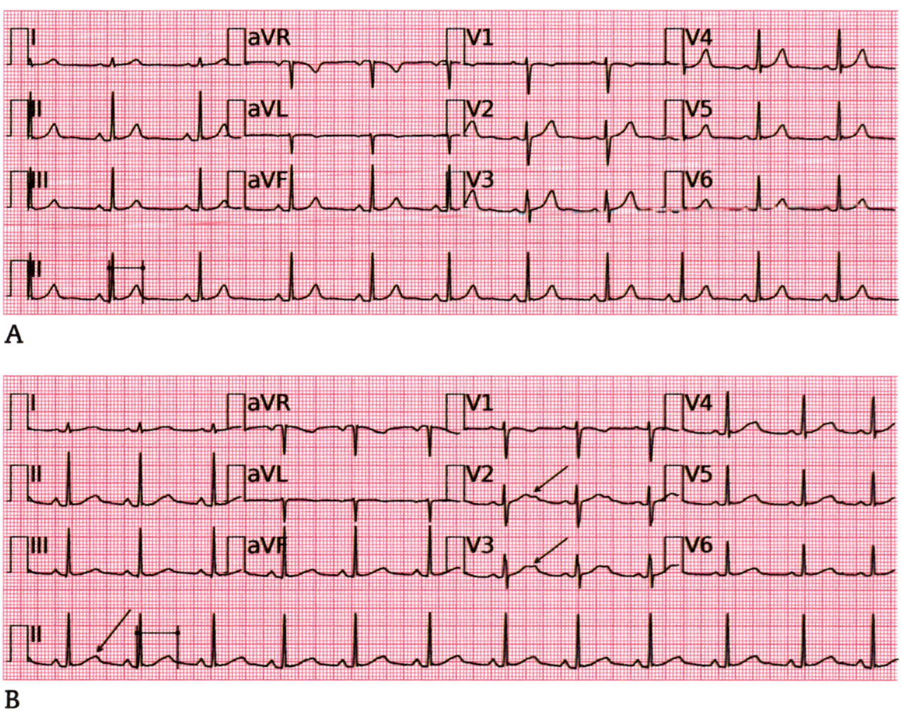

FIGURE 10.10. **A.** Electrocardiogram from clinical trial participant before administration of dofetilide. Caliper, normal QT interval (QTc = 397 ms) and normal T wave amplitude. **B.** Electrocardiogram from the same participant after receiving dofetilide. Caliper, prolonged QT interval (QTc = 490 ms) and decreased T wave amplitude (arrow), sometimes with T wave notching (arrow in V2 and V3). From PhysioNet.[14,15]

Sotalol

Sotalol has both class 2 (β-adrenergic block) and 3 (potassium channel block) drug effects and may therefore produce SA and AV nodal suppression and also prolongation of the QTc interval. **Figure 10.11** shows the ECG of a patient with a history of atrial fibrillation and syncope receiving sotalol. The heart rate is approximately 50 beats/min (β-blocking effect), and the QT interval is prolonged (predominantly due to potassium channel blockade). **Figure 10.12** shows the ECG of a patient on sotalol where the potassium channel block contributes to the development of torsades de pointes ventricular arrhythmia.

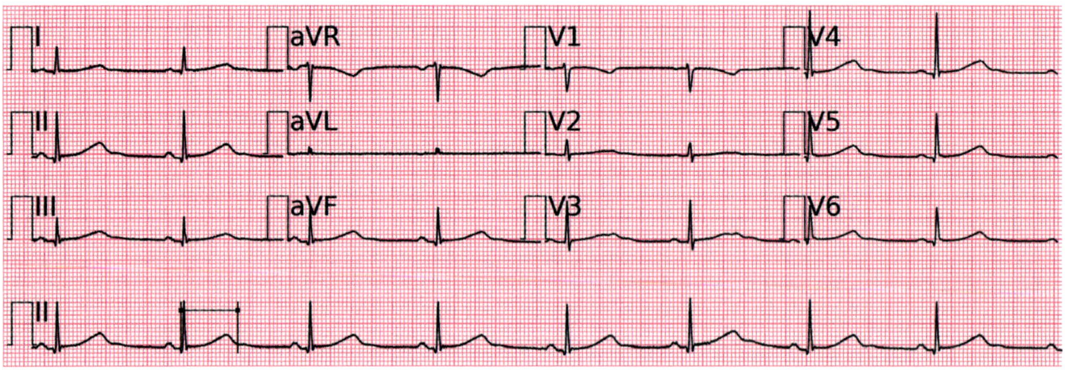

FIGURE 10.11. A 12-lead ECG of a patient with a history of atrial fibrillation and syncope receiving sotalol. The ECG shows a slow heart rate (approximately 50 beats per minute) and the caliper indicates QT prolongation (approximately 560 ms, QTc = 527 ms). Reused with permission from the Telemetric and Holter ECG Warehouse.[16]

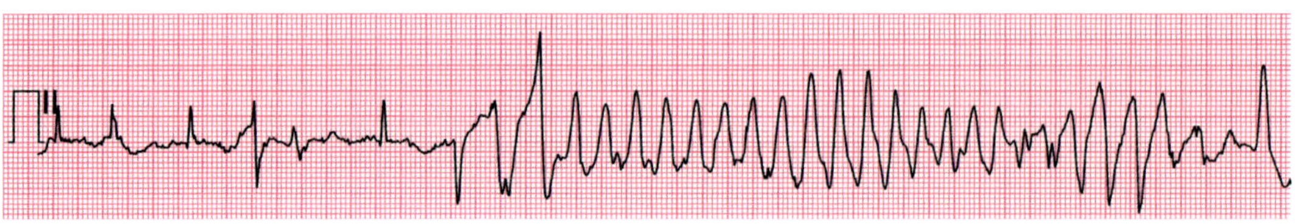

FIGURE 10.12. Rhythm strip (Lead II) showing initiation of torsades de pointes ventricular arrhythmia. Reused with permission from the Telemetric and Holter ECG Warehouse.[17]

Amiodarone

Amiodarone is a commonly used drug and has class I, II, and III effects. Its characteristics in multiple classes gives amiodarone wide utility in treating tachyarrhythmias arising from various mechanisms.

Class IV Drugs

Drugs in class IV of the Vaughan Williams classification system block calcium channels. As a result of this calcium channel blockade, they slow both SA and AV nodal functions. Their effects are, therefore, similar to those of drugs in class II. **Figure 10.13** shows the ECGs of a healthy volunteer on *diltiazem*. Before administration, the ECG is normal (**Figure 10.13A**). After administration of diltiazem (**Figure 10.13B**), the main ECG changes include a prolongation of the PR-interval (first-degree AV block) and incremental AV block up to the point of second-degree AV block (Wenckebach or type I Mobitz).

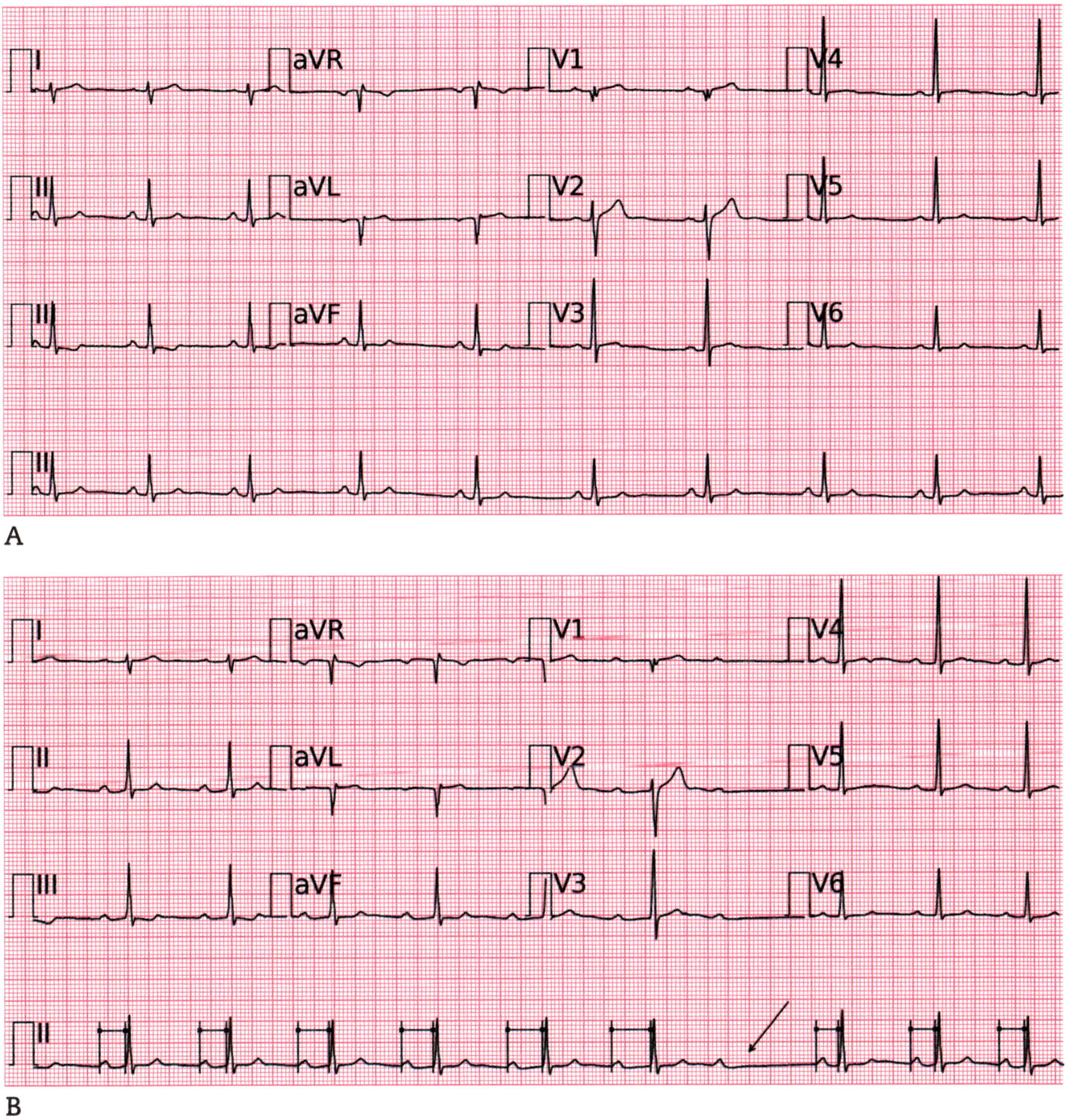

FIGURE 10.13. **A.** Electrocardiogram from clinical trial participant before administration of diltiazem. Normal PR interval. **B.** Electrocardiogram from the same clinical trial participant after receiving diltiazem who develops second-degree atrioventricular block (Wenckebach/type I Mobitz). Calipers show increasing prolongation of the PR interval followed by a P-wave that does not conduct to the ventricles causing a missed QRST complex (arrow), followed by a short PR that begins lengthening with subsequent beats. From PhysioNet.[18]

Other Drugs

Some other commonly used drugs are not included in the Vaughan Williams classification but have significant antiarrhythmic effects.

Digitalis

Digitalis is used to slow the ventricular rate in atrial tachyarrhythmias and sometimes used to treat heart failure. Digitalis preparations can cause characteristic ECG changes termed **digitalis effect** because the recovery or repolarization of the myocardial cells occurs earlier than it normally does (**Figure 10.14**).

Some Electrocardiogram Effects of Digitalis on QRS-T

1. "Coved" ST-segment depression
2. A flattened T wave
3. A decreased QTc interval

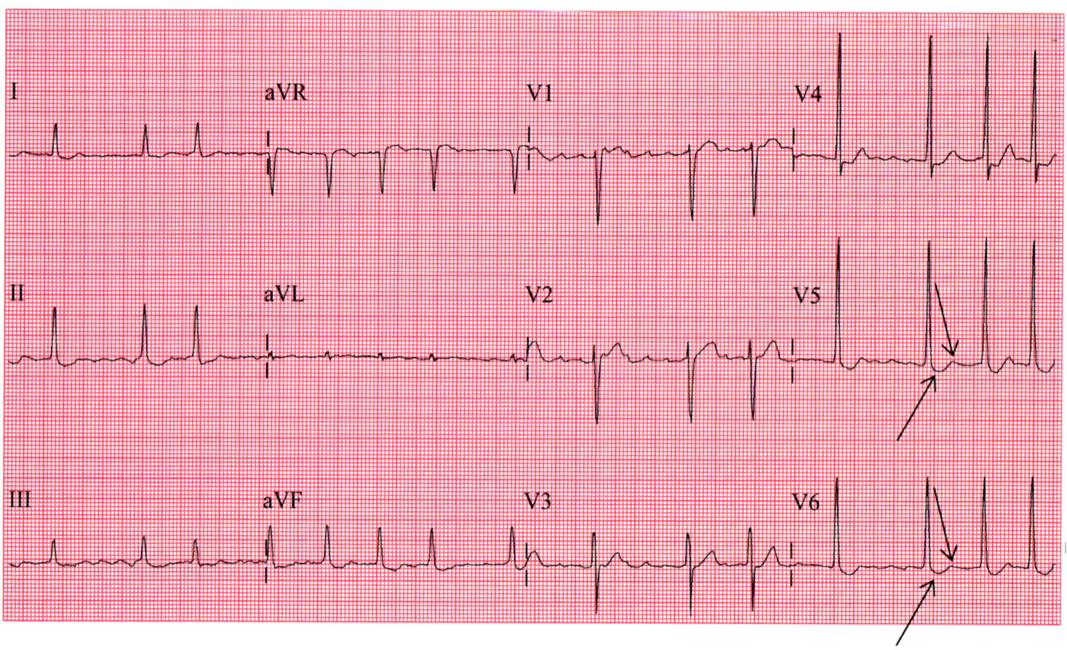

FIGURE 10.14. A 12-lead ECG from a 71-year-old woman on long-term digitalis management for atrial fibrillation. Arrows, coved ST segments and flattened T waves.

Occasionally, the ST-J point is depressed, mimicking subendocardial myocardial ischemia. **Figure 10.15** illustrates this mimicry of subendocardial myocardial ischemia from a patient with congestive heart failure. The ECG changes, including ST-segment depression, developed at the time of administering digitalis loading doses. This extreme example of digitalis effect is usually seen only in those leads with tall R waves. In this case, the digitalis effect may be due (at least in part) to repolarization abnormalities seen in the presence of left-ventricular hypertrophy. Another manifestation of digitalis effect is the vagally mediated slowing of AV nodal conduction (see Chapter 18). In sinus rhythm, digitalis causes a slight increase in the PR interval; in atrial fibrillation, digitalis causes a decrease in the ventricular rate.

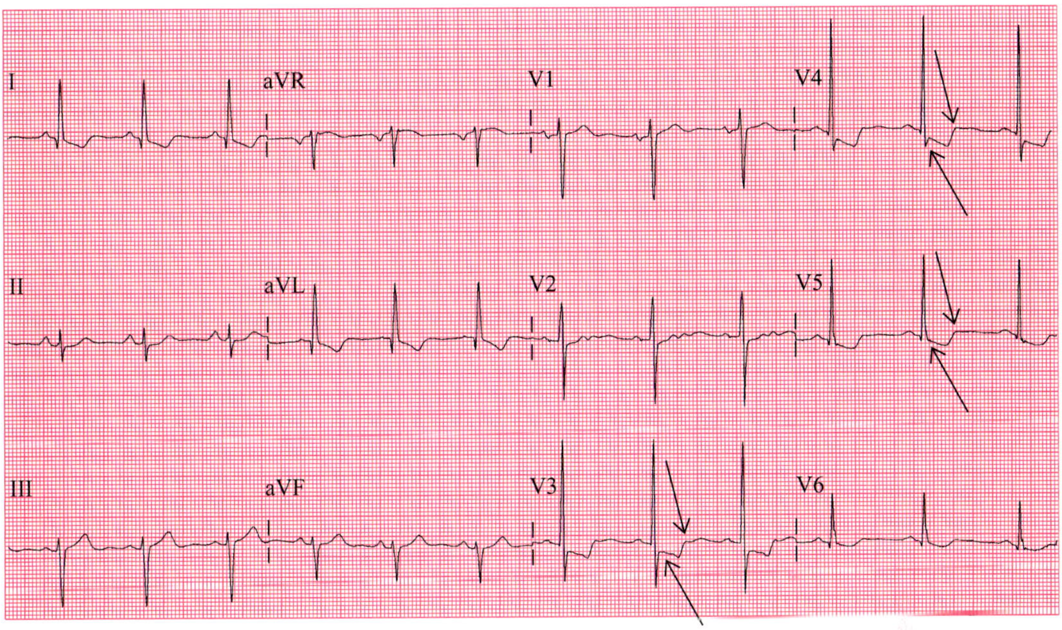

FIGURE 10.15. A 12-lead ECG from a 77-year-old woman with congestive heart failure. The ECG changes, including ST-segment depression, developed at the time of administration of the digitalis loading dosages. Arrows, marked ST-segment depression with decreased T wave amplitude.

Ivabradine

Ivabradine reduces the heart rate by inhibiting the HCN channel-mediated pacemaker current (I_f) in the sinoatrial node. It can be used in heart failure and inappropriate sinus tachycardia. It may cause bradycardia that is usually asymptomatic and can prolong the PR interval.

Adenosine

Adenosine is an activator of the adenosine 1 (A1) receptor chiefly located in the atrioventricular (AV) node. It also shortens the atrial effective refractory period. It is used in the termination of the AV node–dependent tachycardias and can cause sinus bradycardia, apart from the intended AV block.

CHAPTER 10 SUMMARY ILLUSTRATION

Electrolyte Abnormalities

Hypokalemia

- Flat/inverted/notched T waves, prominent U waves, prolonged QTc
- Increased P wave amplitude and width, PR prolongation
- Premature beats and tachyarrhythmia (torsades de pointes)

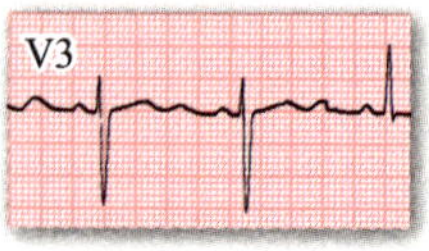

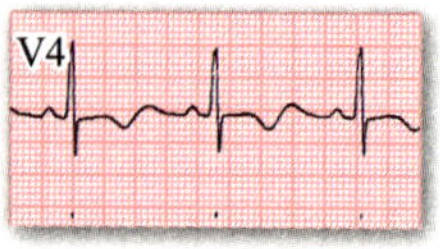

Hyperkalemia

- Tall, peaked T waves
- P wave flattening, PR prolongation, sine wave appearance

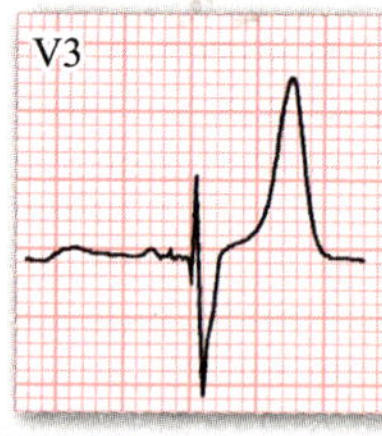

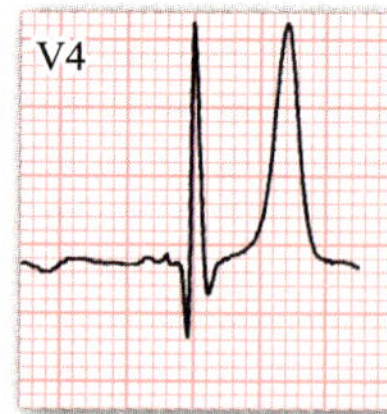

Hypocalcemia

Prolonged QTc, potential inverted T waves

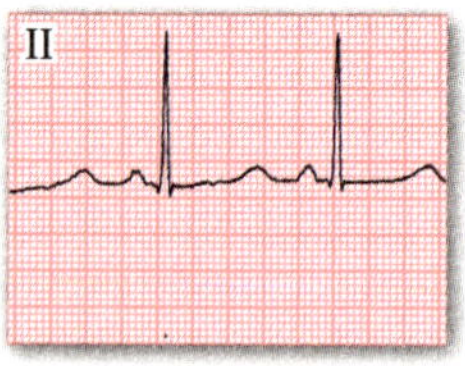

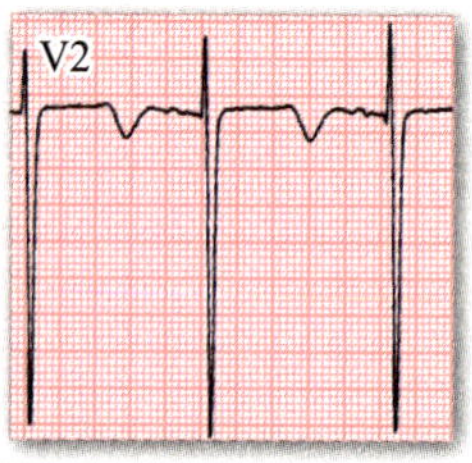

Hypercalcemia

Short QTc, biphasic T waves in some leads

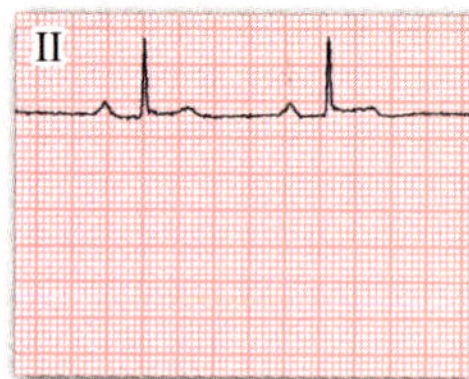

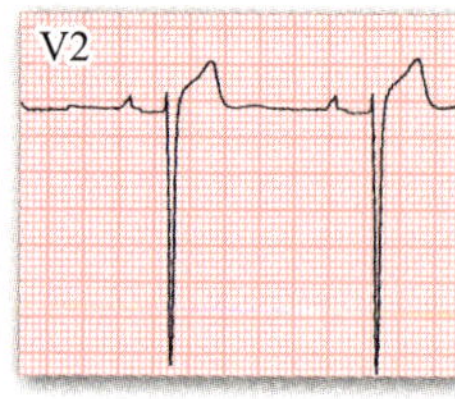

Drug Effects

Quinidine

- Prolonged QTc
- Decreased T-wave amplitude and increased U-wave amplitude
- (QRS prolongation)

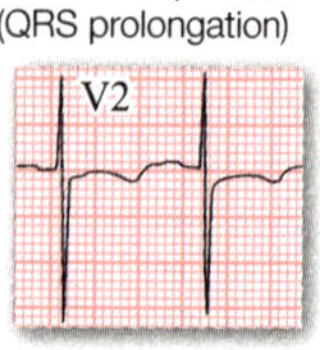

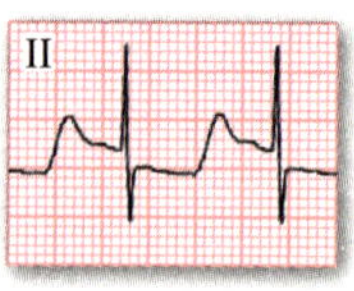

Lidocaine

- Usually unaltered
- (QTc shortening)

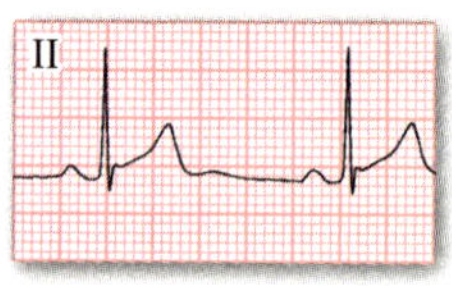

Dofetilide

- Prolonged QTc
- Decreased T-wave amplitude and increased U-wave amplitude

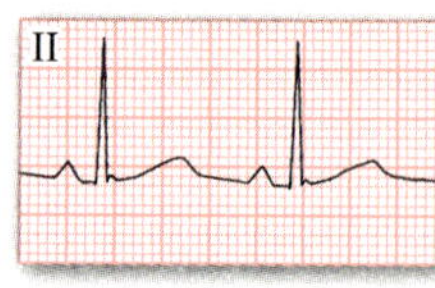

Sotalol

- Slow heart rate
- Prolonged QTc
- Decreased T-wave amplitude and increased U-wave amplitude

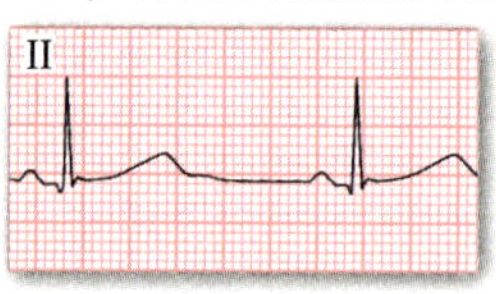

Diltiazem

- Slow heart rate
- PR prolongation/AV-block
- This patient developed second-degree AV block (Wenckebach or type I Mobitz)

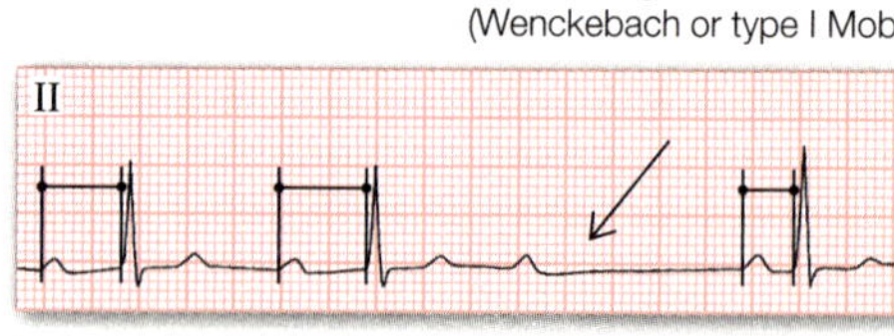

Digitalis

- "Coved" ST-segment depression
- T-wave flattening
- Decreased QTc
- (ST-J depression)

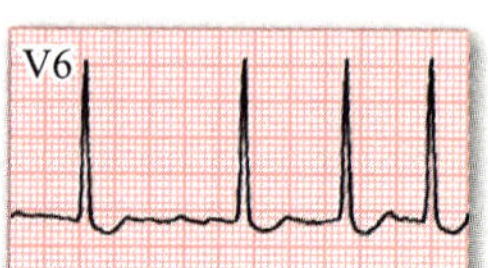

Torsades de Pointes

- Prolonged QTc in sinus beats
- Short-long-short R-R interval cycle prior to initiation
- Twisting of QRS complexes around isoelectric line
- High heart rate once torsades de pointes initiates
- Prolonged QRS

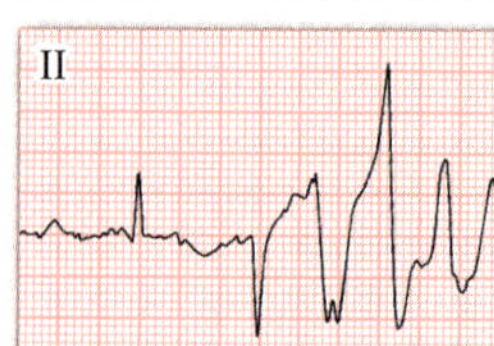

Abbreviation: AV, atrioventricular.

Glossary

Amiodarone: a drug possessing characteristics of several of the Vaughan Williams classes (I, II, III) and clinical usefulness in several types of tachyarrhythmias, both supraventricular and ventricular.

Arrhythmia: any cardiac rhythm other than regular sinus rhythm.

Atrial fibrillation: the arrhythmia produced by multiple circuits in the atria and characterized by irregular multiform F waves.

Digitalis: a drug that occurs naturally in the foxglove plant and is used both to increase contraction of the cardiac muscle and decrease conduction through the AV node.

Diltiazem: a drug that is a nondihydropyridine calcium channel blocker and can decrease heart rate, block conduction in the AV node, lower high blood pressure, and relieve angina pectoris.

Dofetilide: a drug that prolongs repolarization and is used for rhythm control in treating atrial fibrillation or atrial flutter.

Hypercalcemia: an abnormally increased level of serum calcium (Ca^{++}), with a serum Ca^{++} concentration >10.5 mg/100 mL.

Hyperkalemia: an abnormally increased level of serum potassium (K^+), with a serum K^+ concentration >5 mEq/L.

Hypocalcemia: an abnormally decreased level of Ca^{++}, with a serum Ca^{++} concentration <8.5 mg/100 mL.

Hypokalemia: an abnormally decreased level of K^+, with a serum K^+ concentration <3.5 mEq/L.

Osborn waves: abnormal ECG waveforms caused by hypothermia and sometimes seen in cases of extreme hypercalcemia.

Procainamide: a compound related to the local anesthetic procaine that is used in the treatment of reentrant tachyarrhythmias.

Quinidine: a drug that occurs naturally in the bark of the cinchona tree and prolongs myocardial recovery time and protects against some tachyarrhythmias. Quinidine and other related drugs, however, may also produce tachyarrhythmias by marked prolongation of recovery time.

Sotalol: a drug that prolongs repolarization and can be used to treat ventricular tachycardia, atrial fibrillation, and atrial flutter. Sotalol also slows the heart rate due to its β-adrenergic-blocking properties.

Torsades de pointes: a variety of ventricular tachycardia resulting from marked prolongation of the ventricular recovery time. The term is French for "twisting of the points" or of the directions of the QRS complexes in groups that alternate between positive and negative orientation.

Disclaimer

This book chapter reflects the views of the authors and should not be construed to represent the US Food and Drug Administration's views or policies.

References

1. Salerno DM, Asinger RW, Elsperger J, Ruiz E, Hodges M. Frequency of hypokalemia after successfully resuscitated out-of-hospital cardiac arrest compared with that in transmural acute myocardial infarction. *Am J Cardiol.* 1987;59:84-88.
2. Surawicz B. The interrelationship of electrolyte abnormalities and arrhythmias. In: Mandel WJ, ed. *Cardiac Arrhythmias: Their Mechanisms, Diagnosis, and Management.* Philadelphia, PA: JB Lippincott; 1980:83.
3. Krikler DM, Curry PV. Torsade de pointes, an atypical ventricular tachycardia. *Br Heart J.* 1976;38:117-120.
4. Surawicz B. Relationship between electrocardiogram and electrolytes. *Am Heart J.* 1967;73:814-834.
5. Ettinger PO, Regan TJ, Oldewurtel HA. Hyperkalemia, cardiac conduction, and the electrocardiogram: a review. *Am Heart J.* 1974;88:360-371.
6. Sekiya S, Ichikawa S, Tsutsumi T, Harumi K. Nonuniform action potential durations at different sites in canine left ventricle. *Jpn Heart J.* 1983;24:935-945.
7. Bashour TT. Spectrum of ventricular pacemaker exit block owing to hyperkalemia. *Am J Cardiol.* 1986;57:337-338.
8. Nierenberg DW, Ransil BJ. Q-aTc interval as a clinical indicator of hypercalcemia. *Am J Cardiol.* 1979;44:243-248.
9. Douglas PS, Carmichael KA, Palevsky PM. Extreme hypercalcemia and electrocardio-

graphic changes. *Am J Cardiol.* 1984;54: 674-675.
10. Sridharan MR, Horan LG. Electrocardiographic J wave of hypercalcemia. *Am J Cardiol.* 1984; 54:672-673.
11. Vaughan Williams EM. Classification of antiarrhythmic drugs. In: Sandoe E, Flensted-Jensen E, Olsen KH, eds. *Cardiac Arrhythmias.* Sodertalje, Sweden: Astra; 1970:449-472.
12. Roden DM. Drug-induced prolongation of the QT interval. *N Engl J Med.* 2004;350: 1013-1022.
13. Watanabe Y, Dreifus LS. Interactions of quinidine and potassium on atrioventricular transmission. *Circ Res.* 1967;20:434-446.
14. PhysioNet. ECG effects of dofetilide, moxifloxacin, dofetilide+mexiletine, dofetilide+lidocaine and moxifloxacin+diltiazem in healthy subjects. PhysioNet Web site. https://physionet.org/physiobank/database/ecgdmmld/. Accessed June 7, 2019.
15. PhysioNet. ECG effects of ranolazine, dofetilide, verapamil, and quinidine in healthy subjects. PhysioNet Web site. https://physionet.org/physiobank/database/ecgrdvq/. Accessed June 7, 2019.
16. Telemetric and Holter ECG Warehouse. E-OTH-12-0068-010. Cardiac patients with and without a history of drug-induced torsades de pointes. Telemetric and Holter ECG Warehouse Web site. http://thew-project.org/Database/E-OTH-12-0068-010.html. Accessed June 7, 2019.
17. Telemetric and Holter ECG Warehouse. E-OTH-12-0006-009. Recorded "torsades de pointes" event. Telemetric and Holter ECG Warehouse Web site. http://thew-project.org/Database/E-OTH-12-0006-009.html. Accessed June 7, 2019.
18. PhysioNet. CiPA ECG Validation Study. PhysioNet Web site. https://physionet.org/physiobank/database/ecgcipa/. Accessed June 7, 2019.

Reference to the South Asian Edition

A. Lei M, Wu L, Terrar DA, Christopher L, Huang H. Modernized classification of cardiac antiarrhythmic drugs. *Circulation.* 2018;138:1879–1896.

To view digital content associated with this chapter please access lww.co.in. Instructions are located on the inside front cover.

11 Miscellaneous Conditions

DOUGLAS D. SCHOCKEN, TOBIN H. LIM,
DAVID G. STRAUSS, NATARAJAN K U,
AND NISCHAL HEGDE

Introduction

This chapter concludes the section on abnormal wave morphology by presenting various miscellaneous cardiac and noncardiac conditions whose diagnosis may be established or confirmed by interpretation of the electrocardiogram (ECG). This chapter begins with the nonischemic cardiomyopathies.

The subsequent sections include the ECG waveform changes associated with abnormalities of the pericardial lining of the heart and abnormalities related to lungs. Conditions affecting other parts of the body, including the brain and endocrine glands, are considered in the final section.

Cardiomyopathies

Cardiomyopathy is a general term applied to all heart muscle disease. The primary diagnostic classifications of cardiomyopathy are dilated and nondilated or hypertrophic. They may also be classified as "ischemic" and "nonischemic" depending on the role of coronary artery disease in their etiology. Emphasis in this chapter is placed on ECG findings in nondilated and hypertrophic cardiomyopathy. Ischemic cardiomyopathy may either be potentially reversible (hibernation) or irreversible (infarction). The ECG changes of ischemia, injury, and infarction are discussed in Chapters 6 to 9.

Hypertrophic cardiomyopathy is a common nonischemic cardiomyopathy that occurs when a hypertrophied ventricle either fails to maintain or interferes with normal function. The hypertrophy may either be secondary to pressure overload (see Chapter 4) or may be a primary cardiac condition. Primary hypertrophic cardiomyopathy may involve both ventricles, one entire ventricle, or only a portion of one ventricle.

A common localized variety of this condition is hypertrophic obstructive cardiomyopathy, in which the hypertrophied interventricular septum dynamically obstructs the aortic outflow tract during systole, resulting in subaortic stenosis. Hypertrophic obstructive cardiomyopathy is associated with many different ECG manifestations, few of which are typical and may include arrhythmias (see Chapters 13–20). A spectrum of ECG changes may occur in hypertrophic cardiomyopathy regardless of whether or not the problem is localized to the septum, as illustrated in **Figure 11.1**.[1]

Key Features of Electrocardiogram in Hypertrophic Cardiomyopathy

1. Typical left-ventricular hypertrophy (tall precordial R waves in leads V_2-V_5; see Chapter 4)
2. Deep, narrow Q waves in the leftward-oriented leads (aVL and V6) due to the depolarization vector of hypertrophied septum. This may disappear with the onset of LBBB.
3. Left atrial enlargement (including increased terminal P-wave negativity in lead V_1; see Chapter 4).

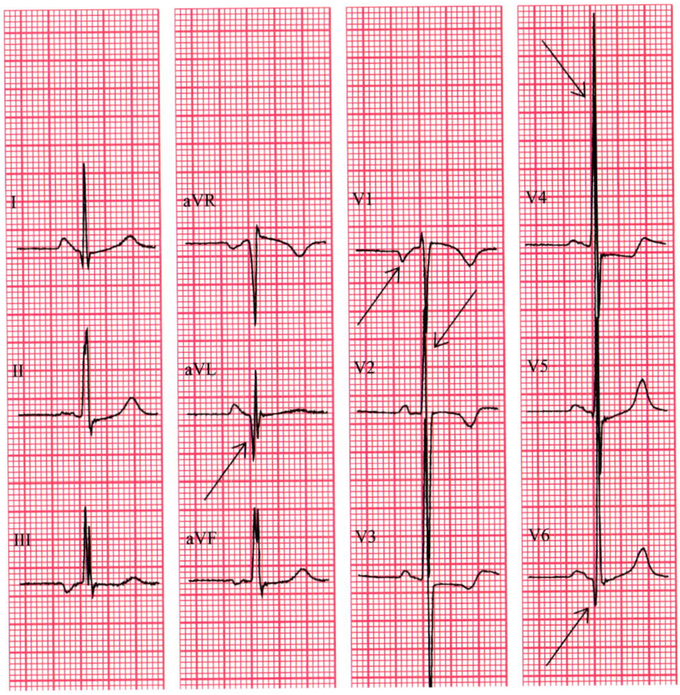

FIGURE 11.1. Arrows, waveforms most characteristic of hypertrophic obstructive cardiomyopathy. ECG shows the following features: 1. Tall 'R' waves in lateral precordial leads with deep 'S' wave in right-oriented leads. 2. Deep narrow 'Q' waves in leads V_6 and aVL, left atrial enlargement (abnormally large terminal negative component of the 'P' wave in lead V_1).

Infiltrative Cardiomyopathy

Infiltration of ventricular (and sometimes atrial) myocardium may also occur with abnormal deposition of pathologic proteins or other substances either displacing or replacing normal myocardial muscle structure. Although the inclusive illnesses causing infiltrative cardiomyopathy are an enormous list, the more common of these include abnormal and misfolded proteins (amyloidosis), granulomas (sarcoidosis), iron (hemochromatosis), dystrophic myocardial muscle (myotonic dystrophy and its variants), and glycosphingolipids (Fabry disease).

Amyloidosis

An abnormally synthesized and misfolded protein called *amyloid* is deposited in the heart during various disease processes. Its accumulation causes cardiac amyloidosis, which eventually may produce sufficient myocardial dysfunction to cause heart failure or serious arrhythmias. Amyloidosis (and other infiltrative diseases of the heart) may be suspected when the following combination of ECG changes appear[2]:

Electrocardiogram Features Suggesting Infiltrative Disease Involving the Heart

1. Low voltage of all waveforms
2. Marked left-axis deviation typical of left-anterior fascicular block
3. Pseudo infarct changes
4. A prolonged atrioventricular conduction time
5. Intraventricular conduction delay (left-bundle-branch block, right-bundle-branch block, intraventricular conduction delay [nonspecific])

Features 1 and 3 are apparent in this elderly patient's ECG. The patient has severe heart failure but no history of ischemic heart disease (**Figure 11.2**). Note the low voltage in both limb and precordial leads and pseudo-infarct changes; Q waves are typically seen suggesting both inferior and anterior infarcts. Paradoxically, evidence of left-ventricular hypertrophy on transthoracic echocardiogram along with low voltage on ECG provide an important additional clue to the presence of amyloidosis.

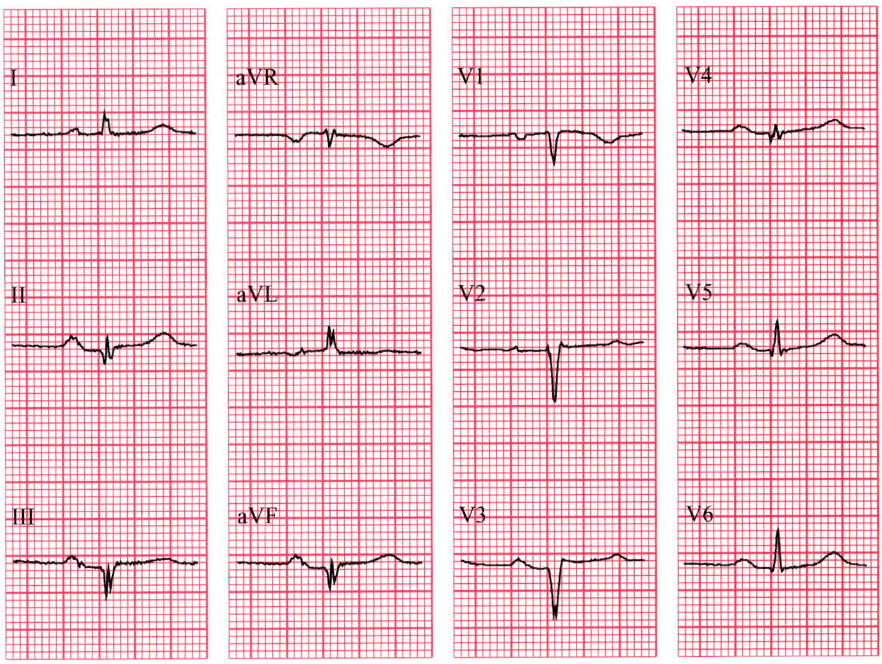

FIGURE 11.2. Electrocardiogram from an elderly patient with heart failure and no history of ischemic heart disease. ECG shows the following features: 1. Low-voltage complexes. 2. Prolonged PR interval of 240 ms. 3. Notched 'P' wave in lead II and abnormally large terminal negative deflection of 'P' in lead V_1, suggesting left atrial enlargement. 4. Poor 'R' wave progression from V_1 to V_3 and 'Q' wave in inferior and anterior leads (pseudo-infarct pattern).

Pericardial Abnormalities

A small, fluid-filled space called the *pericardial sac* separates the heart from the other structures in the thorax. The sac is lined by two layers of connective tissue referred to as the *pericardium*. The innermost of these two layers (visceral pericardium) adheres to the myocardium, and the outer layer (parietal pericardium) encloses the pericardial fluid. These two layers of tissue can become inflamed for many reasons (*pericarditis*). The inflammation usually resolves after an acute phase but may progress to a chronic phase. The acute phase may be complicated by the collection of excess pericardial fluid, a condition termed *pericardial effusion*. Chronic persistence of the inflammatory process may result in thickening and calcification of the pericardial tissues and is called *constrictive pericarditis*.

Acute Pericarditis

Typically, acute pericarditis persists for 3 or 4 weeks, and the ECG changes it produces evolve through two stages. The recordings in **Figure 11.3** are from a patient presenting with the chest pain of acute pericarditis (**Figure 11.3A**) and returning to the clinic 1 month later (**Figure 11.3B**). The characteristic ECG abnormality during the earliest stage of acute pericarditis is *elevation of the ST segments in many leads*, accompanied by upright T waves (see **Figure 11.3A**). *Depression of the PR segment*[3] was also present in half of a series of consecutive patients with acute pericarditis.[4] The ST-segment elevation of acute pericarditis may, however, be confined to only a few leads when the pericarditis is localized such as immediately following open heart surgery. When the ST segments return to the isoelectric level, the ECG may appear normal (see **Figure 11.3B**). In the later phase of recovery from acute pericarditis, the ST segments may return to normal with T-wave inversions that persist for weeks or even months.

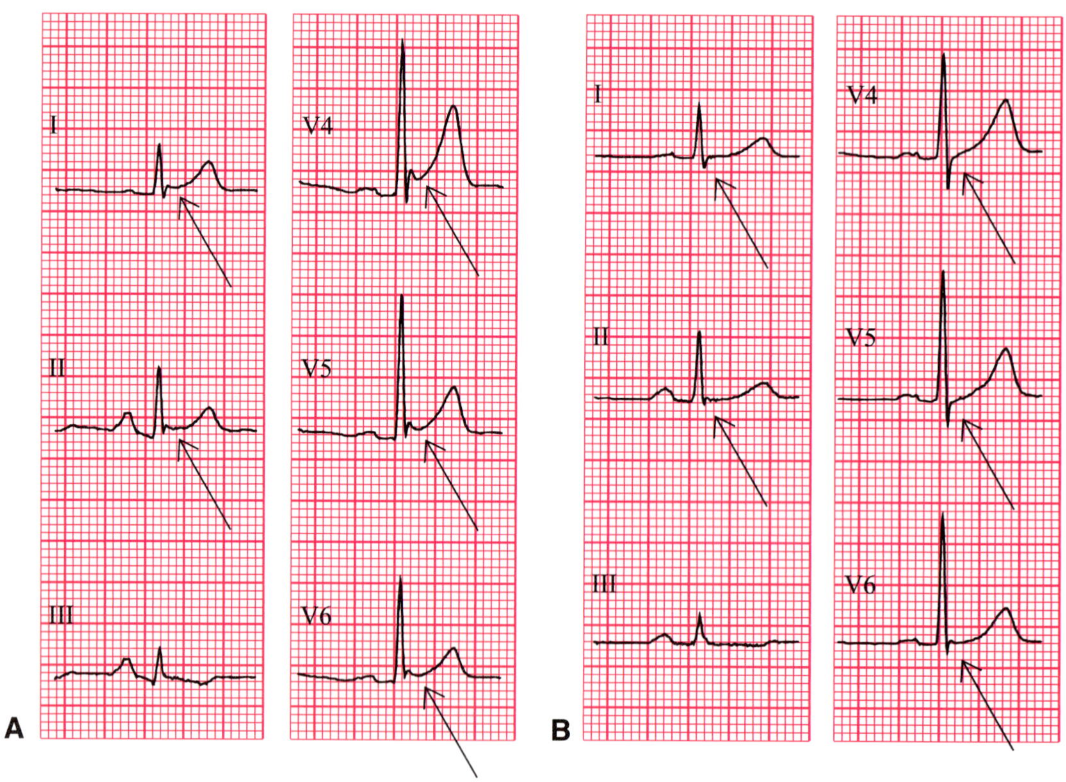

FIGURE 11.3. **A.** Arrows, concave-upward ST-segment elevation with PR-segment depression with tall upright 'T' waves typical of acute pericarditis. **B.** Arrows, resolution of ST-segment and PR segment to isoelectric line after recovery from acute pericarditis.

The differential diagnosis of acute precordial chest pain is quite broad. This differential includes myocardial ischemia; acute pericarditis; acute pulmonary embolism; acute aortic dissection; pneumonia; pleuritis; musculoskeletal injury; ionizing radiation injury; and acute disorders of the esophagus, stomach, gall bladder, and mediastinum. The ECG often plays a crucial role in narrowing this differential diagnosis.

The ST-segment elevation in the first stage of acute pericarditis occurs because the inflammation also involves the immediately adjacent epicardial layer of myocardium, producing an epicardial "injury current" similar to transmural myocardial ischemia discussed in Chapters 6-9. When the epicardial injury is caused by insufficient myocardial perfusion (ie, ischemia), the ST-segment elevation is restricted to the ECG leads that overlie the myocardial region supplied by the obstructed coronary artery. Because pericarditis usually involves the entire epicardium, there is ST-segment elevation in all of the standard leads that are positive leftward and anteriorly and with ST depression in lead aVR. Differentiation between acute pericarditis and acute myocardial ischemia becomes difficult when the pericarditis is localized, creating ST-segment elevation in only a few leads. With ischemia, however, the reciprocal ST-segment shifts seen in the opposite leads are sometimes more marked than those encountered with acute pericarditis.

Figure 11.4 illustrates such an example with a 12-lead ECG from a woman with breast carcinoma and acute chest pain. In both acute pericarditis and acute myocardial infarction, the patient may present with precordial pain. Additional clinical evaluation is necessary to reach the appropriate diagnosis. Serial ECG recordings are extremely useful because the acute epicardial injury current of decreased coronary flow is transient and resolves when the region is either infarcted or reperfused, but the changes of pericarditis persist (without the appearance of new Q waves) until the inflammation resolves.

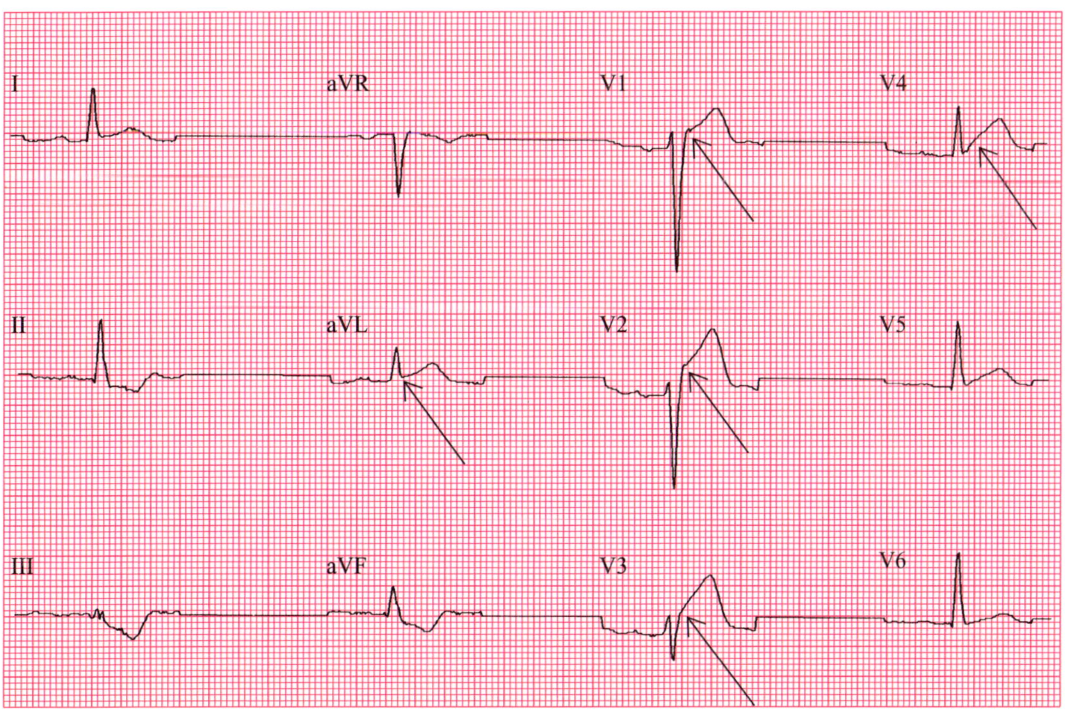

FIGURE 11.4. Electrocardiogram demonstrating findings with acute pericarditis. Arrows, leads with ST-segment elevation. Concave-upward ST-segment elevation with PR-segment depression favors acute pericarditis.

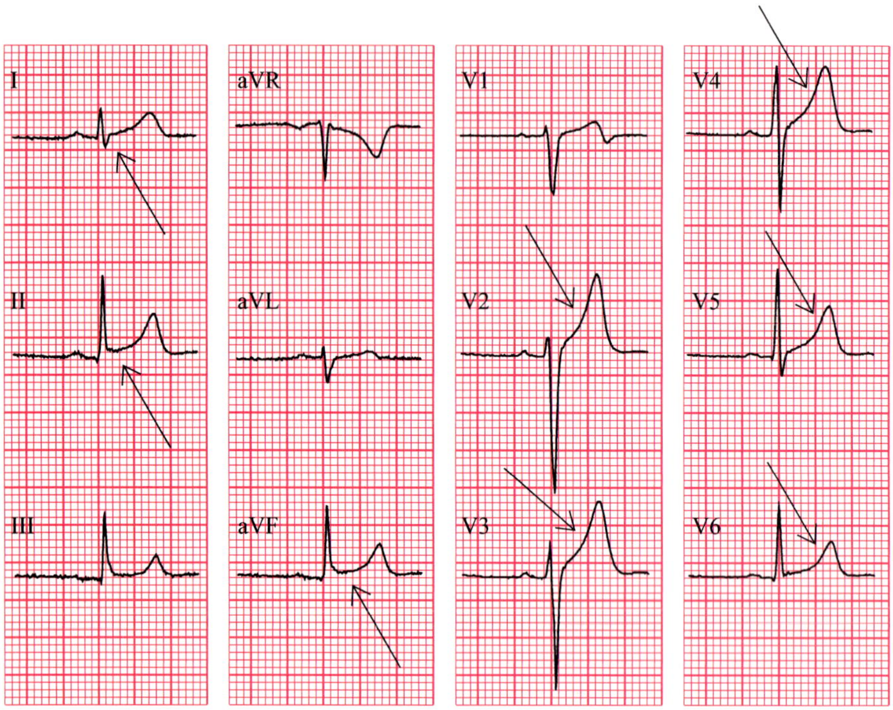

FIGURE 11.5. Acute pericarditis or early repolarization? Arrows, multiple leads with ST-segment elevation. However, absence of PR-segment depression favors early repolarization. Sinus tachycardia is often present in acute pericarditis.

Acute pericarditis also often resembles the normal variant termed *early repolarization* discussed in Chapter 3. **Figure 11.5** presents a typical example of a routine 12-lead ECG recorded from a healthy young man that could represent either early repolarization or the first stage of acute pericarditis. Astute precordial auscultation might disclose a pericardial rub in the latter condition.

A factor on this example that favors a diagnosis of acute pericarditis is the widespread ST elevation, but other factors that favor early repolarization are the increased T-wave amplitudes in several leads and absence of PR depression. This tracing emphasizes the point that it is often not possible to distinguish these very different conditions on the ECG alone. This situation often contributes to a common clinical conundrum requiring more data, more follow-up ECGs, and well-reasoned analysis.

Pericardial Effusion and Chronic Constriction

Small and even moderate amounts of pericardial effusion or constriction may have little or no effect on the ECG. However, a generalized decrease in all of the ECG waveform amplitudes (low voltage) occurs if significant pericardial effusion or thickening develops. These changes probably occur because the cardiac electrical impulses are dampened by the pericardial fluid or fibrotic thickening. Because both of these pathologic conditions have similar effects on the cardiac electrical activity and its transmission to the body surface, they are considered together.

Electrocardiogram Changes Diagnostic of Pericardial Effusion

1. Low voltage
2. Widespread ST-segment elevation or depression
3. Total electrical alternans in cardiac tamponade or large pericardial effusions

These changes are observed in ECG leads V_1 and V_3 recorded from a patient with carcinoma of the lung and malignant pericardial effusion (**Figure 11.6**). *Total electrical alternans* refers to the alternating high and low voltages of all ECG waveforms between cardiac cycles within a given lead.[5,6] One cause of the electrical alternans with large pericardial effusions is thought to be due to the "swinging heart" movement within the massive effusion during successive cardiac cycles. Under these circumstances, progressive restriction of cardiac filling may cause a fall in cardiac output and blood pressure known as *cardiac tamponade.* This problem is a medical emergency requiring immediate removal of pericardial fluid to restore cardiac pumping function.

In addition to these ECG effects, *chronic constrictive pericarditis* may be accompanied by the T-wave inversion characteristic of the second stage of acute pericarditis.[7]

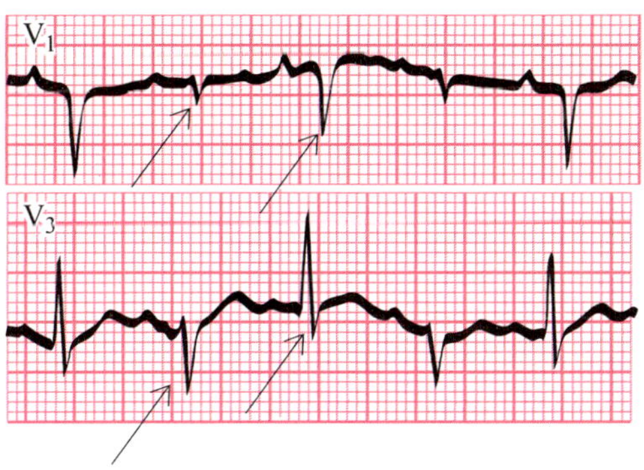

FIGURE 11.6. Electrocardiogram from patient with large pericardial effusion. Arrows, markedly different P-wave and QRS complex waveforms alternating on consecutive cycles.

Pulmonary Abnormalities

When a pulmonary abnormality creates an increased resistance to blood flow from the right side of the heart, systolic or pressure overload (pulmonary hypertension) develops (see Chapter 4). This condition has been termed *cor pulmonale*. This problem can occur either acutely or chronically. The most common cause of acute pulmonary hypertension is pulmonary embolism. Chronic cor pulmonale may be produced by the pulmonary congestion that occurs with left ventricular failure or by the pulmonary hypertension that develops either as a primary disease or as a secondary disease to chronic obstructive pulmonary disease or recurrent pulmonary embolism. Right atrial enlargement (see Chapter 4) commonly occurs with acute and chronic cor pulmonale. In the acute condition, there is right-ventricular (RV) dilation, whereas in the chronic condition, right-ventricular hypertrophy (RVH) occurs and then RV dilatation. Because chronic RVH is discussed in detail in Chapter 4, only acute cor pulmonale is addressed here (see below).

Chronic obstructive pulmonary disease is often characterized by emphysema, in which the lungs become overinflated. This process produces anatomic changes that affect the ECG in unique ways. The ECG changes of pulmonary emphysema may occur alone or in combination with the changes of RVH because emphysema may or may not be accompanied by the obstruction of the airways. When carbon dioxide is unable to be eliminated through the tracheal-bronchial system due to air trapping in the bronchoalveolar bed damaged by emphysema, the resultant hypercapnia (elevated systemic carbon dioxide levels) and respiratory acidosis cause the pulmonary arterial constriction leading to the compensatory RVH that is also termed *chronic cor pulmonale*.

Acute Cor Pulmonale: Pulmonary Embolism

Acute cor pulmonale in the absence of evidence of the changes of RVH owing to chronic cor pulmonale is most commonly seen in pulmonary embolism. Acute cor pulmonale can occur in the presence or absence of chronic changes of RVH. The ECG changes considered here are those in the absence of RVH. The RV distortion produced by an acute outflow obstruction such as pulmonary embolism causes delayed conduction through the right bundle and/or the RV myocardium, resulting in the ECG pattern of incomplete (or even complete) right-bundle-branch block (RBBB) (see Chapter 5). This RV conduction delay shifts the waveforms away from both the inferior (limb leads) and anterior (chest leads), at times mimicking both inferior and anterior infarcts. The shift of the QRS beyond the end of left-ventricular activation produces unopposed late rightward and anterior forces.[8] The rightward direction is represented primarily by an S wave in lead I and the anterior direction by an R′ wave in V_1. In addition, note both the presence of new sinus tachycardia and appearance of diffuse T-wave abnormalities typical of acute pulmonary embolism. **Figure 11.7** presents recordings from before (**Figure 11.7A**) and after (**Figure 11.7B**) sudden dyspnea in an elderly man who had received prostate surgery.

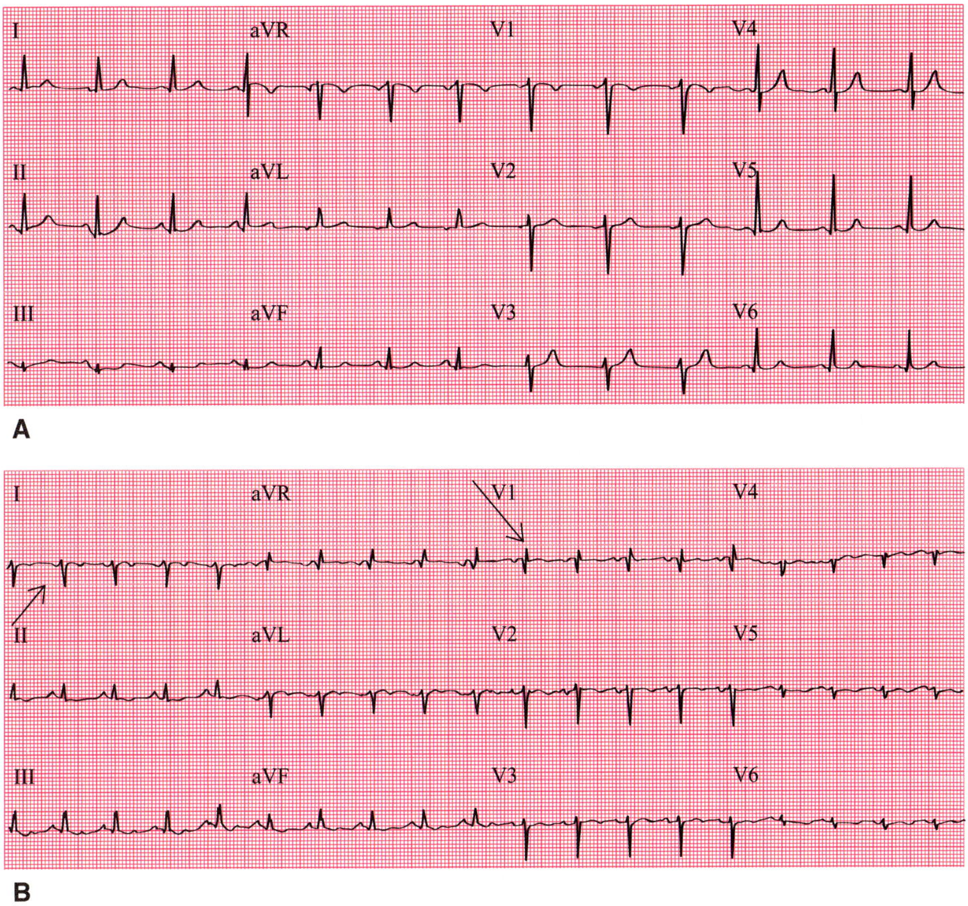

FIGURE 11.7. Sequential electrocardiograms from elderly man. **A.** Preoperative prostate surgery. **B.** Postoperative with acute dyspnea and chest discomfort. Arrows, terminal rightward (I) and anterior (V_1) shift in QRS axis. Other findings here include sinus tachycardia, right-axis deviation, right-ventricular conduction delay, late precordial transition (poor R-wave progression), and diffuse nonspecific T-wave abnormalities.

With acute pulmonary embolism, in the precordial leads, elevated ST segments and inverted T waves are sometimes seen over the right ventricle, whereas S waves may become more prominent over the left ventricle. The typical changes of RBBB may be apparent in lead V_1 (a 12-lead from an elderly woman with a massive pulmonary embolism who exhibits the typical changes of RBBB is illustrated in **Figure 11.8**). All of the ECG changes of the acute cor pulmonale produced by a large pulmonary embolus are seen in **Figure 11.8**. The RBBB is complete with a QRS duration of 120 milliseconds. In addition, there are repolarization changes of T-wave inversion both in leads II, III, and aVF and in leads V_1 through V_4 that accompany RBBB.

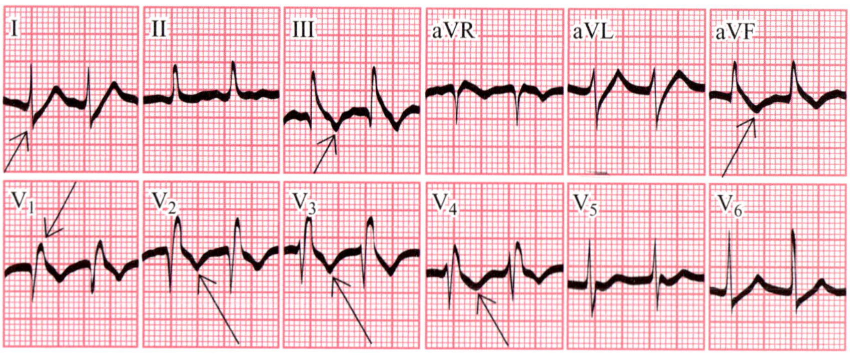

FIGURE 11.8. Electrocardiogram from patient with acute pulmonary embolism. Lead I: arrow, rightward axis shift. Leads II, aVF, and V_2 to V_4: arrows, inverted T waves. Lead V_1: arrow, prominent R′ wave. S1Q3T3 pattern seen ('S' waves in lead I, 'Q' in lead III, and 'T' wave inversion in lead III, typical of acute pulmonary embolism). Incomplete RBBB with 'T' wave inversion is seen in right precordial leads.

Pulmonary Emphysema

Typical Findings in Emphysema[9] With Some Modifications

1. Tall P waves in leads II, III, and aVF
2. Exaggerated atrial repolarization waves producing ≥0.10-mV PR and ST-segment depression in leads II, III, and aVF
3. Rightward shift of the axis of the QRS complex in the frontal plane
4. Decreased progression of the R-wave amplitudes in the precordial leads
5. Low voltage of the QRS complexes, especially in the left precordial leads
6. Vertical orientation of all three major axes (P, QRS, and T)
7. Prominent S waves in leads I, II, and III

Figure 11.9 presents a typical example of pulmonary emphysema with most of these characteristics. Rightward shifts of both the P waves and QRS complexes (negative in lead aVL and only slightly positive in lead I) and a low voltage in the leftward (V_4-V_6) precordial leads are illustrated (see **Figure 11.9**). Note the prominent P waves in II, III, and aVF followed by PR- and ST-segment depression below the TP baseline.

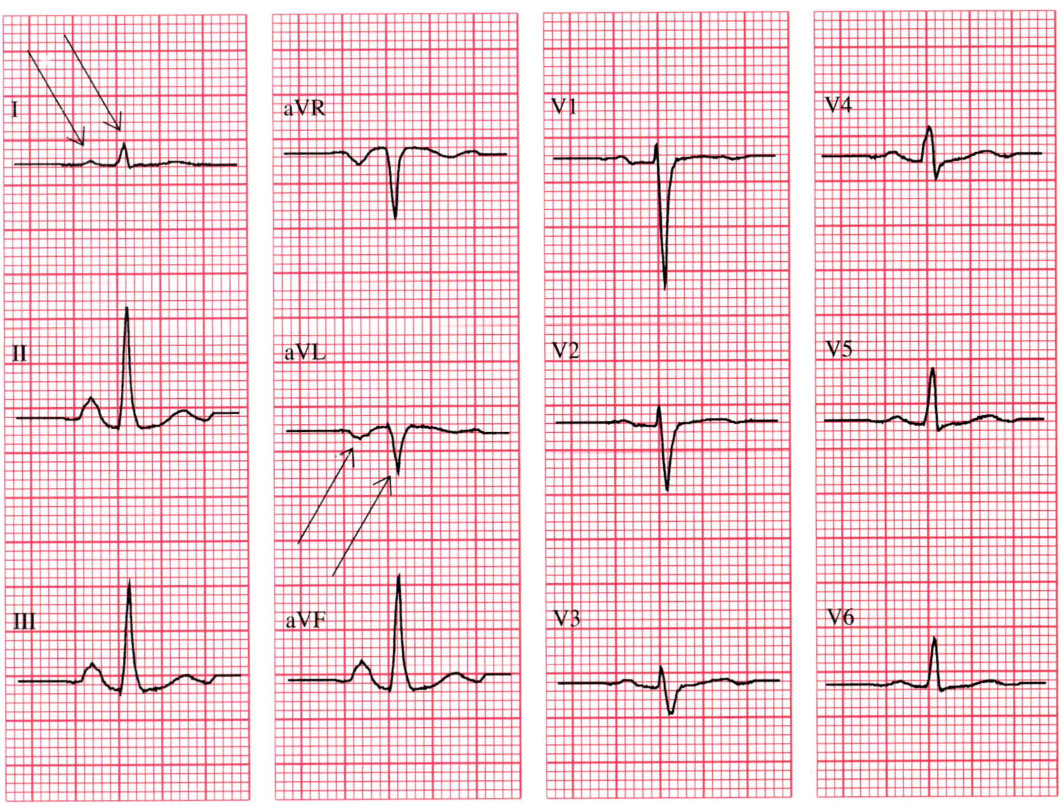

FIGURE 11.9. Electrocardiogram from patient with emphysema. Arrows, rightward axis shift of the P and QRS waveforms.

These ECG changes are produced because the hyperexpanded emphysematous lungs compress the heart, lower the diaphragms, and increase the space between the heart and the recording electrodes. All these effects often produce the vertical downward concordance of the mean axes for all major ECG waves (P, QRS, and T) as seen in the frontal leads, pointing at or close to +90 degrees.

The QRS axis in the frontal plane is occasionally indeterminate (**Figure 11.10**).[10] This occurs because pulmonary emphysema directs the QRS complex posteriorly so that minimal upward or downward deviation swings the frontal plane axis of the complex from +90 degrees to −90 degrees. **Figure 11.10** also illustrates criteria 1, 2, 3, 4, and 7.

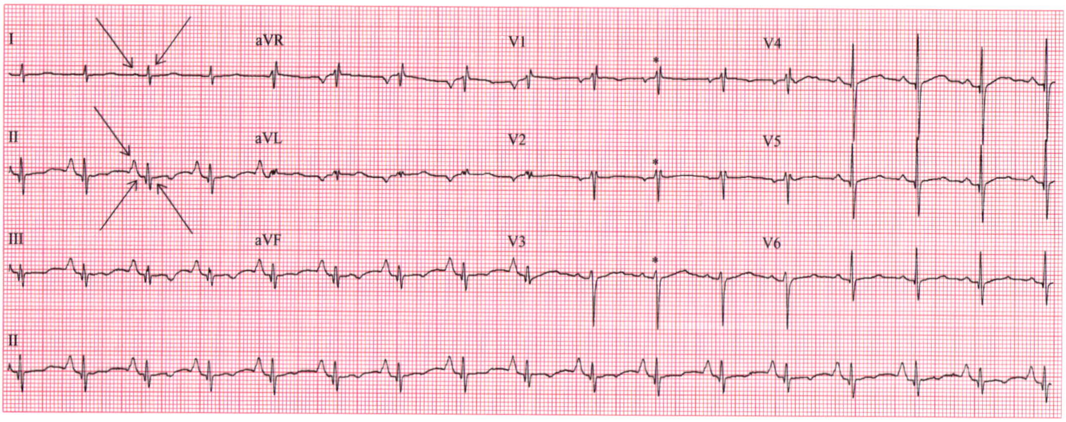

FIGURE 11.10. A 12-lead electrocardiogram recording from a patient with pulmonary emphysema. The arrows in lead I indicate the isoelectric P wave and low-voltage QRS complex, and the arrows in lead II indicate the prominent P wave and PR and ST segments depressed below the TP-segment baseline. Asterisks indicate the absence of properly increased R-wave progression from leads V_1 to V_3.

Selvester and Rubin[11] developed quantitative ECG criteria for both definite and possible emphysema, modified as shown in **Table 11.1**.[12]

These criteria achieve approximately 65% sensitivity for the diagnosis of emphysema and 95% specificity for the exclusion of emphysema in normal control subjects and in patients with congenital heart disease or myocardial infarction.[11] This good performance relative to that of other systems is most likely the result of combining quantitative criteria for the frontal plane P-wave axis with criteria for both the frontal and transverse plane amplitudes of the QRS complex.

Table 11.1.

Electrocardiographic Criteria for Emphysema[a]

Definite Emphysema	Possible Emphysema
A. P axis >+60 degrees in limb leads and either	P axis >+60 degrees in limb leads and either
B. 1. R and S amplitude ≤0.70 mV in limb leads and	1. R and S amplitude ≤0.70 mV in limb leads or
2. R amplitude ≤0.70 mV in V_6 or	2. R amplitude ≤0.70 mV in V_6
C. SV4 ≥ RV4	

Abbreviations: RV4, R wave amplitude in lead V_4; SV4, S wave amplitude in lead V_4.

[a]Reprinted by permission from Springer: Rubin LJ, ed.[12]

Intracranial Hemorrhage

Hemorrhage into either the intracerebral or subarachnoid spaces can produce dramatic changes in the ECG, presumably because of increased intracranial pressure.[13-15] Less severe ECG changes occur with nonhemorrhagic cerebrovascular accidents.[16] The three most common ECG changes in intracranial hemorrhage are the following:

Common Electrocardiogram Changes in Intracranial Hemorrhage

1. Widening and deep inversion of T waves in the precordial leads
2. Prolongation of the QTc interval
3. Bradyarrhythmias

Figure 11.11 presents a 12-lead ECG recording that is a typical example of characteristic 1 above. Additionally, ST elevation or depression can occasionally occur with intracranial hemorrhage, mimicking cardiac ischemia. In some cases, regional wall motion abnormalities are observed in subarachnoid hemorrhage associated with ST elevation, or "neurogenic stunned myocardium."[17] Among less politically correct ECG readers, these deep T-wave inversions have been termed *scrotal T waves*, although the origin of that moniker is (and should remain) obscure.

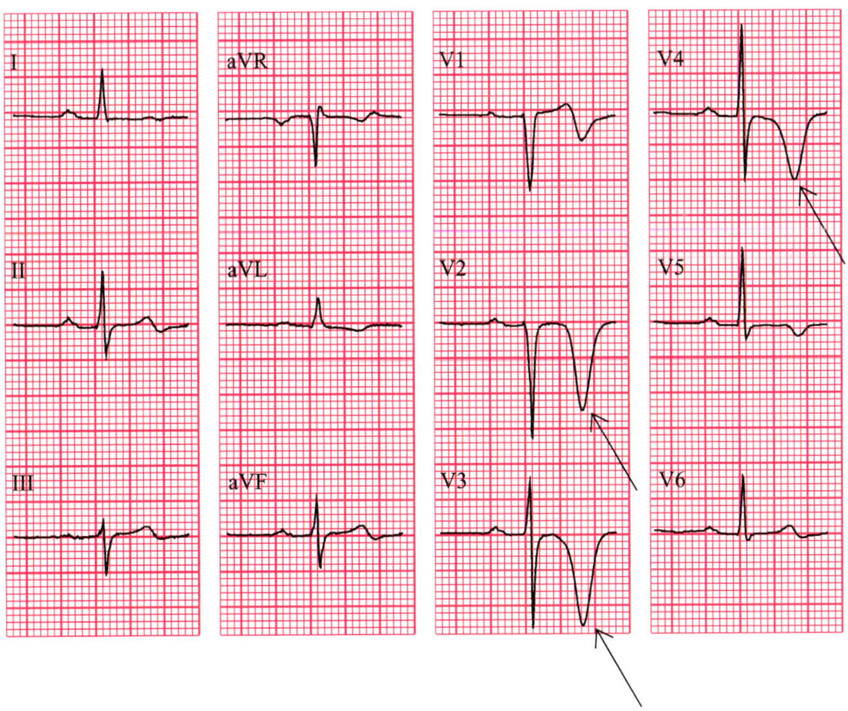

FIGURE 11.11. Electrocardiogram from patient with acute intracranial hemorrhage. Arrows, unusually prominent inverted T waves.

Endocrine and Metabolic Abnormalities

Thyroid Abnormalities

Severe hypothyroidism is termed *myxedema*, and thyroid hormone excess is termed *thyrotoxicosis*. Both conditions are often accompanied by typical changes in ECG waveform morphology. Because the thyroid hormone thyroxin mediates sympathetic nervous activity, hypothyroidism is accompanied by a slowing of the sinus rate (sinus bradycardia). Conversely, the hyperthyroid state is accompanied by an acceleration of the sinus rate (sinus tachycardia).[18] Atrial fibrillation (see Chapter 16) is also a very common manifestation of hyperthyroidism. Similarly, AV conduction may be impaired in hypothyroidism and accelerated in hyperthyroidism.[19]

Hypothyroidism

The diagnosis of hypothyroidism (state of low thyroid function) should be suspected when the following combination of ECG changes is present (**Figure 11.12**):

Electrocardiogram Changes Often Seen in Hypothyroidism

1. Low voltage of all waveforms
2. Inverted T waves without ST-segment deviation in many or all leads
3. Sinus bradycardia

QT prolongation and atrioventricular block or intraventricular conduction delay may also occur. These changes may be related to cardiac deposits of connective tissue typical of myxedema, diminished sympathetic nervous activity, and/or the effect on the myocardium of reduced levels of thyroxin.[20]

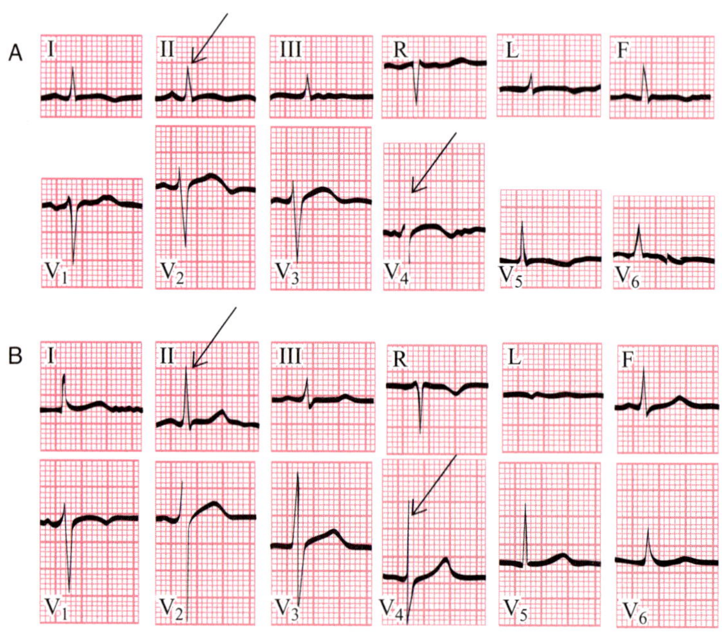

FIGURE 11.12. Electrocardiogram from patient with hypothyroidism, before (**A**) and after (**B**) thyroid replacement therapy. In tracing **A**, note low-voltage QRS (arrows) and nonspecific T-wave abnormalities. In tracing **B**, note the increased QRS voltage (arrows) and normalization of T waves.

Hyperthyroidism

The diagnosis of hyperthyroidism should be suspected when heart rate and the amplitudes of all of the ECG waveforms are increased. This hyperdynamic state stimulates right atrial and left-ventricular enlargement (see Chapter 4). The heart rate is rapid because of the increased levels of thyroxin. The cardiac rhythm may reflect an acceleration of normal sinus impulse formation (sinus tachycardia) or the abnormal atrial tachyarrhythmia known as atrial fibrillation (see Chapter 16). Although the QT interval decreases as the heart rate increases, the corrected QT interval (QTc) may be prolonged.[21]

Hypothermia

Hypothermia has been defined as a rectal temperature of <36°C or <97°F. At these lower temperatures, characteristic ECG changes develop, underscored by the logic that with lower temperatures, things slow down. All intervals of the ECG (including the RR, PR, QRS, and QT intervals) may lengthen. Characteristic Osborn waves appear as deflections at the J point in the same direction as that of the QRS complex.[22] **Figure 11.13** illustrates these changes in an elderly man exposed to cold weather and presented to the hospital with a body temperature of 32.8°C or 91°F.

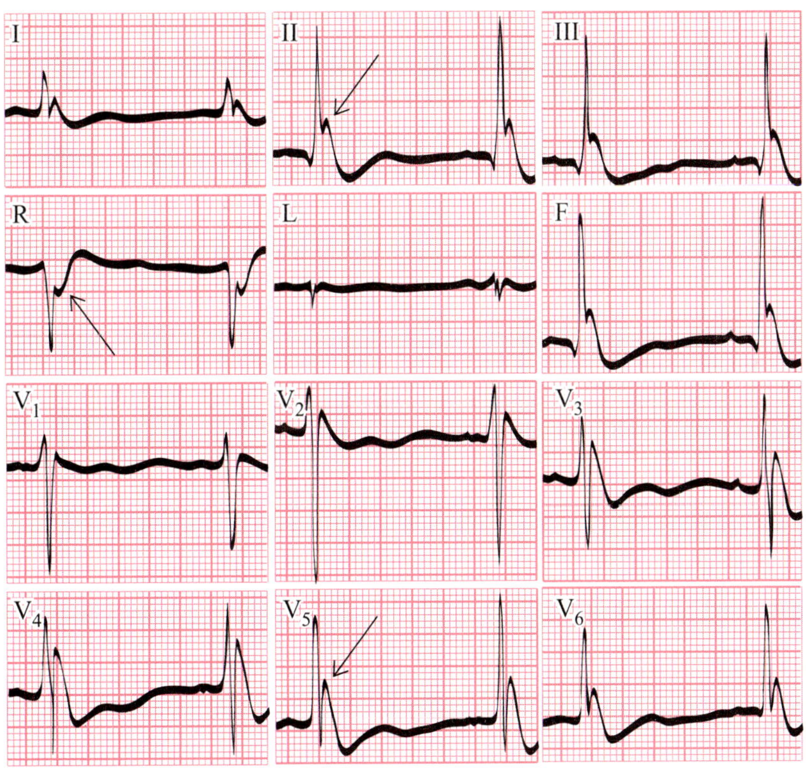

FIGURE 11.13. Electrocardiogram from patient with hypothermia. Arrows, Osborn waves.

Obesity

Obesity has the potential to affect the ECG as noted in the box that follows.

Causes of Electrocardiogram Changes Seen in Obesity

1. Displacing the heart by elevating the diaphragm
2. Increasing cardiac workload
3. Increasing the distance between the heart and the recording electrodes

In a study of >1000 obese individuals, the heart rate, PR interval, QRS interval, QRS voltage, and QTc interval all showed an increase with increasing obesity.[23] The QRS axis also tended to shift leftward. Interestingly, only 4% of this population had low QRS voltage. One study has reported an increased incidence of false-positive criteria for inferior myocardial infarction in both obese individuals and in women in the final trimester of pregnancy (presumably because of diaphragmatic elevation) by visceral adipose tissue or a gravid uterus.[24] One review of this area provides a broader picture of abnormalities that might be encountered with the ECGs of patients with obesity.[25]

Electrocardiogram Changes With Obesity[24]

1. Left shift of all major axes (P, QRS, and T)
2. Increased P-terminal forces in lead V_1
3. Prolongation of the P wave
4. Low QRS voltage
5. Left-ventricular hypertrophy (particularly when criteria are not dependent on precordial voltage)
6. Inferolateral T-wave flattening
7. Prolongation of QTc

CHAPTER 11 SUMMARY ILLUSTRATION

Pericarditis

Acute pericarditis

Diffuse ST-segment elevation, can mimic ST-elevation MI, however does not necessarily localize to a coronary artery region

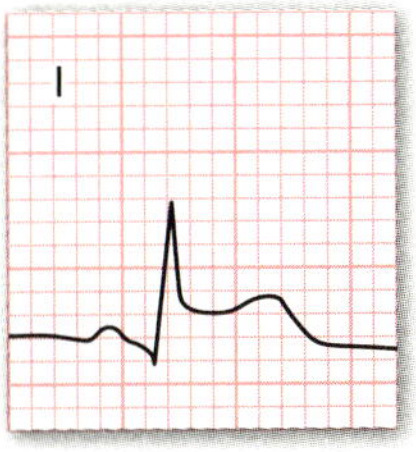

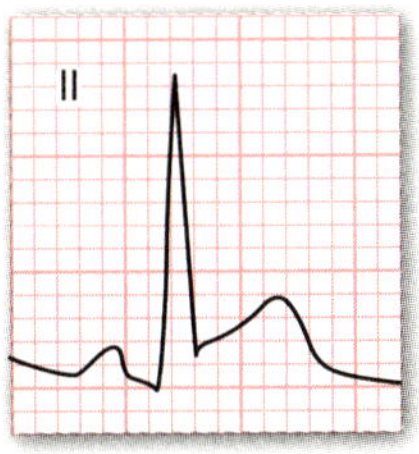

Acute Cor Pulmonale: Pulmonary Embolism

Terminal rightward forces – S in I

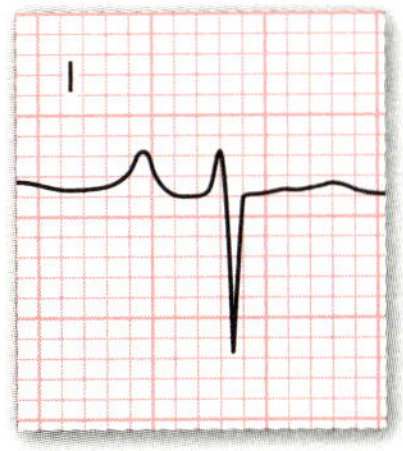

Terminal anterior forces – Late R or R'

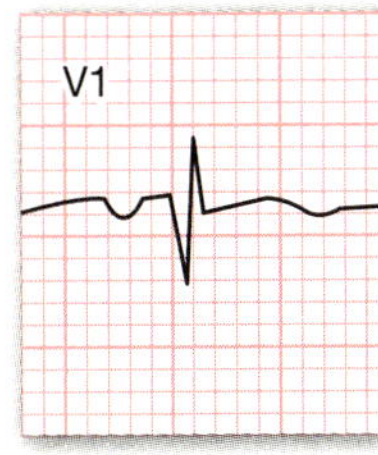

Intracranial hemorrhage

- Prominent inverted T-waves in precordial leads
- Prolonged QTc and bradyarrhythmias

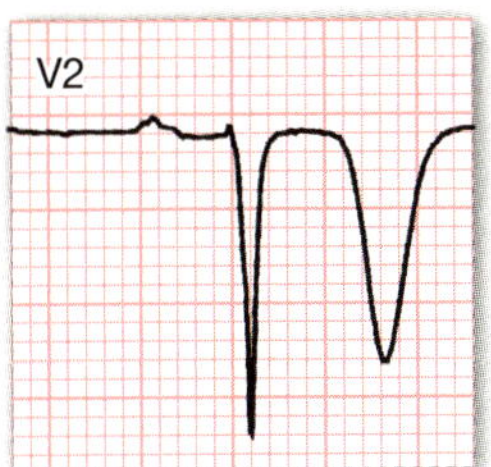

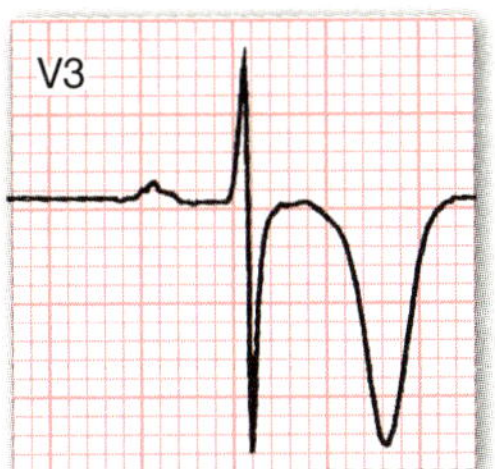

Hypothermia

Osborn wave – elevated J point (in direction of QRS)

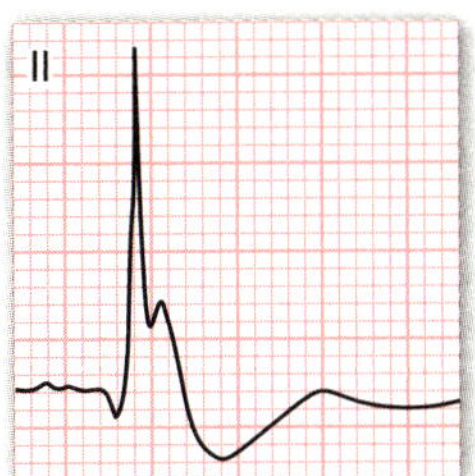

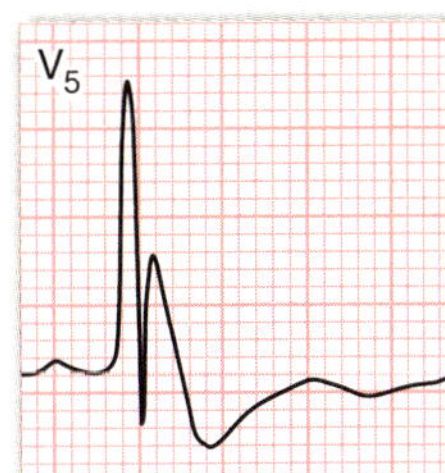

Severe hypothyroidism (myxedema)

Low voltage, inverted T-waves without ST-segment deviation in many leads, sinus bradycardia

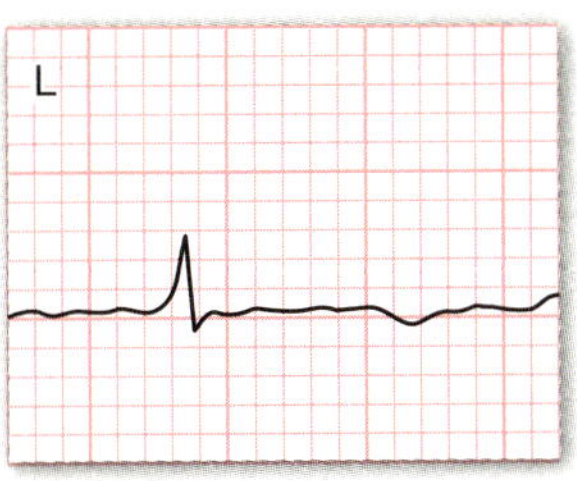

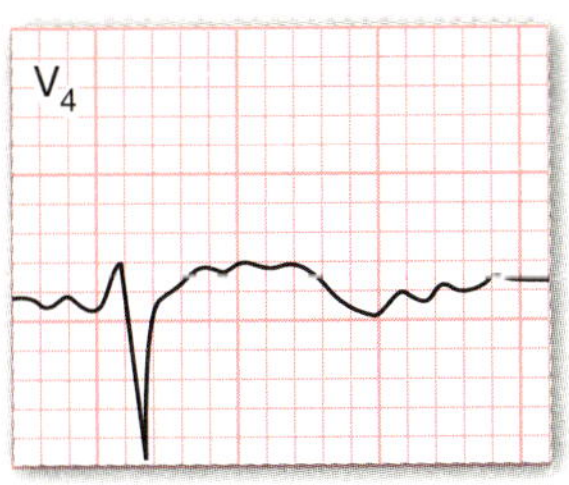

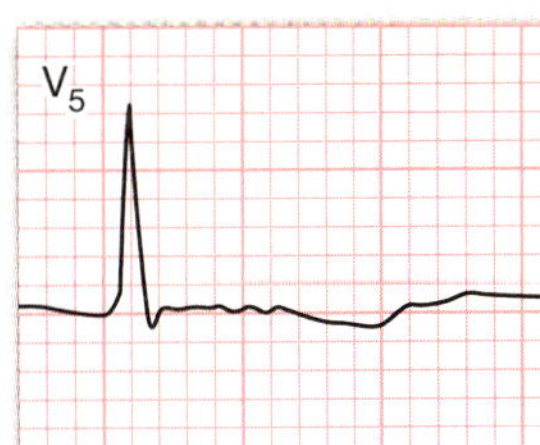

Abbreviation: MI, myocardial infarction.

Glossary

Arrhythmia: any cardiac rhythm other than regular sinus rhythm.

Atrial fibrillation: the tachyarrhythmia at the rapid end of the flutter/fibrillation spectrum produced by macroreentry within multiple circuits in the atria and characterized by irregular multiform F waves. Irregular irregularity is its hallmark.

Constrictive pericarditis: thickening of the pericardium caused by chronic inflammation and resulting in interference with myocardial function, especially in diastole.

Cor pulmonale: an acute or chronic pressure overload of the right side of the heart caused by increased resistance to blood flow through the lungs, characterized by elevated pulmonary artery pressures (pulmonary hypertension). Often caused by chronic obstructive lung disease, acute pulmonary embolism, or left ventricular failure.

Emphysema: a pulmonary disease in which the alveoli are destroyed and the lungs become overinflated.

Hypertrophic cardiomyopathy: a condition in which cardiac function is decreased because of thickened myocardium either obstructing left ventricular outflow or impairing left ventricular diastolic relaxation.

Hypothermia: subnormal temperature of the body defined as temperature <36°C or <97°F.

Low voltage: a total amplitude of the QRS complex that is <0.70 mV in all limb leads and <1.0 mV in all precordial leads.

Myxedema: severe hypothyroidism characterized by a decreased metabolic state, weight gain, coarse voice, firm and inelastic edema; dry skin and hair; and loss of mental and physical vigor.

Osborn waves: abnormal ECG waveforms caused by hypothermia.

Pericardial effusion: an increase in the amount of fluid in the pericardial sac.

Pericardial sac: the fluid-filled space between the two layers of the pericardium.

Pericarditis: acute or chronic inflammation of the pericardium.

Pericardium: the two-layered membrane that encloses the heart and the roots of the great blood vessels.

Pulmonary embolism: the sudden obstruction of a pulmonary artery by a dislodged clot or fat originating from the legs or the pelvic region.

Sinus tachycardia: an acceleration of the normal sinus rhythm beyond the upper limit of 100 beats per minute.

Subaortic stenosis: narrowing of the outflow passage from the left ventricle proximal to the aortic valve to a degree sufficient to obstruct the flow of blood.

Thyrotoxicosis: severe hyperthyroidism characterized by an increased metabolic condition, hyperdynamic state (increased heart rate and blood pressure), sweating, and protruding eyes.

Total electrical alternans: alternation in the amplitudes of all of the ECG waveforms in successive beats in the presence of a regular cardiac cycle lengths, sometimes associated with large pericardial effusions.

Acknowledgment

We gratefully acknowledge the past contributions of the previous edition's author, Dr. Galen S. Wagner, as portions of that chapter were retained in this revision.

References

1. Maron BJ. The electrocardiogram as a diagnostic tool for hypertrophic cardiomyopathy: revisited. *Ann Noninvasive Electrocardiol.* 2001;6:277-279.
2. Cheng Z, Zhu K, Tian Z, Zhao D, Cui Q, Fang Q. The findings of electrocardiography in patients with cardiac amyloidosis. *Ann Noninvasive Electrocardiol.* 2013;18(2): 157-162.
3. Bhardwaj R, Berzingi C, Miller C, et al. Differential diagnosis of acute pericarditis from normal variant early repolarization and left ventricular hypertrophy with early repolarization: an electrocardiographic study. *Am J Med Sci.* 2013;345(1):28-32.
4. Bruce MA, Spodick DH. Atypical electrocardiogram in acute pericarditis: characteristics and prevalence. *J Electrocardiol.* 1980;13: 61-66.
5. Bashour FA, Cochran PW. The association of electrical alternans with pericardial effusion. *Dis Chest.* 1963;44:146-153.
6. Nizet PM, Marriott HJL. The electrocardiogram and pericardial effusion. *JAMA.* 1966;198:169.
7. Dalton JC, Pearson RJ Jr, White PD. Constrictive pericarditis: a review and long-term follow-up of 78 cases. *Ann Intern Med.* 1956;45:445-458.
8. Wasserburger RH, Kelly JR, Rasmussen HK, Juhl JH. The electrocardiographic pentalogy of pulmonary emphysema. A correlation of roentgenographic findings and pulmonary function studies. *Circulation.* 1959;20: 831-841.
9. Ferrari E, Imbert A, Chevalier T, Mihoubi A, Morand P, Baudouy M. The ECG in pulmonary embolism. Predictive value of negative T waves in precordial leads—80 case reports. *Chest.* 1997;111(3):537-543.
10. Thomas AJ, Apiyasawat S, Spodick DH. Electrocardiographic detection of emphysema. *Am J Cardiol.* 2011;107(7):1090-1092.
11. Selvester RH, Rubin HB. New criteria for the electrocardiographic diagnosis of emphysema and cor pulmonale. *Am Heart J.* 1965;69:437-447.
12. Rubin LJ, ed. *Pulmonary Heart Disease.* Boston, MA: Martinus Nijhoff; 1984:122.
13. Burch GE, Meyers R, Abildskov JA. A new electrocardiographic pattern observed in cerebrovascular accidents. *Circulation.* 1954;9:719-723.
14. Hersch C. Electrocardiographic changes in subarachnoid haemorrhage, meningitis, and intracranial space-occupying lesions. *Br Heart J.* 1964;26:785-793.
15. Surawicz B. Electrocardiographic pattern of cerebrovascular accident. *JAMA.* 1966;197:913-914.
16. Fentz V, Gormsen J. Electrocardiographic patterns in patients with cerebrovascular accidents. *Circulation.* 1962;25:22-28.
17. Kono T, Morita H, Kuroiwa T, Onaka H, Takatsuka H, Fujiwara A. Left ventricular wall motion abnormalities in patients with subarachnoid hemorrhage: neurogenic stunned myocardium. *J Am Coll Cardiol.* 1994;24:636-640.
18. Wald DA. ECG manifestations of selected metabolic and endocrine disorders. *Emerg Med Clin North Am.* 2006;24(1):145-157, vii.
19. Vanhaelst L, Neve P, Chailly P, Bastenie PA. Coronary-artery disease in hypothyroidism. Observations in clinical myxoedema. *Lancet.* 1967;2:800-802.
20. Surawicz B, Mangiardi ML. Electrocardiogram in endocrine and metabolic disorders. *Cardiovasc Clin.* 1977;8: 243-266.
21. Harumi K, Ouichi T, eds. Q-T prolongation syndrome [in Japanese]. In: *Naika Mook.* Tokyo, Japan: Kinbara; 1981:210.
22. Okada M, Nishimura F, Yoshino H, Kimura M, Ogino T. The J wave in accidental hypothermia. *J Electrocardiol.* 1983;16:23-28.
23. Frank S, Colliver JA, Frank A. The electrocardiogram in obesity: statistical analysis of 1,029 patients. *J Am Coll Cardiol.* 1986;7: 295-299.
24. Starr JW, Wagner GW, Behar VS, Walston A II, Greenfield JC Jr. Vectorcardiographic criteria for the diagnosis of inferior myocardial infarction. *Circulation.* 1974;49:829-836.
25. Fraley MA, Birchem JA, Senkottaiyan N, Alpert MA. Obesity and the electrocardiogram. *Obes Rev.* 2005;6:275-281.

To view digital content associated with this chapter please access lww.co.in. Instructions are located on the inside front cover.

12 Congenital Heart Disease

SARAH A. GOLDSTEIN,
RICHARD A. KRASUSKI,
ANAND MANICKAVASAGAM,
AND JOHN ROSHAN

Introduction

Congenital heart disease (CHD) is a heterogeneous group of structural abnormalities of the cardiovascular system that are embryologic in origin and are present from birth. CHD is the most common form of birth defect, with 1% to 2% of all live births affected by moderate to severe structural malformations.[1] Although CHD was once primarily a pediatric disease, survival into adulthood has significantly increased over the past 3 decades due to advances in surgical techniques and medical care. There are now more adults living with CHD than children.[2,3] As the life expectancy of patients with CHD approaches that of the general population, it has become clear that surgical interventions allowing for improved survival are generally not curative, and complications from both underlying structural abnormalities, and the surgical interventions used to treat them, can lead to late complications. The 12-lead electrocardiogram (ECG) is a crucial part of the complete cardiovascular evaluation of a patient with known or suspected CHD. Based on current professional society guidelines, an ECG should be performed at the time of initial assessment as well as serially for the evaluation of new symptoms.[4] This chapter outlines the most common forms of CHD, associated ECG patterns, and common arrhythmic complications.

Atrial Septal Defects

The *atrial septal defect* (ASD), among the most common forms of CHD, is a persistent direct communication between the atria. There are numerous possible locations for ASDs (**Figure 12.1**). The most common type of ASD is the ostium secundum defect (75% of all ASDs) located in the region of the fossa ovalis. Most children born with ASDs are initially asymptomatic, with the defect typically identified later in life either incidentally or due to the presence of a heart murmur or arrhythmia, usually supraventricular. Depending on its location and morphology, the ASD can be repaired either surgically or by transcatheter closure.

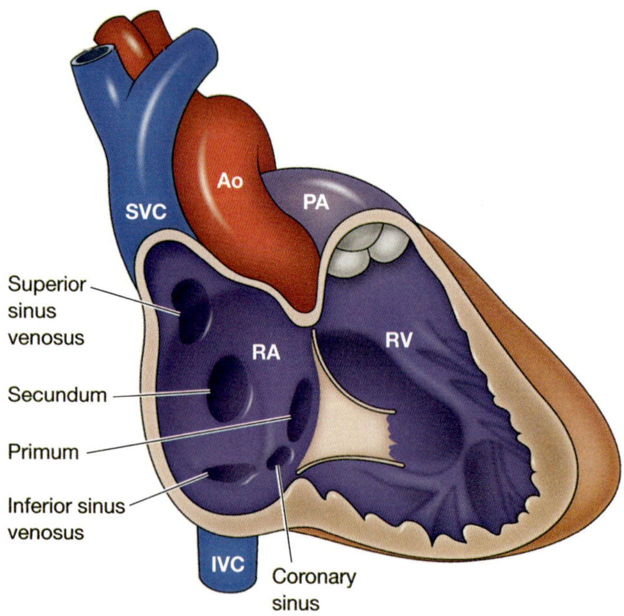

FIGURE 12.1. Anatomic locations of atrial septal defects. Ao, aorta; IVC, inferior vena cava; PA, pulmonary artery; RA, right atrium; RV, right ventricle; SVC, superior vena cava.

In patients with an ASD, the ECG can help shed light on the type of defect and the degree of associated hemodynamic derangement. P-wave morphology is most commonly normal in patients with ASDs. When right atrial enlargement is present due to chronic left-to-right shunting, a peaked and tall P wave in lead II and an increased initial positive P-wave deflection in lead V_1, consistent with right atrial enlargement, may be observed. In most ASD cases, the P-wave axis is normal. The exception is seen in patients with a superior sinus venosus defect. This defect often physically occupies the site of the sinus node, necessitating atrial activation to originate from an ectopic site that is inferiorly located. In superior sinus venosus defects, the P wave is typically inverted in leads II, III, and aVF and upright in aVL.

A hallmark of the ECG in patients with an ASD is an rSR′ morphology of the QRS complex in the right precordial leads (**Figure 12.2**). The right-ventricular outflow tract is the last area of the heart to undergo depolarization. The enlargement and hypertrophy of this area that can occur as a result of chronic right ventricular volume and/or pressure overload associated with left-to-right shunting leads to a longer than normal delay in depolarization. Sequelae of ASDs such as *pulmonary hypertension* can also be responsible for abnormal QRS terminal forces in leads V_1 and V_2, as well as a slightly increased QRS duration.

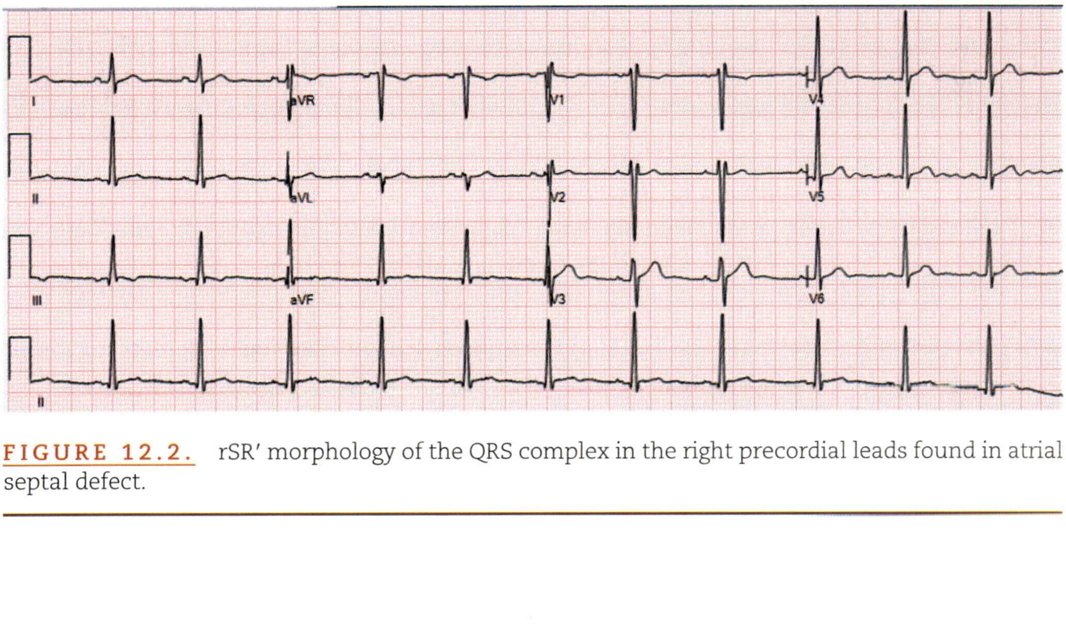

FIGURE 12.2. rSR′ morphology of the QRS complex in the right precordial leads found in atrial septal defect.

The *crochetage pattern*, a notch near the apex of the R wave in the inferior limb leads, is named after its resemblance to the hook of a crochet needle (**Figure 12.3**). This finding is highly specific for the presence of a secundum ASD with significant left-to-right shunting, particularly when present in all three inferior leads.[5,6]

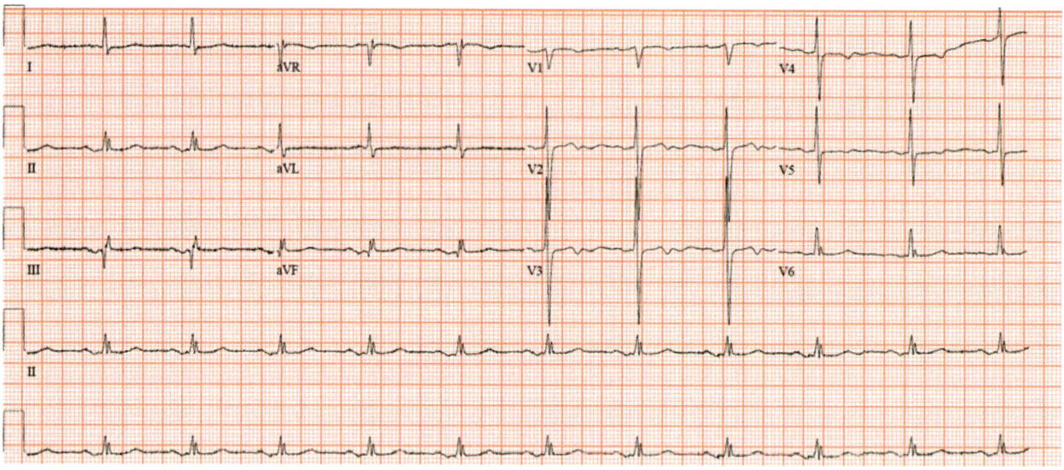

FIGURE 12.3. Crochetage pattern.

Depending on the type of ASD present, the QRS axis may be normal or deviated to the right or left. Right axis deviation is typically observed with ostium secundum defects, whereas left axis deviation is more suggestive of ostium primum defects (**Figure 12.4**).[7] Ostium primum defects are also called atrioventricular septal defects. This is because they do not result from a defect in the atrial septum but instead from the absence of the atrioventricular septum. This leads to posterior displacement of the AV node near the coronary sinus os with the His bundle shifted inferiorly to lie along the inferior rim of the defect. The posteriorly displaced left bundle divides into a short left posterior fascicle that supplies the posterobasal aspect of the LV leading to its early activation. The left anterior division is increased in length with fewer fibers resulting in a delayed activation of the anterosuperior LV. This results in counterclockwise depolarization with rS in inferior leads. The RBBB present on the ECG in an ostium primum ASD is because of delay in RV activation owing to the very long right bundle resulting from the inferoposterior displacement of the conduction system.[A]

Patients with ASDs, particularly those with unrepaired defects or defects repaired later in life, are at risk for atrial tachyarrhythmias. Macroreentrant atrial arrhythmias (such as atrial flutter) are most common. An increased incidence of atrial fibrillation, however, occurs compared to the general population. In uncorrected patients, typical atrial flutter is most commonly seen, whereas atypical flutter is more common in surgically repaired patients.[8] See also Chapter 16. The incidence of atrial arrhythmias increases with age, affecting around 20% of adults with ASDs.[9]

Bradyarrhythmias are a less common complication of ASDs. Sinus node dysfunction generally occurs in superior sinus venosus defects. Likewise, based on its location, ostium primum defects, part of the family of endocardial cushion defects that occur commonly (but not exclusively) in patients with Down syndrome, are associated with abnormal placement of the atrioventricular (AV) node. These ostium primum defects may lead to varying degrees of AV conduction disturbances.

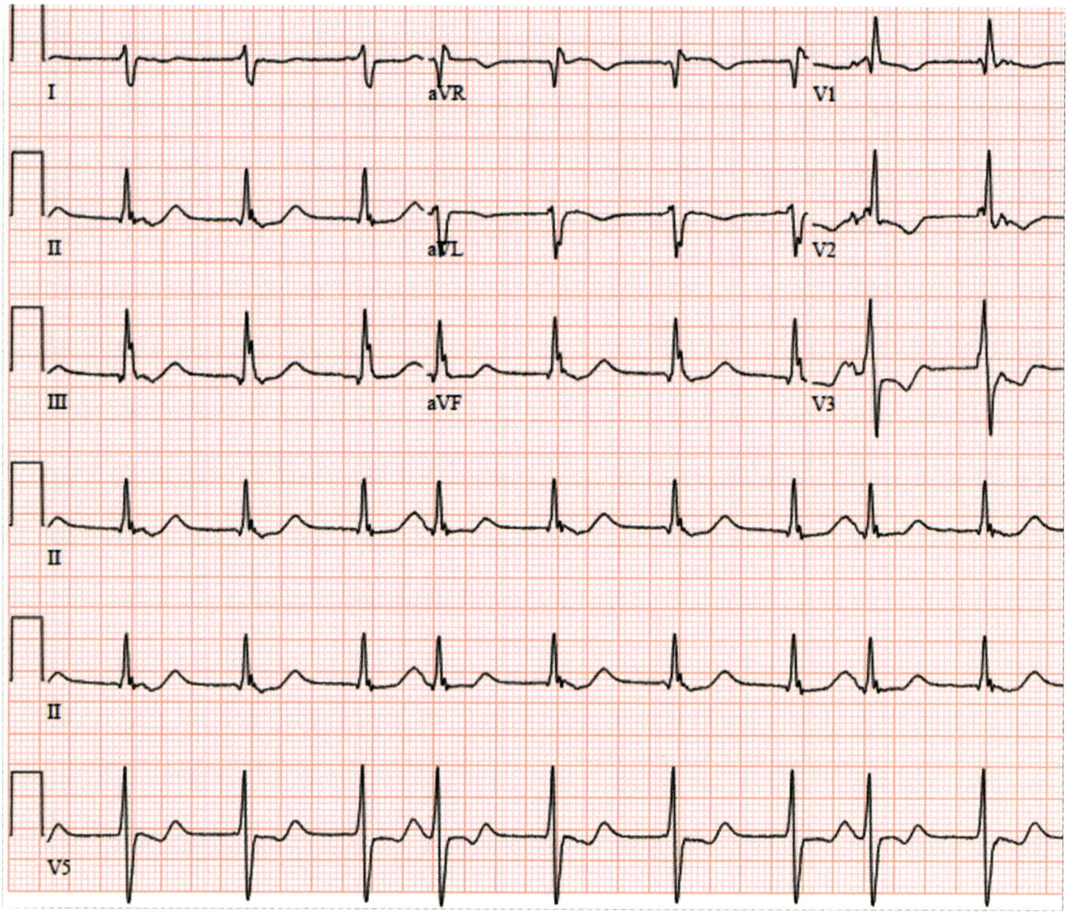

A

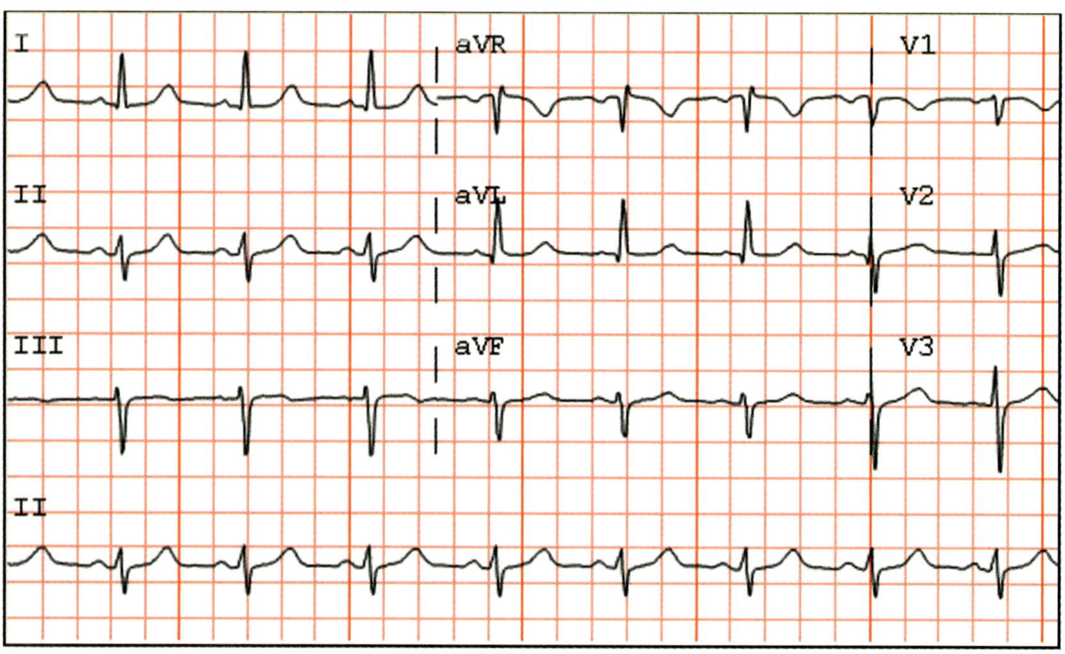

B

FIGURE 12.4. RAD, right axis deviation (**A**) versus LAD, left axis deviation (**B**) seen in secundum and primum defects, respectively.

Ventricular Septal Defect

The *ventricular septal defect* (VSD), a direct and persistent communication between the ventricles, is the second most common congenital morphologic malformation, accounting for around 30% of all CHD cases.[10] As with ASDs, there are multiple possible locations for VSDs (**Figure 12.5**). Perimembranous VSDs are most common (80% of all cases), located adjacent to the membranous portion of the ventricular septum. The majority of VSDs are discovered by the detection of a murmur in childhood. Patients who become symptomatic may develop varying degrees of heart failure, depending on the VSD size, location, and other associated abnormalities (such as *tetralogy of Fallot* [TOF]). Many small VSDs close spontaneously and can be managed conservatively, whereas large VSDs and those affecting the ventricular outlet septum typically require surgical intervention early in life. VSDs with significant left-to-right shunting that are not repaired can lead to pulmonary hypertension, right-to-left shunting, and hypoxia, a complication known as *Eisenmenger syndrome*.

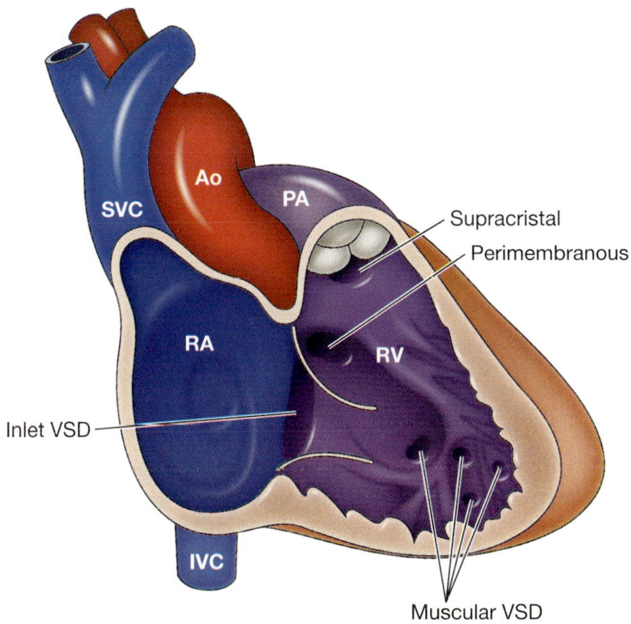

FIGURE 12.5. Anatomic locations of ventricular septal defects. Ao, aorta; IVC, inferior vena cava; PA, pulmonary artery; RA, right atrium; RV, right ventricle; SVC, superior vena cava.

Unlike in patients with an ASD, the ECG does not shed light on the anatomic location of the VSD except in the case of inlet VSD seen along with an ostium primum ASD in endocardial cushion defects, also known as atrioventricular septal defects. Here, the QRS axis is leftward ranging from moderate to extreme. The posteroinferior displacement of the atrioventricular conduction tissues, in conjunction with the loss of ventriculoseptal myocardium, results in this ECG feature.[B]

The ECG in VSD is influenced by the size of the defect, the degree of resultant shunting, and the presence of pulmonary hypertension. Patients with small VSDs and minimal shunting typically have a normal ECG. When the VSD is large and associated with significant and unrestricted left-to-right shunting of blood, ECG abnormalities are typically present. Left atrial enlargement resulting from increased pulmonary blood flow, and consequently increased pulmonary venous return, can lead to notched bifid P waves in the limb leads, as well as a deep, broad terminal negative component of the P wave in lead V_1. Biventricular hypertrophy can occur, with large RS complexes in lead V_2 through V_5, a finding known as *Katz-Wachtel phenomenon* (**Figure 12.6**).[11] In patients with Eisenmenger syndrome, right axis deviation and isolated right-ventricular hypertrophy are typically present on ECG.

Isolated premature ventricular contractions (PVCs), couplets, and multiform PVCs are the most common rhythm disturbances in patients with isolated VSDs. Ventricular ectopy increases in frequency with elevation in pulmonary arterial pressure.[12] In the case of severe right-ventricular hypertrophy or with Eisenmenger syndrome, nonsustained and sustained ventricular arrhythmias can occur.

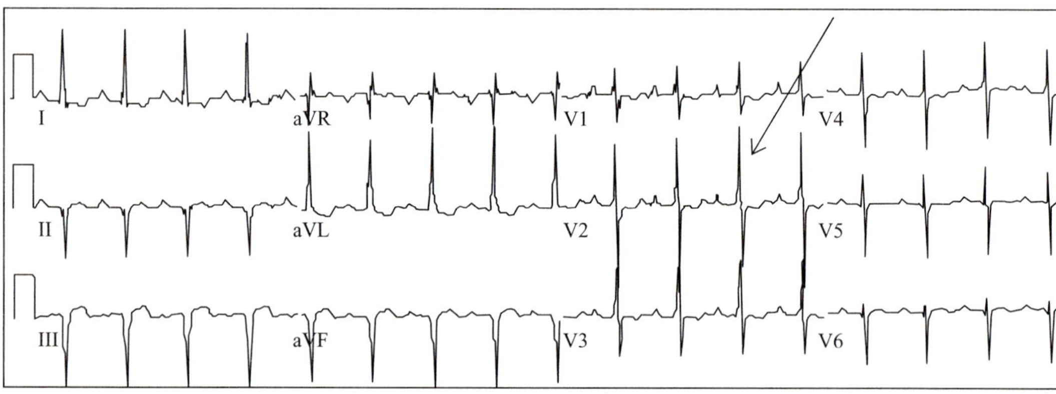

FIGURE 12.6. Katz-Wachtel phenomenon, *arrow* (biventricular hypertrophy).

Patent Ductus Arteriosus

Patent ductus arteriosus (PDA) is present when the ductus arteriosus, a normal communication between the aorta and pulmonary artery that is important for fetal circulation, fails to close after birth. The presence of a PDA allows for shunting of oxygenated blood from the aorta into the pulmonary artery, producing left-to-right shunting. This shunting creates a continuous "machinery-like" cardiac murmur (present in both systole and diastole). When unrepaired, significant shunting can lead to pulmonary hypertension and Eisenmenger syndrome.

Most patients with a small PDA do not have abnormalities on ECG. When unrestricted left-to-right shunting through a large PDA is present, ECG will show features of left ventricular volume overload and left atrial enlargement due to increased blood flow through the left heart. With the development of pulmonary hypertension and Eisenmenger syndrome, right axis deviation and right-ventricular hypertrophy appear on ECG.

Pulmonary Stenosis

Obstruction to the right ventricular outflow can occur above, below, or at the level of the pulmonary valve. *Pulmonary stenosis* (PS) can be part of a constellation of congenital abnormalities or may be an isolated finding. Patients with PS typically present with a heart murmur at birth. Whether a patient requires invasive intervention is generally dependent on the severity of stenosis.

In patients with mild PS, the ECG may be normal. Patients with more severe PS develop right-ventricular hypertrophy, reflected in the ECG by an R/S ratio greater than 1 in lead V_1 or R wave amplitude greater than 7 mm in the same lead. PS gradient of more than 100 has a tall R and insignificant to absent S in V1, while for gradients between 75 and 100, the s in V1, though less than R, is appreciable. For PS gradients less than 75, the R and S are comparable in V1 with the R becoming smaller than the S when there is no gradient.[C] In some cases of severe PS, the R wave amplitude can approach 20 mm or greater. Severe PS can also be associated with right atrial enlargement manifesting as tall and peaked P waves, particularly in lead II. If a pure R wave is present in V1 or V4R in patients aged between 2 and 20 years, the right ventricular pressure can be estimated by multiplying the R wave in millimeters by 5.[D]

Aortic Stenosis

Congenital obstruction of the left ventricular outflow can occur due to a sub- or supra-aortic membrane or a congenitally abnormal or dysplastic aortic valve. The most common cause of congenital left ventricular outflow obstruction seen in adults is due to the presence of a *bicuspid aortic valve*. Although most bicuspid aortic valves typically do not cause obstruction early in life, the valve may become progressively calcified over time, leading to decreased mobility and restricted flow.

Left-ventricular hypertrophy is the most common ECG abnormality seen in patients with left ventricular outflow obstruction. ST depression and T wave inversions can also be present, resulting from significant left-ventricular hypertrophy.

Coarctation of the Aorta

Coarctation of the aorta is a narrowing of the aorta typically located near the aortic attachment of the ligamentum arteriosum (a remnant of the ductus arteriosus), just distal to the great vessels. Patients typically present with upper extremity hypertension and radial-femoral pulse delay. Collateral blood flow can lead to rib notching seen on chest radiograph as well as a murmur over the left upper back. As in other forms of left-sided obstruction, the ECG in adults with unrepaired coarctation of the aorta typically demonstrates left-ventricular hypertrophy.

Tetralogy of Fallot

Tetralogy of Fallot (TOF) is the most common cyanotic congenital heart lesion, affecting 3% to 10% of all patients born with CHD.[13] It is characterized by right ventricular outflow tract obstruction, interventricular communication (VSD), right-ventricular hypertrophy, and an overriding aorta with displacement toward the right heart. TOF is typically diagnosed by fetal ultrasound or echocardiogram in the first days of life. Complete surgical repair, which typically includes closure of the VSD and relief of right ventricular outflow obstruction, is generally pursued within the first year of life and leads to excellent long-term outcomes in most cases. Many repairs result in pulmonic valve regurgitation that can worsen over time and may require further intervention in adulthood. Right-ventricular hypertrophy typically resolves following relief of outflow obstruction.

The P waves in patients with unrepaired TOF are typically broad and peaked in lead II consistent with right atrial enlargement. Right axis deviation, tall R waves in leads III, aVF and aVR, and deep S waves in leads I, aVL and V_2-V_6 are present in the setting of right-ventricular hypertrophy (see Chapter 4). These changes eventually normalize after corrective surgery. In about 48% of cases, the monophasic R in V1 abruptly drops in V2 [rS pattern] only to pick up in amplitude thereafter. This is because of the activation of the trabecular wall of the RV that underlies V2.[E]

The most common abnormality seen on the ECG in patients with repaired TOF is right bundle branch block (see Chapter 5). The QRS prolongation can be profound and occurs due to chronic right ventricular volume and pressure overload (**Figure 12.7**).[14] Extreme QRS prolongation (>180 ms) has been identified as an independent risk factor for sudden cardiac death (SCD) due to ventricular arrhythmia.[15] Other features associated with increase SCD risk include unexplained cardiac syncope, severe pulmonary regurgitation, and nonsustained ventricular tachycardia. Atrial arrhythmias are an important late complication of TOF, occurring in 10% of patients.[15] The ECG typically demonstrates the "saw-tooth" P-wave pattern characteristic of typical atrial flutter. The incidence of atypical atrial flutter increases after surgical repair of TOF and accounts for about 30% of all atrial arrhythmias seen post surgery.[F]

The lifelong incidence of ventricular tachycardia and SCD after surgical repair of TOF is around 12% and 8%, respectively.[15] Monomorphic ventricular tachycardia is most common, and typically involves right ventricular outflow tract scar. Of all patients with CHD, those with TOF are the most common recipients of implantable cardioverter defibrillators.[15]

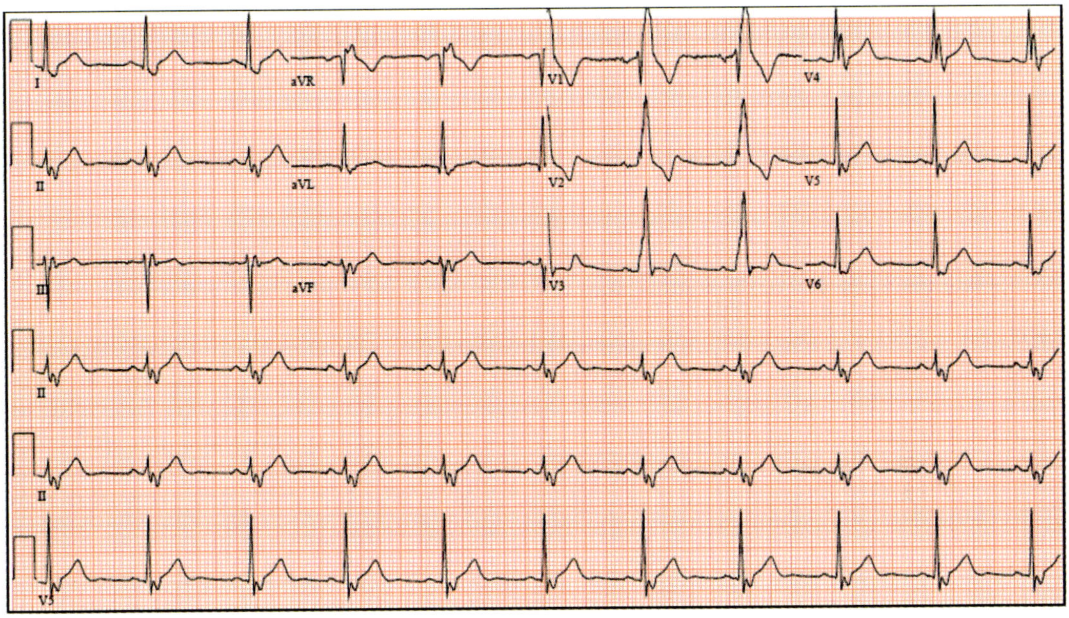

FIGURE 12.7. Right bundle branch block with QRS duration >180 ms.

Ebstein Anomaly

Ebstein anomaly is characterized by displacement of the tricuspid valve (TV) leaflets toward the right ventricular apex (**Figure 12.8**). This abnormal placement of the TV leaflets results in enlargement of the right atrium due to atrialization of the proximal right ventricle, varying degrees of tricuspid regurgitation, and right ventricular dysfunction. Fetal exposure to lithium, a medication used to treat bipolar disorder, increases the risk of developing this anomaly.[16] The most common presenting symptoms in adolescents and adults is arrhythmia.

The ECG in patients with Ebstein anomaly is rarely normal, even in the case of mild disease. The P waves are usually very tall and peaked, characterized as Himalayan P waves, representative of aberrant conduction through the enlarged right atrium.[17] The P waves are most prominent in leads II, III, aVF, and V_1 and can be taller than the R wave in lead II. The PR interval is often prolonged, the result of abnormal conduction through the enlarged right atrium. Usually, there is right bundle branch block pattern and the QRS axis is inferior. QRS may be splintered and polyphasic due to delayed activation in the atrialized right ventricle.

Atrial arrhythmias are common in patients with Ebstein anomaly. Right-sided accessory pathways with AV reentrant tachycardia (Wolff-Parkinson-White syndrome) are classically associated with this form of CHD, occurring in around 25% of cases.[18] Absence of right bundle branch block or presence of left axis deviation in a patient with Ebstein indicates the presence of right-sided accessory pathways. See also Chapter 19, Ventricular Preexcitation. Ventricular arrhythmias are uncommon in Ebstein anomaly.

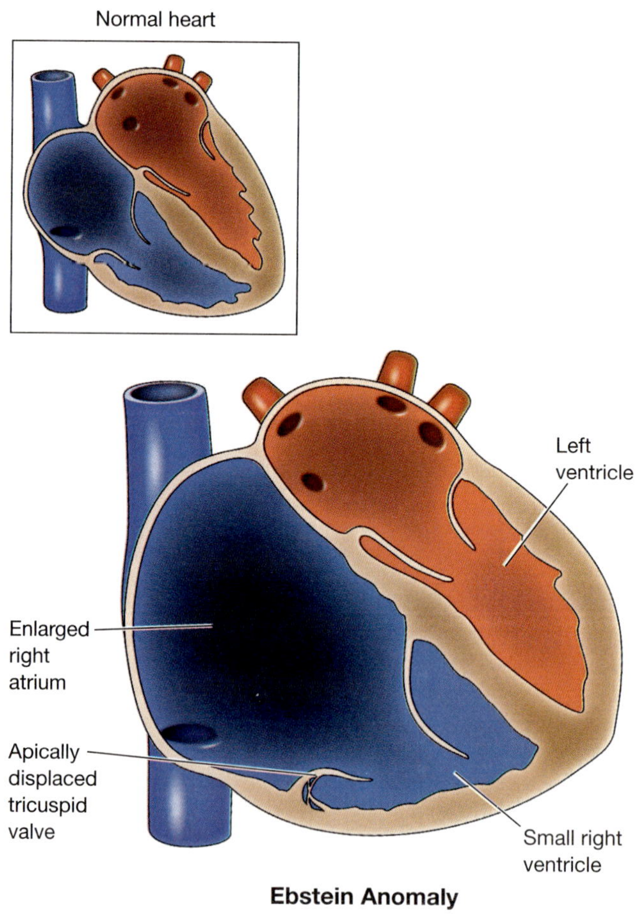

FIGURE 12.8. Ebstein anomaly.

Congenitally Corrected Transposition of the Great Arteries

In normal development, the ventricles and great vessels are concordant, with the aorta originating from the left ventricle and the pulmonary artery from the right ventricle. *Transposition of the great arteries* (TGA) is characterized by ventriculoarterial discordance. The pulmonary artery arises from the morphologic left ventricle and the aorta from the morphologic right ventricle. Congenitally corrected TGA (L-TGA) occurs in the setting of both ventriculoarterial and atrioventricular discordance (**Figure 12.9**). Patients with isolated congenitally corrected TGA do not commonly require surgical intervention.

Bradyarrhythmias are the most common rhythm disturbance seen in patients with L-TGA. More than 75% of patients with L-TGA exhibit some degree of AV block, with a 30% overall lifetime incidence of complete heart block.[19] This high incidence of AV block in L-TGA is related to the abnormal position of the AV node resulting from the atypical alignment of the atria and ventricles.

Complete Transposition of the Great Arteries

With complete transposition (D-TGA), there is ventriculoarterial discordance with preservation of the typical atrioventricular relationship. This ventriculoarterial discordance leads to the pulmonary and systemic circulations existing in parallel, as opposed to in sequence (see **Figure 12.9**). Immediate survival after birth is dependent on the presence of a shunt to connect the two parallel but separate circuits. Infants, therefore, require surgical intervention very early in life.

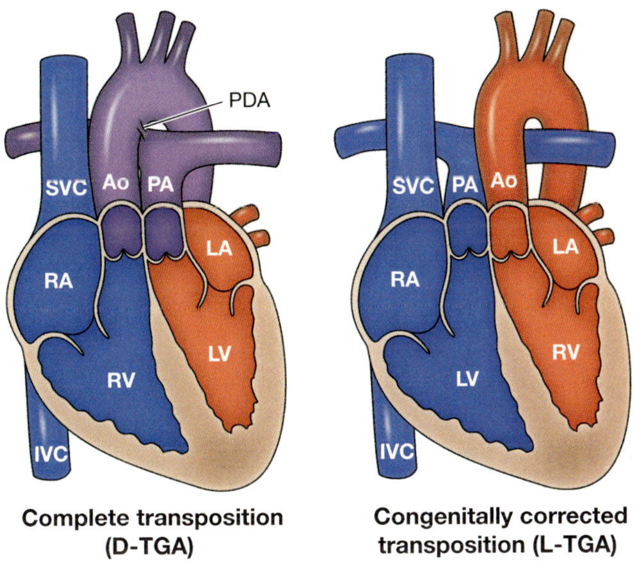

FIGURE 12.9. Complete transposition versus congenitally corrected transposition. Ao, aorta; D-TGA, dextro-transposition of the great arteries (complete transposition of the great arteries); IVC, inferior vena cava; LA, left atrium; LV, left ventricle; PA, pulmonary artery; RA, right atrium; RV, right ventricle; SVC, superior vena cava.

Surgery for D-TGA has evolved significantly over the past 80 years. The *Senning and Mustard procedures*, involving atrial baffling to divert blood to the opposite ventricle, were common until the 1980s. These operations, also termed atrial switch procedures, resulted in a systemic right ventricle and were therefore complicated by high rates of systemic right ventricular failure. More recently, the arterial switch procedure, which allows for restoration of a systemic left ventricle, has become the standard repair.

Sinus node dysfunction is common following the atrial switch procedure. Ectopic atrial and junctional rhythms are frequently seen. Because the atrioventricular relationship is preserved, the AV node is normally positioned. The PR interval is therefore typically normal. The QRS complex morphology is dependent on the type of surgical repair used. In the setting of the arterial switch procedure, the ECG is typically normal. Following the atrial switch procedure, however, ECG findings consistent with right-ventricular hypertrophy and right axis deviation develop over time, a consequence of the right ventricle supporting the systemic circulation.

Twenty years after the atrial switch procedure, the most common late arrhythmic complications include sinus node dysfunction (in 60%) and atrial fibrillation/flutter (in 24%).[20] Although not the most common arrhythmic complication, malignant ventricular arrhythmia is the leading causes of late mortality in patients with D-TGA who have undergone the atrial switch procedure, with a lifetime prevalence of 2% to 15%.[21] High-risk features for SCD in this group include prior VSD closure, unexplained syncope, atrial tachycardia, systemic ventricular dysfunction, and severe tricuspid regurgitation.[22] Transvenous implantable cardioverter defibrillator placement can be challenging, particularly in the setting of baffle stenosis. Subcutaneous implantable cardioverter defibrillators have emerged as an effective and safe alternative to transvenous devices in these patients.[23]

Fontan Circulation

Some forms of CHD, such as *tricuspid atresia* and *hypoplastic left heart syndrome*, result in only one fully developed ventricle. Palliation of these "single-ventricle" patients can be achieved through a series of surgical procedures to directly connect vena caval blood return into the pulmonary arterial circulation. The final stage of this process is referred to as the Fontan procedure, which was first performed for management of tricuspid atresia in 1971.[24] The classic Fontan connection involves direct anastomosis of the right atrium to the pulmonary artery (**Figure 12.10**). Because of frequent complications including thrombosis and atrial arrhythmias, the procedure has evolved over time. Subsequent iterations include the lateral tunnel or an extracardiac conduit. The lateral tunnel is an intra-atrial baffle that directs flow from the inferior vena cava to the pulmonary artery through the lateral portion of the right atrium. The extracardiac conduit is a direct connection between the inferior vena cava and the pulmonary artery via a prosthetic tube that is positioned outside the heart.

Findings on baseline ECG in patients with *Fontan circulation* are highly heterogeneous and depend on the underlying congenital lesion as well as the type of Fontan connection. Arrhythmias are the most frequent cardiac event reported in patients with Fontan circulation. Supraventricular tachycardia is common, affecting up to 60% of patients following Fontan palliation, and is associated with significant morbidity and mortality.[25] The incidence of supraventricular tachycardia is dependent on Fontan type. Patients with a classic Fontan are at highest risk for the development of supraventricular arrhythmias due to progressive and severe enlargement of the involved atrium. Patients who have an extracardiac Fontan have the lowest risk of atrial arrhythmias because the atrium is bypassed and, therefore, protected from high Fontan flow.[26] Sinus node dysfunction is also frequently found in patients with Fontan circulation, as is chronotropic incompetence; both of these sinus node problems are associated with fatigue and exercise intolerance. Epicardial atrial pacemaker placement has been shown to alleviate both of these complications.[27]

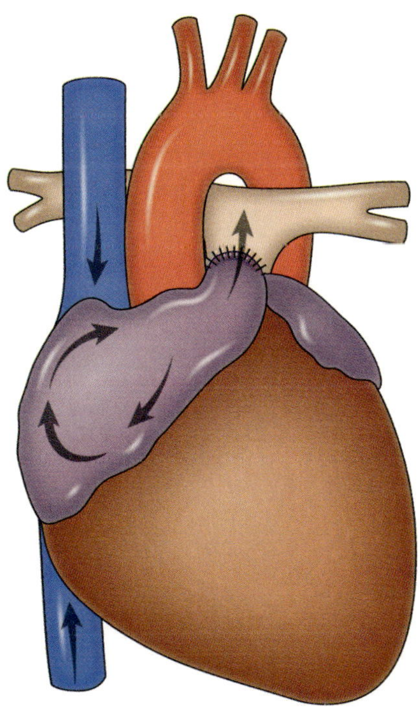

FIGURE 12.10. Classic Fontan.

CHAPTER 12 SUMMARY ILLUSTRATION

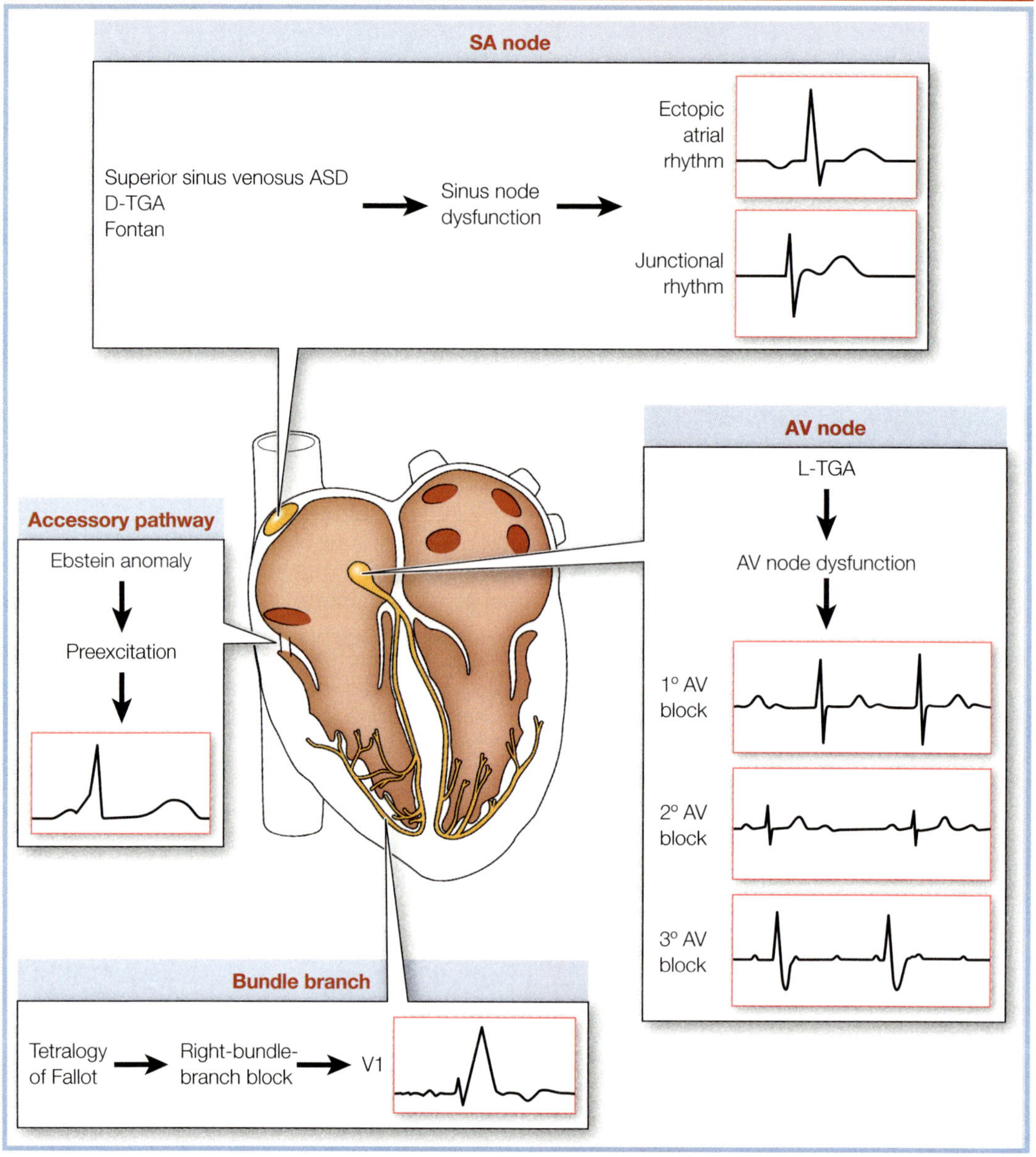

Abbreviations: ASD, atrial septal defect; AV, atrioventricular; D-TGA, D-transposition of the great arteries (complete transposition of the great arteries); L-TGA, L-transposition of the great arteries (congenitally corrected transposition of the great arteries); SA, sinoatrial.

Glossary

Aortic stenosis: narrowing and obstruction of the left ventricular outflow tract, either above, below, or at the level of the aortic valve.

Atrial septal defect: a persistent direct communication between the atria.

Bicuspid aortic valve: a structural anomaly in which the aortic valve is composed of two leaflets instead of three.

Coarctation of the aorta: narrowing of the aorta typically located near the aortic attachment of the ligamentum arteriosum (remnant of the ductus arteriosus), just distal to the great vessels.

Congenital heart disease: a heterogeneous group of structural abnormalities of the cardiovascular system that are embryologic in origin and are present from birth.

Crochetage pattern: a notch near the apex of the R wave in the inferior limb leads that is named after its resemblance to the hook of a crochet needle and associated with atrial septal defects.

Ebstein anomaly: congenital displacement of the tricuspid valve leaflets toward the right ventricular apex.

Eisenmenger syndrome: pulmonary hypertension, right-to-left shunting, and hypoxia resulting from chronic, prior significant left-to-right shunting.

Fontan circulation: surgical procedure used to directly connect blood flow from the inferior vena cava to the pulmonary arterial circulation; useful in patients who are born with only one ventricle.

Hypoplastic left heart syndrome: diminutive left ventricle and small left-sided cardiac and vascular structures.

Katz-Wachtel phenomenon: ECG evidence of biventricular hypertrophy, with large RS complexes in leads V_2 through V_5.

Patent ductus arteriosus: a shunt that is present when the ductus arteriosus, a normal communication between the aorta and pulmonary artery that is important for fetal circulation, fails to close after birth.

Pulmonary hypertension: elevated blood pressure in the pulmonary arteries.

Pulmonary stenosis: narrowing and obstruction of the right ventricular outflow tract, either above, below, or at the level of the pulmonary valve.

Senning and Mustard procedures: atrial baffling to divert blood to the opposite ventricle; a palliative surgical approach to correct transposition of the great arteries.

Tetralogy of Fallot: a constellation of congenital anomalies including right ventricular outflow tract obstruction, interventricular communication (VSD), right-ventricular hypertrophy, and an overriding aorta with displacement toward the right heart.

Transposition of the great arteries: a congenital anomaly characterized by ventriculoarterial discordance—the pulmonary artery arises from the morphologic left ventricle and the aorta from the morphologic right ventricle.

Tricuspid atresia: congenital agenesis or absence of the tricuspid valve.

Ventricular septal defect: a direct and persistent communication between the ventricles.

References

1. Hoffman JI, Kaplan S. The incidence of congenital heart disease. *J Am Coll Cardiol.* 2002;39:1890-1900.
2. Khairy P, Ionescu-Ittu R, Mackie AS, Abrahamowicz M, Pilote L, Marelli AJ. Changing mortality in congenital heart disease. *J Am Coll Cardiol.* 2010;56:1149-1157.
3. Marelli AJ, Mackie AS, Ionescu-Ittu R, Rahme E, Pilote L. Congenital heart disease in the general population. Changing prevalence and age distribution. *Circulation.* 2007;115:163-172.
4. Stout KK, Daniels CJ, Aboulhosn JA, et al. 2018 AHA/ACC guideline for the management of adults with congenital heart disease: a report of the American College of Cardiology/American Heart Association Task Force on Clinical Practice Guidelines. *Circulation.* 2019;139:e698-e800.
5. Heller J, Hagège AA, Besse B, Desnos M, Marie FN, Guerot C. "Crochetage" (notch) on R wave in inferior limb leads: a new independent electrocardiographic sign of atrial septal defect. *J Am Coll Cardiol.* 1996;27:877-882.
6. Shen L, Liu J, Li JK, et al. The significance of crochetage on the R wave of an electrocardiogram for the early diagnosis of pediatric secundum atrial septal defect. *Pediatr Cardiol.* 2018;39:1031-1035.
7. Fournier A, Young ML, Garcia OL, Tamer DF, Wolff GS. Electrophysiologic cardiac function before and after surgery in children with atrioventricular canal. *Am J Cardiol.* 1986;57:1137-1141.
8. Delacretaz E, Ganz LI, Soejima K, et al. Multi atrial maco-re-entry circuits in adults with repaired congenital heart disease: entrainment mapping combined with three-dimensional electroanatomic mapping. *J Am Coll Cardiol.* 2001;37:1665-1676.

9. Gatzoulis MA, Freeman MA, Siu SC, Webb GD, Harris L. Atrial arrhythmia after surgical closure of atrial septal defects in adults. *N Engl J Med.* 1999;340:839-846.
10. Egbe A, Uppu S, Lee S, Stroustrup A, Ho D, Srivastava S. Temporal variation of birth prevalence of congenital heart disease in the United States. *Congenit Heart Dis.* 2015;10:43-50.
11. Elliott LP, Taylor WJ, Schiebler GL. Combined ventricular hypertrophy in infancy: vectorcardiographic observations with special reference to the Katz-Wachtel phenomenon. *Am J Cardiol.* 1963;11:164-172.
12. Liberman L, Kaufman S, Alfayyadh M, Hordof AJ, Apfel HD. Noninvasive prediction of pulmonary artery pressure in patients with isolated ventricular septal defect. *Pediatr Cardiol.* 2000;21:197-201.
13. Apitz C, Webb GD, Redington AN. Tetralogy of Fallot. *Lancet.* 2009;374:1462-1471.
14. D'Andrea A, Caso P, Sarubbi B, et al. Right ventricular myocardial activation delay in adult patients with right bundle branch block late after repair of tetralogy of Fallot. *Eur J Echocardiogr.* 2004;5:123-131.
15. Gatzoulis MA, Balaji S, Webber SA, et al. Risk factors for arrhythmia and sudden cardiac death late after repair of tetralogy of Fallot: a multicentre study. *Lancet.* 2000;356:975-981.
16. Zalzstein E, Koren G, Einarson T, Freedom RM. A case-control study on the association between first trimester exposure to lithium and Ebstein's anomaly. *Am J Cardiol.* 1990;65:817-818.
17. Iturralde P, Nava S, Sãlica G, et al. Electrocardiographic characteristics of patients with Ebstein's anomaly before and after ablation of an accessory atrioventricular pathway. *J Cardiovasc Electrophysiol.* 2006;17:1332-1336.
18. Ho SY, Goltz D, McCarthy K, et al. The atrioventricular junctions in Ebstein malformation. *Heart.* 2000;83:444-449.
19. Warnes CA. Transposition of the great arteries. *Circulation.* 2006;114:2699-2709.
20. Gelatt M, Hamilton RM, McCrindle BW, et al. Arrhythmia and mortality after the Mustard procedure: a 30-year single-center experience. *J Am Coll Cardiol.* 1997;29:194-201.
21. Kammeraad JA, van Deurzen CH, Sreeram N, et al. Predictors of sudden cardiac death after Mustard or Senning repair for transposition of the great arteries. *J Am Coll Cardiol.* 2004;44:1095-1102.
22. Al-Khatib SM, Stevenson WG, Ackerman MJ, et al. 2017 AHA/ACC/HRS guideline for management of patients with ventricular arrhythmias and the prevention of sudden cardiac death: executive summary: a report of the American College of Cardiology/American Heart Association Task Force on Clinical Practice Guidelines and the Heart Rhythm Society. *Heart Rhythm.* 2018;15:e190-e252.
23. Moore JP, Mondesert B, Lloyd MS, et al. Clinical experience with the subcutaneous implantable cardioverter-defibrillator in adults with congenital heart disease. *Circ Arrhythm Electrophysiol.* 2016;9. pii: e004338.
24. Fontan F, Baudet E. Surgical repair of tricuspid atresia. *Thorax.* 1971;26:240-248.
25. Giannakoulas G, Dimopoulos K, Yuksel S, et al. Atrial tachyarrhythmias late after Fontan operation are related to increase in mortality and hospitalization. *Int J Cardiol.* 2012;157:221-226.
26. d'Udekem Y, Iyengar AJ, Galati JC, et al. Redefining expectations of long-term survival after the Fontan procedure: twenty-five years of follow-up from the entire population of Australia and New Zealand. *Circulation.* 2014;130(11, suppl 1):S32-S38.
27. Villain E. Indications for pacing in patients with congenital heart disease. *Pacing Clin Electrophysiol.* 2008;31(suppl 1):S17-S20.

References to the South Asian Edition

A. Boineau JP, Moore EN, Patterson DF. Relationship between the ECG, ventricular activation, and the ventricular conduction system in ostium primum ASD. *Circulation* 1973;48:556-564.
B. Feldt RH, DuShane JW, Titus JL. The atrioventricular conduction system in persistent common atrioventricular canal defect: Correlations with electrocardiogram. *Circulation* 1970;42:437-444.
C. DePasquale N, Burch GE. The electrogram and ventricular gradient in isolated congenital pulmonary stenosis. *Circulation* 1960;21:181-187.
D. Rudolph AM. Congenital Diseases of the Heart. *Chicago: Yearbook Medical*, 1974.
E. Pileggi F,Bocanegra I, Tranchesi I, et al. The electrocardiogram in tetralogy of Fallot: a study of 142 cases. *Am Heart J* 1960;59:667-680.
F. MS de Groot, Lukac P, Schalij MJ et al. Long-term outcome of ablative therapy of post-operative atrial tachyarrhythmias in patients with tetralogy of Fallot: a European multicentre study. *Europace.* 2012; 14: 522-527.

SECTION V

Abnormal Rhythms

13 Introduction to Arrhythmias

ZAK LORING, DAVID G. STRAUSS,
DOUGLAS D. SCHOCKEN,
JAMES P. DAUBERT, AND
KARTIKEYA BHARGAVA

"Every self-respecting arrhythmia has three different interpretations."

HJL Marriott

Introduction to Arrhythmia Diagnosis

The term *arrhythmia* is very general, referring to all rhythms other than regular sinus rhythm. Even the slight variation in sinus rate caused by altered autonomic balance during the respiratory cycle is termed *sinus arrhythmia*. The term *dysrhythmia* has been proposed by some as an alternative, but *arrhythmia*, meaning "imperfection in a regularly recurring motion," is the commonly accepted term for rhythms other than regular sinus rhythm. The presence of an arrhythmia does not necessarily reflect cardiac disease, as indicated by the broad array of abnormal rhythms that commonly occur in healthy individuals of all ages. Arrhythmias are primarily classified according to their rate (**Table 13.1**). Usually, the atria and ventricles have the same rates. There are, however, many different atrial/ventricular relationships among the cardiac arrhythmias:

Table 13.1.

Cardiac Arrhythmias Classified According to Atrial/Ventricular Rate and Relationships

	Atrial and Ventricular Association	Atrial vs Ventricular Rate	Chamber of Origin of Rhythm	Example
1	a. Associated	A=V	Atria	Atrial tachycardia with 1 to 1 AV conduction
	b. Associated	A=V	Ventricles	Ventricular tachycardia with 1 to 1 VA conduction
2	Associated	A>V	Atria	Atrial tachycardia with 2 to 1 AV conduction
3	Associated	A<V	Ventricles	Ventricular tachycardia with 2 to 1 VA conduction
4	Independent *(AV dissociation)*	a. A=V *(isorhythmic AV dissociation)*	Dual rhythm	Junctional rhythm with isorhythmic AV dissociation
		b. A>V	Atrial rhythm – atria	Atrial flutter with complete AV block with ventricular escape rhythm
		c. A<V	Ventricular rhythm – ventricular/AV junction	Ventricular tachycardia with AV dissociation and underlying sinus rhythm

A = atrial, V = ventricular; AV = atrioventricular; VA = ventriculoatrial.

When the atrial and ventricular rhythms are associated but have differing rates, the rhythm is named according to the rate of the chamber (atrial or ventricular) from which it originates (eg, when a rapid atrial rhythm is associated with a slower ventricular rate, the name "atrial tachyarrhythmia" is used). When the atrial and ventricular rhythms are dissociated, names should be given to both of the rhythms (eg, sinus rhythm with ventricular tachyarrhythmia).

The term *bradyarrhythmia* is used to identify any rhythm with a rate <60 beats/min, and *tachyarrhythmia* is used to identify any rhythm with a rate >100 beats/min. There are also many arrhythmias with rates that fall within these "normal" limits. In contrast to the general terms *bradyarrhythmia* and *tachyarrhythmia*, the terms *bradycardia* and *tachycardia* refer to specific arrhythmias such as sinus bradycardia and sinus tachycardia. The two important aspects of arrhythmias that are basic to their understanding are their mechanism and their site of origin.

Mechanisms That Produce Arrhythmias

1. Problems of impulse formation (automaticity)
2. Problems of impulse conduction (block or reentry)

In this chapter, we explore the common mechanisms for arrhythmias and present a practical approach to electrocardiogram (ECG) diagnosis of their site of origin. The following chapters continue this exploration in more detail.

Problems of Automaticity

Arrhythmias caused by problems of automaticity can originate in any cell in the pacemaking and conduction system that is capable of spontaneous depolarization. Such cells are termed *pacemaker cells.*

Location of Pacemaker Cells

1. Sinus node
2. Purkinje cells scattered through the atria
3. Common (His) bundle
4. Right and left bundle branches
5. Purkinje cells in the fascicles and peripheral ventricular endocardial network

See Chapter 1, **Figure 1.7**.

While all these pacemaker cell types are capable of setting the cardiac rate, the cells with the fastest rate determine the overall cardiac rate and rhythm due to *overdrive suppression* of slower automatic foci. Normally, the automaticity of the sinus node exceeds that of all other parts of the pacemaking and conduction systems, allowing it to control the cardiac rate and rhythm. This fact is important because of both the location of the sinus node and its relationship to the parasympathetic and sympathetic components of the autonomic nervous system (see Chapter 3).

A site below the sinus node can initiate the cardiac rhythm either because it usurps control from the sinus node by accelerating its own automaticity or because the sinus node abdicates its role by decreasing its automaticity. The term *ectopic* is often applied to rhythms that originate from any site other than the sinus node. Cardiac cells function as pacemakers by forming electrical impulses called *action potentials* via the process of spontaneous depolarization (**Figure 13.1** and **Animation 13.1**). When the automaticity of cardiac cells is severely impaired, the therapeutic use of an artificial pacemaker may be required (see Chapter 21).

The mechanism by which a tachyarrhythmia continues determines the treatment required for its management. Accelerated automaticity can best be treated by eliminating the cause of the acceleration rather than by treating the acceleration itself. When the accelerated automaticity originates from the sinus node, the cause is virtually always increased sympathetic nervous activity resulting from systemic conditions such as exertion, anxiety, fever, anemia, decreased cardiac output, or thyrotoxicosis. When the accelerated automaticity originates from another location, the most common causes are ischemia, chronic pulmonary disease, and digitalis toxicity. Therefore, both accelerated sinus automaticity and nonsinus (*ectopic*) automaticity are treated by addressing the responsible systemic condition.

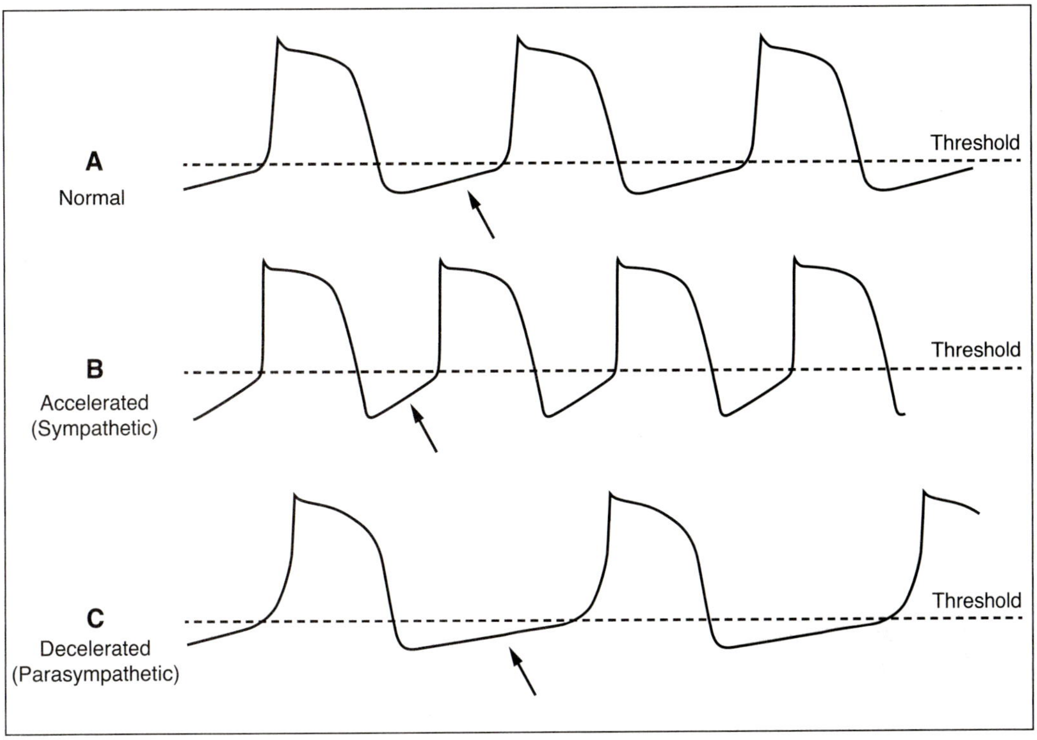

FIGURE 13.1. Schematic action potentials of a pacemaking cell. **A.** Normal sinus rhythm. **B.** Excess sympathetic activity increases the slope of the slow spontaneous depolarization, creating an accelerated rhythm, as in sinus tachycardia. **C.** Excess parasympathetic activity decreases the slope of the slow spontaneous depolarization, creating a decelerated rhythm, as in sinus bradycardia. Arrows indicate the slow spontaneous depolarization in all three conditions. See **Animation 13.1**.

Problems of Impulse Conduction: Block

The term *block* is used to refer to the situation in which conduction is slowed or fails to occur at all (eg, atrioventricular [AV] block, see Chapter 18; or bundle-branch block, see Chapter 5). Cardiac impulses can be either partly blocked, causing conduction delay (eg, a prolonged PR interval in first-degree AV block), or totally blocked, causing conduction failure (eg, third-degree AV block). With a partial block of impulses, there is no change in the rate of the affected site, but with a total block of impulses, a bradyarrhythmia can be produced in the affected site. *Either partial or total block can occur at any site within the pacemaking and conduction system and primarily affects the tissue distal to that site.*

To view the animation(s) and video(s) associated with this chapter please access lww.co.in. Instructions are located on the inside front cover.

Problems of Impulse Conduction: Reentry

Although conduction abnormalities sufficient to produce block can occur only within the pacemaking and conduction systems, uneven or inhomogeneous conduction can occur in any part of the heart. This inhomogeneous spread of electrical impulses can result in an impulse falling into a *reentry circuit* in an area that has just previously been depolarized and repolarized.[1] Reentry produces transmission of the impulse in a path resembling a circle (or any other closed shape), which continues as long as the impulse encounters receptive cells, resulting in a single premature beat, multiple premature beats, a non-sustained tachyarrhythmia, or even a sustained tachyarrhythmia.

Prerequisites to the Development of Reentry

1. An available circuit with two potential pathways of conduction separated by nonconducting tissue
2. A difference in the refractory periods of the two pathways (limbs) in the circuit
3. Conduction that is sufficiently slow somewhere in the circuit to allow the remainder of the circuit to recover its responsiveness by the time the impulse returns

In **Figure 13.2**, the diagrams represent three different situations with an available circuit (reentry prerequisite 1) regarding the homogeneity of pathway receptiveness to impulse conduction: (A) Both limbs of the pathway are receptive—the left and right limbs have completed the recovery process and are receptive to the entering impulse; no reentry occurs; (B) both limbs of the pathway are refractory—the left and right limbs are still refractory (because of the persisting depolarized state) to being reactivated by the entering impulse, no reentry occurs; (C_1) one limb of the pathway is receptive and the other is refractory due to differences in refractory periods (reentry prerequisite 2); and (C_2) the left limb of the pathway is refractory and the right limb is receptive. By the time the impulse reaches the distal end of the left limb (by traveling down the right limb), it is able to reenter because repolarization has been completed (reentry prerequisite 3). The impulse continues to cycle within the reentry circuit as long as it encounters receptive cells, thus producing a reentrant tachyarrhythmia. These concepts are also illustrated in **Animation 13.2**.

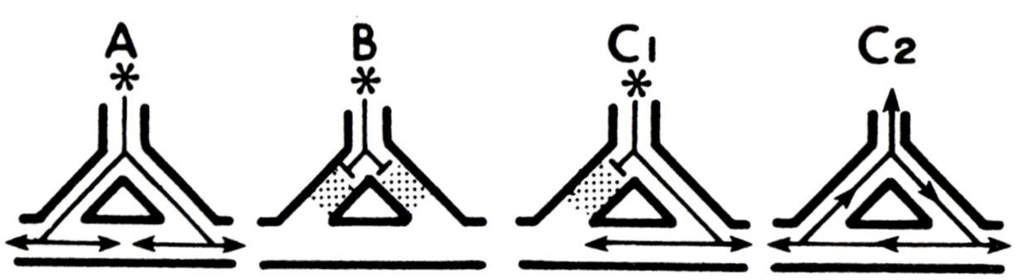

FIGURE 13.2. Asterisks indicate sites of impulse formation, arrows indicate the directions of impulse conduction, perpendicular lines indicate block of impulse conduction, and shaded areas indicate areas that have not yet completed the repolarization process. See **Animation 13.2**.

An example of the development of a *reentry circuit* in the presence of an accessory AV conduction pathway is presented in **Figure 13.3**. During sinus rhythm (**Figure 13.3A**), both the AV node and the bundle of Kent (an accessory muscle bundle capable of conducting impulses) have had time to recover from their previous activation. Impulses from the atria are able to activate the ventricle through both the bundle of Kent (preexciting the ventricle and causing a *delta wave* as shown in beat A on the ECG tracing) and the AV node (capturing the remainder of the ventricle via the specialized conduction system reflected by the narrowing of the QRS after the *delta wave* in beat A). The premature atrial beat in **Figure 13.3B** encounters persisting refractoriness in the nearby bundle of Kent but encounters receptiveness in the more distant AV node, a situation analogous to that shown in **Figure 13.2** (C_1). By the time the impulse reaches the distal end of the bundle of Kent, it is no longer refractory and leads to the development of a *reentry circuit* (**Figure 13.3C**) analogous to that in **Figure 13.2** (C_2). *Reentry circuits* vary in size from a local area of myocardial fibers (see **Figure 13.2** [C_2]) to the entire atrial and ventricular chambers (see **Figure 13.3C** and **Animation 13.3**).

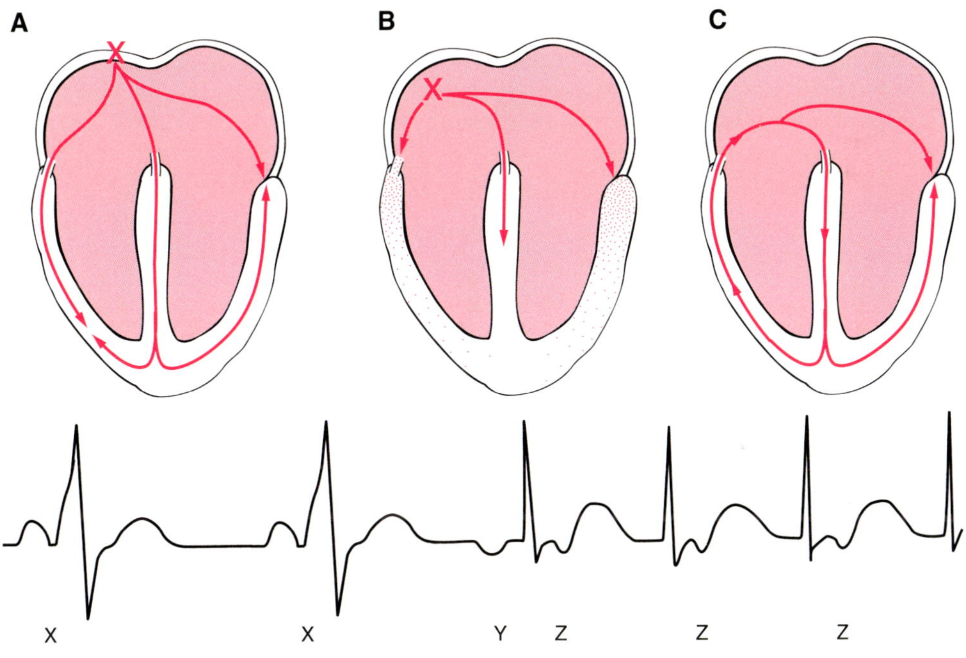

FIGURE 13.3. Top. The presence of a Kent bundle is indicated by the open space between the right atrium and ventricle and the atrioventricular node by the open space at the summit of the interventricular septum. X, site of the pacemaker in the sinus node (**A**) and in the right atrium (**B**). The reentrant circuit overdrive suppresses all pacemaking cells in **C**. The arrows indicate the directions of impulse conduction. Bottom. The corresponding electrocardiogram, indicating sinus rhythm with a normal P wave immediately followed by the QRS complex, indicating ventricular preexcitation (X); an inverted P wave preceding the QRS complex, indicating an atrial premature beat (APB) without preexcitation (Y); and inverted P waves following the QRS complexes, indicating a reentrant tachycardia, namely atrioventricular reciprocating tachycardia (Z). See **Animation 13.3**. (Modified from Wagner GS, Waugh RA, Ramo BW. *Cardiac Arrhythmias*. New York, NY: Churchill Livingstone; 1983:13. Copyright © 1983 Elsevier. With permission.)

The term *microreentry* describes the mechanism that occurs when a reentry circuit is too small for its activation to be represented by a waveform on the surface ECG. The impulses formed within the reentry circuit spread through the surrounding myocardium just as they would spread from an automatic or pacemaking site. The P waves and QRS complexes on the ECG are produced by this passive spread of activation through the atria and ventricles. Microreentry commonly occurs in the AV node and in the ventricles (see Chapter 16).

The term *macroreentry* describes the mechanism that occurs when a reentry circuit is large enough for its own activation to be represented on the surface ECG (see **Figure 13.3C**). Cycling of the activating impulse through the portion of the circuit contained in the right atrium and its spread through the uninvolved left atrium is represented by the inverted P wave (annotated C on the third, fourth, and fifth beats of the ECG tracing). Cycling of the impulse through the portion of the circuit contained in the right ventricle (see **Figure 13.3C**) and its spread through the uninvolved left ventricle via the specialized conduction system is represented by the narrow QRS complex.

There are also forms of macroreentry in which the reentry circuit is entirely within either the atrial or ventricular myocardium, resulting in sawtooth-like P waves (see Chapter 16) or bizarre broad QRS complexes (see Chapter 17), respectively, on surface ECG.

In attempting to treat reentry, it is important to understand its mechanism. For any reentry circuit to perpetuate itself, the advancing head of the recycling impulse must not catch up with the refractory tail (a consequence of reentry prerequisite 3, shown in **Figure 13.4A**).

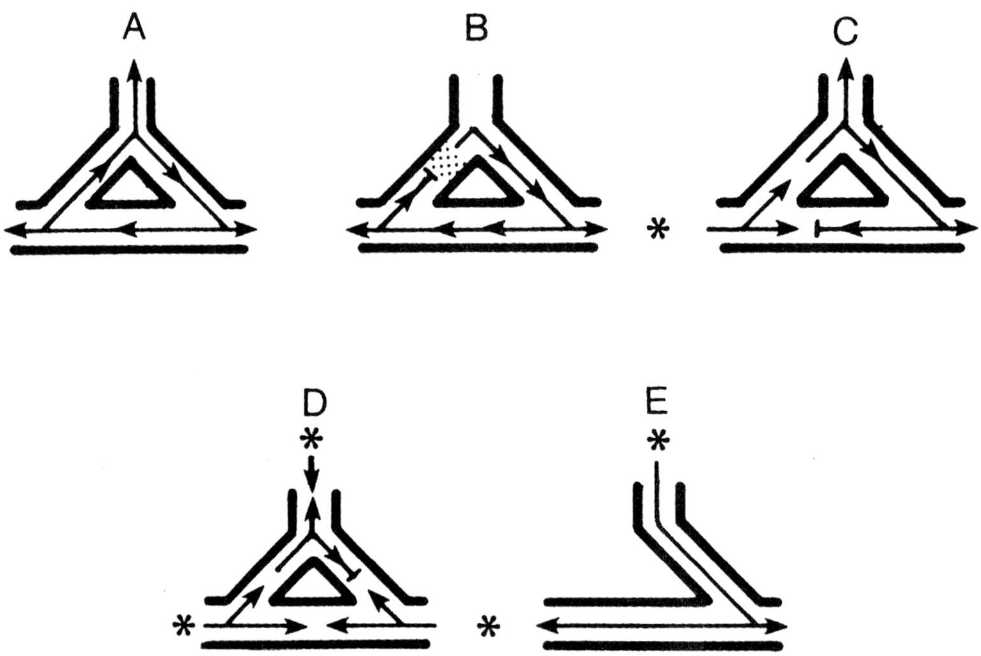

FIGURE 13.4. The diagram illustrating reentry (**A**) and the four mechanisms of termination (**B-E**). Asterisks, arrows, perpendicular lines, and shaded areas have the same meanings as in **Figure 13.2**. The asterisk in **C** indicates an ectopic site of impulse formation, the three asterisks in **D** indicate impulse reception from all sides initiated by the precordial electric shock, and the single asterisk in **E** indicates sinus node impulse formation. See **Animation 13.4**.

Thus, there must always be a gap of nonrefractory cells between the head and the tail of the recycling impulse. A sustained reentrant tachyarrhythmia can be terminated as follows:

Methods for Terminating Sustained Reentrant Tachyarrhythmias
See Animation 13.4

1. Administering drugs that accelerate conduction of the impulse in the reentry circuit so that it encounters an area that has not yet recovered (**Figure 13.4B**). Termination also results if a drug prolongs the recovery time.
2. Introducing an impulse from an artificial pacemaker that depolarizes (captures) a receptive part of the *reentry circuit*, thereby rendering it nonreceptive to the returning reentrant impulse (**Figure 13.4C**).
3. Delivering a precordial electrical shock, termed *cardioversion*, that captures all receptive parts of the heart simultaneously, including those in the reentry circuit, rendering the circuit nonreceptive to the returning impulse (**Figure 13.4D**).
4. Performing surgical or catheter ablation of one limb of the tissue required for the *reentry circuit*. For example, ablation of the accessory atrioventricular pathway in a patient with ventricular preexcitation (**Figure 13.4E**).

Approach to Arrhythmia Diagnosis

Understanding the mechanisms outlined earlier is helpful to understanding how to diagnose arrhythmias by the ECG. In this section, we outline a systematic approach to the diagnosis of arrhythmias. **Chapter 13 Summary Illustration** (shown later in this chapter) illustrates the diagnostic schema we use to approach arrhythmia diagnosis.

Dr. Marriott created his own approach to the diagnosis of arrhythmias over the course of developing the first eight editions of *Practical Electrocardiography*. We include some of his diagnostic "pearls" written in his own voice in the boxes accompanying this section.

The first diagnostic step is also the simplest: Determine the rate. As outlined in Chapter 3, normal sinus rhythm has rate limits of 60 to 100 beats/min (with slight irregularity due to respiratory variation). In addition to classification by general chamber of origin as discussed earlier, arrhythmias can be grouped into *tachyarrhythmias* (fast) or *bradyarrhythmias* (slow). Although arrhythmias can also occur within the normal heart rate range of 60 to 100 beats/min, often, there is either a *tachyarrhythmia* or *bradyarrhythmia* at some level within the heart despite a "normal" ventricular rate.

Bradyarrhythmias

As discussed previously, the mechanisms that produce arrhythmias are either problems of impulse formation (automaticity) or problems of impulse conduction (block or reentry). We begin by discussing problems of impulse conduction.

Dr. Marriott's Approach: "Know the Causes"

The first step in any medical diagnosis is to know the causes of the presenting symptom. For example, if you want to be a superb headache specialist, the first step is to learn the 50 causes of a headache—which are the common ones, which are the uncommon ones, and how to differentiate between them. This is because "you see only what you look for, you recognize only what you know." Knowing the causes of the various cardiac arrhythmias is part of the equipment that you carry with you and are prepared to use when faced with an unidentified arrhythmia.

Normal sinus rhythm originates in the sinoatrial (SA) node from where it activates the right and the left atria and also travels down to the AV node. After a brief delay in the AV node, the impulse continues down the His bundle into the left and right bundle branches and finally activates the endocardial surface of both the left and the right ventricles via the extensive Purkinje fiber network in a rapid and coordinated manner. Problems of conduction block can occur at any of the sites along this path of cardiac conduction system.

The origin of the impulse in the SA node is not visualized on the ECG, and only when the impulse has exited and activated the atria, a P wave is formed. A block or delay at the level of the SA node can result in a *bradyarrhythmia* due to SA exit block in which the impulses do not exit the SA node or do so with a delay resulting in delayed activation of the atria and disruption of the regularly appearing P waves found in normal sinus rhythm.

At the level of AV node or His bundle, block or delay results in impulses not entering the specialized conduction system and thus delays electrical activation of the ventricles. This is seen on the ECG as resulting in an abnormal relationship between the atrial and ventricular activation (P waves and QRS complexes).

Block or delay in conduction in the bundle branches results in impulses activating the left and right ventricles asynchronously. The ventricle that is not activated via the rapid, specialized conduction system takes more time to depolarize, resulting in a wide QRS complex.

Increased automaticity can also result in *bradyarrhythmias*. Ectopic impulses can interrupt or interfere with normal conduction and result in slowing of the ventricular rate. Premature ectopic impulses from the atrium (premature atrial complexes), His bundle (premature junctional complexes) and ventricular myocardium (premature ventricular complexes) can interfere with normal conduction by depolarizing elements of the conduction system early, leaving them refractory and unable to conduct the impulses from the sinus node when they arrive.

Dr. Marriott's Approach: "Who's Married to Whom"

Establish relationships by asking yourself, "Who's married to whom?" This is often the crucial step in arriving at a firm diagnosis in a case of arrhythmia. **Figure 13.5** illustrates this principle in its simplest form. A junctional escape rhythm is dissociated from sinus bradycardia. On three occasions, there are bizarre early beats with a qR configuration that look similar to ventricular premature beats, but the fact that they are seen only when a P wave is emerging beyond the preceding QRS complex tells us that they are "married to" the preceding P waves. This therefore establishes the beats as conducted or capture beats with atypical right-bundle-branch block aberration.

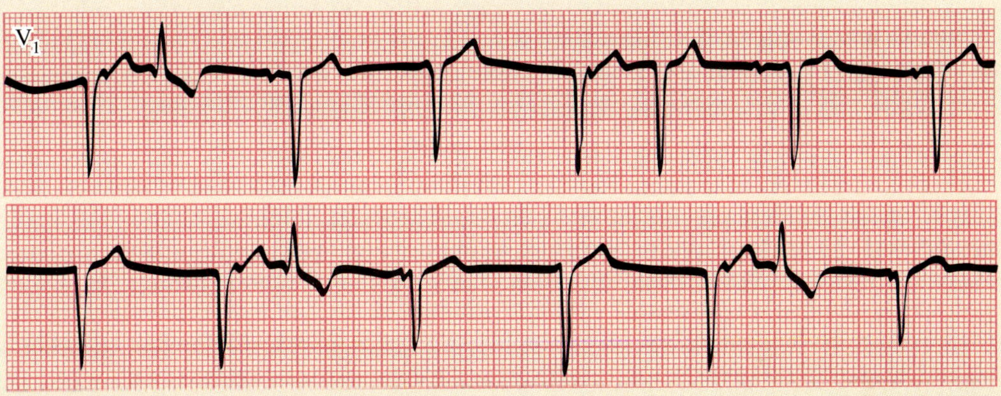

FIGURE 13.5. The rhythm strips are continuous. All of the early QRS complexes, but only some of the later QRS complexes, are preceded by P waves. The use of calipers reveals dissociation between the atria (which have a regular rate of about 50 beats/min) and the ventricles (the later QRS complexes have a regular rate of about 60 beats/min). The presence of P waves before each early QRS complex suggests intermittent capture of the ventricular rhythm by the atrial rhythm.

The diagnostic approach to *bradyarrhythmias* is to examine the conduction from the sinus node through the ventricular myocardium and evaluate whether there are signs of block or delay at any step along the way. If impulse conduction through each step appears to be normal, evaluate for the presence of ectopy that may be interfering with normal conduction. The specifics of each *bradyarrhythmia* are explored in more depth in Chapter 18.

Tachyarrhythmias

The most clinically important distinction in diagnosing *tachyarrhythmias* is determining whether the source of the arrhythmia is coming from the ventricular myocardium (ventricular) or from above the ventricle (supraventricular tachyarrhythmia). Whereas wide complex tachycardias can be caused by both ventricular tachycardia and supraventricular tachycardia (SVT, the discrimination between these rhythms is discussed in depth in Chapter 16), narrow complex tachycardias are usually supraventricular. Several ECG features help diagnose the mechanism or type of SVT.

Dr. Marriott's Approach: "Milk the QRS Complex"

When a specific arrhythmia confronts you, you should first "milk" the QRS complex. There are two reasons for this. The first is an extension of the Willie Sutton law: "I robbed banks because that's where the money is." Second, milking the QRS complex keeps us in the healthy frame of mind of giving priority to ventricular behavior. It matters comparatively little what the atria are doing as long as the ventricles are behaving normally. If the QRS complex is of normal duration in at least two leads of the ECG, then the rhythm is supraventricular. If the QRS complex is wide and bizarre, you are faced with the decision of whether this is of supraventricular origin with ventricular aberration, whether it is of ventricular origin, or if it preexcited. If you know your QRS waveform morphology, you know what to look for and you will recognize it if you see it.

Regularity is a key branch point when evaluating supraventricular tachyarrhythmias. Arrhythmias originating in the atria like atrial fibrillation or multifocal atrial tachycardia are usually irregular, whereas reentrant tachycardias like atrial flutter or AV node-dependent tachycardias (SVT) are typically very regular as are monomorphic ventricular tachycardias.

Because of *overdrive suppression*, the site of origin for an arrhythmia has the highest rate. In many arrhythmias, the atria and ventricle conduct at the same rate; however, if either one is observed to have a higher rate than the other, the faster chamber is typically the driver of the arrhythmia unless there is AV dissociation. Thus, it is imperative to pay close attention to the relationship between P waves and QRS complexes.

Dr. Marriott's Approach: "Cherquez le P" and "Mind Your Ps"

In one's search for P waves, there are several clues and caveats to bear in mind. One technique that may be useful is to employ an alternate lead placement (see Chapter 2) with the positive electrode at the fifth right intercostal space close to the sternum and the negative electrode on the manubrium. This [alternative lead placement] sometimes greatly magnifies the P wave, rendering it readily visible when it is virtually indiscernible in other leads. If it succeeds, this technique is much kinder to the patient than introducing an atrial wire or an esophageal electrode to corral elusive P waves.

Another clue to the detection of P waves is contained in the "Bix rule," named after the Baltimore cardiologist Harold Bix, who observed that "whenever the P waves of an SVT are halfway between the ventricular complexes, you should always suspect that additional P waves are hiding within the QRS complex."

The next caveat in identifying the source of an arrhythmia is to "mind your Ps." This means to be wary of things that look like P waves and P waves that look like other things. This particularly applies to P-like waves that are adjacent to QRS complexes, which may turn out to be part of the QRS complexes. This is a trap for someone who suffers from the "P-preoccupation syndrome," to whom anything that looks like a P wave is a P wave.

The relationship between the atrial and ventricular activation can also help discriminate between different types of SVT. Conduction of impulses through the AV node is somewhat regulated due to a phenomenon known as *decremental conduction*, by which conduction through the AV node slows when it is stimulated at faster rates. Conduction through abnormal connections of the atria and ventricles (eg, via an accessory muscle bundle) is not regulated in this way. Understanding the relative conduction time between ventriculoatrial (VA) conduction and AV conduction can provide clues as to the mechanism of arrhythmia and narrow down the differential diagnosis. This relationship is often revealed on the ECG by comparing the RP interval (VA conduction time) to the PR interval (AV conduction time).

Dr. Marriott's Approach: "Dig the Break"

Whenever a regular rhythm is difficult to identify, it is always worthwhile to seek and focus on any interruption in the regularity—a process that can be condensed into the three words: "Dig the break." It is at a break in the rhythm that you are most likely to find the solution to the source of an arrhythmia. For example, in the beginning strip of **Figure 13.6**, where the rhythm is regular at a rate of 200 beats/min, it is impossible to know whether the tachyarrhythmia is atrial or junctional. A third possibility is that the small positive waveform is part of the QRS complex and not a P wave at all. Further along the strip, there is a break in the rhythm in the form of a pause. The most common cause of a pause is a nonconducted atrial premature beat, and this culprit is indicated by the arrow. As a result of the pause, the mechanism of the arrhythmia is immediately obvious. When the rhythm resumes, the returning P wave is in front of the first QRS complex, indicating that the tachyarrhythmia is evidently an atrial tachycardia.

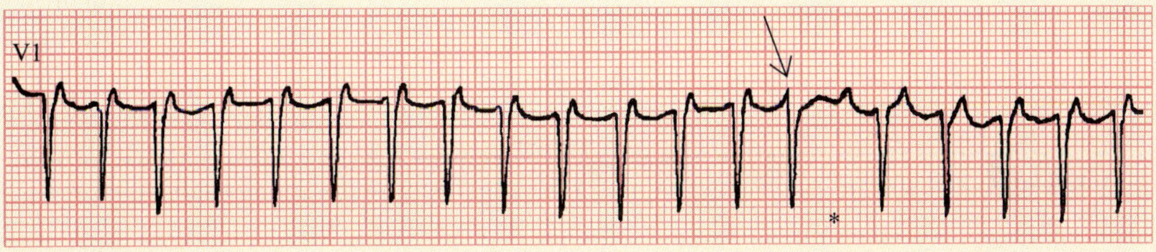

FIGURE 13.6. At the beginning of the rhythm strip, the small positive waveform following the large negative QRS waveform could be (1) a part of a wide QRS complex, (2) a retrograde P wave closely following a narrow QRS complex, or (3) an anterograde P wave with prolonged conduction to a narrow QRS complex. This sequence is broken during the 14th cycle (arrow), where the beginning of a small positive waveform is seen preceding the large negative QRS waveform, and in the 15th cycle, there is no QRS complex (asterisk). The pause (asterisk) produced by the blocked premature atrial beat is terminated by a normally conducted (PR interval ≤ 0.20 second) beat.

Ladder Diagrams

Ladder diagrams are often helpful for understanding difficult arrhythmias. These diagrams have rows for indicating atrial (A), AV junction, and ventricular activation (see **Figure 13.8A**). Additional rows can be added as needed to diagram more complex arrhythmias. The ladder diagram should be constructed directly under or on a photocopy of the ECG recording in two sequential stages as follows:

Tips for Building Ladder Diagrams

1. Include what you can see (eg, draw lines to represent the visible P waves and QRS complexes).
2. Add what you cannot see (eg, connect the atrial and ventricular lines to represent atrioventricular or ventriculoatrial conduction and draw lines to represent any missing P waves at regular PP intervals between visible P waves).

The online version of the book contains multiple animated figures that further explain ladder diagrams and apply them to the following arrhythmia topics:

- **Animation 13.5** Introduction to Tachyarrhythmias
- **Animation 13.6** Tachyarrhythmias: Enhanced Automaticity
- **Animation 13.7** Tachyarrhythmias: Micro Re-Entry
- **Animation 13.8** Tachyarrhythmias: Macro Re-Entry
- **Animation 13.9** Termination of Re-Entrant Tachyarrhythmia
- **Animation 13.10** Atrial and Ventricular Macro Re-Entry Spectra

Figure 13.7B provides an illustration of the use of ladder diagrams to understand a cardiac arrhythmia with varying PR intervals and varying QRS complex morphologies. In the first stage of the diagram, all visible P waves and QRS complexes have been represented. Note the reversed slope representing the premature wide QRS complex, indicating the likelihood that it originated from the ventricles. When the lines representing AV conduction are added in the second stage, the prolonged PR interval following the third P wave is indicated by a slant to represent a conduction delay. The ventricular premature beat must have traveled retrogradely into the AV junction so that the next sinus impulse found the junction *relatively refractory*.

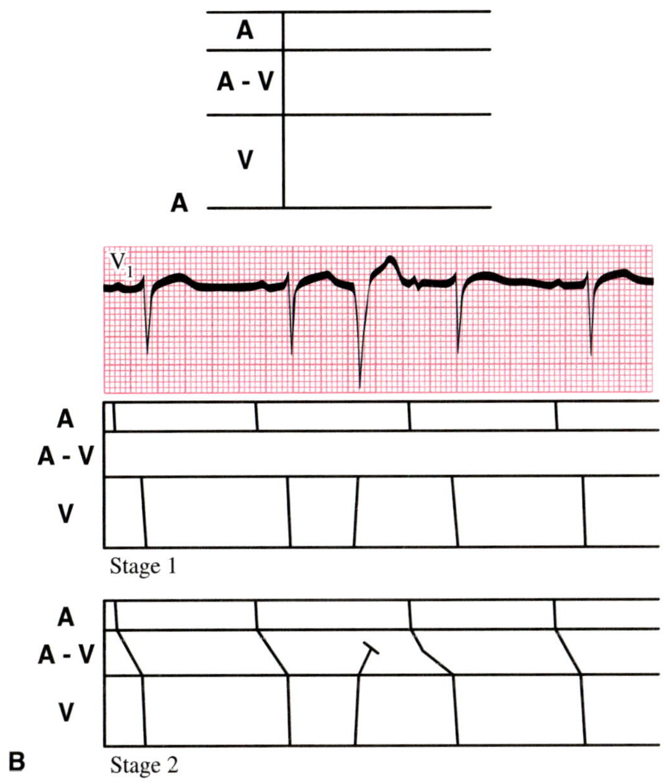

FIGURE 13.7. **A.** The format by which ladder diagrams are constructed: Spaces are provided for representing atrial (A), atrioventricular junctional (A-V), and ventricular (V) activation. The two stages of construction of a ladder diagram: Stage 1 involves the use of slanted lines to include the duration of the obvious waveforms representing both atrial and ventricular activation. The forward or backward slope of the slanted lines indicates the presumed direction of spread of activation. **B.** Stage 2 involves constructing lines in the AV junctional space to connect the atrial and ventricular lines to represent the presumed direction of the spread of junctional activation. These lines are terminated and capped with short perpendicular lines to indicate the presumed failure of impulse conduction.

In subsequent chapters, ladder diagrams are used as visual aids to understand mechanisms of arrhythmias. **Figure 13.8A-D** presents four examples to indicate how various symbols may be used to represent aberrant ventricular conduction (see **Figure 13.8A**), junctional rhythm (see **Figure 13.8B**), ventricular rhythm (see **Figure 13.8C**), and dissociation between atrial and ventricular rhythms (see **Figure 13.8D**).

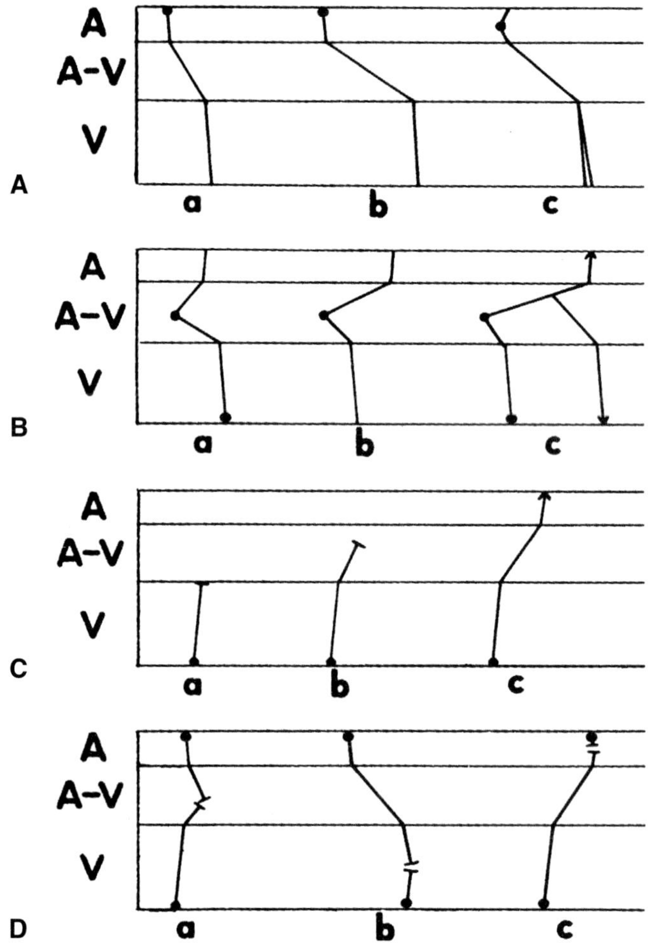

FIGURE 13.8. Solid circles indicate the site of impulse formation, split lines indicate aberrant conduction, pointed arrow heads and line slope (left to right) indicate impulse direction, and flat arrow heads indicate impulse block. **A.** A normal sinus beat (a) encounters prolonged atrioventricular (AV) conduction (b) and is then replaced by an ectopic atrial beat that encounters both prolonged AV conduction and aberrant ventricular conduction (indicated by the split line) (c). **B.** AV-junctional beats with progressively longer retrograde conduction times to the atria: in a, the P wave precedes the QRS complex, but in b, it follows the QRS complex. In c, the retrograde conduction time is so long that a second QRS complex is generated. **C.** Ventricular beats with progressively greater penetration into the AV junction: no conduction (a), partial conduction (b), and complete retrograde ventricular-atrial conduction (c). **D.** In a, there is complete AV dissociation; in b, AV conduction results in "fusion" during the QRS complex; and in c, ventricular-atrial conduction results in fusion during the P wave.

Summary

When evaluating a tachyarrhythmia, key elements of the ECG to focus on include the following:

Elements Useful in Evaluating Tachyarrhythmias

1. Wide or narrow QRS complexes
2. Regular or irregular
3. P wave rate and axis
4. PR and RP intervals
5. What happens when the rhythm is interrupted or terminates?

Integrating this information with an understanding of the mechanisms of arrhythmia will allow the electrocardiographer to either diagnose an arrhythmia or create a focused and informed differential diagnosis.

Dr. Marriott's Approach: "Pinpoint the Primary Diagnosis"

A final piece of advice from Dr. Marriott:

Pinpoint the primary diagnosis. One must never be content to let the diagnosis rest on a secondary phenomenon such as AV dissociation, escape, or aberration. Each of these is always secondary to some primary disturbance in rhythm that must be sought out and identified.

Clinical Methods for Detecting Arrhythmias

There has been enormous growth in technology applied to cardiology in general and the diagnosis and management of arrhythmias, in particular. These methods should not substitute for but rather complement the astute collection of a detailed history from the patient and a competent and complete physical examination of the patient.

The introduction of coronary care units in the early 1960s stimulated rapid advances in the diagnosis and treatment of cardiac arrhythmias. In the coronary care unit, patients who have either arrhythmias, or a high risk of developing arrhythmias because of conditions such as acute myocardial infarction, are continuously monitored (see Chapter 2). A modified chest lead V_1 is commonly used as the display lead because it provides both a good view of atrial activity and of differentiation between right and left ventricular activity (**Figure 13.9**).[2] Often, however, multiple leads are displayed on both bedside and central surveillance monitors to provide multiple views of the cardiac electrical activity to facilitate rapid and accurate rhythm interpretation.

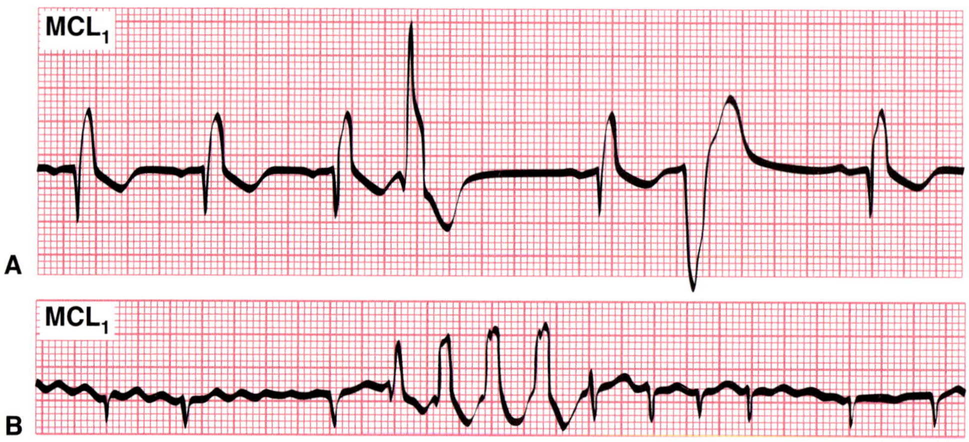

FIGURE 13.9. **A.** Right-bundle-branch block during sinus rhythm and both lead V_1-positive (fourth beat) and lead V_1-negative (sixth beat) ventricular premature beats (see Chapter 15). **B.** The basic rhythm is atrial fibrillation, with most beats conducted normally; however, beats 4 through 7 are not conducted through the right bundle (*aberrantly conducted*). Note the typical triphasic appearance of the initial wide QRS complex. MCL_1, modified chest lead V_1.

Ambulatory Electrocardiogram Monitoring

A method for continuous ECG monitoring of ambulatory patients in their own environment was developed in the 1960s by Holter.[3] The patient is attached via chest electrodes to a portable recorder that records one to three ECG leads for 24 hours. The patient keeps a diary of activities so that symptoms, activity, and cardiac rhythm can be correlated. Thus, the patient is monitored during situations that actually occur in real-life situations. Holter monitoring is used to identify any correlation between an arrhythmia and symptoms such as palpitations, dizziness, syncope, or chest pain (**Figure 13.10**).

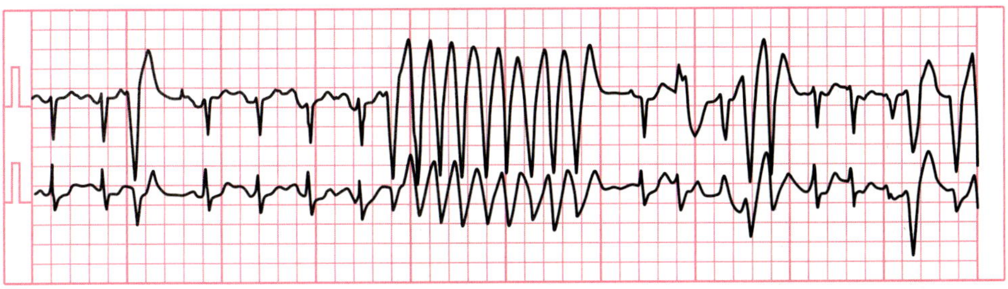

FIGURE 13.10. Holter recording of modified chest leads V_1 and V_5 revealing ventricular premature beats and ventricular tachycardia in a 57-year-old man with dyspnea and palpitations following hospital discharge for an acute myocardial infarction.

Ambulatory monitoring of arrhythmias has evolved substantially since the time of the original Holter monitor (which weighed 75 lb [34.1 kg] and used a large reel-to-reel tape recorder). The expansion of ambulatory monitoring technologies was driven in part due to the increased need to identity asymptomatic atrial fibrillation as a potential source for cryptogenic stroke.[4] Modern ambulatory ECG monitors can record continuously or intermittently and are used for short- or long-term monitoring. Selection of the type of ambulatory monitoring device is dictated by clinical need.[5]

Continuous Monitors (Holter Monitors)

Current Holter technology allows for recording and storage of data from a two- or three-lead ECG system with data collected continuously. These devices are typically used for short-term monitoring as they record for 24 to 48 hours; however, some newer devices can record up to 16 days of ECG data (**Figure 13.11**). This type of monitoring is ideal for evaluation of arrhythmias that occur frequently enough to be captured on such a brief monitor.

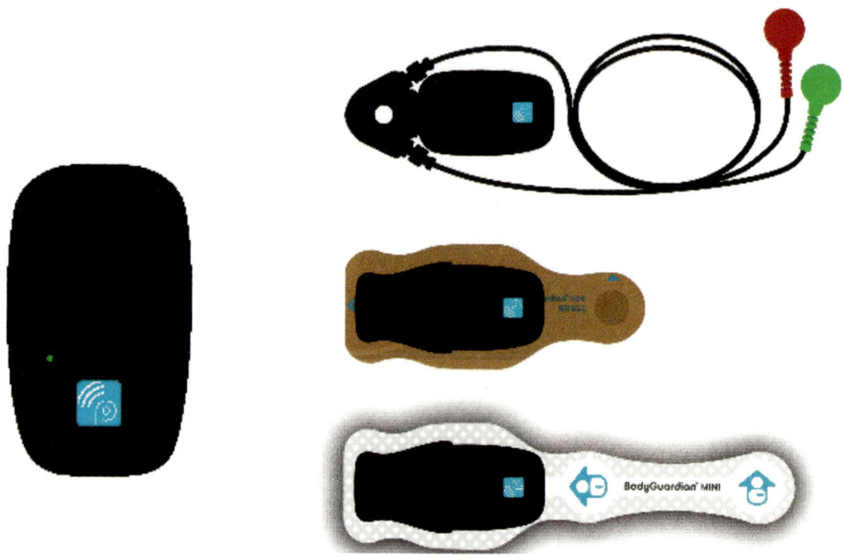

FIGURE 13.11. Example of continuous ambulatory monitor: BodyGuardian MINI Preventice Solutions, Inc. (BodyGuardian is a registered trademark of Preventice Solutions, Inc.)

Holter monitoring is also of value in specific cardiac diseases or in conditions in which information about the heart's rhythm is important for prognosis and management. These conditions include ischemic heart disease, mitral valve prolapse, cardiomyopathy, SA node dysfunction, conduction disturbances, evaluation of pacemaker function, or Wolff-Parkinson-White syndrome. In addition, Holter monitoring may be of value in assessing the therapeutic effect of antiarrhythmic drugs and adjusting drug dosages. In this context, however, it is important to realize that the frequency of an arrhythmia may have day-to-day variation of up to 90%[6] and that a marked and consistent reduction in the incidence of the arrhythmia must occur before its successful treatment can be assumed. Disadvantages of continuous monitors include issues with noncompliance with symptom logs, the absence of real-time data analysis, and patient discomfort with wearing an external monitor for many days, although there have been many advances in material design to adapt to patients with sensitive skin.

Intermittent Patient- or Event-Activated Recorders

Event monitors provide intermittent monitoring of cardiac rhythm that is directed by the patient's experience (**Figure 13.12**). The ECG data is measured continuously, but only recorded when activated by the patient. Once activated, the device records electrocardiographic activity for a fixed amount of time after the activation. Postevent monitors are applied by the patient only after symptom development, whereas external loop devices are worn continuously and can record electrocardiographic data both after the activation time as well as recall data from directly prior to activation (via "looping memory"). Data are then transmitted to a central monitoring station for analysis.

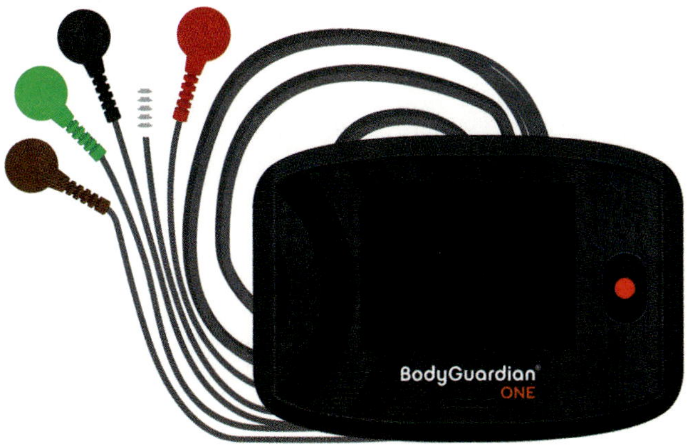

FIGURE 13.12. Example of intermittent patient- or event-activated recorder: BodyGuardian One Preventice Solutions, Inc. (BodyGuardian is a registered trademark of Preventice Solutions, Inc.)

These devices are typically less cumbersome and allow for ambulatory monitoring over longer periods. They are ideal for patients who have symptomatic events that allow them to trigger the devices appropriately. Because they require patient interaction, these devices may not work well for arrhythmias that are associated with altered consciousness or syncope or for patients who lack the technologic prowess to operate the device and transmit the recordings.

Real-time Continuous Event Recorders (Mobile Telemetry)

Real-time continuous event recorders allow for prolonged monitoring of ambulatory electrocardiography in near real time (**Figure 13.13**). They are smaller in size as intermittent event-activated recorders but automatically transmit data to a centralized analysis center. The device transmits data if it detects an arrhythmia or if activated by the patient, which is analyzed by technicians in near real time. The ease of use and continuous nature of this technology has resulted in it having a higher diagnostic yield more than 2.5 times that of an intermittent event-activated recorder.[7]

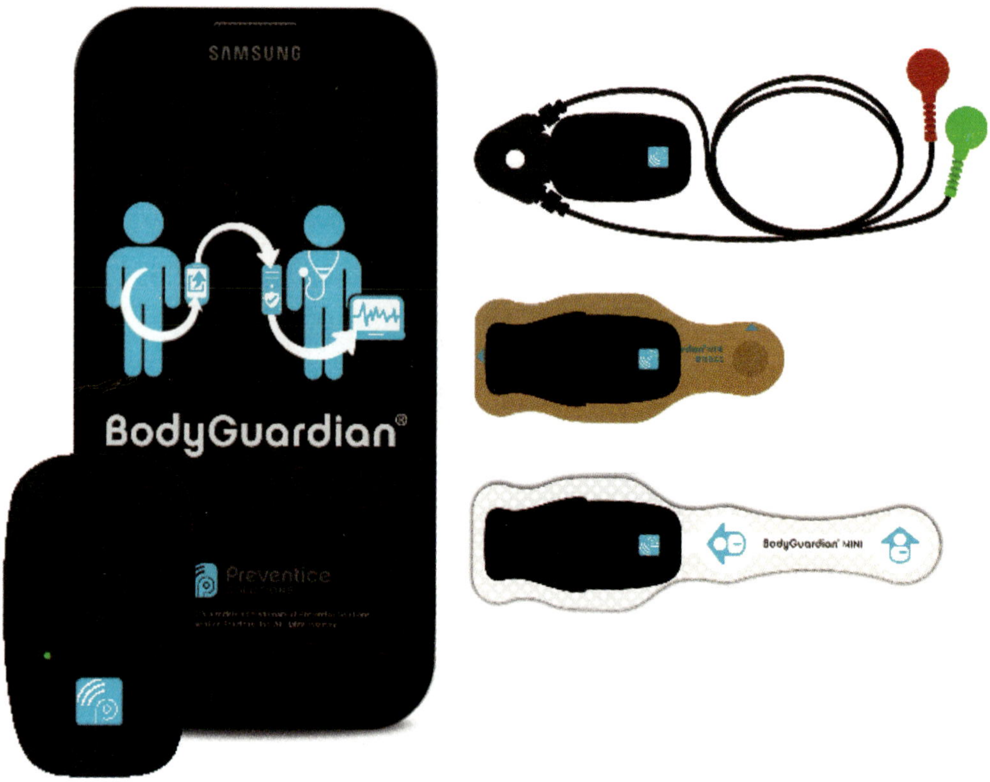

FIGURE 13.13. Example of near real-time mobile cardiac telemetry: BodyGuardian MINI PLUS Preventice Solutions, Inc. (BodyGuardian is a registered trademark of Preventice Solutions, Inc.)

Implantable Loop Recorders

For prolonged ambulatory monitoring, implantable loop recorders provide an attractive option as they can record data for up to 3 years (**Figure 13.14**). These devices are subcutaneously inserted and record a single-lead ECG, which can be transmitted automatically or by patient activation to the patient's provider. The newest versions of these devices are small and not externally visible for most patients.

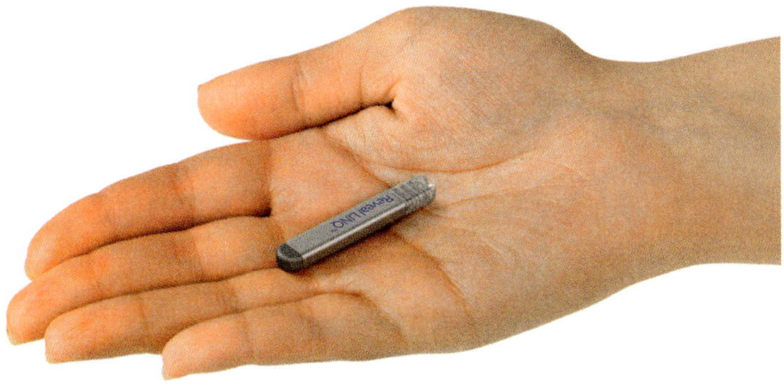

FIGURE 13.14. Example of implantable loop recorder: Medtronic Reveal LINQ Implantable Loop Recorder. (Reproduced with permission of Medtronic, Inc.)

Mobile and Wearable Technology

Novel technologies continue to emerge that may allow broader access to ambulatory electrocardiographic monitoring. Smartwatch and smartphone-based technology such as KardiaBand (AliveCor, Mountain View, CA) allows for patient-initiated, single-lead or six-lead ECG recordings to be obtained and generates an automated interpretation of the cardiac rhythm.[8] Some of the newer smartwatches (eg, Apple watch) can notify and alert the wearer to a potential arrhythmia and also prompt him/her to record a single-lead ECG with the watch itself. The watch can diagnose some of the arrhythmias such as atrial fibrillation. Also, the ECG can be sent to the physician or service provider to confirm the diagnosis and advise further management.[A] How these mobile technology monitors should be integrated into clinical care is an area of ongoing research.[B]

Invasive Methods of Recording the Electrocardiogram

Because monitoring systems via electrodes on the body surface provide access only to electrical activity from the atrial and ventricular myocardia, a definitive rhythm diagnosis is often not possible. The atrial activity may be obscured during a tachyarrhythmia because of superimposed QRS complexes and T waves. When the use of alternate body surface sites for electrodes fails to reveal atrial activity, either transesophageal or intra-atrial recording may be necessary. **Figure 13.15** illustrates the ability of intra-atrial recording to reveal diagnostic atrial activity when none is clearly visible on the body surface. The atrial flutter-fibrillation is confirmed in this patient.

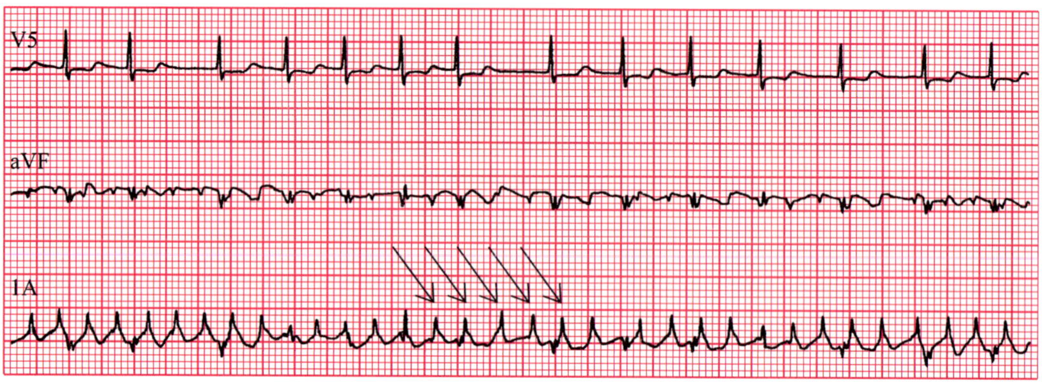

FIGURE 13.15. Simultaneous recording from surface leads V_5 (top) and aVF (middle) and from an intra-atrial electrode (IA) (bottom) from an 81-year-old woman with congestive heart failure. An irregularly irregular ventricular rhythm is apparent in lead V_5, and intermittent atrial activity can be detected in lead aVF. The diagnosis of the rapid atrial rhythm (flutter-fibrillation) with variable atrioventricular block is confirmed by the intra-atrial recording, with arrows indicating the atrial rate of 330 beats/min.

An even more definitive rhythm diagnosis can be obtained by positioning a multipolar catheter across the tricuspid valve, providing direct access to recording from the common or His bundle as a part of invasive electrophysiological study.[9-11] With a more proximal electrode in the right atrium, simultaneous recording from multiple intracardiac locations is possible (**Figure 13.16**). This diagnostic information is clinically important when AV block is present, and differentiation between AV nodal versus His-Purkinje location cannot be inferred from the surface ECG. Moreover, a tachyarrhythmia mechanism can be ascertained by studying the intracardiac electrograms and the features of the tachycardia and performing various diagnostic pacing maneuvers during the same electrophysiological study. If the tachyarrhythmia is not present during the study, it can be induced by stimulation of the atrium and/or ventricle.

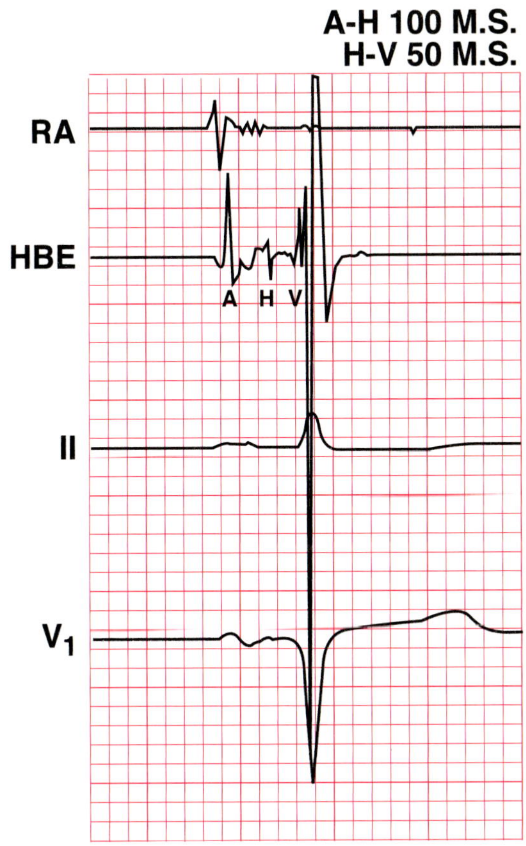

FIGURE 13.16. Electrograms from the right atrium (RA) and His bundle (HBE) are presented, along with recordings from standard leads II and V_1. The atrium-to-His (A-H) interval of 100 milliseconds and His-to-ventricle (H-V) interval of 50 milliseconds combine to form the 150 milliseconds PR interval. M.S., milliseconds. (Reprinted from Wagner GS, Waugh RA, Ramo BW. *Cardiac Arrhythmias*. New York, NY: Churchill Livingstone; 1983:117. Copyright © 1983 Elsevier. With permission.)

Recording from the His bundle provides division of the PR interval into its two components: from the atria through the AV node to the His bundle (atrium-to-His interval) and from the His bundle to the ventricles (His-to-ventricle interval). This method provides direct identification of the site of an AV block (**Figure 13.17**).[12] His bundle recordings have provided proof for many of the originally assumed electrocardiographic principles discussed in later chapters.

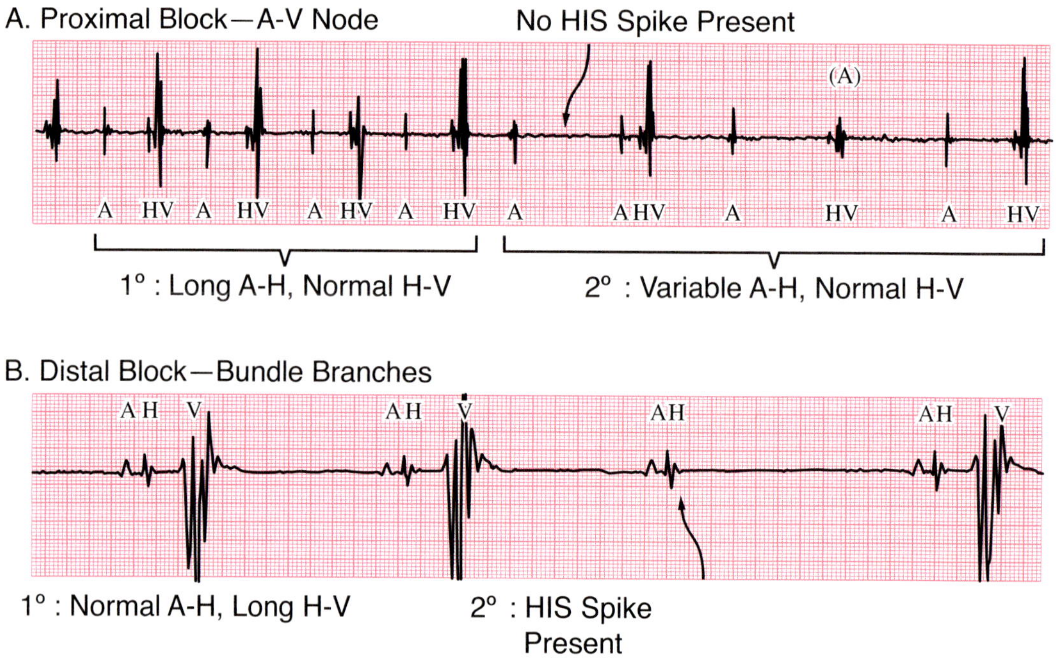

FIGURE 13.17. His bundle electrograms from two patients with initial delay and then complete failure of atrioventricular (AV) conduction. Conduction delays proximal (**A**) and distal (**B**) to the His bundle are indicated by the relationships among atrial (A), His (H), and ventricular (V) spikes. In **A**, during the initial slowly conducted beats (1-4), the A-H time is long but the H-V time is normal; however, in **B**, during the initial slowly conducted beats (1-2), the A-H time is normal and the H-V time is long. When AV conduction fails to occur in **A** (during the fifth cardiac cycle), no His activation occurs; however, when AV conduction fails to occur in **B** (during the third cardiac cycle), the His activation is present (arrow). Slow AV conduction resumes at the end of both **A** and **B**. (Reprinted from Wagner GS, Waugh RA, Ramo BW. *Cardiac Arrhythmias*. New York, NY: Churchill Livingstone; 1983:119. Copyright © 1983 Elsevier. With permission.)

CHAPTER 13 SUMMARY ILLUSTRATION

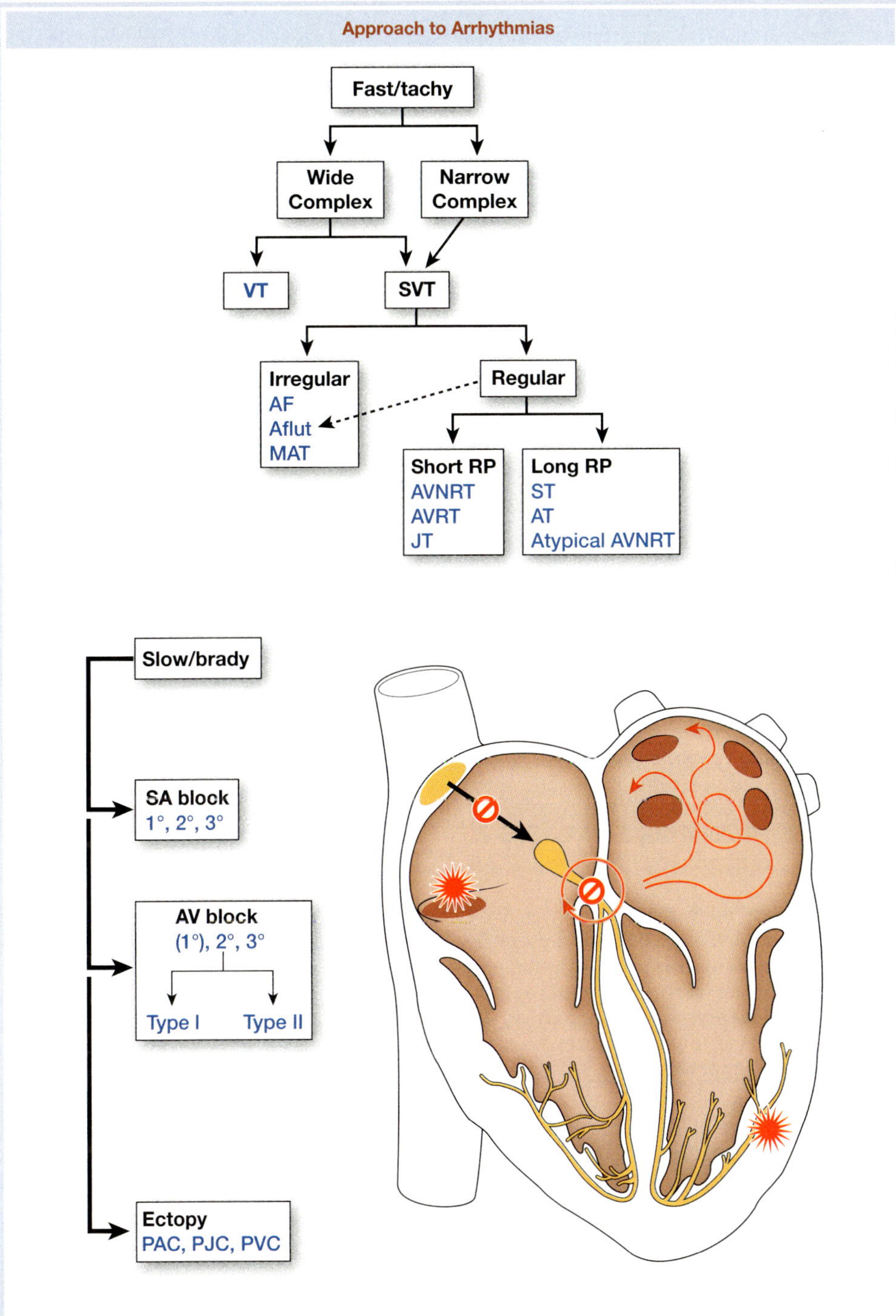

Abbreviations – AFL: atrial flutter; AT: atrial tachycardia; AV: atrioventricular; AVNRT: atrio ventricular nodal reentrant tachycardia; AVRT: atrio ventricular reciprocating (or reentrant) tachycardia; PAC: premature atrial contraction; SN: sinus node; SVT: supraventricular tachycardia

Glossary

Aberrant conduction: intermittent abnormal intraventricular conduction of a supraventricular impulse due to unequal refractoriness of the bundle branches, usually resulting in wider QRS than normal (>120 ms).

Atrial flutter: an AV node independent tachyarrhythmia produced by macroreentry in the atria characterized by regular, uniform flutter waves occurring at rates of 250 to 350 per minute.

Automaticity: the ability of specialized cardiac cells to achieve spontaneous depolarization and function as "pacemakers" to form new cardiac-activating impulses.

AV dissociation: a condition of independent beating of the atria and ventricles, caused either by block of the atrial-activating impulse in the AV junction or by interference with conduction of the atrial-activating impulse by a ventricular impulse.

Block: either a delay (first degree), partial failure (second degree), or total failure (third degree) of impulse conduction through a part of the heart.

Bradyarrhythmia: any rhythm with a ventricular rate of <60 beats/min.

Cardioversion: application of a synchronized electric shock to restore a normal heartbeat.

Decremental conduction: slowed conduction in response to more rapid stimulation.

Delta wave: a slurred upstroke in the QRS complex due to slow cell-to-cell conduction of ventricular myocardium due to preexcitation.

Dysrhythmia: a synonym (by usage) for arrhythmia.

Ectopic: an electrical focus that depolarizes prior to being activated by normal sinus rhythm.

Inhomogeneous conduction: the phenomenon in which the wave front of cardiac activation spreads unevenly through a part of the heart because of varying refractoriness from previous activation, creating the potential for impulse reentry.

Isorhythmic dissociation: AV dissociation, with the atria and ventricles beating at the same or almost the same rate.

Junctional: a term referring to the cardiac structures that electrically connect the atria and ventricles and normally including the AV node and common (His) bundle.

Macroreentry: recycling of an impulse around a circuit that is large enough for its own activation to be represented on the surface ECG.

Microreentry: the recycling of an impulse around a circuit that is too small for its own activation to be represented on the surface ECG.

Overdrive suppression: the phenomenon by which the pacemaker activity with the highest frequency dominates other latent pacemaker centers.

Pacemaker cells: specialized cardiac cells that are capable of automaticity.

Palpitation: perception of heart beating in other than normal fashion for that patient. May be described by the patient as a skipped beat, racing, fluttering, or pounding.

Premature beat: a beat that occurs before the time when the next normal beat would be expected to appear.

Reentry circuit: a circuitous course traveled by a cardiac impulse, created by reentry, and having the potential for initiating premature beats and tachyarrhythmias.

Relatively refractory: a term referring to cells that have only partly recovered from their previous activation and are therefore capable of slow conduction of another impulse.

Spontaneous depolarization: the ability of a specialized cardiac cell to activate by altering the permeability of its membrane to a sufficient degree to attain threshold potential without any external stimulation.

Tachyarrhythmia: any rhythm with a rate of >100 beats/min.

Acknowledgment

We gratefully acknowledge the past contributions of the previous edition's author, Dr. Galen S. Wagner, as portions of that chapter were retained in this revision.

References

1. Hoffman BF, Cranefield PF, Wallace AG. Physiological basis of cardiac arrhythmias. *Mod Concepts Cardiovasc Dis*. 1966;35:103.
2. Marriott HJL, Fogg E. Constant monitoring for cardiac dysrhythmias and blocks. *Mod Concepts Cardiovasc Dis*. 1970;39:103-108.
3. Holter NJ. New method for heart studies. *Science*. 1961;134:1214-1220.
4. Liao J, Khalid Z, Scallen C, Morillo C, O'Donnell M. Noninvasive cardiac monitoring for detecting paroxysmal atrial fibrillation or flutter after acute ischemic

stroke: a systematic review. *Stroke*. 2007;38: 2935-2940.
5. Zimetbaum P, Goldman A. Ambulatory arrhythmia monitoring: choosing the right device. *Circulation*. 2010;122:1629-1636.
6. Michelson EL, Morganroth J. Spontaneous variability of complex ventricular arrhythmias detected by long-term electrocardiographic recording. *Circulation*. 1980;61: 690-695.
7. Rothman SA, Laughlin JC, Seltzer J, et al. The diagnosis of cardiac arrhythmias: a prospective multi-center randomized study comparing mobile cardiac outpatient telemetry versus standard loop event monitoring. *J Cardiovasc Electrophysiol*. 2007;18: 241-247.
8. Bumgarner JM, Lambert CT, Hussein, AA et al. Smartwatch algorithm for automated detection of atrial fibrillation. *J Am Coll Cardiol*. 2018;29;71(21):2381-2388.
9. Damato AN, Lau SH. Clinical value of the electrogram of the conduction system. *Prog Cardiovasc Dis*. 1970;13:119-140.
10. Goldreyer BN. Intracardiac electrocardiography in the analysis and understanding of cardiac arrhythmias. *Ann Intern Med*. 1972;77:117-136.
11. Vadde PS, Caracta AR, Damato AN. Indications for His bundle recordings. *Cardiovasc Clin*. 1980;11:1-6.
12. Pick A. Mechanisms of cardiac arrhythmias: from hypothesis to physiologic fact. *Am Heart J*. 1973;86:249-269.

References to the South Asian Edition

A. Turakhia MP, Desai M, Hedlin H, et al. Rationale and design of a large-scale, app-based study to identify cardiac arrhythmias using a smartwatch: The Apple Heart Study. *Am Heart J*. 2019;207:66-75.

B. Marcus GM. The Apple Watch can detect atrial fibrillation: so what now? *Nat Rev Cardiol* 2020;17(3):135-136.

To view digital content associated with this chapter please access lww.co.in. Instructions are located on the inside front cover.

14

Premature Beats

JAMES P. DAUBERT, AIMÉE ELISE HILTBOLD, FREDRIK HOLMQVIST, AND DEBABRATA BERA

Premature Beat Terminology

Normal sinus rhythm, defined as an electrical signal originating in the sinus node, can be interrupted by a premature electrical signal from either the atria or ventricles. These premature electrical signals are referred to as premature beats (PB) for the remainder of this chapter. An alternate term for "beat" is "contraction," with both terms referring to the mechanical event initiated by the early QRS complex on the electrocardiogram (ECG) recording. It should be noted, however, that not all PB originating in the atria result in a QRS complex. In fact, it is not uncommon for such electrical activity to find the specialized conduction system refractory. When a PB results in a QRS complex, that QRS can either have a normal or abnormal configuration and is either preceded or not preceded by a P wave, which can also have a normal or abnormal appearance and axis. Other terms frequently used for the term "premature beat," include "premature contraction," "early beat," "extrasystole," "premature systole," and *ectopic beat.*

The individual who has a PB may or may not experience a sensation referred to as a *palpitation*. Palpitations can result from several physiologic phenomena including pauses, irregularity, tachycardia, and contraction of atria against closed valves. Most commonly, however, if the PB affects the specialized conduction system or renders the myocardium refractory, a palpitation is felt during the next on-time beat because of the increased ventricular contraction strength caused by the higher volume of blood that enters the ventricles during the delay following the PB. **Figure 14.1** illustrates the following sequence of events that occur as a result of a single PB:

What Happens When a Premature Beat Occurs?

1. The premature beat (PB) occurs earlier than the next sinus rhythm beat.
2. The presence of the PB often prevents the occurrence of the next normal beat, particularly in the chamber in which it originated.
3. If the specialized conduction system and/or myocardium are made refractory by the PB, there is a pause following the PB until the next normal beat occurs.

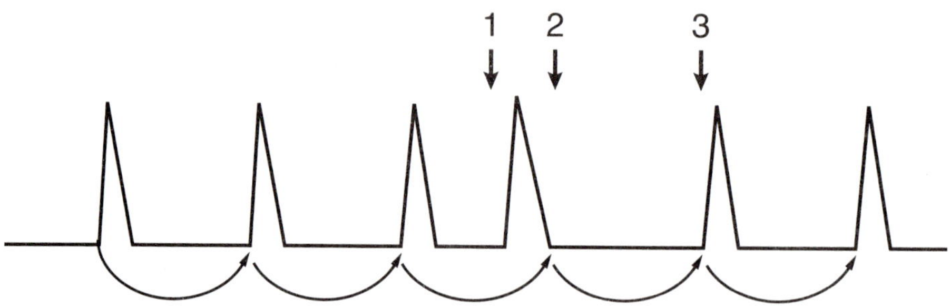

FIGURE 14.1. The timing of a regular underlying rhythm is indicated by the curved lines with arrows. A premature beat interrupts this rhythm (1), preventing the occurrence of the next normal beat (2); however, the following normal beat occurs at the expected time (3).

Table 14.1.

Terminology of Quantities of Premature Beats

Number of Consecutive Beats	Term
1	A premature beat
2	A pair or a *couplet*
3-30 s continuous	Nonsustained tachycardia
>30 s continuous	Sustained tachycardia

A single PB is potentially the first beat of a sustained tachyarrhythmia ("tachycardia"). That single PB may be followed by any number of similarly appearing beats to which the terms in the following two paragraphs are applied (**Table 14.1**). Sustained and nonsustained tachycardias will be discussed in other chapters.

When a PB follows every normal beat, the term *bigeminy* is used; when a PB follows every second normal beat, the term *trigeminy* is used. The PBs may originate from any part of the heart other than the sinoatrial (SA) node including any part if the atria, ventricles, or associated venous structures such as the pulmonary veins or superior vena cava. They are generally classified as either *supraventricular premature beats* (SVPBs), which originate above the ventricles including from the atrioventricular (AV) node or His bundle, or *ventricular premature beats* (VPBs; **Figure 14.2**). This distinction is useful because beats

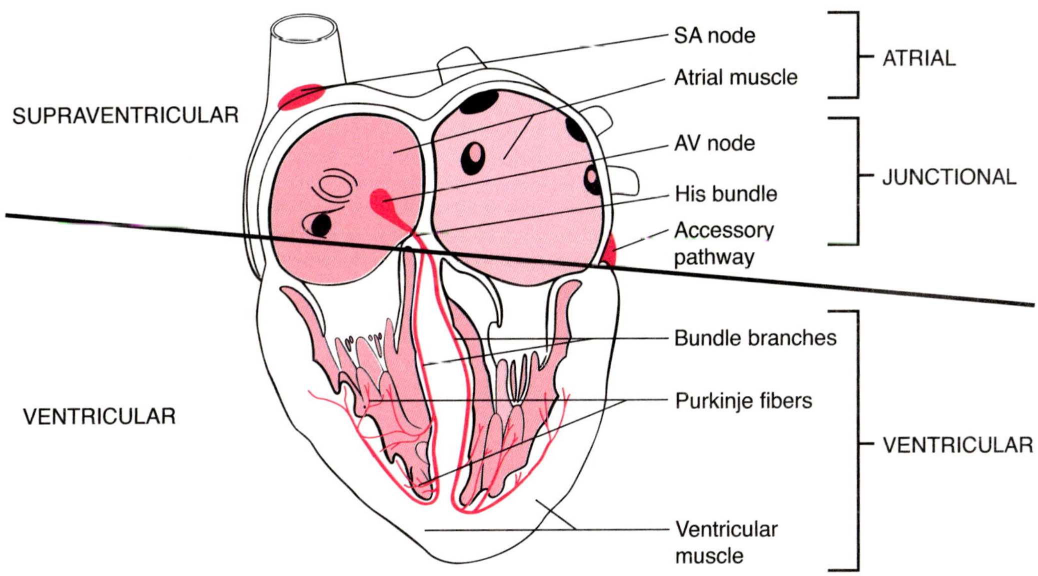

FIGURE 14.2. The anatomic parts of the supraventricular and ventricular areas are indicated. Note the red band connecting the left atrium and left ventricle on the epicardial surface, which represents an accessory pathway. AV, atrioventricular; SA, sinoatrial. (Modified from Netter FH. *The Ciba Collection of Medical Illustrations*. Summit, NJ: Ciba-Geigy; 1978:49. *Heart*; vol 5, with permission.)

originating from anywhere above the branching of the His bundle (SVPBs) are capable of producing either a normal or abnormal QRS complex depending on whether they are conducted normally or *aberrantly* through the intraventricular conduction system. Aberrancy in conduction (wider than normal QRS complex) from SVPBs occurs when part of the ventricular specialized conduction system is refractory to the incoming electrical signal. The PBs originating from beyond the branching of the His bundle (VPBs), however, can produce only an abnormally appearing QRS complex because they do not have equal access to both the right and left bundle branches. In other words, the QRS complex for VPBs is always abnormally prolonged, but the QRS for an SVPB may be of normal duration or may be prolonged (aberrant).[1-6]

The SVPBs include *atrial premature beats* (APBs) and *junctional premature beats* (JPBs). The JPBs are those originating from the AV node or His bundle. The term junctional is used instead of "nodal" because it is impossible to distinguish beats originating within the AV node from those originating in the His bundle. Normally, the AV junction consists of only the AV node and the His bundle as shown in **Figure 14.2**.

Differential Diagnosis of Wide Premature Beats

When SVPBs produce abnormally prolonged or wide QRS complexes, identification of their supraventricular versus ventricular origin may be facilitated by observing the effect on the regularity of the underlying sinus rhythm (**Figure 14.3**). A VPB typically does not disturb the sinus rhythm in the atrium because it is usually not conducted retrogradely through the slowly conducting AV node back to the SA node (see **Figure 14.3A**). In this case, although the SA node discharges on time, its impulse cannot be conducted antegrade to the ventricles because of refractoriness associated with the preceding VPB. The pause (see **Figure 14.3A**) between the VPB and the following conducted beat is termed a *compensatory pause* because it compensates for the prematurity of the VPB. If the SA node is not retrogradely affected by the VPB, the interval from the sinus QRS prior to the VPB to the sinus QRS following the VPB is equal to two sinus cycles. (In the less common scenario, when a VPB does retrogradely conduct to the atria and affects the sinus node, the pause will not be exactly compensatory, similar to what is described for an SVPB below.)

In contrast to a VPB (see **Figure 14.3A**), an SVPB usually does disturb the sinus rhythm. Unlike the VPB, which typically does not affect the sinus node, the SVPB can easily be conducted into the SA node, depolarizing it ahead of schedule and causing the following cycle to occur also in advance of when it otherwise would have fired. The pause between the SVPB and the following sinus beat is therefore less than compensatory. This shorter pause is apparent because the interval from the sinus beat before the SVPB to the sinus beat after the SVPB is less than the duration of two sinus cycles (curved arrows in **Figure 14.3B**). When, however, the SVPB prematurely discharges the SA node, that depolarization occasionally suppresses SA nodal automaticity. This *overdrive suppression* may delay the formation of the next sinus impulse for so long that the resulting pause is compensatory, or even longer than compensatory. Thus, as mentioned above, although these are good general rules, the compensatory pause must not be relied on as the sole indicator of ventricular origin of a wide PB.

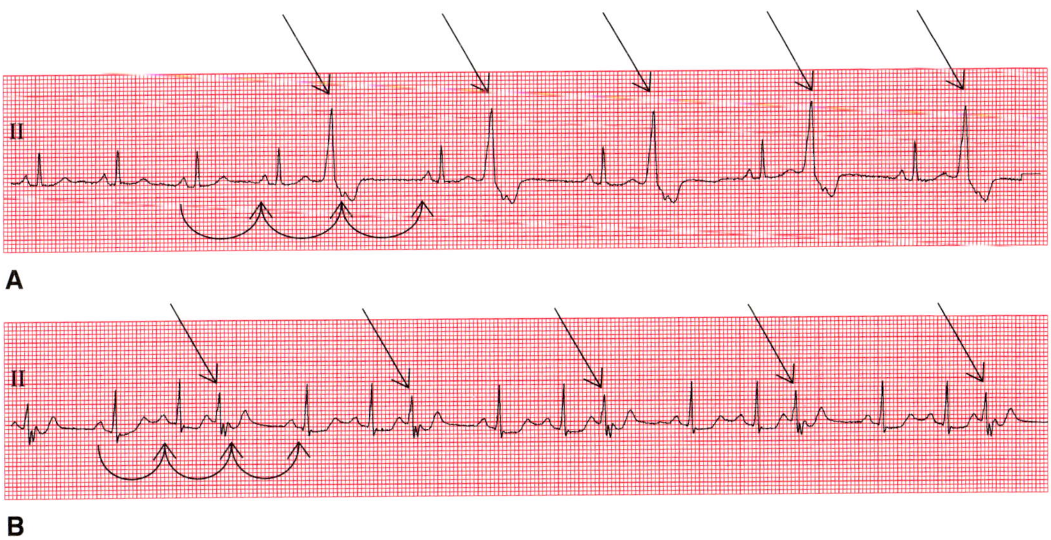

FIGURE 14.3. **A.** Ventricular premature beat. **B.** Supraventricular premature beat. The straight arrows indicate the premature wide QRS complexes in **A** and **B**. The curved arrows show the baseline *PP interval*. Note that in **A**, the P wave after the ventricular premature beat occurs "on time." The PP interval surrounding the ventricular premature beat is exactly twice the normal PP interval. However, in **B**, the (sinus) P wave after the supraventricular premature beat falls earlier than the last curved arrow. The PP interval surrounding the supraventricular premature beat is less than twice the normal PP interval.

Mechanisms of Production of Premature Beats

The PBs may be caused by the one of several mechanisms, including reentry, automaticity, or triggered activity (see Chapter 13). It is usually difficult to determine the mechanism of PBs unless two or more occur in succession. Fortunately, the mechanism of a PB is usually not clinically critical (**Figure 14.4**).

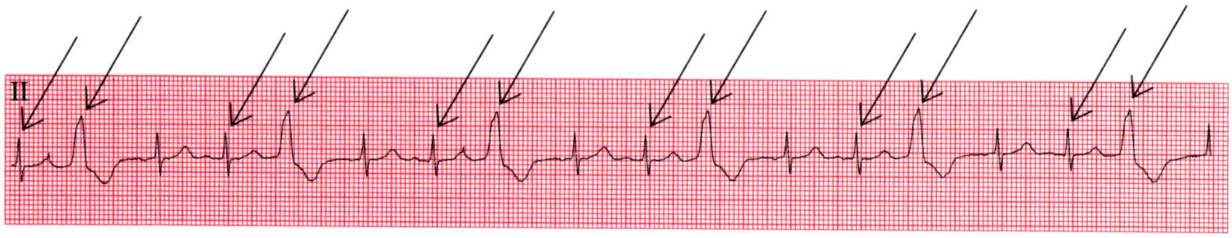

A

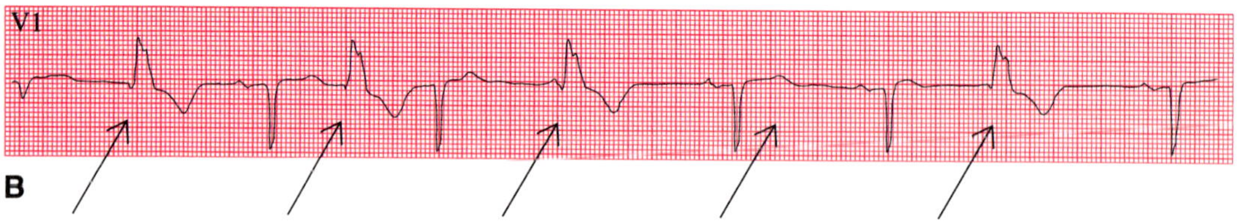

B

FIGURE 14.4. **A.** Premature beats with a fixed *coupling interval* to the prior normal complex; this could be due to reentry or possibly triggered activity. Every third complex is a ventricular premature beat, or the rhythm is ventricular trigeminy. **B.** A constant interectopic interval (with one complex "missing" due to ventricular refractoriness). This sequence can occur due to parasystole.[7] Parasystole has been postulated to be also modulated or variable in interval.[8]

Atrial Premature Beats

The Usual Features of Atrial Premature Beats

1. A premature and abnormal-appearing P wave, although those originating high on the crista terminalis, may look similar to a sinus P wave.
2. A QRS complex identical to that of the normal sinus beats is most often seen. Some APBs, however, exhibit aberrancy, or a prolonged, abnormal QRS complex usually due to block in either the right- or left-bundle-branch block because of refractoriness.[9]
3. A following interval that is less than compensatory because of the premature activation of the SA node and resetting of its timing cycle

Usually, these characteristics hold true, but "deceptions" occur (particularly when the APB is most premature) so that no one characteristic is completely reliable. In **Figure 14.5A**, the premature P waves appear normal; in **Figure 14.5B**, the premature QRS complexes are not always similar to those of the normal sinus beats.

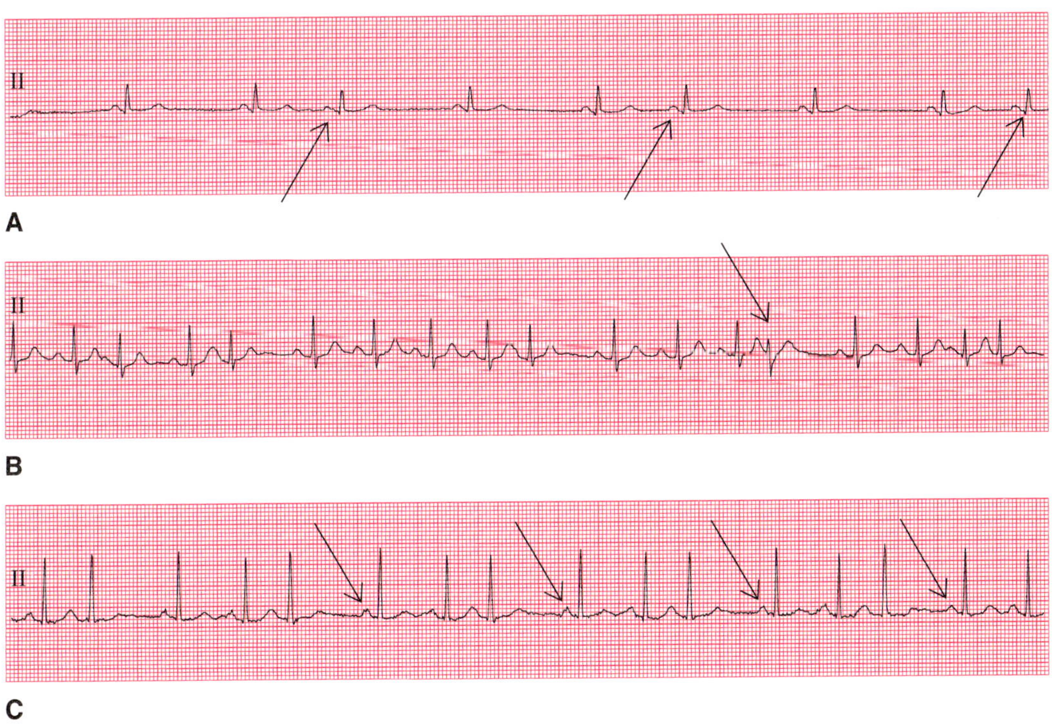

FIGURE 14.5. Three-lead II rhythm strips. Arrows indicate normal-appearing premature P waves in **A**, the aberrant QRS resulting from the earliest of the three atrial premature beats (APBs) in **B**, and the timing of the fully compensatory pause resulting from the early APBs in **C**. Note the abnormal T wave due to superimposed APB P wave before arrow in **B**.

Common Electrocardiogram "Deceptions" in Recognizing Atrial Premature Beats

1. The P wave may be unrecognizable because it occurs during the previous T wave (see **Figure 14.5B,C**). This "P on T" usually results in an abnormal appearing T wave, at least in one or more ECG leads.
2. The QRS complex may show aberrant ventricular conduction (see **Figure 14.5B**).
3. The pause between the APB and the following P wave is compensatory, probably because of the extreme prematurity of the APB and the overdrive suppression of the sinus node (see **Figure 14.5C**).

It is extremely rare to have all three of these deceptions appear at the same time. Therefore, with care, one can usually identify an APB.

When an APB follows every sinus beat, this is termed atrial bigeminy (**Figure 14.6A**); when it follows every two consecutive sinus beats, the result is atrial trigeminy (**Figure 14.6B**).

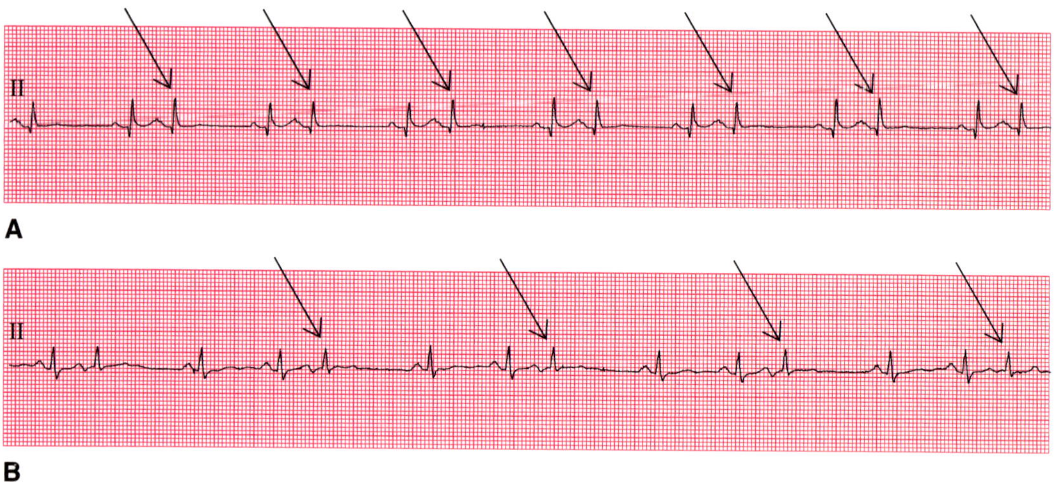

FIGURE 14.6. In **A**, every normal sinus beat and, in **B**, every second normal sinus beat is coupled through constant PP intervals to atrial premature beats. The QRS complexes resulting from these atrial premature beats are indicated by the arrows in the lead II rhythm strips.

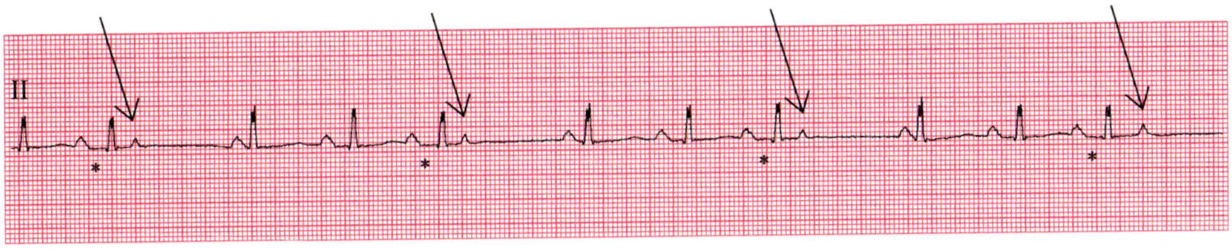

FIGURE 14.7. Nonconducted premature P waves are indicated by arrows, but even some on-time P waves have some conduction delay as indicated by prolonged PR intervals (asterisks).

When APBs occur very early (a short coupling interval), some parts of the heart may not have had time to complete their recovery from the preceding normal activation. This incomplete recovery may result in failure of the premature atrial activation to cause any ventricular activation. Indeed, the most common cause of an unexpected atrial pause is a nonconducted APB (**Figure 14.7**). It is better to refer to such beats as "nonconducted" rather than "blocked" because, by definition, "block" implies an abnormal condition. The APBs fail to be conducted only because they occur so early in the cycle that the AV node is still in its normal refractory period. It is important to differentiate normal (physiologic) from abnormal (pathologic) nonconduction to avoid mistakenly treating a normal physiologic response with an unneeded pacemaker.

> "The most common cause of a pause is a non-conducted APB."
>
> HJL Marriott

Nonconducted APBs that occur in a bigeminal pattern can be difficult to identify (**Figure 14.8**). If the premature P waves are obscured by the T waves of the preceding normal beats, and if the earlier T waves during the regular sinus rhythm are not available for comparison, then the rhythm is often misdiagnosed as sinus bradycardia.

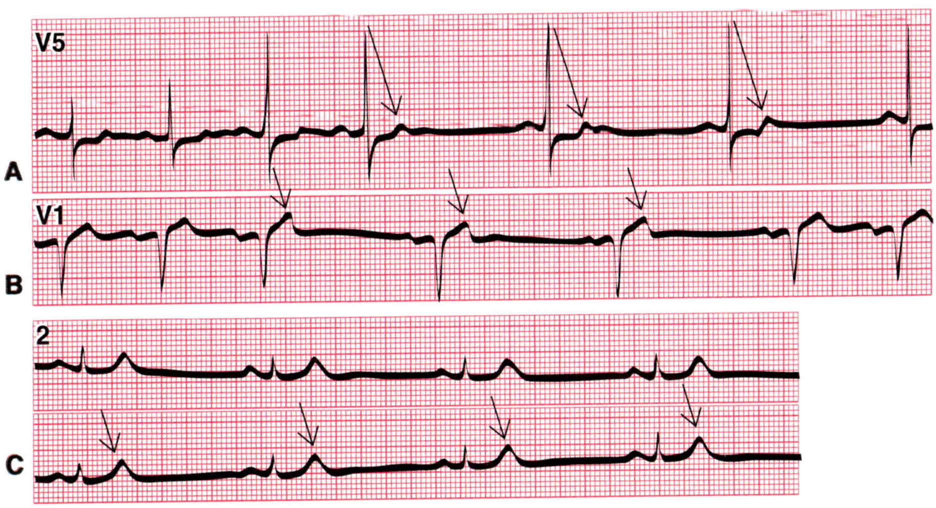

FIGURE 14.8. **A,B.** T waves preceding the pauses (arrows) appear different from usual. **C.** There are suspicious peaks on the T waves (arrows), but there are no "usual" T waves available for comparison.

When APBs occur very early in the cardiac cycle of normal beats, they may have other effects on conduction to the ventricles (**Figure 14.9**). In **Figure 14.9A**, there is prolonged AV conduction, whereas in **Figure 14.9B** there is both slightly prolonged AV conduction and there is also aberrant intraventricular conduction. In **Figure 14.9B**, there are varying coupling intervals (PP intervals) between normal sinus beats and APBs. When the PP interval is long, the premature PR interval is normal, but when the PP interval is short, the premature PR interval is prolonged. This inverse relationship occurs because of the uniquely long relative refractory period of the AV node: The longer the duration from its most recent activation, the better is the node able to conduct the following impulse and vice versa. This concept is vital to use of the ECG to differentiate a nodal versus Purkinje location of AV block.

When an early APB traverses the AV junction but encounters refractoriness in one of the bundle branches or fascicles, aberrant ventricular conduction occurs (see **Figure 14.9B**). The morphology of the QRS complex will be altered and may resemble a VPB. Remembering the previously mentioned clues for differentiating between APBs with aberrancy and VPBs and looking for the preceding P wave and/or finding that the pause between the APB and the next sinus beat is less than compensatory usually establishes the diagnosis of an APB.

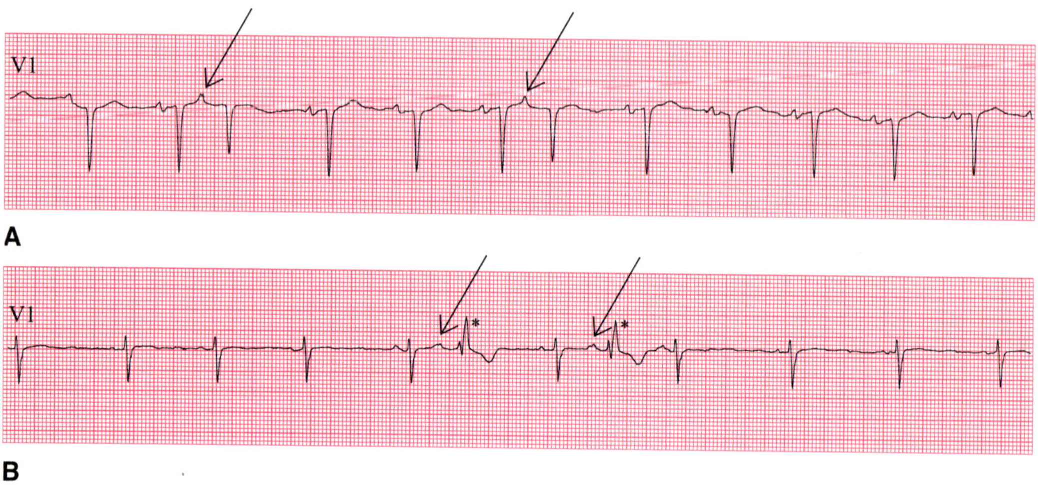

FIGURE 14.9. Recordings of lead V_1 illustrate other varieties of physiologic conduction delays that may occur when the atrioventricular (AV) node alone (**A**) or both the AV node and the right bundle branch (**B**) have not had time to fully recover from their preceding normal activation. Arrows indicate prolonged AV nodal conduction in **A** and **B**, and asterisks indicate right-bundle-branch aberrancy in **B**.

The APBs may occur so early that even parts of the atria have not completed their refractory periods or parts of the conduction system such as the fast AV nodal pathway may block. During this time (the *vulnerable period*), the APB may initiate a reentrant atrial tachyarrhythmia such as AV nodal reentrant tachycardia (AVNRT) due to block in the fast AV nodal pathway and activation down the slow pathway with subsequent retrograde activation through the fast pathway, atrial flutter typically involving activation around the tricuspid annulus, or the nearly totally disorganized rhythm of atrial fibrillation (**Figure 14.10**). In this instance, the APB becomes the first beat of atrial flutter/fibrillation. The APBs may occur in patients with normal hearts or mild to advanced heart disease. Frequent APBs are associated with atrial fibrillation and thus a risk of stroke.[2]

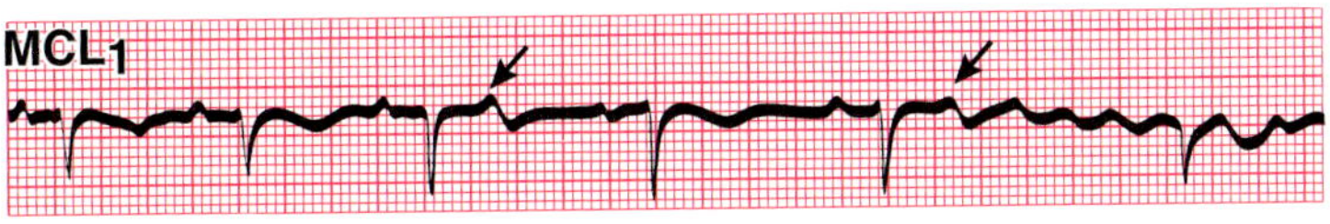

FIGURE 14.10. Arrows indicate two early atrial premature beats with PP intervals of 0.40 second (400 ms). The second atrial premature beat initiates atrial fibrillation.

Junctional Premature Beats

The PBs arising in the AV junction and conducting to the ventricles may retrogradely activate the atria before, during, or after ventricular activation. Thus, the retrograde P wave may be seen preceding or following the QRS complex or may be buried within the QRS complex. These variations are illustrated in **Figure 14.11**.

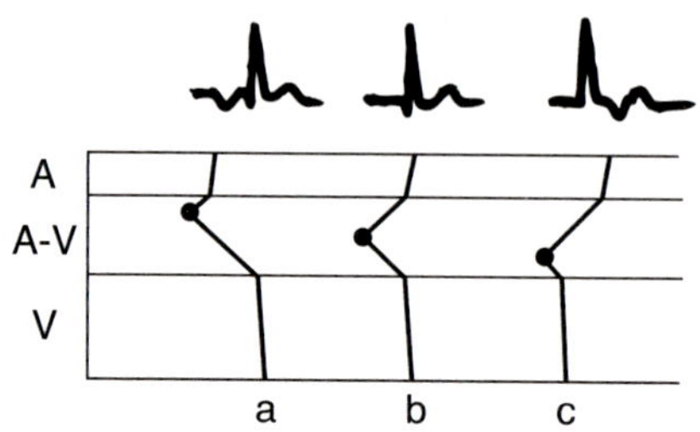

FIGURE 14.11. Three impulses (a, b, c) are formed within the atrioventricular (A-V) junction as illustrated in the electrocardiogram recordings and explained in the ladder diagrams. In the ladder diagram, the anatomic site of impulse formation (solid circle) varies, but the A-V nodal conduction velocity is constant, resulting in the varying P-QRS relationships and aberrant ventricular conduction (c). A, atrium; V, ventricle.

The diagnosis of junctional origin of PBs is easiest when a premature normal QRS complex is closely accompanied by an inverted P wave (**Figure 14.12**). As expected, the morphology of the P waves associated with JPBs is markedly different from that of the P waves of normal sinus rhythm. The polarity of the P waves associated with JPBs is approximately opposite that of the P waves of normal sinus rhythm, as is best seen in a lead with base-to-apex orientation, such as lead II. A P wave originating from the AV junction is also inverted in the other inferiorly oriented leads (III, aVF).

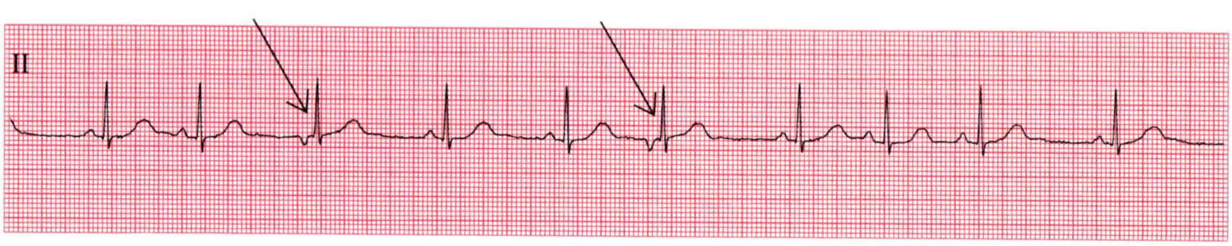

FIGURE 14.12. The contrasting appearances of P waves originating from the sinus node and the atrioventricular junction (arrows) are illustrated in this lead II rhythm strip.

A JPB may be confused with an APB when a premature normal QRS complex is preceded by an abnormal P wave (see **Figure 14.12**). The sinus rhythm is typically reset by an APB but may or may not be reset by a JPB depending on its ability to invade the sinus node and if the JPB conducts to the atrium. The pause following a JPB is often fully compensatory (see **Figure 14.12**).

A JPB may fail to conduct retrogradely to the atrium leading to a premature (usually) narrow QRS without an accompanying P wave (**Figure 14.13**). In addition, a JPB may fail to conduct antegradely to the ventricles, a situation that can be suspected in the setting of other conducted JPBs. These are termed concealed His extrasystoles.[10]

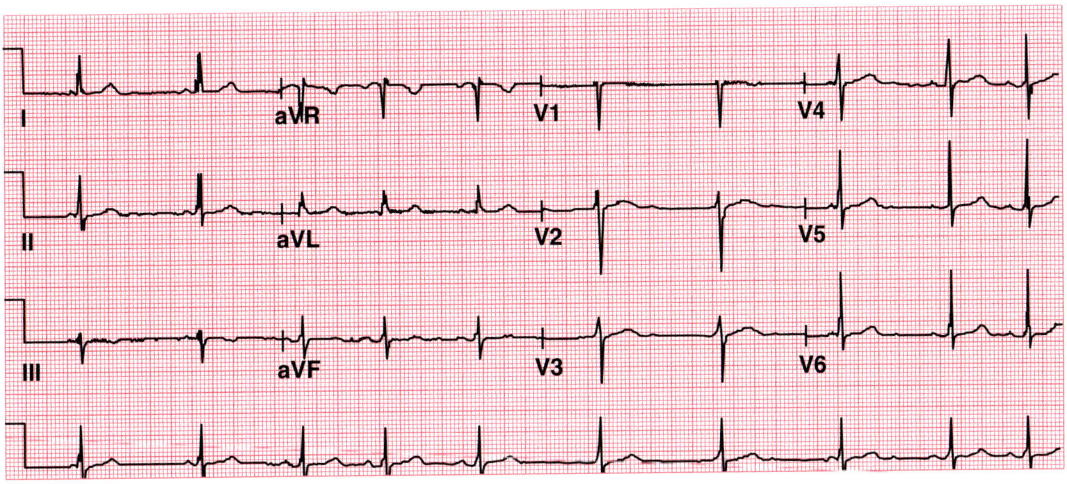

FIGURE 14.13. A 12-lead electrocardiogram with lead II rhythm strip at the bottom is shown. The underlying rhythm, on first glance, appears to be sinus, and the QRS complexes are narrow. Several beats stand out as exceptions, including the sixth and seventh ones. The normal PR interval is seen on the third, fourth, and fifth beats. All the P waves appear identical, but notice that the sinus PP interval varies due to sinus arrhythmia. Look at the most obviously abnormal beats, the sixth and seventh ones. There is not a preceding P wave for these. These are junctional premature beats. On closer examination, the PR interval is abbreviated on the first, second, and eighth beats, too. These are also junctional beats. The sinus P wave is during the initial part of the sixth QRS, slightly earlier for the seventh and just barely in front of the eighth QRS. When the PP interval is longer, the junctional beats emerge. This is an example of sinus rhythm being isorhythmic (nearly the same rate) as junctional rhythm.

A JPB may be confused with a VPB when the premature QRS complex is wide. **Figure 14.14** shows JPBs with differing degrees of right-bundle-branch (RBB) aberration. The retrograde atrial activation is apparent from the P waves following the premature QRS complexes. Although the first PB in each ECG strip cannot be distinguished from a VPB, the fact that the second PB manifests a lesser degree of RBB block is a strong point for aberrant conduction from a JPB.

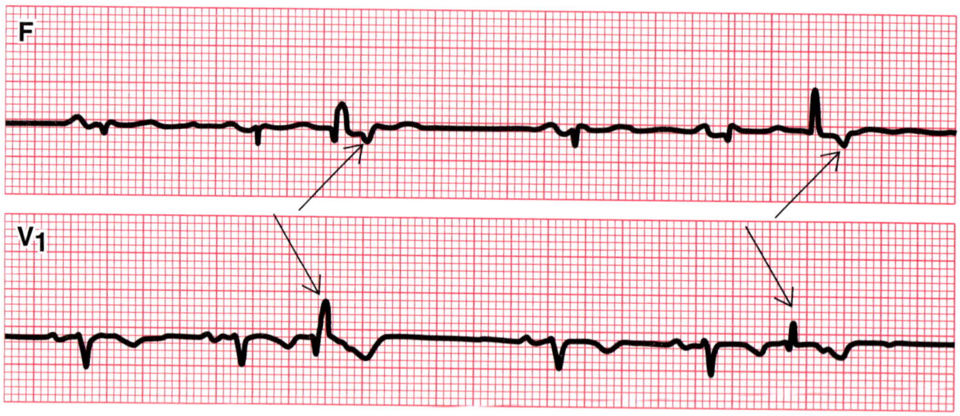

FIGURE 14.14. Lead aVF optimally illustrates the inverted P waves (arrows) in this case of junctional premature beats with right-bundle-branch block aberration. Lead V_1 helps confirm the varying amounts of right-bundle-branch block aberrancy (arrows). The combined contributions of both leads confirm the junctional origin of the premature beats.

Ventricular Premature Beats

The characteristic VPB (**Figure 14.15**) is not preceded by a premature P wave and is represented by a wide and bizarre QRS complex, generally not a typical RBB or left-bundle-branch block pattern. A VPB is usually followed by a compensatory pause because of its inability to conduct retrogradely through the AV node to reset the SA node, although this is not universally true.

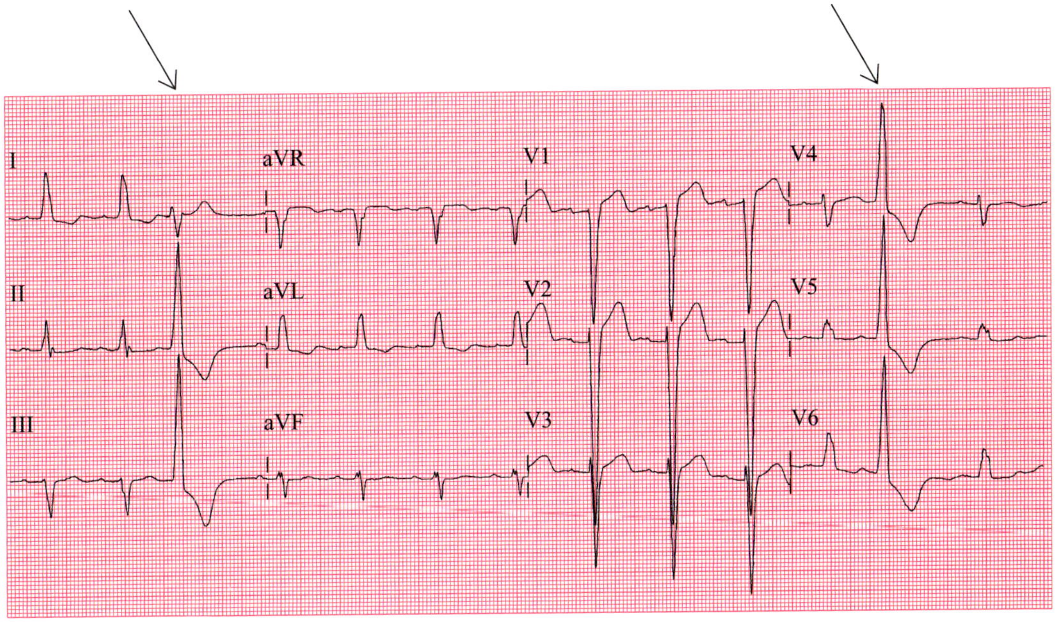

FIGURE 14.15. The views of typical ventricular premature beats (arrows) from multiple, simultaneously recorded electrocardiogram leads. Note that ventricular premature beats occur only during displays of the first and fourth groups of leads.

Exceptions to "Rules" for Interpreting Premature Beats

1. Regarding a preceding premature P wave, a ventricular premature beat (VPB) may be preceded by a premature P wave if both an atrial premature beat and a VPB are present; however, this coincidence is rare.
2. Regarding the appearance of the QRS complex, a VPB, although typically ≥0.12 second (ie, wide), may appear to have a normal duration in any single lead because its initial or terminal component may be isoelectric. A VPB may, by coincidence, appear similar to the normal beats in a single lead, as illustrated in lead V_1 in **Figure 14.16**. It is important to consider two or even three simultaneously recorded leads in determining the origin of a premature beat.
3. Regarding the pause following the VPB, if there is marked variation in the underlying sinus regularity because of sinus arrhythmia, it cannot be determined whether or not a pause is compensatory. When the sinus rhythm is regular, however, there are rare occurrences of a VPB that lacks a following compensatory pause.

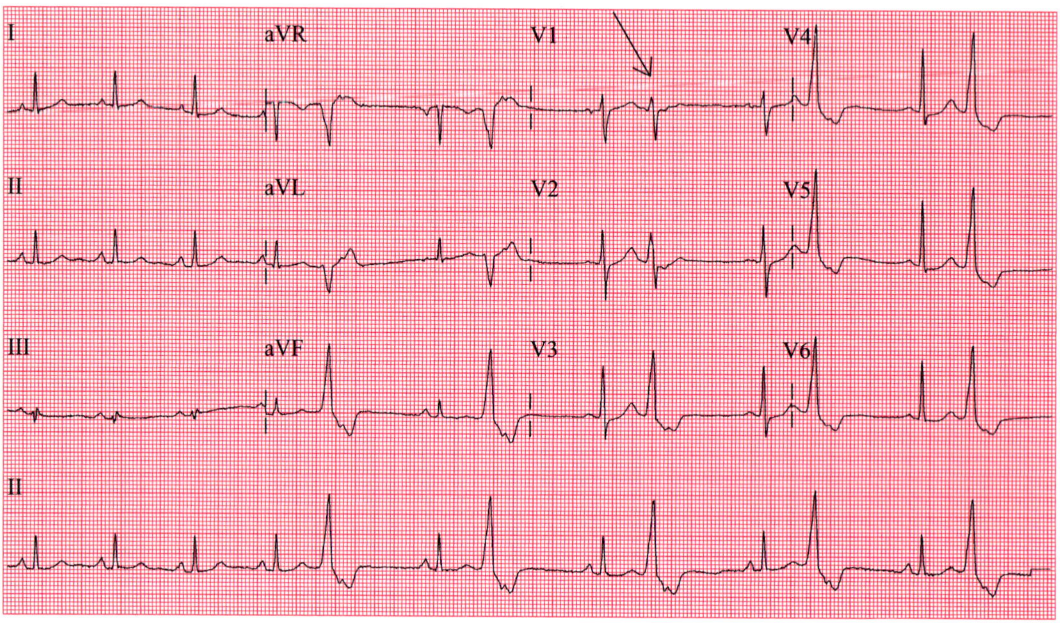

FIGURE 14.16. Multiple ventricular premature beats are obvious in many electrocardiogram leads. However, in lead V_1 (arrow), the QRS complexes of the ventricular premature beats coincidentally appear very similar to those of the normal sinus beats. If only a lead V_1 recording was available, the erroneous diagnosis of atrial premature beats might be made.

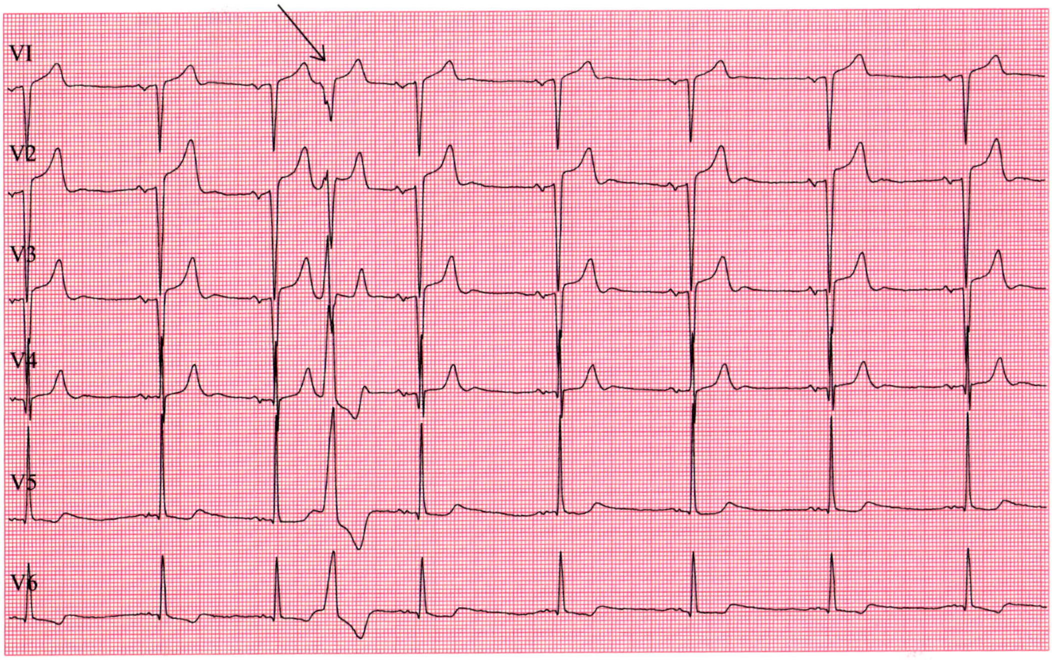

FIGURE 14.17. A single interpolated ventricular premature beat occurs (arrow) between the third and fourth sinus beat. Note the slight sinus irregularity (sinus arrhythmia).

A VPB that lacks a compensatory pause occurs for one of two reasons: (1) the VPB is *interpolated* between consecutive sinus beats or (2) the VPB resets the sinus rhythm. Examples of these two possibilities are seen in **Figures 14.17** and **14.18**.

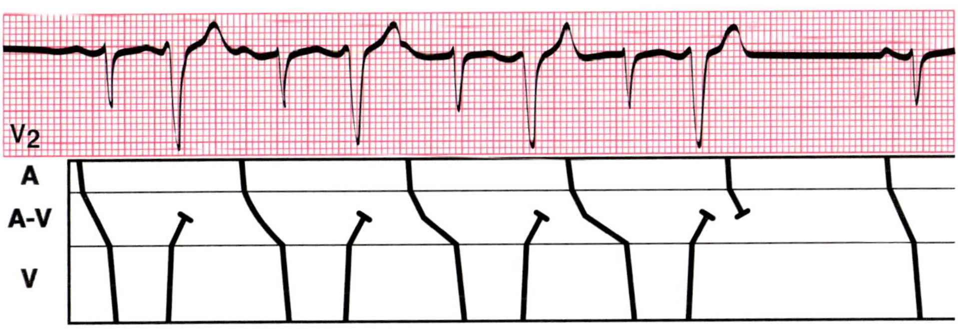

FIGURE 14.18. The ladder diagram indicates the relationships between the P waves and QRS complexes when both anterograde and retrograde activation prevent full recovery of the atrioventricular (A-V) node. A, atrium; V, ventricle.

The Ventricular Premature Beat Is Interpolated Between Consecutive Sinus Beats

When the sinus rate is relatively slow and an early VPB occurs (ie, long before the following sinus impulse), there may be ample time for the AV node and ventricles to complete their refractory periods, thus allowing the next normal sinus impulse to conduct anterogradely. The VPB is said to be interpolated between sinus beats, and there is no pause (see **Figure 14.17**).

The PR interval of the sinus beat following the VPB will be prolonged if the AV node is still partly refractory from its retrograde activation by the VPB. This type of PR prolongation is an example of "concealed conduction" because the absence of both a retrograde P wave and resetting of the sinus rhythm indicates that the impulse produced by the VPB never reached the atria. The concealed retrograde conduction into the AV node from the retrograde direction prevents its complete recovery for the next anterograde impulse, thereby leading to PR prolongation. Depending on timing and AV nodal properties, there may be complete failure of anterograde conduction due to the concealed retrograde conduction (see **Figure 14.18**). As was discussed with regard to APBs, this pause represents a physiologic case of nonconduction in contrast to pathologic AV block.

The Ventricular Premature Beat Resets the Sinus Rhythm

When a VPB is only slightly premature (close to the time of the next sinus impulse), it can pass retrogradely through the AV node because this structure has recovered from the anterograde conduction of the previous sinus beat. The atrial impulse (from the VPB) can then enter the SA node and reset it in much the same way as does an APB. The retrograde P wave generated by the VPB may appear in the T wave or in the ST segment after the VPB (**Figure 14.19**). The pause after the VPB and prior to the next sinus beat is therefore less than compensatory.

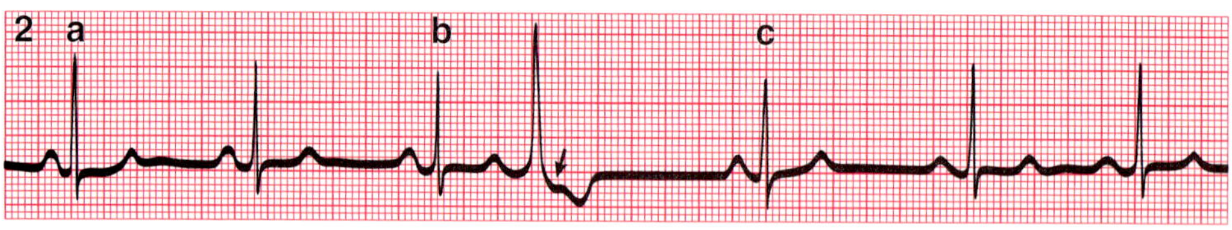

FIGURE 14.19. The arrow points to the retrograde atrial activation by a ventricular premature beat that resets the sinus node, as indicated by the less-than-compensatory pause (the b-c interval is less than the a-b interval).

When a VPB occurs so late that the next sinus P wave has already appeared (**Figure 14.20**), the compensatory pause is not really a pause at all. Only the short PR interval provides a clue that the wide QRS complex is indeed from a VPB. If the PR interval were normal, the incorrect diagnosis would most likely be intermittent bundle-branch block. The pattern of a normal P wave, short PR interval, and wide QRS complex could also be produced by ventricular preexcitation (see Chapter 19).

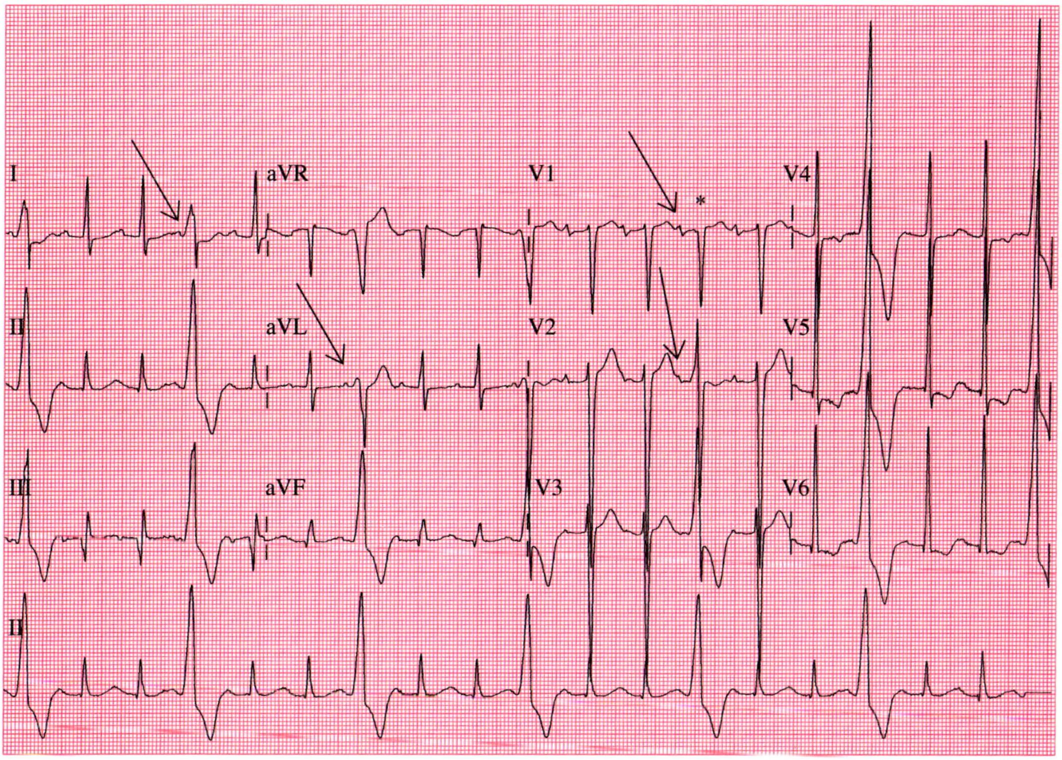

FIGURE 14.20. The ventricular premature beats in this electrocardiogram recording occur so late in the cycle that they follow the P waves of the normal sinus beats (arrows). Note, as in **Figure 14.16**, that the ventricular premature beats appear similar to the normal sinus beats in lead V_1 (asterisk).

Right-Ventricular Versus Left-Ventricular Premature Beats

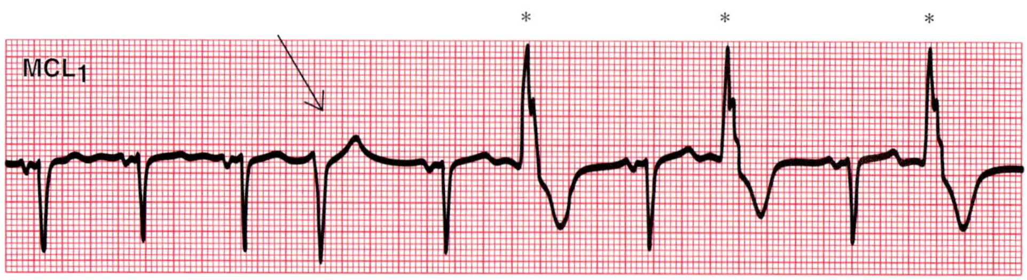

FIGURE 14.21. The use of lead MCL_1 provides identification of the ventricle of origin of the ventricular premature beats (VPBs). The arrow shows the initial VPB (from the right ventricle) producing a long cycle that precipitates another VPB (from the left ventricle), which is shown by the asterisks. This pattern continues, resulting in a bigeminal rhythm.

Figures 14.21 and **14.22** illustrate the contrast between VPBs originating from the right ventricle (*right VPBs*) and those originating from the left ventricle (*left VPBs*).[11] The ventricle of origin of ectopic beats can often best be recognized in lead V_1 (see Chapter 1). If the VPB in lead V_1 is predominantly positive (V_1 positive), the impulse must be traveling anteriorly and rightward from its origin in the posteriorly located left ventricle (**Figure 14.22A**). If the VPB in lead V_1 is predominantly negative (V_1 negative), the impulse must be traveling posteriorly and leftward, usually from its origin in the anteriorly located right ventricle (**Figure 14.22B**).[3] However, VPBs from the ventricular septum may exhibit a negative V_1 morphology.

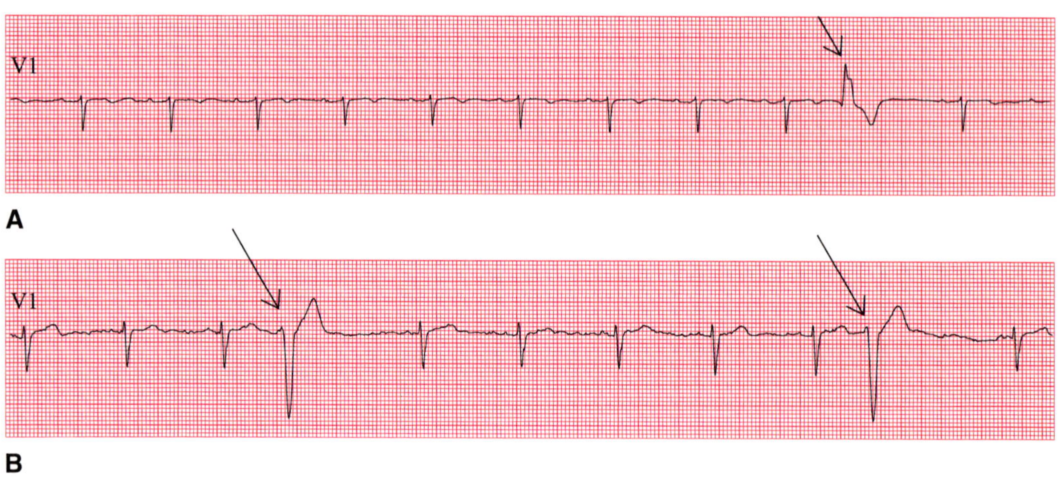

FIGURE 14.22. The contrasting appearances of V_1-positive (left ventricular) (**A**) and V_1-negative (right ventricular) (**B**) ventricular premature beats (arrows).

The differentiation between a right- and left-ventricular origin of VPBs can be clinically useful,[12] but previous associations with or without heart disease have not proven as definitive as once believed (**Figure 14.23**).

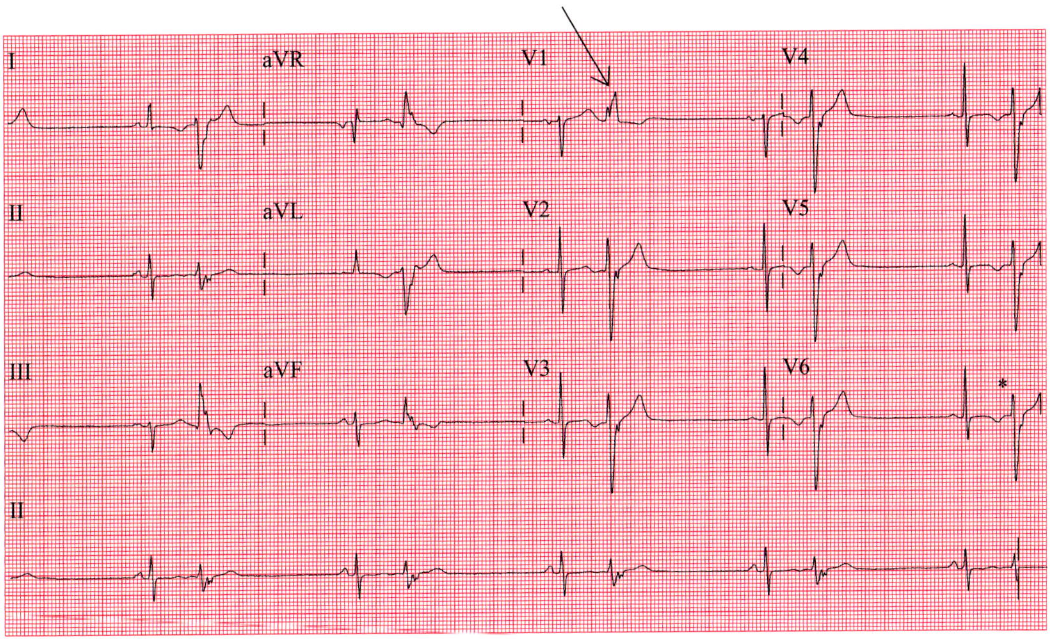

FIGURE 14.23. The monophasic V_1 R wave (arrow) and diphasic V_6 rS wave (asterisk) appearances that typify a ventricular premature beat from the left ventricle.

Right-ventricular outflow tract VPBs, with a negative V_1 (and V_2) complex, a strongly positive complex in the inferior leads (II, III, and aVF), and negative complex in aVL (and usually I) are the most common location for VPBs in patients without serious structural heart disease (**Figure 14.24**).[13] On the other hand, VPBs from this location and with a similar morphology may occur in patients with cardiomyopathy, especially arrhythmogenic right-ventricular cardiomyopathy.[14,15]

VPBs from the left ventricle are common in patients with prior infarction but can occur in patients with other cardiomyopathies, mitral valve prolapse,[16] and in patients without structural heart disease.[17]

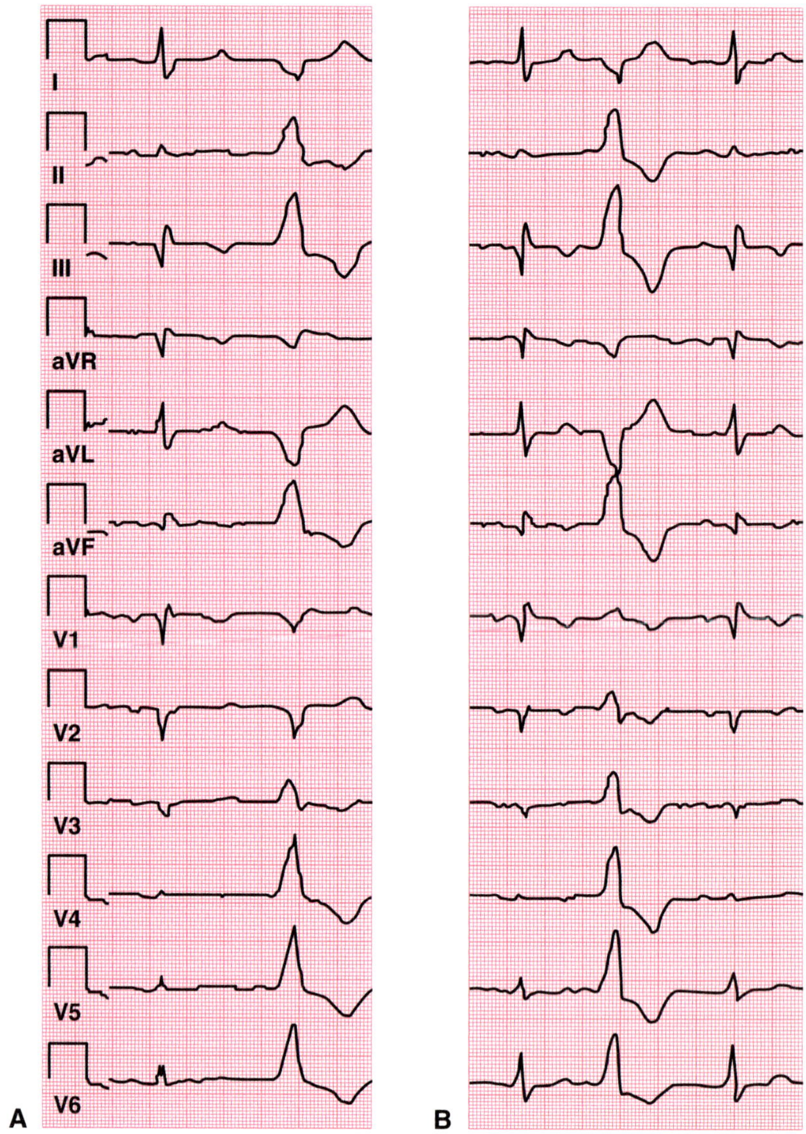

FIGURE 14.24. Outflow tract ventricular premature beats. A 12-lead electrocardiogram with 12-channels of rhythm display format. **A.** The underlying rhythm is sinus with an incomplete right-bundle-branch block. The second beat is a premature ventricular beat with a wide QRS and no preceding P wave. It originates from the right ventricle having a QS wave in V_1 to V_2, specifically from the right-ventricular outflow tract with positive complex in the inferior leads (II, III, and aVF) and negative complex in I and aVL. **B.** The second beat is a premature ventricular beat with a wide QRS and no preceding P wave. It originates from the left ventricle having an R wave in V_1 to V_2, specifically from the left-ventricular outflow tract with positive complex in the inferior leads (II, III, and aVF) and negative complex in I and aVL.

Multiform Ventricular Premature Beats

When VPBs manifest different QRS complex morphologies in the same lead (**Figure 14.25**), they are termed *multiform VPBs*. Because such VPBs are assumed to arise from different foci, they are also called *multifocal VPBs*. It is possible, however, that slight variation in QRS complex morphology produced by VPBs may result from varying intraventricular conduction rather than from varying sites of origin. Multifocal VPBs usually indicate underlying disease such as myocardial ischemia, myocarditis, inflammation, or scar.

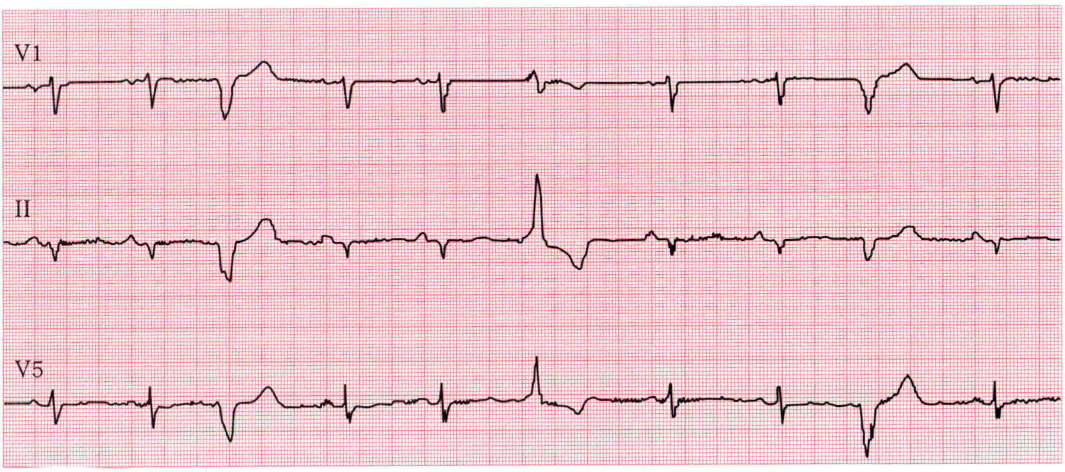

FIGURE 14.25. Multiform ventricular premature beats. Three-lead rhythm strip (V_1, II, V_5, from top to bottom) showing sinus rhythm with three ventricular premature beats (third, sixth, ninth beats) each with a different axis and morphology.

Groups of Ventricular Premature Beats

The definitions of the various groupings of VPBs was provided earlier in this chapter. **Figure 14.26** illustrates the typical appearances of ventricular bigeminy (**Figure 14.26A**), trigeminy (**Figure 14.26B**), and couplets or pairs (**Figure 14.26C**) of VPBs.

"The appearance of couplets applies to sonnet form such as those by Shakespeare. Two VPBs in a row are a pair, not a couplet."

HJL Marriott

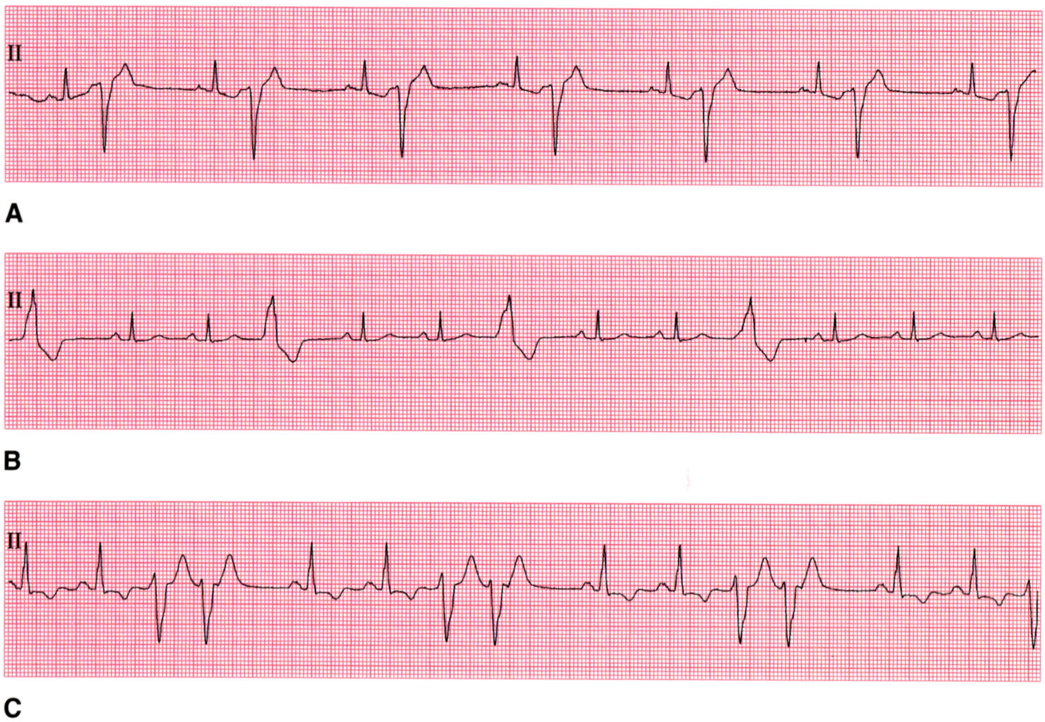

FIGURE 14.26. **A,B.** Frequent single ventricular premature beats (VPBs) in lead II rhythm strips. The VPB morphology in **A** and **B** differs widely. In **A**, the VPBs are bigeminal, whereas in **B**, they are trigeminal (except for the last complex). In **C**, there are ventricular pairs with a morphology similar to that of **A** (at least in the one lead shown).

Vulnerable Period and R-on-T Phenomenon

The peak of the T wave coincides with the vulnerable period in the cardiac cycle. Many studies have focused on VPBs during the T wave as being more ominous.[18,19] Other studies, however, have questioned the threat of *R-on-T VPBs* as compared with later VPBs. In patients with normal hearts, a VPB coinciding with the T wave is rarely of significance. Even in patients with prior infarction, single ventricular extrastimuli rarely induce ventricular tachycardia (VT) or ventricular fibrillation. In patients with long QT syndrome, VPBs timed with the T-wave may initiate runs of polymorphic VT termed torsades de pointes.[20] A form of usually benign right-ventricular outflow tract VPBs with short coupling of the VPB and resultant polymorphic VT has been reported along with very short coupled VPB-initiated ventricular fibrillation.[21,22]

Prognostic Implications of Ventricular Premature Beats

VPBs are nearly ubiquitous. Most people have them more or less frequently, and even continuous ventricular bigeminy is sometimes found in people with otherwise normal hearts.[23,24] These are termed idiopathic VPBs.[13] Regarding symptoms of VPBs, some people never report feeling any of theirs at all. Others feel every VPB and may be very bothered by them. Between these two extremes, there is a wide spectrum of complaints. Indeed, after heart disease has been ruled out, such patients may be reassured regarding a good prognosis. Benign VPBs commonly disappear when the sinus rate increases, such as during exercise. The prognostic significance of exercise-induced VPBs (or VT), however, is variable.[25] Patients with a high burden of VPBs (ie, greater than about 15%-20% of total beats) may develop new or worsening ventricular systolic dysfunction; elimination of the VPBs with medication or catheter ablation may restore normal ventricular function.[26]

Many studies have been directed at evaluating the prognostic significance of VPBs during and after acute myocardial infarction. During the acute phase of infarction, VPBs are very common. In patients who have survived myocardial infarction, frequent and multiform VPBs as well as nonsustained VT have been shown to increase the risk of sudden death.[27-29]

CHAPTER 14 SUMMARY ILLUSTRATION

Atrial premature beat

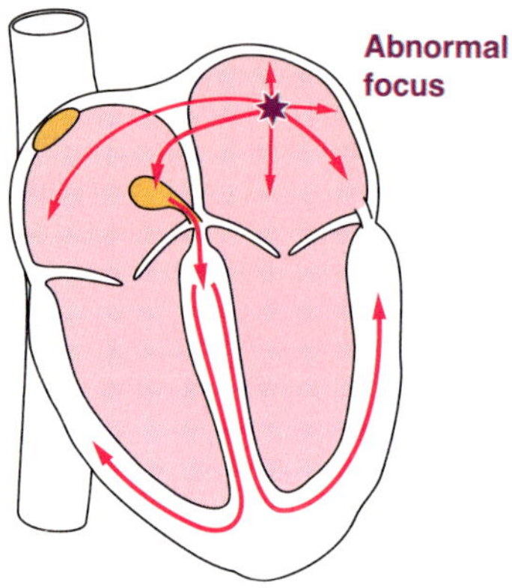

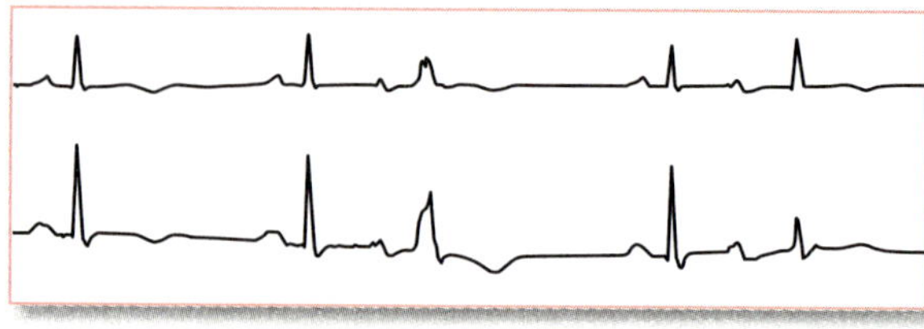

- Different P-wave morphology often noted
- QRS usually narrow (unless conducts with BBB or over AP)
- Usually less than compensatory pause

Junctional premature beat

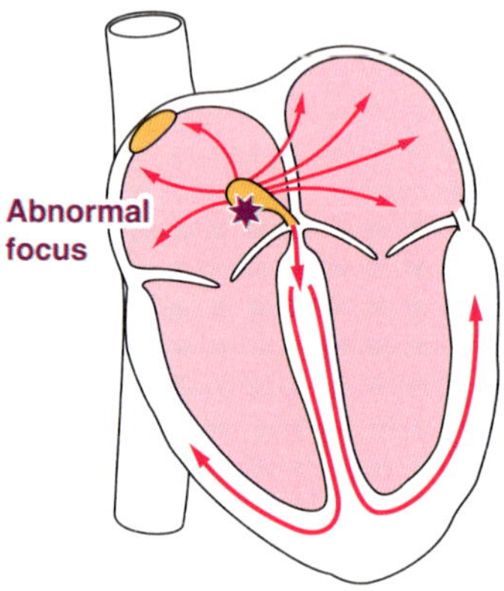

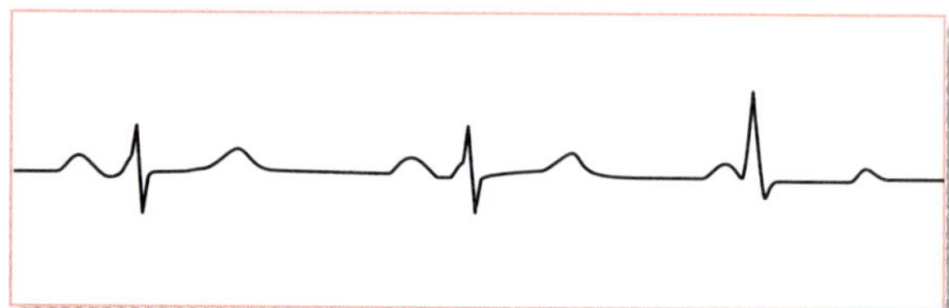

- QRS usually narrow (unless conducts with BBB or over AP)
- No preceding P-wave*
- P-wave inverted and usually in QRS or after it
- Usually less than compensatory pause

*** Two sinus beats are followed by a junctional premature beat; note the markedly abbreviated PR interval which is not physiologic for this patient.**

Ventricular premature beat

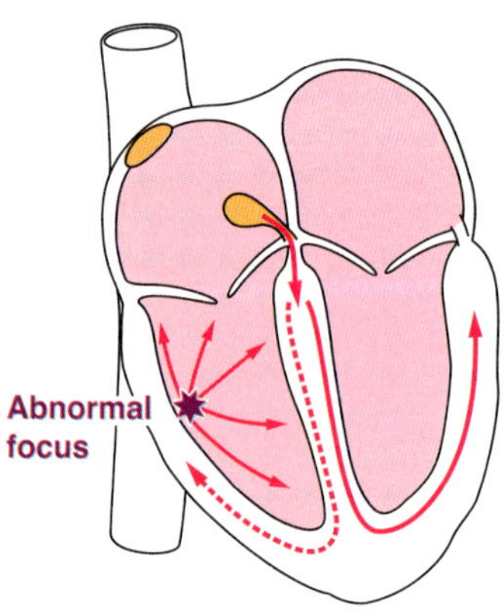

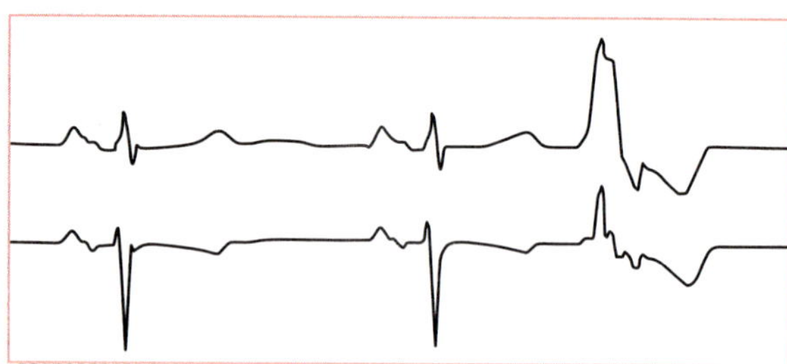

- Wide, abnormal QRS unlike typical BBB
- No preceding P-wave**
- Compensatory pause usually present

**** Rarely a P-wave may precede a VPB, but the PR interval will be shorter than the usual PR interval because the two events are unrelated**

Abbreviations: AP, accessory pathway; BBB, bundle-branch block; VPB, ventricular premature beat.

Glossary

Aberrantly: being conducted abnormally (usually through the ventricular conduction system).

Atrial premature beat: a P wave produced by an impulse that originates in the atria and appears before the expected time of the next P wave generated from the sinus node.

Bigeminy: a rhythm pattern in which every sinus beat is followed by a PB.

Compensatory pause: the long cycle length (pause) following a PB completely "compensates for" the short cycle length preceding the PB. This is identified when the interval between the beginning of the P waves of the sinus beats preceding and following a PB is equal to two PP intervals of sinus beats not associated with PBs.

Couplet (or pair): two consecutive PBs.

Coupling intervals: the periods between normal sinus beats and PBs. With APBs, the PP′ is the coupling interval, and with JPBs and VPBs, the QRS-QRS′ is the coupling interval.

Ectopic beat: a beat arising in any location other than the sinus node.

Interpolated: occurring between normal beats.

Junctional premature beat: a P wave and QRS complex produced by an impulse that originates in the AV node or His bundle and appears before the expected time of the next P wave and QRS complex generated from the sinus node.

Left VPBs: PBs originating from the left ventricle, usually with a V_1-positive morphology but sometimes with a V_1-negative morphology when originating from the ventricular septum.

Multifocal VPBs: VPBs originating from two or more different ventricular locations.

Multiform VPBs: VPBs with two or more different morphologies in a single ECG lead.

Overdrive suppression: a decrease in the rate of impulse formation resulting from premature activation of the pacemaking cells.

Palpitation: the physical awareness of a heartbeat.

PP interval: the interval between consecutive P waves.

Right VPBs: PBs originating from the right ventricle, always with a V_1-negative morphology.

R-on-T VPB: a VPB that occurs so prematurely that it occurs during the T wave of the previous beat.

Supraventricular premature beat: either an APB or a JPB.

Trigeminy: a rhythm pattern in which every second sinus beat is followed by a PB.

Ventricular premature beat: a QRS complex produced by an impulse originating from the ventricles and appearing before the expected time of the next QRS complex generated from the sinus node or other basic underlying rhythm.

Vulnerable period: the time in the cardiac cycle, before complete repolarization, when a reentrant tachyarrhythmia may be induced by the introduction of a premature impulse.

References

1. Cantillon DJ. Evaluation and management of premature ventricular complexes. *Cleve Clin J Med.* 2013;80:377-387.
2. Huang BT, Huang FY, Peng Y, et al. Relation of premature atrial complexes with stroke and death: systematic review and meta-analysis. *Clin Cardiol.* 2017;40:962-969.
3. Bagliani G, Della Rocca DG, De Ponti R, Capucci A, Padeletti M, Natale A. Ectopic beats: insights from timing and morphology. *Card Electrophysiol Clin.* 2018;10: 257-275.
4. Gorenek B, Fisher JD, Kudaiberdieva G, et al. Premature ventricular complexes: diagnostic and therapeutic considerations in clinical practice: a state-of-the-art review by the American College of Cardiology Electrophysiology Council. *J Interv Card Electrophysiol.* 2020;27:5-26.
5. Mond HG, Haqqani HM. The electrocardiographic footprints of atrial ectopy. *Heart Lung Circ.* 2019;28:1463-1471.
6. Rosenbaum MB. Classification of ventricular extrasystoles according to form. *J Electrocardiol.* 1969;2:289-297.
7. Pick A. Parasystole. *Circulation.* 1953;8: 243-253.
8. Jalife J, Antzelevitch C, Moe GK. The case for modulated parasystole. *Pacing Clin Electrophysiol.* 1982;5:911-926.
9. Gozensky C, Thorne D. Rabbit ears: an aid in distinguishing ventricular ectopy from aberration. *Heart Lung.* 1974;3:634-636.
10. Cannom DS, Gallagher JJ, Goldreyer BN, Damato AN. Concealed bundle of His extrasystoles simulating nonconducted atrial premature beats. *Am Heart J.* 1972;83:777-779.
11. Swanick EJ, LaCamera F Jr, Marriott HJ. Morphologic features of right ventricular ectopic beats. *Am J Cardiol.* 1972;30:888-891.
12. Lewis S, Kanakis C, Rosen KM, Denes P. Significance of site of origin of premature ventricular contractions. *Am Heart J.* 1979;97: 159-164.

13. Lerman BB. Mechanism, diagnosis, and treatment of outflow tract tachycardia. *Nat Rev Cardiol.* 2015;12:597-608.
14. Marcus FI, McKenna WJ, Sherrill D, et al. Diagnosis of arrhythmogenic right ventricular cardiomyopathy/dysplasia: proposed modification of the task force criteria. *Circulation.* 2010;121:1533-1541.
15. Towbin JA, McKenna WJ, Abrams DJ, et al. 2019 HRS expert consensus statement on evaluation, risk stratification, and management of arrhythmogenic cardiomyopathy. *Heart Rhythm.* 2019;16:e301-e372.
16. Miller MA, Dukkipati SR, Turagam M, Liao SL, Adams DH, Reddy VY. Arrhythmic mitral valve prolapse. *J Am Coll Cardiol.* 2018;72:2904-2914.
17. Latchamsetty R, Yokokawa M, Morady F, et al. Multicenter outcomes for catheter ablation of idiopathic premature ventricular complexes. *JACC Clin Electrophysiol.* 2015;1:116-123.
18. Adgey AA. The Belfast experience with resuscitation ambulances. *Am J Emerg Med.* 1984;2:193-199.
19. Engel TR, Meister SG, Frankl WS. The "R-on-T" phenomenon: an update and critical review. *Ann Intern Med.* 1978;88: 221-225.
20. Viskin S, Alla SR, Barron HV, et al. Mode of onset of torsade de pointes in congenital long QT syndrome. *J Am Coll Cardiol.* 1996;28:1262-1268.
21. Leenhardt A, Glaser E, Burguera M, Nürnberg M, Maison-Blanche P, Coumel P. Short-coupled variant of torsade de pointes. A new electrocardiographic entity in the spectrum of idiopathic ventricular tachyarrhythmias. *Circulation.* 1994;89: 206-215.
22. Viskin S, Rosso R, Rogowski O, Belhassen B. The "short-coupled" variant of right ventricular outflow ventricular tachycardia: a not-so-benign form of benign ventricular tachycardia. *J Cardiovasc Electrophysiol.* 2005;16:912-916.
23. Kennedy HL, Whitlock JA, Sprague MK, Kennedy LJ, Buckingham TA, Goldberg RJ. Long-term follow-up of asymptomatic healthy subjects with frequent and complex ventricular ectopy. *N Engl J Med.* 1985;312:193-197.
24. Ataklte F, Erqou S, Laukkanen J, Kaptoge S. Meta-analysis of ventricular premature complexes and their relation to cardiac mortality in general populations. *Am J Cardiol.* 2013;112:1263-1270.
25. Corrado D, Drezner JA, D'Ascenzi F, Zorzi A. How to evaluate premature ventricular beats in the athlete: critical review and proposal of a diagnostic algorithm [published online ahead of print September 3. 2019]. *Br J Sports Med.* doi:10.1136/bjsports-2018-100529.
26. Latchamsetty R, Bogun F. Premature ventricular complex-induced cardiomyopathy. *JACC Clin Electrophysiol.* 2019;5:537-550.
27. Moss AJ, Davis HT, DeCamilla J, Bayer LW. Ventricular ectopic beats and their relation to sudden and nonsudden cardiac death after myocardial infarction. *Circulation.* 1979;60:998-1003.
28. Ruberman W, Weinblatt E, Goldberg JD, Frank CW, Shapiro S. Ventricular premature beats and mortality after myocardial infarction. *N Engl J Med.* 1977;297:750-757.
29. Bigger JT Jr, Weld FM. Analysis of prognostic significance of ventricular arrhythmias after myocardial infarction. Shortcomings of Lown grading system. *Br Heart J.* 1981;45:717-724.

15 Supraventricular Tachyarrhythmias

KEVIN P. JACKSON, JAMES P. DAUBERT,
ANINDYA GHOSH, AND
ULHAS PANDURANGI M

Introduction

Supraventricular tachycardia (SVT) is an umbrella term used to describe cardiac arrhythmias occurring in the upper cardiac chambers (His bundle and above) with atrial rates greater than 100 beats/min. Types of SVT include sinus tachycardia, focal and *multifocal atrial tachycardia*, junctional tachycardia, atrioventricular (AV) nodal reentrant tachycardia (AVNRT), various forms of accessory pathway–mediated reentrant tachycardias (especially orthodromic AV reentrant tachycardia or AVRT), and macroreentrant atrial arrhythmias including *atrial flutter* and *atrial fibrillation*. *Paroxysmal* supraventricular tachycardia (PSVT) is a subset of SVT that is characterized by a regular, rapid tachycardia with abrupt onset and termination. The PSVT usually occurs in young people without underlying heart disease and is generally considered benign. Although in middle-aged or older patients AVNRT is the most common cause of PSVT, in younger patients there is equal prevalence between AVNRT and accessory pathway–mediated tachycardia. Women have twice the risk of men of developing PSVT during their lifetimes.

The three predominant mechanisms of PSVT are altered automaticity, triggered activity, and reentry (**Figure 15.1**). Altered automaticity is the mechanism for sinus tachycardia and for junctional tachycardia. Triggered activity is the most common mechanism for ectopic atrial tachycardia as well as single or repetitive premature beats, which may be an initiating factor in reentrant arrhythmias.[1] For reentrant arrhythmias such as AVNRT or AV reentrant tachycardia (AVRT) to initiate and sustain, there needs to be the presence of two

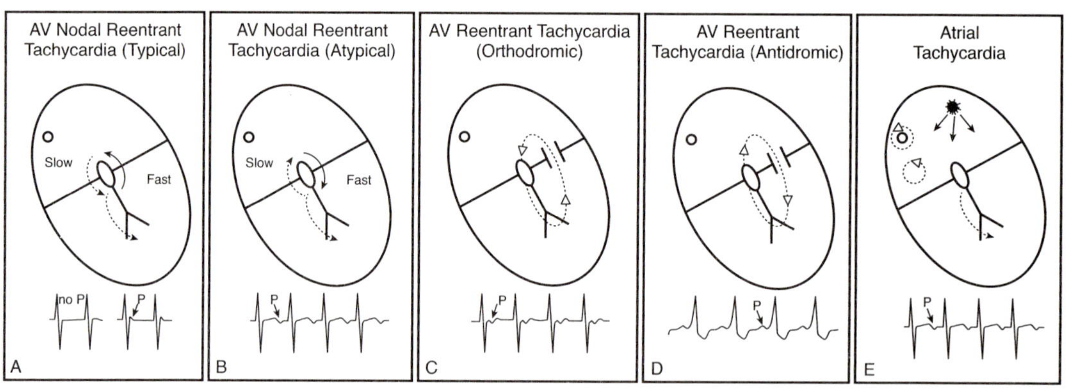

FIGURE 15.1. The mechanism and typical electrocardiogram findings of the five varieties of paroxysmal supraventricular tachycardia are illustrated. **A.** For typical atrioventricular (AV) nodal reentrant tachycardia, antegrade conduction is down a slow AV nodal pathway and retrograde conduction up a fast AV nodal pathway. The P waves may be hidden within the QRS complex or may be visible just after the R or S wave. **B.** For atypical AV nodal reentrant tachycardia, antegrade conduction is down a fast AV nodal pathway (or a slow AV nodal pathway) and retrograde conduction is up a slow AV nodal pathway. **C.** For orthodromic AV reentrant tachycardia, antegrade conduction is typically down the AV node with retrograde conduction up an accessory pathway. There is a short RP interval with P waves visible shortly after the QRS complex. **D.** For antidromic AV reentrant tachycardia, antegrade conduction is down an accessory pathway with retrograde conduction up the AV node. **E.** For atrial tachycardia, the morphology and axis of the P wave is variable depending on the location and mechanism of tachycardia. (Reprinted/modified with permission from Ferguson JD. Contemporary management of paroxysmal supraventricular tachycardia. *Circulation*. 2003;107[8]:1096–1099.)

electrophysiologically heterogenous pathways of conduction with unidirectional block in one of the pathways (**Figure 15.2**).

During sustained AVNRT, the reentrant circuit uses dual AV nodal pathways (slow and fast). The presence of an accessory AV conduction pathway creates the potential for the development of reentry circuits in which the impulses travel in either the normal or reverse direction through the AV node and His-Purkinje system. Reentry via an accessory pathway as one limb and the AV node as the other limb is the common mechanism of AVRT. The term *orthodromic reentrant tachycardia* (ORT) is used when the impulse proceeds in the normal antegrade direction down the AV node, and the term *antidromic reentrant tachycardia* (ART) is used when the impulse proceeds in the reverse direction. Reentry utilizing two accessory pathways (also known as duodromic tachycardia) is possible but rare.

Animation 15.1 shows additional information on the relationship between intracardiac conduction between the atria and ventricles and the surface ECG during sinus rhythm, AVNRT, ORT and ART.

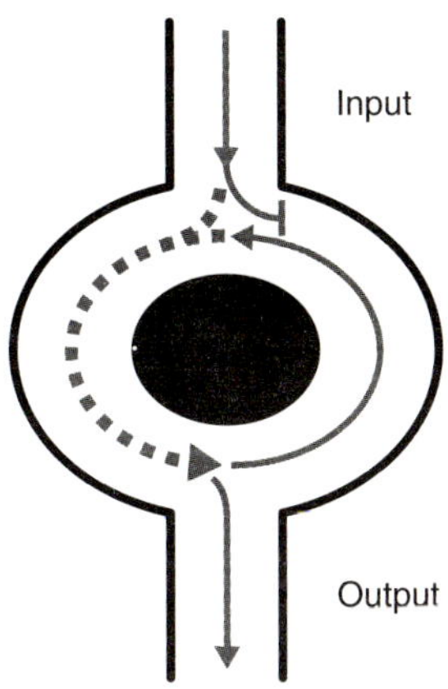

FIGURE 15.2. Formation and conduction of the cardiac impulse through a reentry circuit. The condition for reentry occurs when two distinct conduction pathways are present. Unidirectional block down one pathway allows conduction down the alternative pathway. If repolarization has occurred once the impulse reaches the "turn around" point, reentry ensues.

To view the animation(s) and video(s) associated with this chapter please access lww.co.in. Instructions are located on the inside front cover.

Differential Diagnosis of Supraventricular Tachycardia

Classification of SVT can be made based on the suddenness of onset and regularity of the rhythm (**Table 15.1**).

Table 15.1.

Common Mechanisms of SVT

Onset	Regularity	Arrhythmia
Gradual	Regular	Sinus tachycardia Inappropriate sinus tachycardia
Gradual	Irregular	Multifocal atrial tachycardia
Sudden	Regular	AV nodal reentrant tachycardia AV reentrant tachycardia Atrial tachycardia Atrial flutter
Sudden	Irregular	Atrial fibrillation

Abbreviations: AV, atrioventricular; SVT, supraventricular tachycardia.

Observance of the onset or termination should differentiate normal, physiologic sinus tachycardia from reentrant PSVT as the enhanced automaticity of sinus tachycardia gradually accelerates and decelerates in contrast with the abrupt behavior of reentrant tachyarrhythmias (**Figure 15.3**). Careful analysis of the onset of tachycardia can provide further clues as to the mechanism of PSVT. For example, a premature atrial contraction that results in a sudden prolongation of the PR interval with onset of tachycardia is the common initiation of typical (slow-fast) AVNRT (**Figure 15.4**), although it does not rule out other mechanisms.

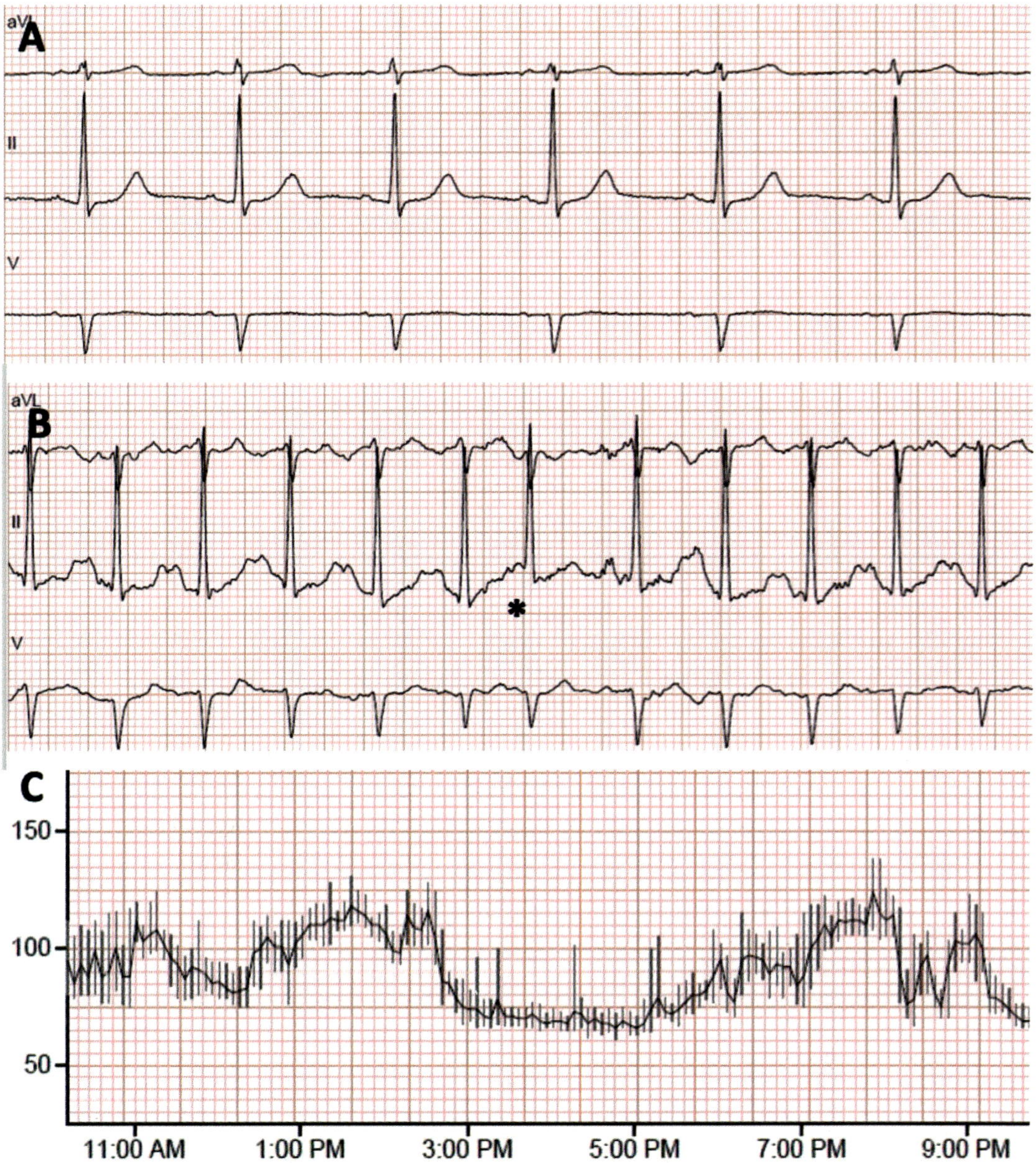

FIGURE 15.3. The gradual onset of sinus tachycardia is demonstrated. **A.** During rest, sinus P waves are seen preceding each QRS complex. **B.** During symptomatic tachycardia, notching is seen in the T wave; however, the origin of atrial activation is difficult to determine. A premature atrial contraction (asterisk) results in separation of the subsequent T and P waves revealing atrial activity originating from the sinus node. **C.** Heart rate trend confirms gradual onset and offset of the rhythm, consistent with sinus tachycardia.

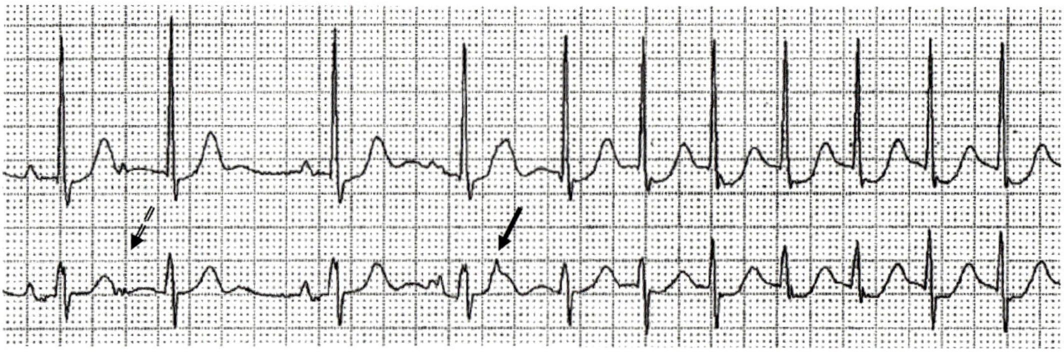

FIGURE 15.4. Two-lead rhythm strip demonstrating the initiation of tachycardia. The first premature atrial contraction (dashed arrow) causes prolongation of the PR interval but does not initiate tachycardia. An earlier premature atrial contraction (solid arrow) causes PR prolongation with initiation of typical (slow-fast) atrioventricular nodal reentrant tachycardia.

Analysis of the P-wave axis and morphology as well as the relationship between atrial and ventricular activity during SVT can further clarify the mechanism. Therefore, obtaining a 12-lead electrocardiogram (ECG) when feasible is critical. Reentrant SVT utilizing the AV node as the retrograde limb will have a narrow, superiorly directed P wave, distinct from the inferiorly directed sinus P wave. When P waves are not easily seen due to the rapidity of the tachycardia or other factors, maneuvers such as *carotid sinus massage* can help elucidate the mechanism of SVT.[2] The typical responses of atrial tachycardia, atrial flutter, and AVNRT to *vagal maneuvers* are presented in **Figure 15.5**. All three tachyarrhythmias are rapid and narrow (QRS complex duration <0.12 s), with atrial activity either apparent after the T waves or absent. Atrial tachycardia (**Figure 15.5A**) and atrial flutter (**Figure 15.5B**) are unaffected by the maneuver, but the atrial activity and diagnosis is made clear by the increased AV nodal block. The abrupt termination of the arrhythmia seen in **Figure 15.5C** is a typical response of AVNRT. The increase in parasympathetic activity terminates AVNRT by prolonging the AV nodal refractory period, causing the impulse to block in

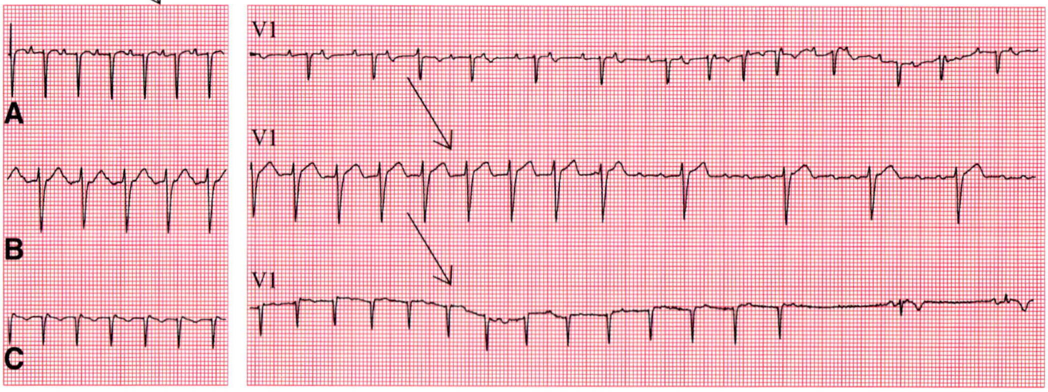

FIGURE 15.5. Lead V_1 rhythm strips from three patients with various supraventricular tachyarrhythmias. Arrows above the rhythm strips indicate the onset of carotid sinus massage in these typical examples of the responses of atrial tachycardia (**A**), atrial flutter (**B**), and atrioventricular nodal reentrant tachycardia (**C**).

one pathway of the circuit. AVRT would respond similarly. When the arrhythmia fails to respond to parasympathetic stimulation and the diagnosis remains uncertain, a pharmacologic intervention with adenosine, intravenous β-blockers, or intravenous calcium channel blocker may be used.[3]

The relationship of the P wave to the QRS complex is helpful in distinguishing the mechanism of SVT. The P wave should precede each QRS complex in sinus tachycardia and atrial tachycardia, and changes in P-P intervals precede and predict changes in R-R intervals. For AVNRT and orthodromic AVRT, the atrium is activated retrogradely through the AV node or accessory pathway, respectively. The R-P relationship on ECG or rhythm strip can be used to distinguish these arrhythmias. Because the circuit of AVNRT is contained within the AV node, the P waves and QRS complexes usually occur simultaneously. During typical (slow-fast) AVNRT, there are often no visible P waves (**Figure 15.6**), or P waves are seen just after the QRS complex. In the latter case, the retrograde P wave appears as a "pseudo S wave" of the QRS complex in leads II, III, and aVF or "pseudo r′ wave" in lead V_1 (**Figure 15.7**). Because the reentry circuit in orthodromic reentrant tachycardia is longer (includes both the atrium and ventricle), the P waves and QRS complexes cannot occur simultaneously and P waves are seen distinctly after the QRS complex (**Figure 15.8**). The classification based on the R-P intervals divides SVTs (with visualized P waves) as short and long R-P tachycardias (short when RP< PR and long when RP > PR). Possibilities when encountering a short R-P tachycardia include typical AVNRT, orthodromic AVRT, and atrial tachycardia with a prolonged PR interval. A long R-P tachycardia could be atypical AVNRT, atrial tachycardia, and orthodromic AVRT using a decrementally conducting pathway.

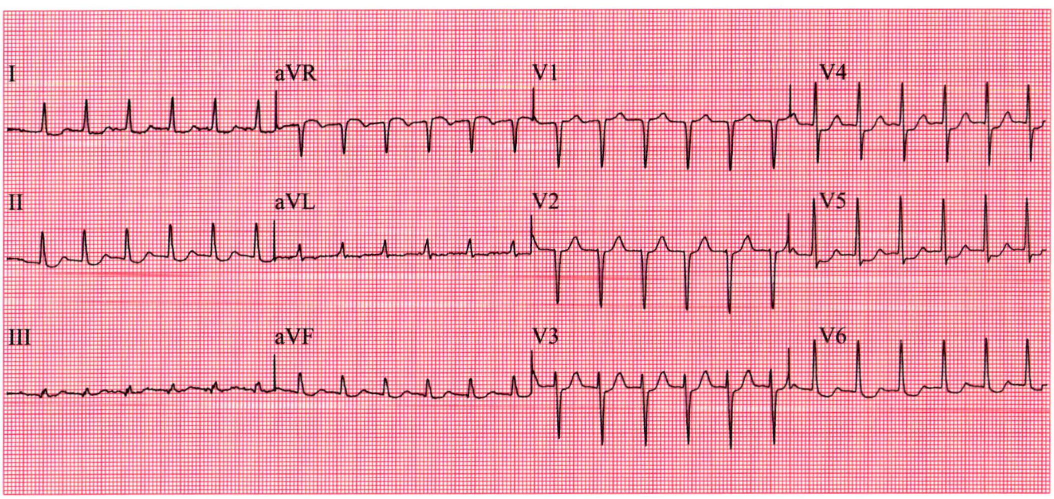

FIGURE 15.6. Twelve-lead electrocardiogram recording from a 20 year-old woman who presented to the emergency department with sudden onset of weakness and palpitations. A rapid, regular, narrow tachycardia without visible P waves often indicates typical atrioventricular nodal reentrant tachycardia as the mechanism of tachycardia.

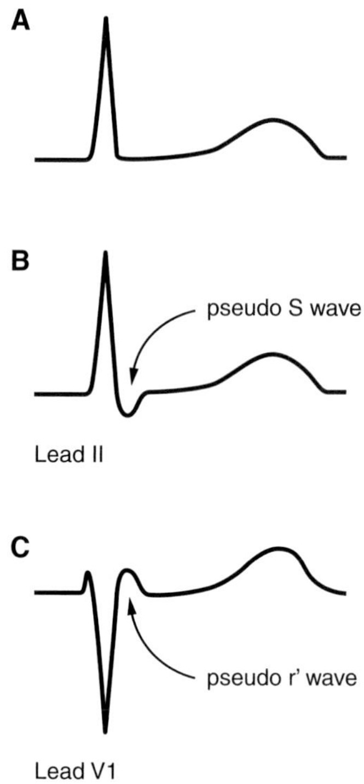

FIGURE 15.7. Typical short R-P relationship during atrioventricular nodal reentry tachycardia. **A.** In most cases, the atrium and ventricle activate simultaneously and P waves are not visible. Alternatively, P waves may be visible at the end of the QRS complex either as a pseudo S wave (**B**) in electrocardiogram lead II or a pseudo r′ wave (**C**) in electrocardiogram lead V_1.

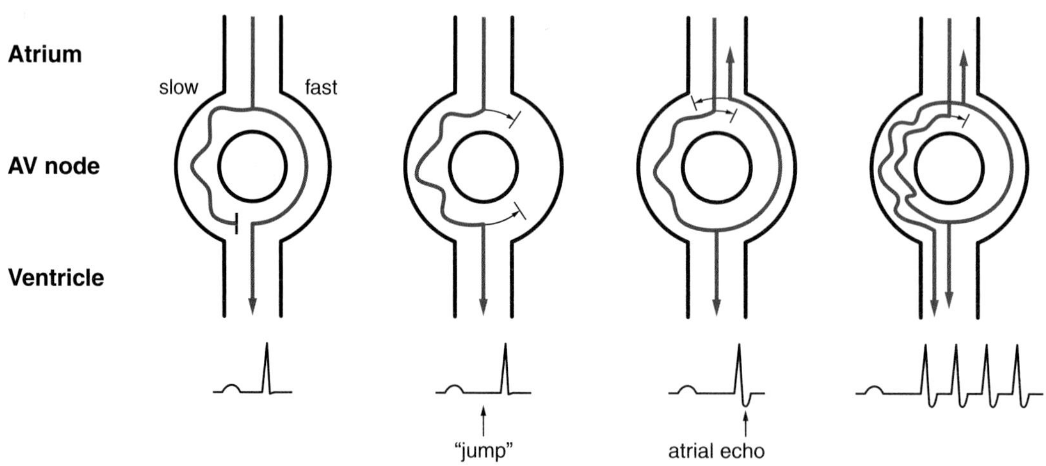

FIGURE 15.8. The mechanism of atrioventricular (AV) nodal reentry tachycardia involves a circuit utilizing a fast and slow AV node pathway. In the baseline state, the sinus impulse is preferentially conducted through the AV node via the fast pathway. A well-timed premature atrial beat finds the fast pathway refractory and conduction "jumps" to the slow AV nodal pathway. The impulse conducts retrograde through the fast pathway resulting in an atrial echo. If the refractory period of the slow pathway has recovered, tachycardia perpetuates.

Sinus Tachycardia

The rate of cardiac impulse formation from the sinoatrial (SA) node is regulated by the balance between the parasympathetic and sympathetic divisions of the autonomic (or involuntary) nervous system. An increase in parasympathetic activity decreases the rate of impulse formation, whereas an increase in sympathetic activity increases the rate. The sympathetic nervous system becomes activated by any condition that requires "fight or flight." The sinus tachycardia that results is therefore a physiologic response to the body's needs rather than a pathologic cardiac condition. By this principle, treatment of the tachyarrhythmia should be directed at correcting the underlying condition and not at suppression of the SA node itself. Maximal sympathetic stimulation can increase the heart rate produced by the SA node to 200 beats/min or, rarely, 220 beats/min in younger individuals. The generally accepted formula for maximal sinus rate is 220 beats/min subtracted by age. The rate rarely exceeds 160 beats/min in nonexercising adults.

In sinus tachycardia, there is normally one P wave for every QRS complex, but coexisting abnormalities of AV conduction may alter this relationship. The PR interval is shorter than during normal sinus rhythm because the increased *sympathetic tone* that produces the sinus tachycardia also speeds AV nodal conduction. The QRS complex is usually normal in appearance but can be abnormal either because of a fixed intraventricular conduction disturbance (such as bundle-branch block, hypertrophy, or myocardial infarction) or because the rapid rate of activation does not permit time for full recovery of the intraventricular conduction system before the arrival of the next impulse. **Figure 15.9** demonstrates sinus tachycardia with left-bundle-branch block. Conduction block is proven to be due to rate-related aberrancy when it disappears during carotid sinus massage–induced sinus slowing or AV block and returns when the rate gradually increases following the massage.

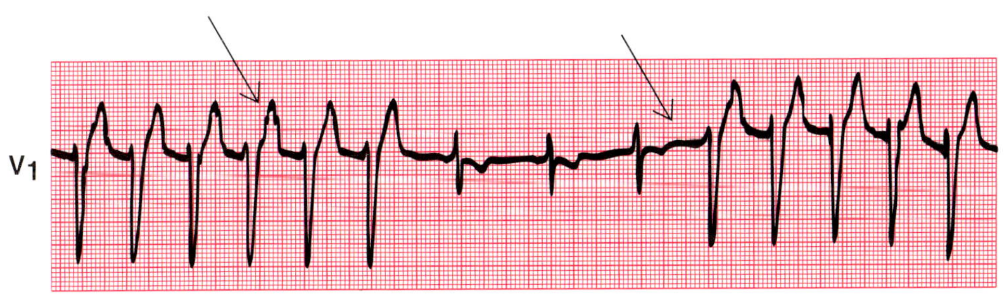

FIGURE 15.9. Lead V_1 rhythm strip with arrows indicating the beginning and ending of carotid sinus massage. (Reprinted from Wagner GS, Waugh RA, Ramo BW. *Cardiac Arrhythmias*. New York, NY: Churchill Livingstone; 1983:140. Copyright © 1983 Elsevier. With permission.)

A common clinical problem is the differentiation of sinus tachycardia from a reentrant tachyarrhythmia. Automatic atrial rhythms such as sinus tachycardia have a gradual onset and termination because they result from acceleration of automaticity in the cells of the pacemaking and conduction system. This is apparent on the ECG as a gradual decrease in the interval between cardiac cycles (the P-P interval) during the period of onset and a gradual increase during the period of termination of a tachyarrhythmia. In **Figure 15.10**, there is a tachyarrhythmia during exercise at a rate of 140 beats/min, with no visible P waves and wide (V_1-negative) QRS complexes (0.14 s). When the exercise is stopped, the rate gradually slows and P waves emerge from the ends of each of the T waves, indicating that the rhythm is sinus tachycardia with left-bundle-branch block.

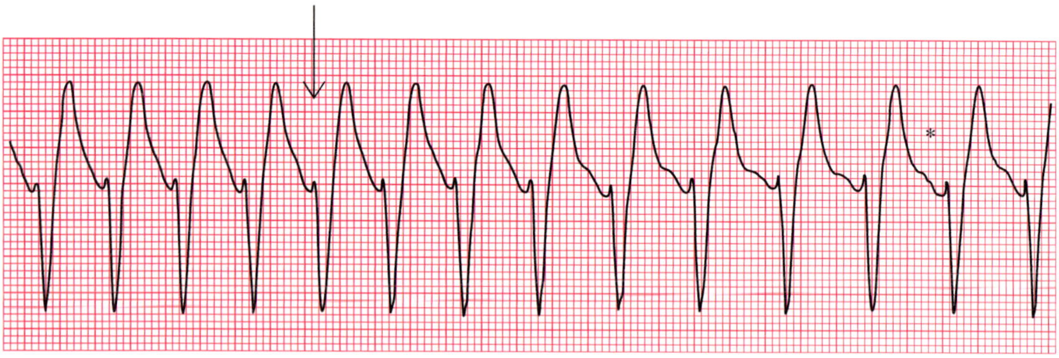

FIGURE 15.10. Lead V_1 rhythm strip. Arrow indicates the time at which exercise was stopped, and asterisk indicates the P wave emerging from the T wave. (Reprinted from Wagner GS, Waugh RA, Ramo BW. *Cardiac Arrhythmias*. New York, NY: Churchill Livingstone; 1983:145. Copyright © 1983 Elsevier. With permission.)

Atrial Tachycardia

Atrial tachycardia is usually a regular, focal arrhythmia originating in the atrium outside of the sinus node. Generally, the arrhythmia spreads centrifugally from the focus. The mechanism is a most often triggered activity involving calcium loading of the myocardial cell, although automaticity is not uncommon. Alternatively, atrial tachycardia can be a very small, so called microreentrant circuit. The latter is common in scarred atrial tissue, such as from prior catheter ablation. The atrial rate is generally regular, although it commonly exhibits gradual acceleration after onset and deceleration (prolongation of the P-P interval) before spontaneous termination. The rate is most often 130 to 240 beats/min but can be slower or faster.[4] Atrial tachycardia may exhibit one to one AV conduction but intermittent block or 2:1 block is common; only the atrium is required for perpetuation of the tachycardia. An AV block can be precipitated by carotid sinus massage or by adenosine injection as shown in **Figure 15.11**.

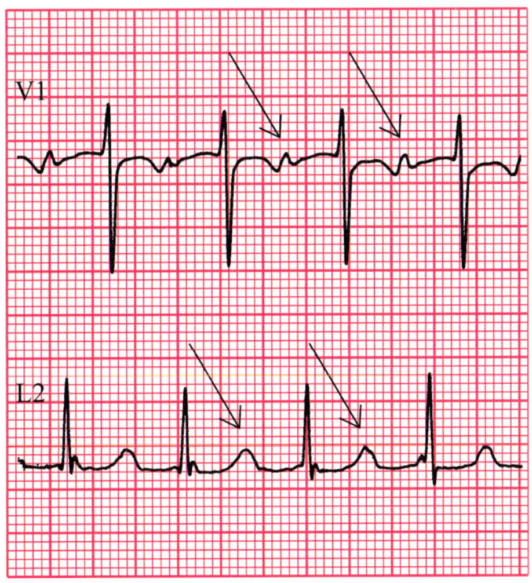

A

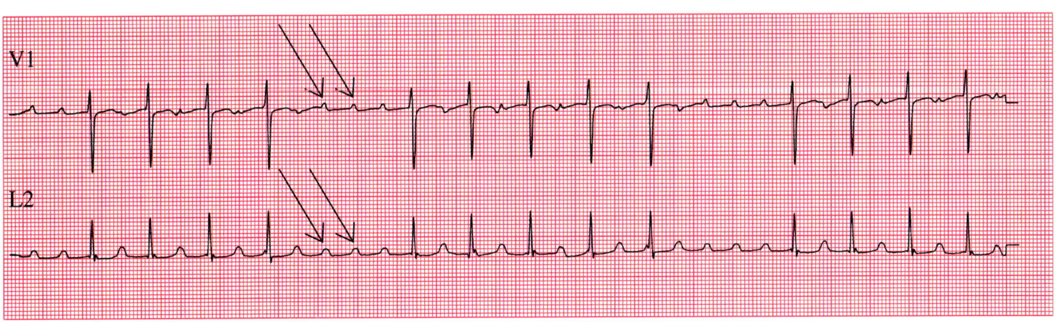

B

FIGURE 15.11. Lead II (L2) and V_1 rhythm strips from a woman presenting with shortness of breath who was found to have idiopathic cardiomyopathy. Arrows indicate similar-appearing P waves in L2 and V_1 in the presenting condition (**A**) and during carotid sinus massage (**B**).

The P-wave morphology is constant and usually differs substantially from the sinus P wave unless the focus is very near the SA node in the high right atrium. **Figure 15.12A,B** shows the expected P-wave morphology for common sites of atrial tachycardia originating in the right atrium and left atrium, respectively.[5] Multifocal atrial tachycardia exhibits at least three P-wave morphologies and is irregular; it is classically seen in chronic obstructive lung disease (**Figure 15.13**). Aside from managing the underlying condition, treatment is challenging, but verapamil has been reported to be beneficial.

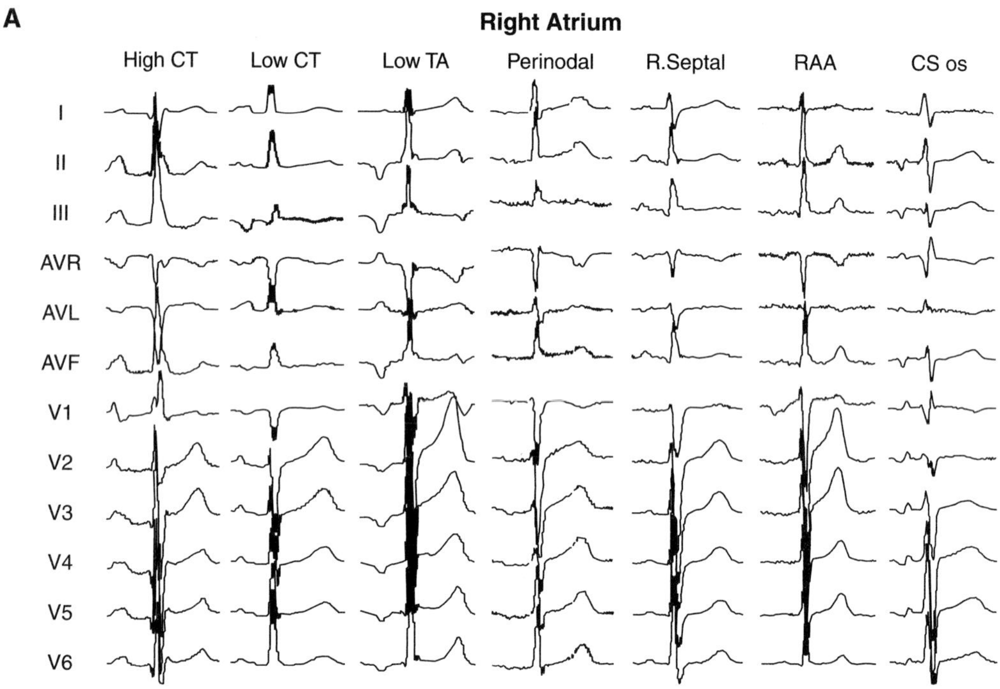

FIGURE 15.12. Typical P-wave morphologies from the common sites of origin of atrial tachycardia within the right atrium (**A**) and left atrium (**B**). CS, coronary sinus; CT, crista terminalis; LAA, left atrial appendage; LIPV, left inferior pulmonary vein; LSPV, left superior pulmonary vein; MA, mitral annulus; RAA, right atrial appendage; RIPV, right inferior pulmonary vein; RSPV, right superior pulmonary vein; TA, tricuspid annulus. *(continued)*

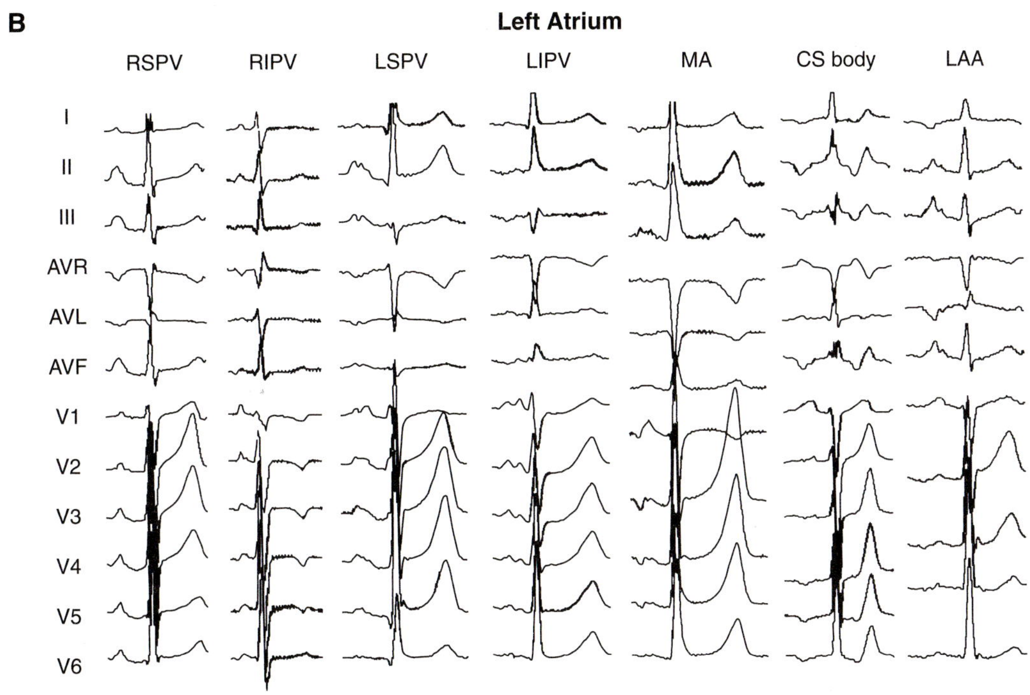

FIGURE 15.12. *(continued)*

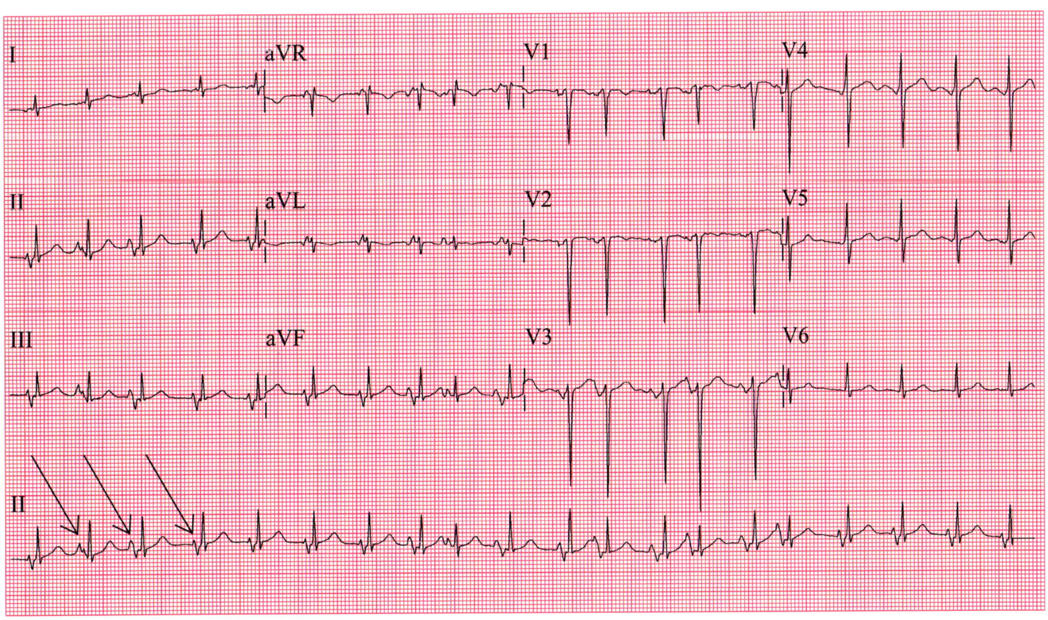

FIGURE 15.13. A 12-lead electrocardiogram and lead II rhythm strip from a 53-year-old woman with severe pulmonary emphysema. Arrows indicate marked variation in P-wave morphology in the rhythm strip.

Atrial flutter and macroreentrant atrial tachycardia

Atrial flutter (AFl) is a reentrant arrhythmia, with a regular pattern and at a rate above 240 bpm without an isoelectric line between atrial deflections in the ECG. The typical form (counterclockwise cavotricuspid-dependent flutter) usually shows a sawtooth pattern in inferior ECG leads with negative waves in II, III, and aVF and positive waves in V1. In the presence of rapid conduction, the flutter waves may not be seen. Adenosine administration or vagal maneuvers may unmask the flutter in this case (**Figure 15.14**).

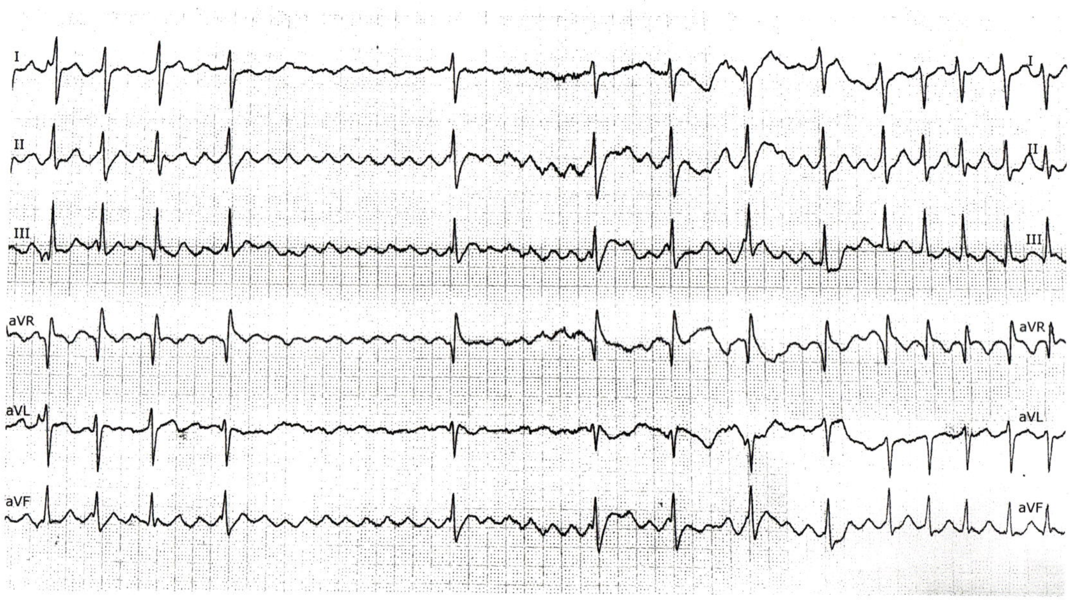

FIGURE 15.14. A six-lead (limb) electrocardiogram rhythm strip during narrow complex tachycardia with adenosine causing AV nodal block and unmasking the flutter P waves.

Junctional Tachycardia

Junctional tachycardia (**Figure 15.15**) is usually due to accelerated (enhanced) automaticity in either the AV node or the His bundle and has a rate exceeding 100 beats/min, usually 100 to 130 beats/min. The QRS is typically narrow, but it can present with rate-related or fixed bundle-branch block. *Accelerated junctional rhythm* is essentially the same rhythm, but the rate is 60 to 100 beats/min. Junctional tachycardia should be differentiated from AVNRT and from AVRT, which also use the "junction" (ie, the AV node and His bundle).

Patients may be symptomatic with palpitations, fatigue, or dizziness due to loss of AV synchrony. The P waves are most often retrograde and therefore inverted in the inferior ECG leads and follow the QRS by a variable time period. However, depending on the antegrade and retrograde conduction properties, the P waves may be superimposed on the QRS or even slightly precede it. The rate will vary with sympathetic and parasympathetic tone or exogenous agents. Junctional tachycardia will be precipitated or accelerated by epinephrine or isoproterenol or other sympathomimetic agents; atropine or adenosine will slow it. A related condition is junctional ectopic tachycardia that is seen primarily in pediatric and congenital heart patients, especially postsurgical; it is difficult to control and frequently exhibits a much more rapid tachycardia.[6] Another related condition is that of single junctional extrasystolic impulses, also called His extrasystolic beats. These are single ectopic beats originating in the AV node or His bundle, thus usually having a narrow QRS and lacking a preceding P wave.

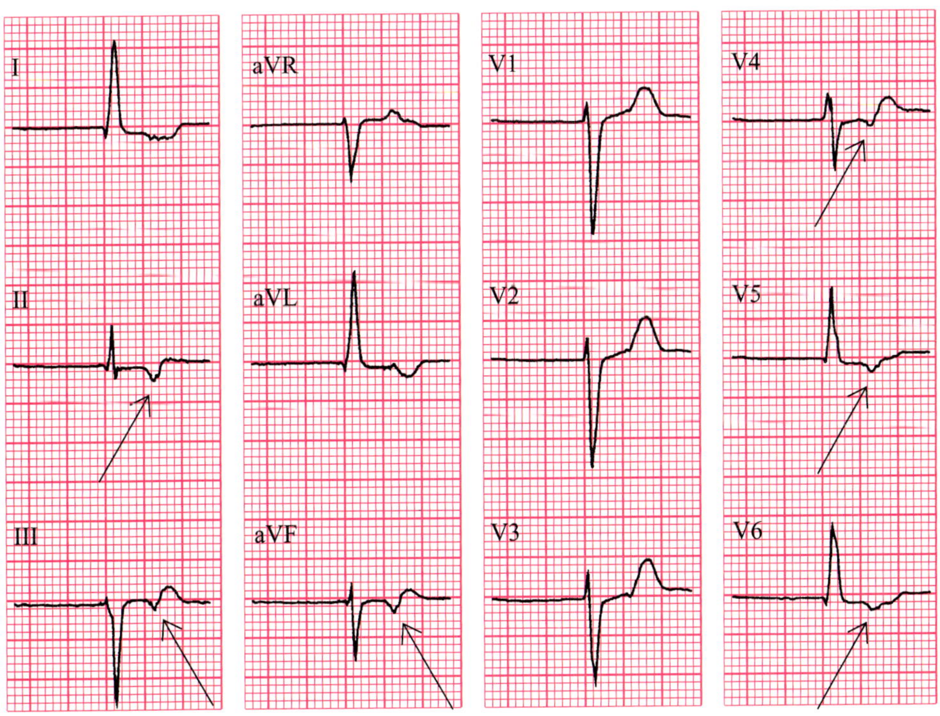

FIGURE 15.15. A 12-lead electrocardiogram from a healthy 51-year-old woman. Arrows indicate retrograde P waves associated with junctional beats.

Atrioventricular Nodal Reentrant Tachycardia

AVNRT is caused by a reentrant loop that involves the AV node and the atrial tissue (see **Figure 15.8**). In persons with this type of tachycardia, the AV node has two pathways, one of which conducts rapidly and the other slowly. During the baseline state, the sinus impulse preferentially conducts to the ventricle via the rapidly conducting fast pathway. The slower pathway, which lies parallel to the tricuspid valve, remains "dormant" as the electrical impulse meanders through and collides with the wavefront from fast pathway conduction. The baseline ECG is therefore unremarkable (normal PR interval) except in the rare situation where there is preferential conduction through the slow AV node pathway (**Figure 15.16**).

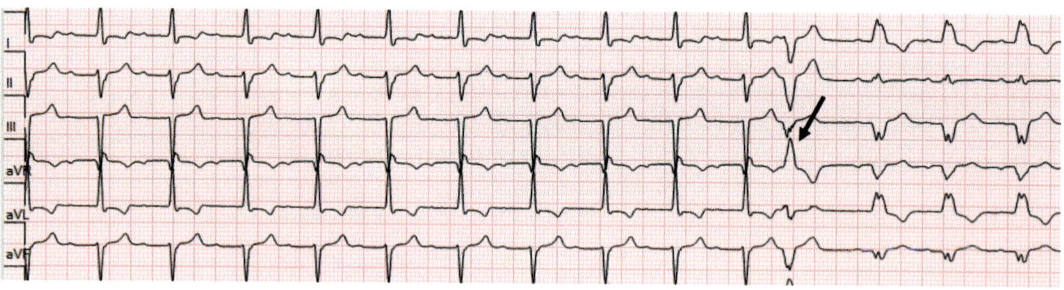

FIGURE 15.16. Continuous recording of six limb-lead electrocardiogram in a patient with manifest slow and fast atrioventricular nodal pathways during sinus rhythm. The PR interval is long as the sinus impulse conducts through the slow atrioventricular node pathway. The fast pathway is refractory due to retrograde penetration from this impulse. A premature ventricular contraction (arrow) "peels back" the refractoriness of the fast pathway allowing the sinus impulse to "jump" back to the fast pathway with normalization of the PR interval.

Although the conduction time through the fast pathway is short, its refractory period is long in comparison to the slow pathway. When a well-timed premature atrial contraction enters the AV nodal tissue with the fast pathway in the refractory state, the impulse will "jump" to the slow pathway. This is manifested on the surface ECG with a sudden prolongation of the PR interval (**Figure 15.17**). By the time the impulse reaches the distal AV node, the fast pathway has completed its refractory period and reentry is possible. The impulse will travel retrograde to the atrium via the fast pathway resulting in an atrial *echo beat*. Tachycardia perpetuates during typical AVNRT with antegrade conduction down the slow pathway and retrograde conduction up the fast pathway.

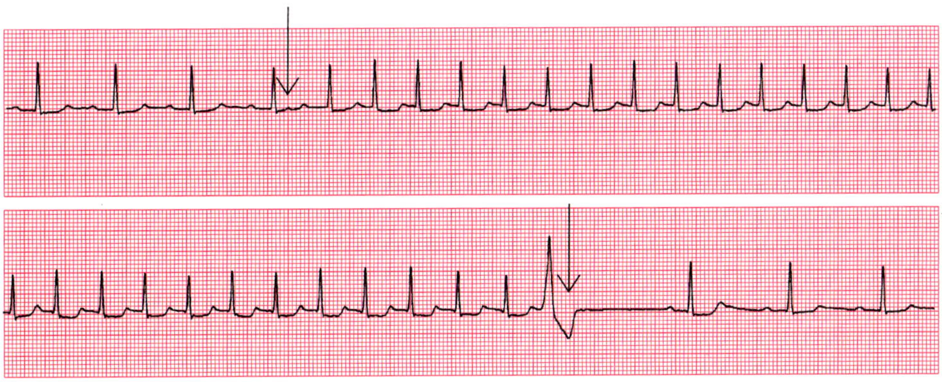

FIGURE 15.17. Continuous recording in lead II of a 52-year-old woman with typical (slow-fast) atrioventricular nodal reentrant tachycardia. A premature atrial contraction (arrow) "jumps" to the slow pathway as evidenced by a sudden prolongation of the PR interval. Tachycardia is initiated and perpetuated until a premature ventricular contraction (arrow) causes concealed penetration of the atrioventricular node and terminates tachycardia.

During sustained typical AVNRT, the retrograde P wave is often hidden by the QRS complex because atrial activation via the fast pathway occurs simultaneously with activation of the ventricles via the His-Purkinje system. The P wave is either invisible, as in **Figure 15.7A**, or is seen just emerging from the terminal part of the QRS complex, as in **Figure 15.7B**. Less commonly, AVNRT occurs in the "atypical" form, where antegrade conduction is via the fast pathway and retrograde conduction via the slow pathway. In this situation, the RP relationship is long and P wave activity may be seen just prior to the QRS complex (**Figure 15.18**). Tachycardia is often initiated with a premature ventricular contraction (PVC) as retrograde activation of the atrium "jumps" to the slow pathway. Finally, patients may present with intermediate forms of atypical AVNRT with conduction via multiple slow pathways.

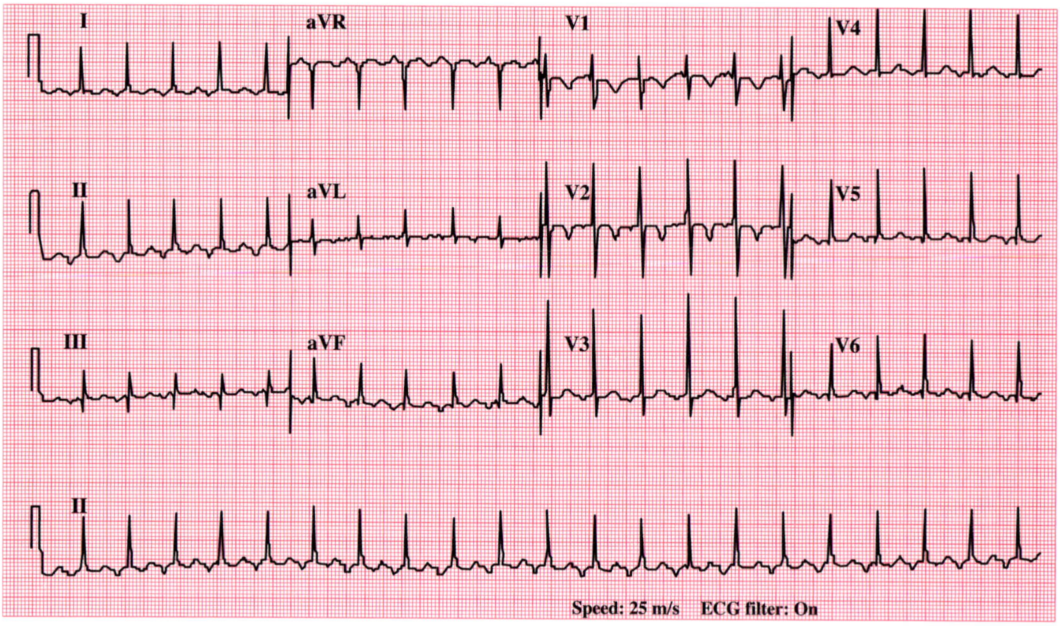

FIGURE 15.18. A standard 12-lead electrocardiogram in a patient with atypical (fast-slow) atrioventricular nodal reentrant tachycardia. There is a long RP interval with retrograde atrial activity seen just before the onset of the QRS complex.

Accessory Pathway–Mediated Tachycardia

In the normally developed heart, the only electrically conducting structures between the atria and ventricles are the AV node and the His bundle. However, congenitally anomalous accessory pathways (Kent bundles), either located centrally in the region of the AV node and His bundle or peripherally, may serve as part of the circuit of PSVT. Accessory pathways may conduct antegradely only from atrium to ventricle, retrogradely only from ventricle to atrium or in both directions. When an accessory pathway conducts in the antegrade direction, it can be identified by ECG evidence of ventricular preexcitation during sinus rhythm (**Figure 15.19**). Ventricular preexcitation and the Wolff-Parkinson-White syndrome are discussed separately in Chapter 19.

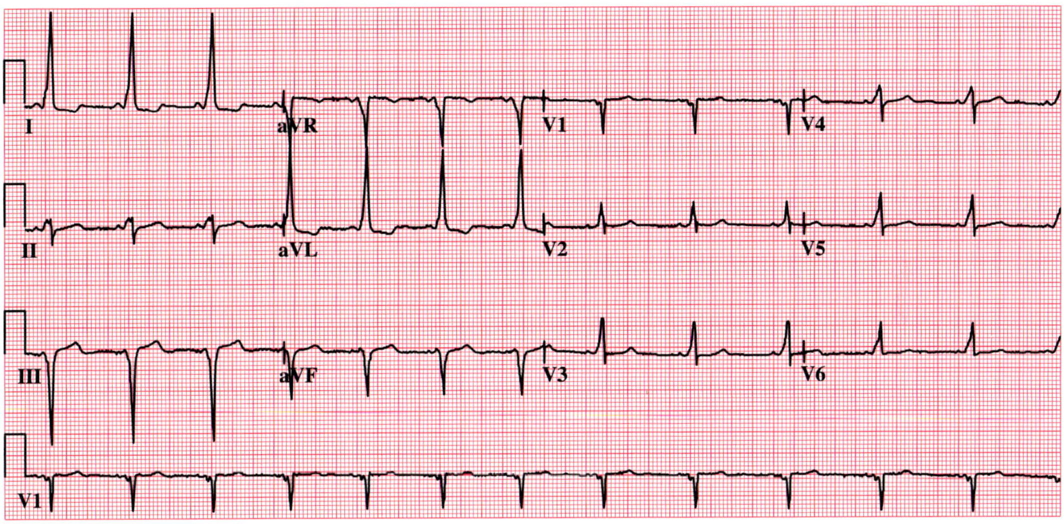

FIGURE 15.19. A standard 12-lead electrocardiogram in a patient with manifest preexcitation (Wolff-Parkinson-White pattern) in sinus rhythm.

Individuals with accessory pathways are at risk for developing PSVT. The two major varieties of tachycardia are orthodromic reentrant tachycardia (ORT) and antidromic reentrant tachycardia (ART) where conduction to the ventricles is via the AV node or accessory pathway, respectively (**Figure 15.20**). Rarely, two or more accessory pathways are present and antegrade or retrograde AV nodal conduction is entirely absent during tachycardia.

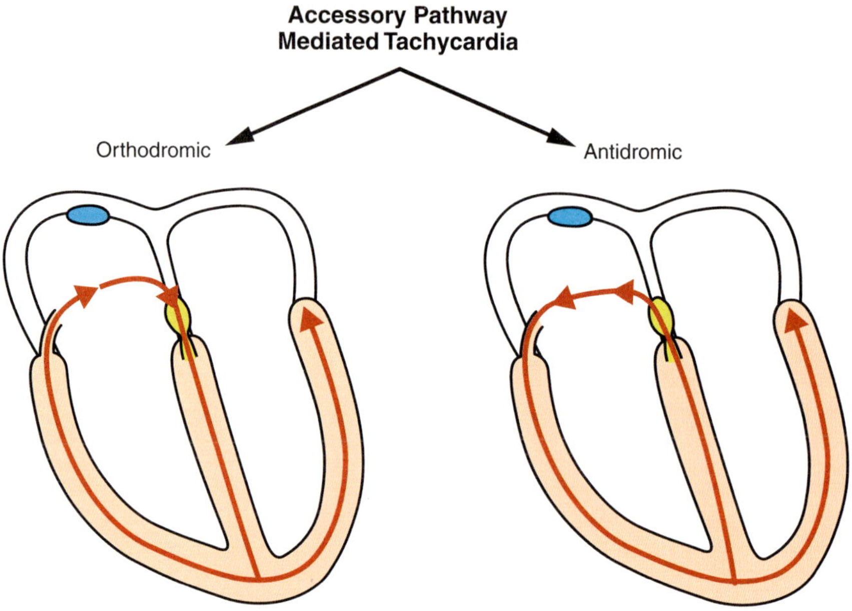

FIGURE 15.20. The two major mechanisms of accessory-mediated tachycardia are shown. During orthodromic reentrant tachycardia, the impulse is carried antegrade from the atrium to the ventricle via the atrioventricular node and retrograde through the accessory pathway. The QRS complex during tachycardia is narrow unless bundle-branch block is present. During antidromic reentrant tachycardia, the impulse is carried antegrade from the atrium to the ventricle via the accessory pathway and retrograde through the atrioventricular node. The QRS complex is very wide and abnormal due to maximal preexcitation.

A common form of accessory pathway-mediated tachycardia is ORT. During tachycardia, antegrade conduction from the atrium to the ventricle is via the AV node and His-Purkinje system and therefore the QRS complex is narrow. The exception to this is when left bundle or right bundle branch aberration is present, often at the onset of ORT (**Figure 15.21**). The retrograde limb of the circuit (ventricle to atrium) is via the accessory pathway. In 50% of patients with ORT, the accessory pathway is "concealed" and incapable of antegrade conduction. In this situation, the resting 12-lead ECG is normal (no preexcitation). ORT accounts for approximately 35% of PSVT and should be differentiated from atypical AVNRT and atrial tachycardia, which also present with a long RP interval on ECG. Pacing maneuvers in the electrophysiology laboratory during tachycardia can distinguish between these mechanisms.

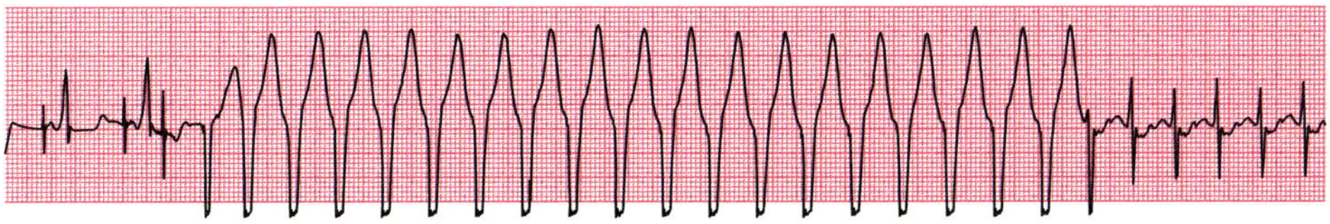

FIGURE 15.21. Lead II electrocardiogram of arrhythmia induction in a patient with orthodromic reentrant tachycardia via a left lateral accessory pathway. Left-bundle-branch block is present at the onset of tachycardia. With resolution of left-bundle-branch block aberrancy, the tachycardia cycle length accelerates due to more rapid conduction through the normal His-Purkinje system.

When antegrade conduction from atrium to ventricle during tachycardia is via the accessory pathway and retrograde conduction via the AV node, the tachycardia mechanism is referred to as ART. The QRS complex during tachycardia will be wide due to maximal ventricular preexcitation and may be confused for ventricular tachycardia as is shown in **Figure 15.22**. The presence of preexcitation on a prior sinus rhythm ECG clarifies the diagnosis. Patients with antegrade accessory pathway conduction in sinus rhythm (Wolff-Parkinson-White pattern) may present with ART, ORT, or other preexcited tachycardias. **Figure 15.23** demonstrates the sudden onset of SVT with a narrow QRS complex in a patient with evident preexcitation during sinus rhythm. There are distinct retrograde P waves during tachycardia with a long RP interval consistent with a diagnosis of ORT.

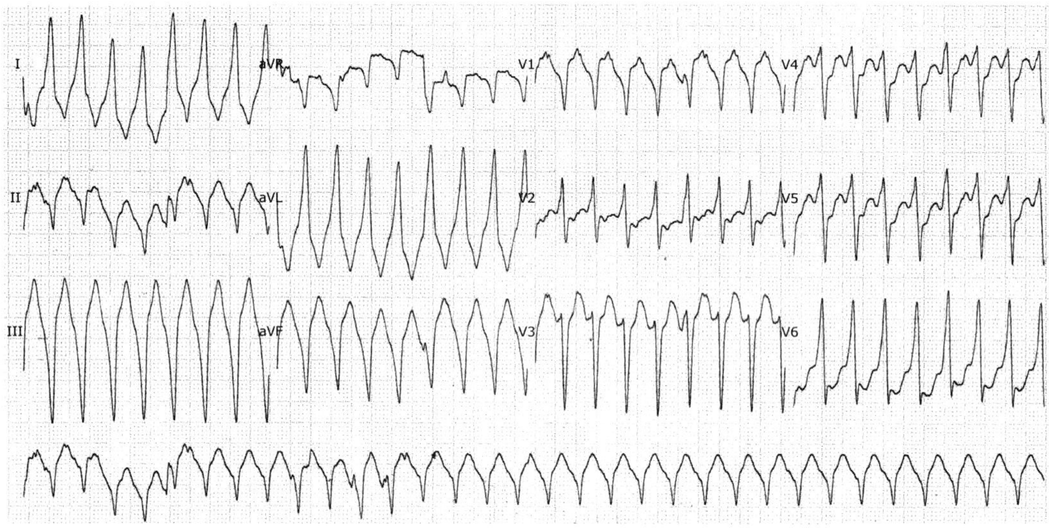

FIGURE 15.22. A 12-lead electrocardiogram from a 35-year-old man symptomatic with recurrent syncope having wide complex regular tachycardia with rate 250 bpm with a distinct P and delta waves (V1) suggesting antidromic tachycardia as the mechanism. Sinus rhythm ECG shows evidence of preexcitation.

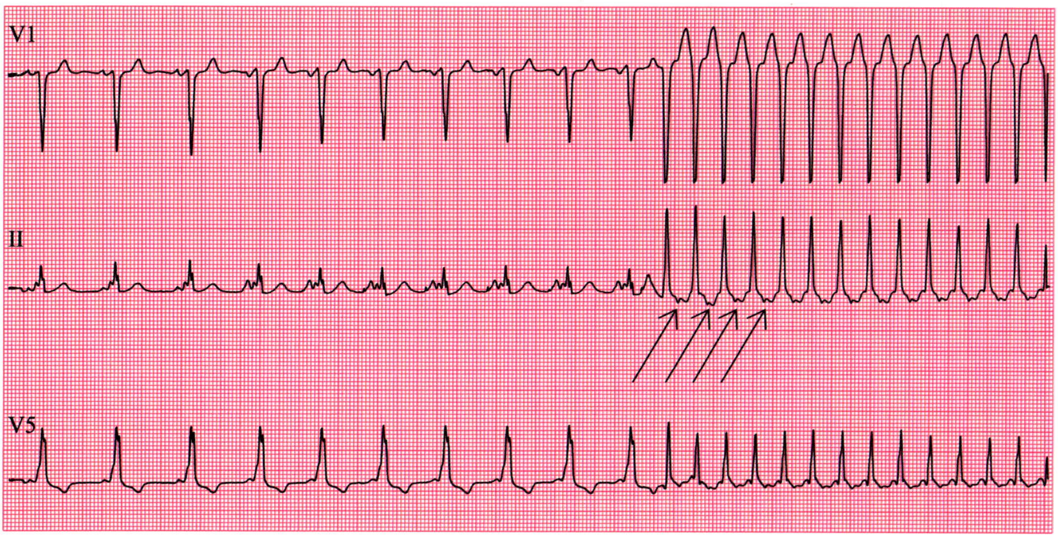

FIGURE 15.23. A three-lead electrocardiogram rhythm strip during sinus rhythm and the abrupt onset of orthodromic atrioventricular bypass tachycardia. Arrows indicate the retrograde P waves visible in lead II.

Electrical Alternans during SVT

Electrical alternans, typically seen in a large pericardial effusion with cardiac tamponade due to pendular movement of the heart in a fluid-filled pericardium, can also be encountered in fast SVT. In general, the presence of electrical alternans during SVT has been considered to be suggestive of AVRT. However, it may be a function of the heart rate rather than the mechanism of the SVT and may also occur during AVNRT.[A]

CHAPTER 15 SUMMARY ILLUSTRATION

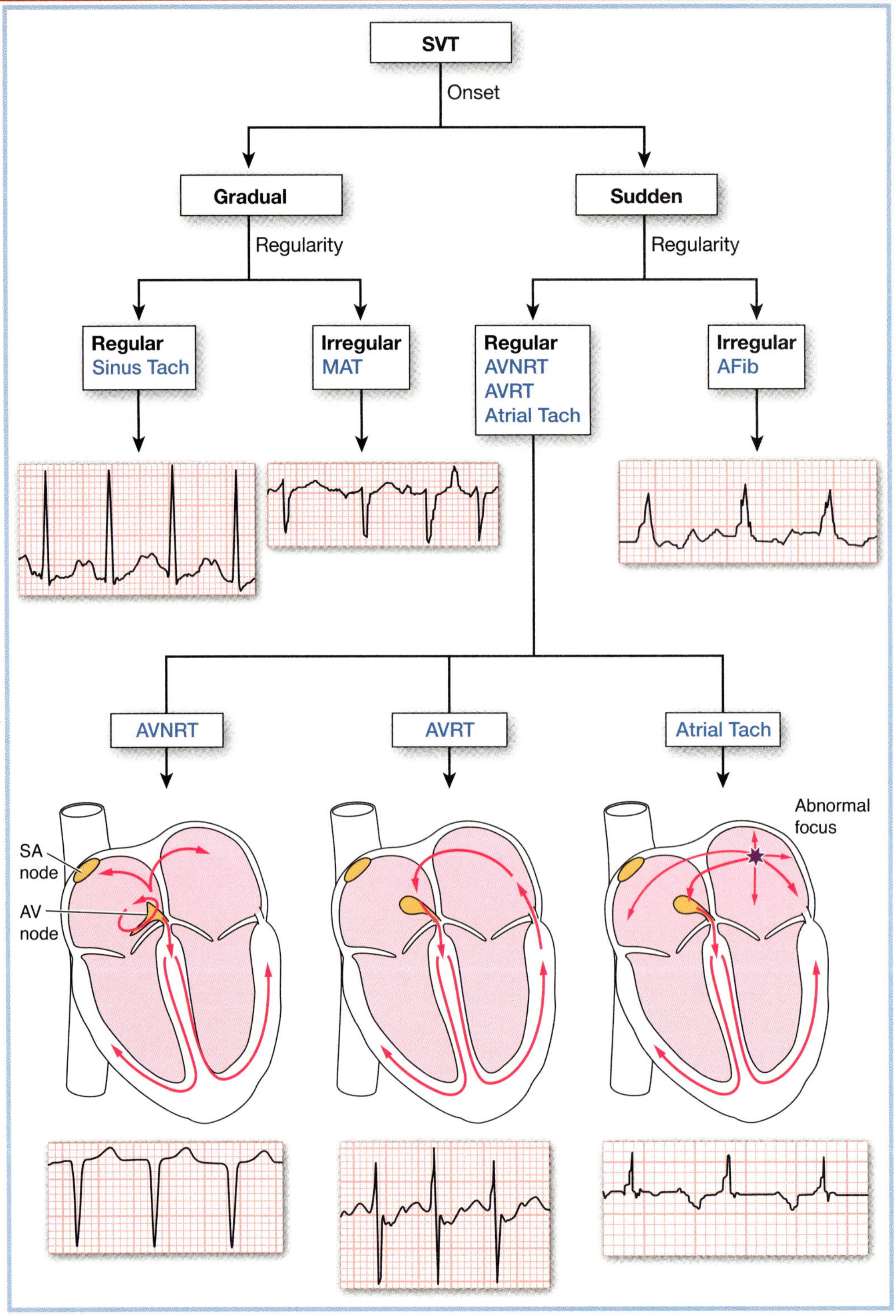

Abbreviations: AFib, atrial fibrillation; atrial tach, atrial tachycardia; AVNRT, atrioventricular nodal reentrant tachycardia; AVRT, atrioventricular reentrant (or "reciprocating") tachycardia; MAT, multifocal atrial tachycardia; sinus tach, sinus tachycardia; SVT, supraventricular tachycardia.

Glossary

Accelerated atrial rhythm: tachyarrhythmia caused by an increase of automaticity in atrial pacemaking cells.

Accelerated junctional rhythm: tachyarrhythmia caused by an increase of automaticity in the pacemaking cells of the His bundle.

Accelerated rhythm: an increase in a particular cardiac rhythm above its normal limit.

Accelerated ventricular rhythm: tachyarrhythmia caused by an increase of automaticity in pacemaking cells of the bundle branches and their fascicles.

Antidromic tachycardia: a reentrant tachycardia of the AV-bypass variety produced by macroreentry in which the causative impulse recycles sequentially through an accessory pathway, ventricle, AV node, and atrium.

Atrial fibrillation: the tachyarrhythmia produced by reentry within multiple circuits in the atria and is characterized by irregular multiform f waves.

Atrial flutter: the tachyarrhythmia produced by macroreentry within a single circuit in the atria and is characterized by regular uniform F waves.

AV reentrant tachycardia: a tachycardia produced by macroreentry, which includes the AV node along with the atrium, ventricle, and an accessory pathway.

AV nodal reentrant tachycardia: a tachycardia produced by microreentry within the AV node.

Calcium antagonist: a drug that diminishes calcium entry into cells and slows conduction through the AV node.

Carotid sinus massage: manual stimulation of the area of the neck that overlies the bifurcation of the carotid artery to increase parasympathetic nervous activity.

Chaotic atrial tachycardia: another term used for multifocal atrial tachycardia.

Coarse fibrillation: fibrillation marked by prominent f waves in some of the ECG leads.

Concealed accessory pathway: a Kent bundle that is capable only of VA conduction and is therefore incapable of producing ventricular preexcitation.

Concealed conduction: nonconducted atrial impulses that depolarize part of the AV node and thereby make it refractory to following impulses.

Digitalis toxicity: an arrhythmia produced by digitalis.

Echo beat: an atrial premature beat produced by reentry within the AV node.

Electrical cardioversion: use of transthoracic electrical current to terminate a reentrant tachyarrhythmia, such as those in the atrial flutter/fibrillation spectrum.

Fast-slow AV nodal tachycardia: a tachycardia of the AV nodal variety produced by microreentry in which the impulse travels down the fast pathway and up the slow pathway.

Fine fibrillation: either minute f waves or no atrial activity at all in any of the ECG leads.

f waves: the irregular, multiform atrial activity characteristic of fibrillation.

F waves: the regular, uniform, sawtooth-like atrial activity characteristic of flutter.

Irregularly irregular: a term describing an irregular rhythm with no discernible pattern to the sequence of ventricular beats.

Lone fibrillation: atrial fibrillation occurring in an individual who shows no evidence of cardiac disease.

Multifocal atrial tachycardia: a rapid rhythm produced by increased automaticity in pacemaking cells located at multiple sites within the atria.

Orthodromic tachycardia: a tachycardia of the accessory pathway AV-bypass variety produced by macroreentry in which the impulse recycles sequentially through the AV node, ventricle, an accessory pathway, and atrium.

Pacemaker: a cell in the heart or an artificial device that is capable of forming or generating an electrical impulse.

Paroxysmal: a term referring to an arrhythmia of sudden occurrence.

Paroxysmal atrial tachycardia with block: a tachyarrhythmia, commonly caused by digitalis toxicity, in which a rapid atrial rhythm is accompanied by failure of some of the atrial impulses to be conducted through the AV node to the ventricles.

Retrograde atrial activation: spread of an activating impulse from the AV junction through the atrial myocardium and toward the SA node.

Slow-fast AV nodal tachycardia: a tachycardia of the AV nodal variety produced by microreentry in which the impulse travels down the slow pathway and up the fast pathway.

Slow ventricular tachycardia: another term used for an accelerated ventricular rhythm.

Sympathetic tone: the relative amount of sympathetic nervous activity as compared with the amount of parasympathetic activity.

Vagal maneuver: an intervention that increases parasympathetic activity in relation to the amount of sympathetic activity.

Acknowledgment

We gratefully acknowledge the past contributions of the previous edition's author, Dr. Galen S. Wagner, as portions of that chapter were retained in this revision.

References

1. Ip JE, Liu CF, Thomas G, Cheung JW, Markowitz SM, Lerman BB. Unifying mechanism of sustained idiopathic atrial and ventricular annular tachycardia. *Circ Arrhythm Electrophysiol.* 2014;7(3):436-444.
2. Link MS. Clinical practice. Evaluation and initial treatment of supraventricular tachycardia. *N Engl J Med.* 2012;367(15): 1438-1448.
3. Page RL, Joglar JA, Caldwell MA, et al. 2015 ACC/AHA/HRS guideline for the management of adult patients with supraventricular tachycardia: a report of the American College of Cardiology/American Heart Association Task Force on Clinical Practice Guidelines and the Heart Rhythm Society. *J Am Coll Cardiol.* 2016;67(13): e27-e115.
4. Saoudi N, Cosio F, Waldo A, et al. Classification of atrial flutter and regular atrial tachycardia according to electrophysiologic mechanism and anatomic bases: a statement from a joint expert group from the working group of Arrhythmias of the European Society of Cardiology and the North American Society of Pacing and Electrophysiology. *J Cardiovasc Electrophysiol.* 2001;12(7):852-866.
5. Kistler PM, Roberts-Thomson KC, Haqqani HM, et al. P-wave morphology in focal atrial tachycardia: development of an algorithm to predict the anatomic site of origin. *J Am Coll Cardiol.* 2006;48(5):1010-1017.
6. Wasmer K, Eckardt L. Management of supraventricular arrhythmias in adults with congenital heart disease. *Heart.* 2016;102(20): 1614-1619.

Reference to the South Asian Edition

A. Pulignano G, Patruno N, Urbani P, Greco C, Critelli G. Electrophysiological significance of QRS alternans in narrow QRS tachycardia. *Pacing Clin Electrophysiol.* 1990;13(2):144-150. doi:10.1111/j.1540-8159.1990.tb05063.x

To view digital content associated with this chapter please access lww.co.in. Instructions are located on the inside front cover.

16 Atrial Fibrillation and Flutter

JONATHAN P. PICCINI,
JAMES P. DAUBERT,
TRISTRAM D. BAHNSON,
NARAYANAN NAMBOODIRI K K,
AND SAI KIRAN KAKARLA

Pathophysiology of Atrial Fibrillation and Atrial Flutter

Atrial fibrillation (AF) and *atrial flutter* (AFL) are the most commonly encountered supraventricular arrhythmias in clinical practice. AF is characterized by chaotic and disorganized electrical activation of the atrial tissue involving multiple unstable "functional" wavelets of reentry to produce disorganized atrial activation with consequent irregularly irregular ventricular conduction.[1] AFL, in contrast to AF, is an organized macroreentrant rhythm that results from a stable activating *wavefront* traveling around a fixed nonconducting region of either atrium. Risk factors include, but are not limited to, hypertension, sleep apnea, diabetes, obesity, and cardiovascular disease such as coronary artery disease, hypertension, mitral or tricuspid regurgitation, pulmonary hypertension, and heart failure. Atrial arrhythmias also increase in frequency with age because the exposure to these risk factors increases with age producing "age-related" changes in atrial tissue.

Both AF and AFL share common risk factors that predispose to impaired and heterogenous atrial conduction, which allows for initiation and maintenance of the arrhythmias.

Coumel's triangle of arrhythmogenesis summarizes different contributors of AF.[A]

1. Trigger factor or initiator: Most commonly, the triggers are ectopic beats arising from pulmonary vein or its antrum. Other non-pulmonary vein triggers include ectopy from superior vena cava, coronary sinus or vein of Marshall, crista terminalis, etc. Rarely, atrioventricular nodal reentry or atrioventricular reentry can be triggers, especially in young adults.[B]
2. The arrhythmogenic substrate or sustainer of AF: Electrical remodeling, which causes shortening and dispersion of action potential duration (APD); downregulation of ICa2+ channel, which alters the calcium homeostasis; and structural remodeling of LA lead to LA fibrosis.
3. The modulation factors of which the most common is the autonomic nervous system.

Functional reentry during AF refers to a pattern of wavefront propagation where the leading edge of the advancing wavefront impinges on partially refractory tissue as it moves around a barrier of completely refractory tissue. In comparison, "classic" reentry, which underlies AFL, involves a single abnormal activation wavefront moving around a fixed nonconducting obstacle such as the atrioventricular valve annuli. This kind of reentry is also called "macroreentry."

AF and AFL can both occur in the same individual. Moreover, AF can "organize" into AFL, and AFL can "degenerate" into AF.[2] In the case of typical AFL, abnormal atrial activation proceeds counterclockwise around the tricuspid annulus as viewed from the ventricle (**Video 16.1**), as discussed in more detail below. Typical AFL can be recognized on electrocardiogram (ECG) due to regular and uniform "flutter waves" without long atrial diastolic intervals in most ECG leads consistent with stable continuous atrial activation, which is the hallmark of macroreentry (**Figure 16.1**).

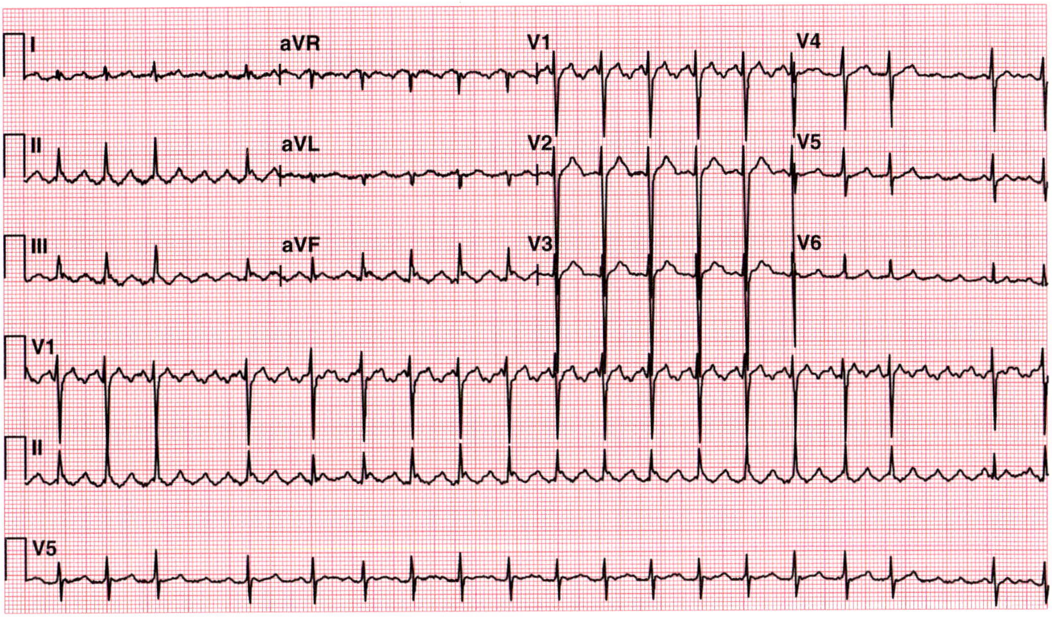

FIGURE 16.1. Twelve-lead electrocardiogram and lead V_1, II, V_5 rhythm strips from a 68-year-old man 1 day after cholecystectomy. The patient had a long history of poorly treated hypertension. There are several notable features on this electrocardiogram. Most notable is the variable atrioventricular conduction of the macroreentrant atrial rhythm. The F waves are negative in the inferior limb leads (leads II, III, and aVF) and positive in lead V_1. Note that the RR intervals are always multiple of the FF intervals as is characteristic in atrial flutter.

To view the animation(s) and video(s) associated with this chapter please access lww.co.in. Instructions are located on the inside front cover.

In the case of AF (**Figure 16.2**), atrial activation is dynamic and chaotic, mediated by multiple simultaneous reentrant wavelets most of which are continually changing. Such atrial activation leads to continuous and disordered activation of the atrial myocardium and highly variable *F waves* on the ECG except for leads V_1 and V_2, which often reveal relatively stable reentrant wavelets during AF in the interatrial septum.

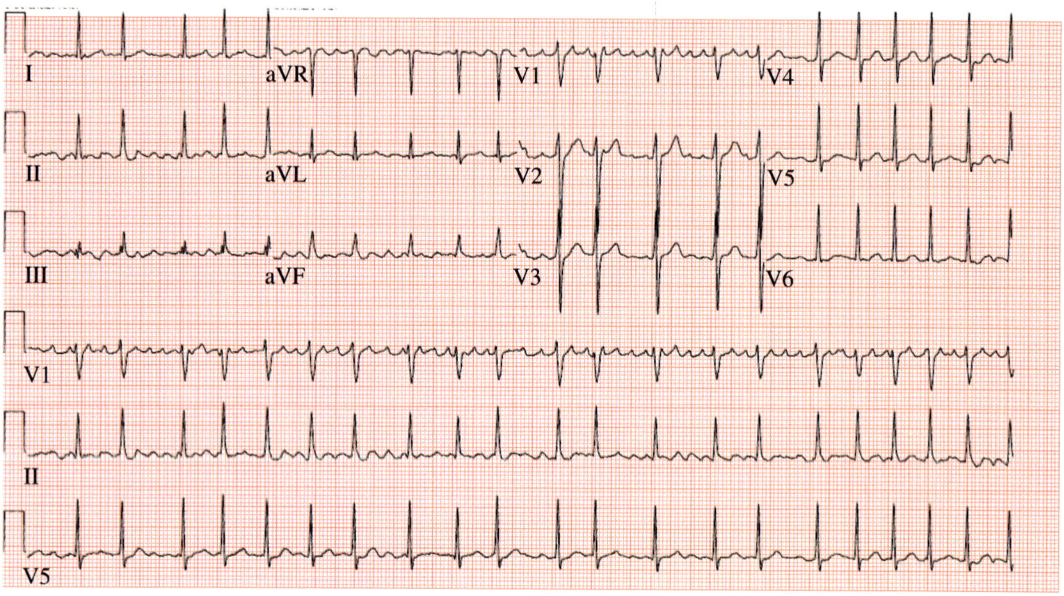

FIGURE 16.2. This figure depicts coarse atrial fibrillation. The F waves in leads V_1 and V_2 appear discrete and regular and could be mistaken for atrial flutter; however, the cycle length (CL) of less than 160 milliseconds is too fast for atrial flutter. The organized activity in leads V_1 and V_2 represents a stable wavelet of reentry in the region of the intra-atrial septum during the time this electrocardiogram was recorded. Other leads show fluctuating F-wave morphology, and the ventricular response is irregularly irregular, confirming the diagnosis of atrial fibrillation.

The sine qua non of AF is appearance of an irregularly irregular ventricular response (see **Chapter 16 Summary Illustration**; top panel; **Figures 16.2** and **16.3**). As rapid and irregular atrial activations bombard the atrioventricular node, refractoriness of the AV node tissue prevents most of the atrial impulses from conducting down to the ventricles.[3] However, the impulses that do get conducted do so irregularly due to the dynamic nature of the atrial activation wavelets and the AV node refractoriness in response to the AF. Specifically, variable concealed conduction into the AV node produces dynamic AV node refractoriness contributing to the irregularly irregular ventricular response. When examining the ECG in AF, the RR intervals (distance between the QRS complexes) are completely irregular and not reproducible. In the absence of drugs that impair atrioventricular conduction, or intrinsic atrioventricular conduction disease, the ventricular rates in AF are often greater than 100 beats/min. Over time, this rapid ventricular conduction can lead to left ventricular dysfunction, which is called tachycardia-induced cardiomyopathy, which is an important clinical problem.

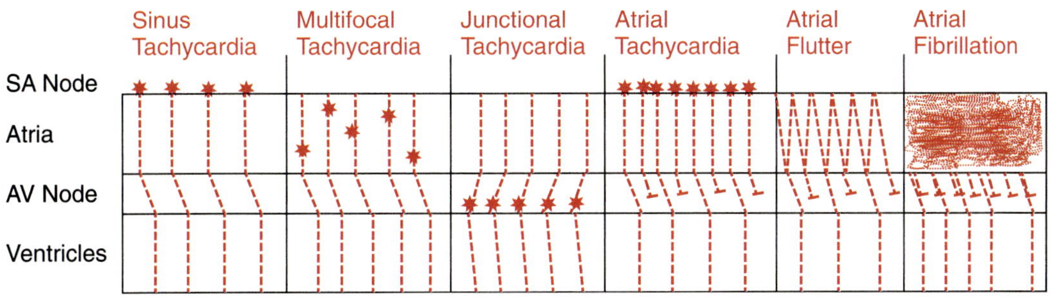

FIGURE 16.3. These ladder diagrams illustrate the mechanisms of conduction in these supraventricular rhythms. The star notes the site of impulse formation in focal or multifocal arrhythmias. Note the absence of focal sites of impulse formation in the case of atrial flutter, which is a self-sustaining macroreentrant rhythm, and atrial fibrillation, which is a rhythm characterized by dynamic and chaotic reentry. Sinus tachycardia, multifocal atrial tachycardia, and junctional tachycardia are all characterized by enhanced automaticity. Atrial tachycardias can be due to several mechanisms, including enhanced automaticity, triggered activity, and microreentry. In this figure, atrial tachycardia and atrial flutter are both depicted with 2:1 atrioventricular (AV) conduction, which appears regular; more variable AV conduction or higher-grade atrioventricular block during atrial tachycardia and atrial flutter can also be seen. Atrial fibrillation, however, is irregularly irregular. SA, sinoatrial.

Twelve-Lead Electrocardiographic Characteristics of Atrial Fibrillation

As previously described, AF is an irregularly irregular rhythm due to chaotic dynamic reentry in the atria. Functional reentrant wavelets during AF are not fixed to a specific location and often demonstrate spatial drift producing continuously changing atrial activation waves (F waves) on the surface ECG. Thus, the key electrocardiographic characteristics of AF include the absence of organized atrial activity and an irregularly irregular ventricular rhythm. So-called "coarse" AF may show pseudo-organization in lead V_1 when there are fewer wavelets of reentry, some of which may be relatively stable to produce the appearance of organized activity in specific ECG leads like V_1 (see **Figure 16.2**). Accordingly, when organized atrial activation cannot be discerned in all ECG leads, or when the morphology of atrial activation waves on the ECGs are not constant over time with a clear reproducible pattern of atrial activation, AF should be suspected rather than AFL. Sometimes in clinical practice, these ECGs are described or labeled as AF/AFL. This is incorrect, and the term should be avoided. AF and AFL may be interrelated and may share substrate, but they are distinct electrophysiologic phenomena.

Careful search for the underlying etiology of AF should be done in every electrocardiogram. Evidence of right atrial enlargement can be seen with Qr pattern in V1, and right ventricular hypertrophy with right axis deviation may be a pointer for pulmonary hypertension.

Although AF is usually irregularly irregular, there are rare instances where AF is accompanied by a regular RR interval due to complete atrioventricular block with a junctional rhythm (**Figures 16.4** and **16.5**). This situation is often encountered in cardiothoracic surgery patients who have postoperative heart block together with AF and who are also on adrenergic agents like epinephrine that foster an accelerated junctional rhythm. AF with a junctional rhythm can also be observed in patients on digoxin, particularly those who have evidence of digoxin toxicity.[4]

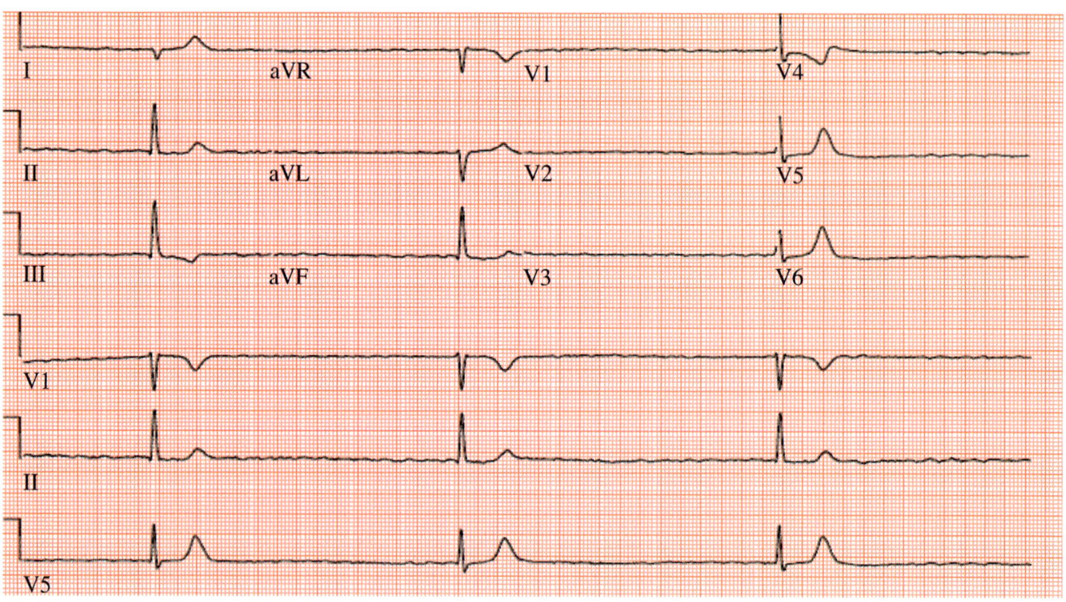

FIGURE 16.4. Patient who presented with syncope after taking an extra metoprolol dose due to palpitations. This shows atrial fibrillation with complete heart block and a junctional rhythm.

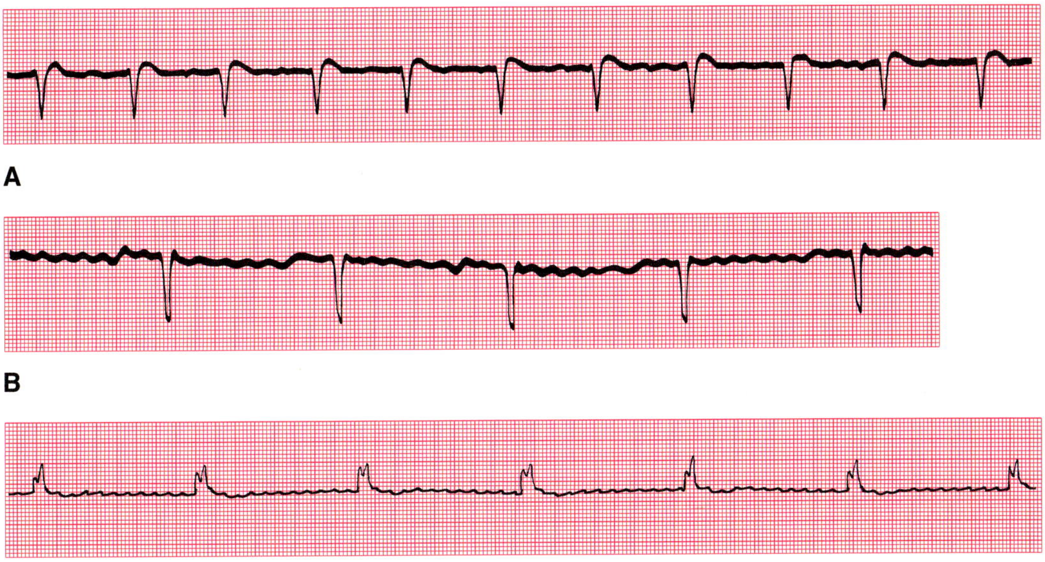

A

B

C

FIGURE 16.5. Note that the ventricular rhythm is regular and the rate varies from accelerated (65 beats/min [**A**]) to within the typical escape range (50 beats/min [**B**]) to a rate in the slow escape range (40 beats/min [**C**]).The proper terminology for each of these conditions would be atrial fibrillation with atrioventricular (AV) dissociation owing to high-degree AV block and accelerated junctional rhythm (**A**), complete AV block with right-ventricular escape rhythm (**B**), and complete AV block with left-ventricular escape rhythm (**C**). At times, the escape site may be below the branching of the common bundle, producing a widened QRS complex.

Finally, it is also important to recognize AF with evidence of preexcitation (**Figures 16.6** and **16.7**). This is important for several reasons. First, these patients may benefit from treatment of their preexcitation with catheter ablation of their accessory pathway. Many of these patients do not have further AF once their accessory pathway is eliminated. Second, when a patient is in AF with preexcitation, administration of atrioventricular nodal-blocking agents is contraindicated as it can facilitate rapid anterograde conduction down the accessory pathway, with subsequent induction of ventricular fibrillation and cardiac arrest.[5]

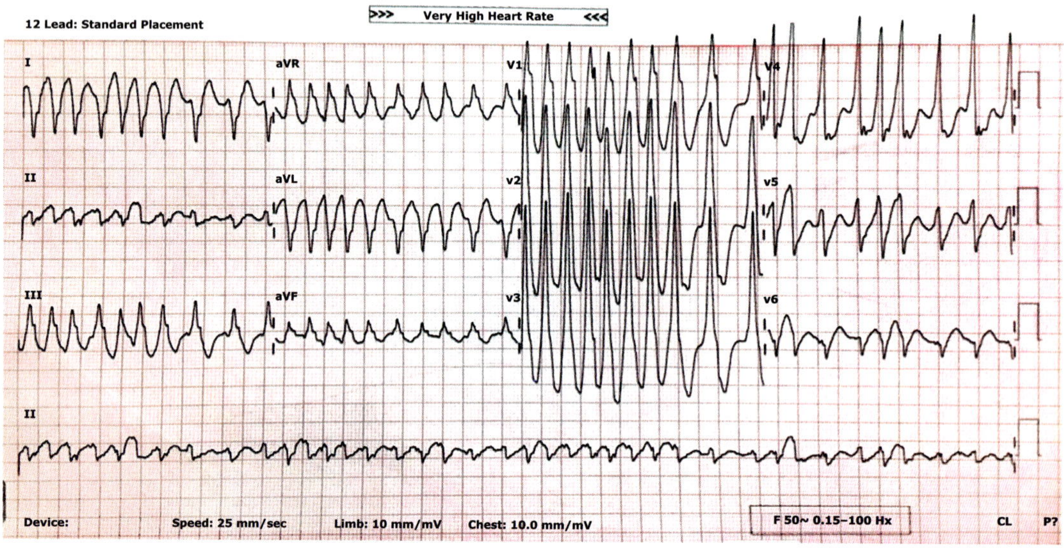

FIGURE 16.6. This ECG is recorded in a young lady who presented with episodes of syncope and palpitation. It shows fast, broad, and irregular tachycardia at a rate of around 240 bpm, with varying degrees of preexcitation across the QRS complexes with varied morphologies. She had a left lateral accessory pathway at mitral annulus.

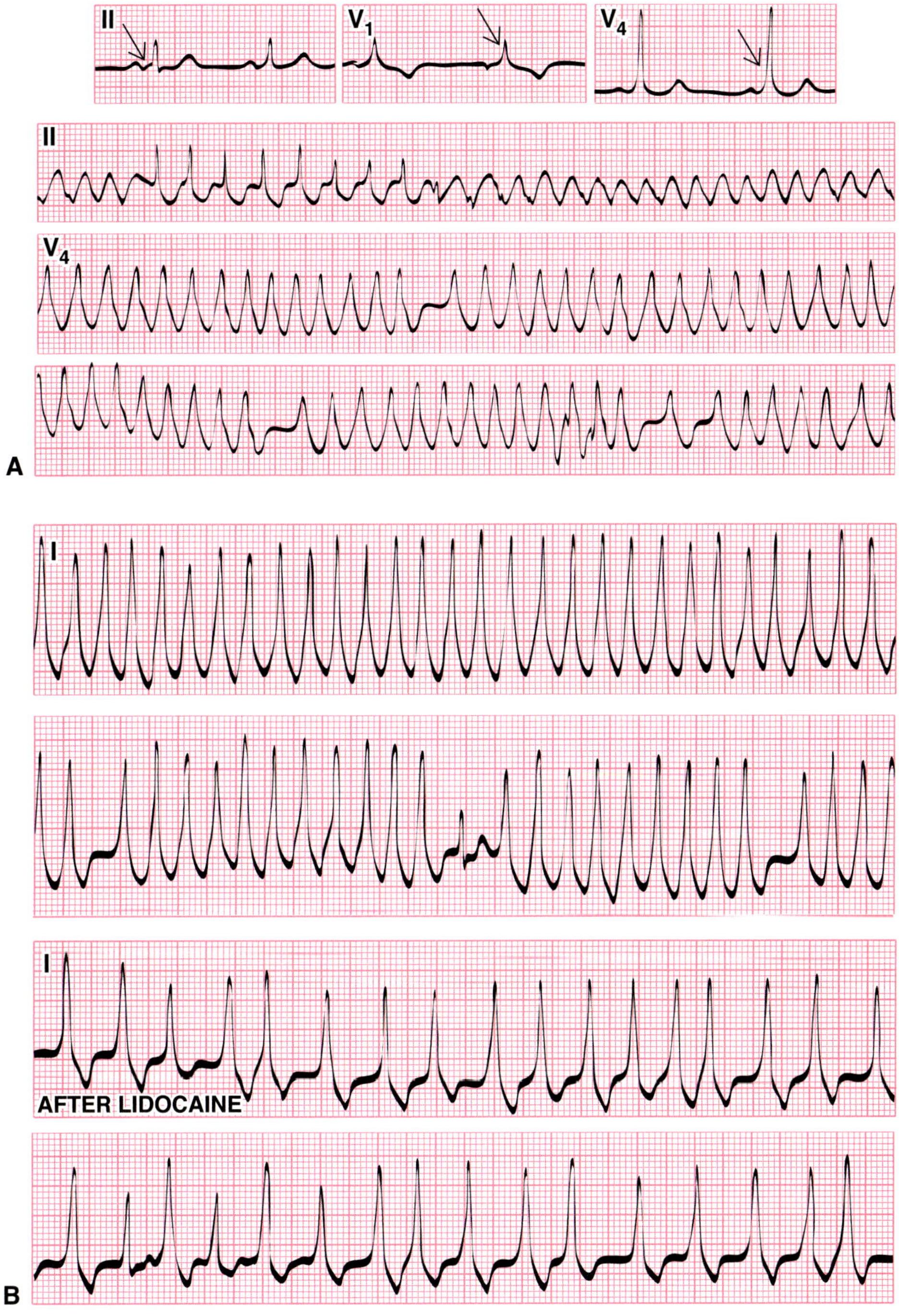

FIGURE 16.7. Electrocardiogram recordings from two teenage patients evaluated in the emergency department with palpitations and weakness and evidence of preexcited atrial fibrillation. **A.** Top, electrocardiogram leads II, V_1, and V_4 with preexcitation during sinus rhythm consistent with an antegrade conducting accessory pathway (arrows, delta waves). Lead II and V_4 rhythm strips show variable degrees of preexcitation during atrial fibrillation with a very rapid ventricular response. **B.** Preexcited atrial fibrillation in the second patient with a very rapid ventricular response with variable QRS morphologies and a single QRS without preexcitation. After lidocaine, the ventricular response rate is slower.

Digitalis and AF

Digitalis is used as a common drug to decrease the AF rate. The arrhythmias of digitalis intoxication arise from two actions of the drug: 1. Delaying atrioventricular (AV) nodal conduction, which is an important therapeutic as well as a potentially toxic effect; and 2. Enhanced automaticity, which is not of any therapeutic value. Simultaneous presence of both phenomena should raise the suspicion of digoxin toxicity.[C]

Most common arrhythmias noted in digitoxicity are ventricular bigeminy and non-paroxysmal atrial tachycardia (secondary to enhanced automaticity) with variable AV conduction (secondary to AV nodal suppression). Similarly, regularization of rhythm in a preexisting AF suggests complete heart block with an automatic junctional rhythm, a combination of these two toxic effects.

Bidirectional ventricular tachycardia and ventricular bigeminy with AF are also seen in cases of digitoxicity. Two arrhythmias that are not commonly seen with digitoxicity are AF with fast ventricular rate and type II second degree AV block.

Rheumatic AF

Incidence of AF in patients with rheumatic heart disease (RHD) is estimated to be about 40%.[D] Factors potentially contributing to the development of AF in this condition are multifactorial. However, it is mediated by atrial fibrosis, which in turn is predominantly determined by hemodynamic factors and progressive dilation of atria. Once present, AF further leads to increase in the degree of LA enlargement. AF is self-sustaining, and the vicious cycle is further perpetuated by drugs and advancing age, hence aptly described as "AF begets AF".[E] The incidence of AF is more common in the later stages of RHD, indicating the mechanistic effects predisposing to it rather than the rheumatic activity itself.[F] Every increment of 5 mm in LA size above 35 mm caused an age- and sex- adjusted hazard ratio of 1.42 for the occurrence of new-onset AF.[G]

It is worthwhile to note that there has been dramatic evolution in the treatment of AF over the last two decades that relate to two key concepts regarding the pathophysiology of AF.[6] The first is that AF is frequently initiated by trigger beats originating in or near the left atrial pulmonary vein muscle sleeves. In **Figure 16.8**, the tracing shows surface ECG leads and intracardiac recordings during initiation of AF. Catheter ablation of these triggers has been shown to be effective in preventing recurrent AF.[7] The second key concept is that there are also factors that increase the likelihood that AF is sustained for long periods of time. These factors include left atrial enlargement, left atrial scar, abnormally slowed atrial conduction velocity, and shortened atrial refractory periods, all of which facilitate multiwavelet functional reentry. In advanced cases of AF, elimination of triggers alone may not eliminate AF, and treatments directed to these other substrate factors are often considered to prevent AF recurrence.

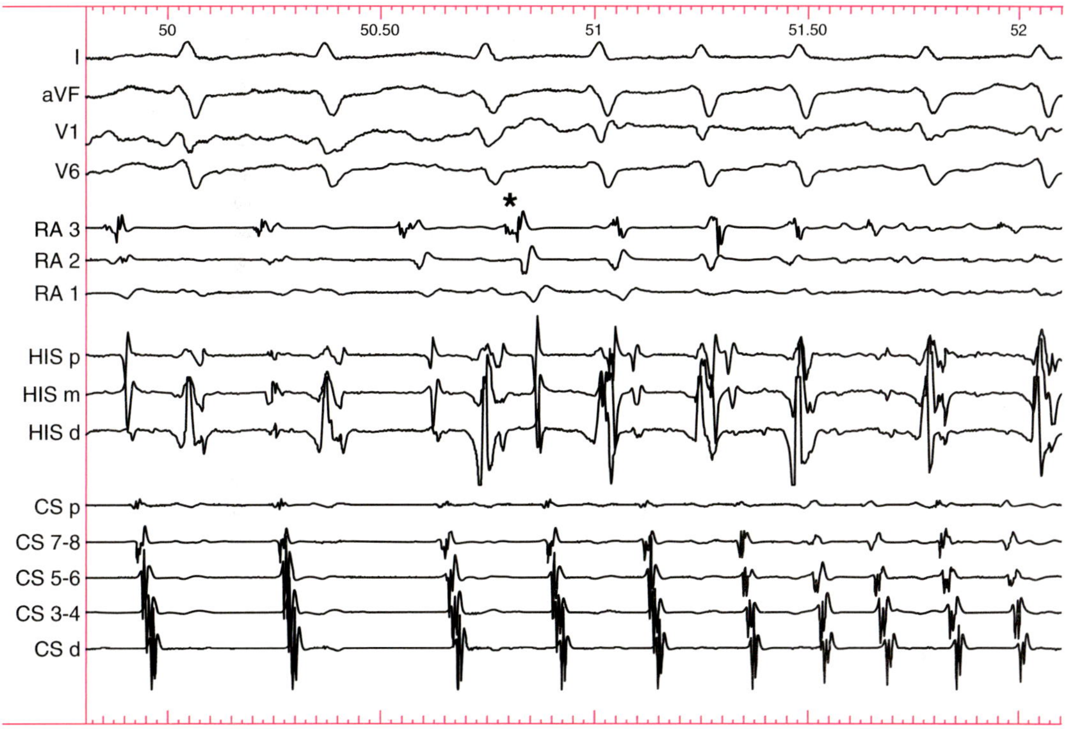

FIGURE 16.8. Electrocardiographic leads and intracardiac electrograms demonstrating the onset of atrial fibrillation (AF) due to a trigger emanating from the superior vena cava. This patient continued to have AF despite prior pulmonary vein isolation. He was found to have triggers inducing AF that originated from the superior vena cava (recordings on channels RA3-RA1). The asterisk denotes the premature beat or trigger that initiates AF. Electrical isolation of the superior vena cava resulted in long-term suppression of his AF.

Atrial Flutter

Broadly speaking, AFL is a stable macroreentrant atrial arrhythmia that can occur in either atrium to produce rapid atrial activation. A common classification of AFL has to do with whether or not the arrhythmia is caused by macroreentry around the tricuspid annulus in the right atrium in a counterclockwise direction; if so, the AFL is termed "typical." Although a characteristic ECG appearance can often allow correct identification of typical AFL (see **Figure 16.1**), this is not always so, and invasive electrophysiologic studies are required to confirm with certainty the mechanism of AFL. Atypical forms of AFL occur when stable macroreentry occurs in the left atrium or in the right atrium apart from typical AFL. The increasing prevalence of heart surgery and left atrial ablation for AF have resulted in an increasing incidence of *atypical atrial flutter*.

Typical Atrial Flutter

The most common form of AFL is typical AFL. This arrhythmia depends on conduction through the cavotricuspid isthmus, which is defined as the atrial tissue that lies between the tricuspid valve annulus and the inferior vena cava. Accordingly, typical AFL is also called counterclockwise cavotricuspid isthmus-dependent flutter. **Video 16.1** reveals the circuit in atypical AFL. Atrial activation spreads up the septum, across the roof, and then down the lateral wall of the right atrium along the crista terminalis before reaching the isthmus again. This activation pattern leads to the diagnostic ECG pattern with F waves that are negative in the inferior leads and positive in lead V_1 (**Figure 16.9**; see also **Figure 16.1**). In clockwise AFL, this pattern is reversed, and the F waves are positive in the inferior leads and negative in V_1. Based on the ECG alone, clockwise cavotricuspid isthmus-dependent AFL can be difficult to distinguish from left AFLs.

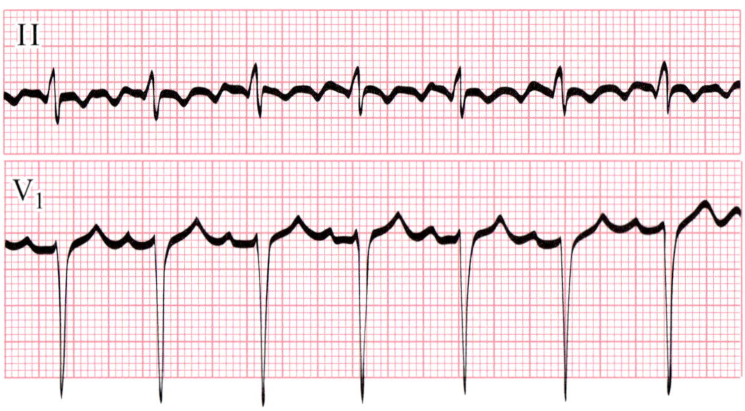

FIGURE 16.9. A two-channel rhythm strip (leads II and V_1) from a woman who presented with new-onset atrial flutter. Her history was notable for chronic obstructive pulmonary disease. The F-wave vector is consistent with typical atrial flutter.

The F waves of AFL typically occur at rates between 200 and 350 beats/min. The ventricular rate is usually regular and always a multiple of the FF interval. In the absence of atrioventricular nodal-blocking agents, AFL often presents with 2:1 conduction but can present with higher degrees of A:V block. Dynamic maneuvers such as carotid sinus massage or administration of bolus dose adenosine that transiently increase A:V block can aid diagnosis by revealing flutter waves hidden during 2:1 conduction due to fusion between flutter waves and the T wave or concealment of flutter waves within the QRS. **Figure 16.10** depicts atypical AFL with both 2:1 conduction and higher-grade A:V block with carotid sinus massage.

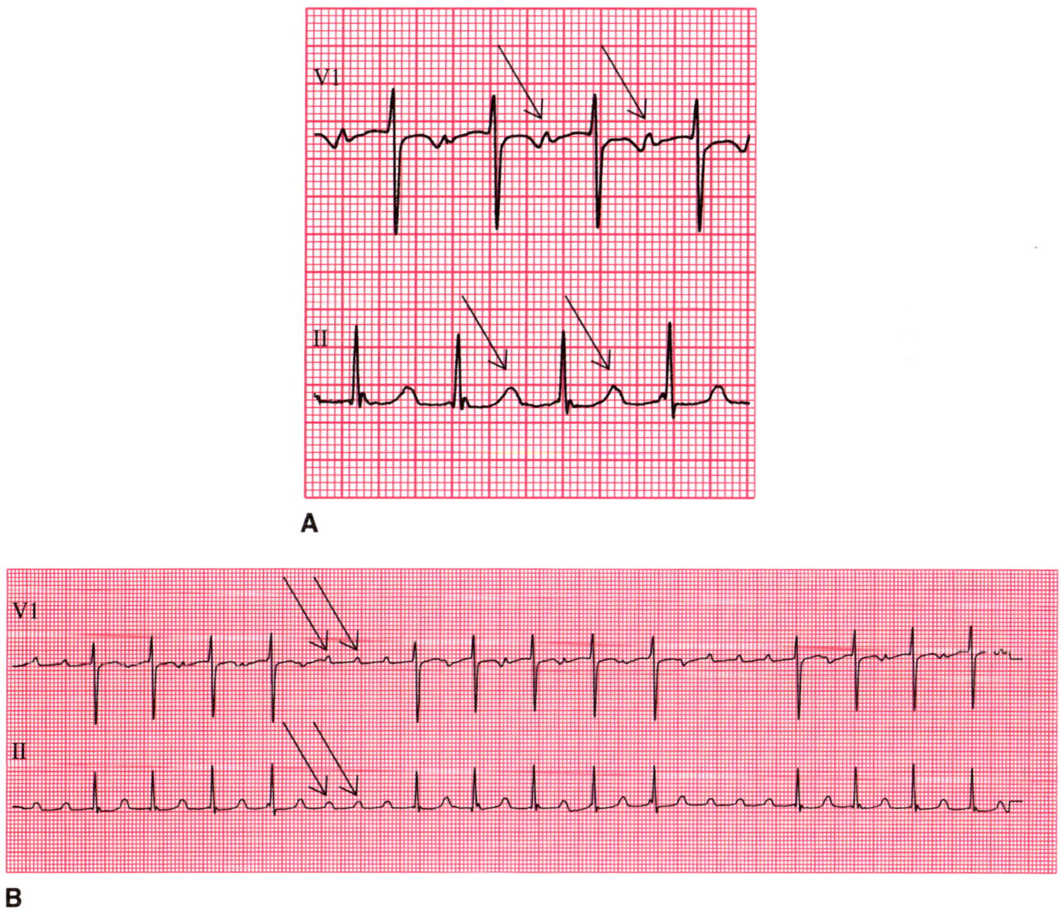

FIGURE 16.10. Leads V1 and II rhythm strips from a patient presented with dyspnea and had a history of idiopathic dilated cardiomyopathy. Arrows annotate the F waves during tachycardia in the presenting condition that are fused with the T wave (**A**) and during carotid sinus massage (**B**). Note the predominance of 2:1 atrioventricular conduction followed by periods of nonconduction to the ventricles with carotid sinus massage.

Due to the fast and regular atrial rate produced by AFL, it can be difficult to slow A:V conduction to less than 2:1 with AV blocker medications when patients have "normal" AV node function without producing hypotension. When AV blocker medications are tolerated and there is preexisting AV node disease, slowing rates to the range of 60 to 80 beats/min (eg, 4:1 conduction) may be associated with periods of even higher-grade AV block manifesting as significant pauses. Given the difficulty in achieving rate control, AFL is often cardioverted. As with AF, antiarrhythmic drugs, and to some extent β-blockers, can reduce the risk of recurrent AFL. Once the potential circuit to sustain AFL has been manifest, it is very likely that AFL will recur. Accordingly, AFL is often treated with catheter ablation due to its highly symptomatic nature and the difficulty in achieving adequate rate control. This is particularly true in the case of typical AFL where the ablation procedure requires right atrial access only, has minimal risk, and provides a high cure rate (>95%). Given that the triggers for AFL and AF are often the same, it is not surprising that patients who had demonstrated AFL are at increased risk of developing AF in the future. The risk of developing AF after AFL is between 25% and 50% over the next 5 to 10 years.[8,9] Of course, as previously mentioned, incessant AFL can itself produce atrial remodeling to favor AF by decreasing atrial refractory periods thereby facilitating degeneration of AFL into AF.

Atypical Atrial Flutter

Atypical AFL circuits can occur virtually anywhere in either the right or the left atrium when trigger beats result in a wavefront of activation moving around morphologically defined obstacles in the atria such as the superior vena cava orifice, the right or left appendage orifices, the pulmonary veins, the mitral annulus, or regions of scar resulting from prior surgery or cardiomyopathic processes. Atypical AFLs (like typical AFL) are "macroreentrant" arrhythmias involving a single wavefront repetitively traveling over a discrete circuit. As previously discussed, the substrate for initiation and maintenance of atypical AFL includes the occurrence of trigger beats that initiate the arrhythmia and factors that cause the time it takes for an activating wavefront to traverse the flutter circuit to be sufficiently long to allow previously activated tissue to recover excitability. In other words, stable reentry can occur when the tachycardia cycle length is longer than the longest refractory period of tissue anywhere in the circuit to allow an initiating activation wavefront to reenter the circuit over and over without encountering refractory tissue.

Atrial enlargement from a variety of disease states and regions of slow conduction within the arrhythmia circuit (eg, from surgery or fibrosis) can result in AFL cycle lengths sufficiently long to allow for stable reentry. The time for a wavefront to traverse the circuit once defines the cycle length of atypical (or typical) AFL. Antiarrhythmic drugs that prolong refractoriness of atrial tissue work by eliminating the "excitable gap" of tissue in front of the advancing AFL wavefront to prevent stable reentry. In contrast, antiarrhythmic drugs that slow conduction can produce conduction block in areas of already impaired conduction, thus terminating AFL. However, in some instances, slowed conduction can also be proarrhythmic by prolonging the flutter cycle length making AFL possible or more stable.

When interpreting ECGs with possible AF or AFL, it is useful to know what medications the patient is taking. Vaughan-Williams class III drugs like sotalol and dofetilide primarily act to delay repolarization (increase refractory periods), class I drugs like flecainide and propafenone primarily slow impulse propagation, and amiodarone has features of both groups. Amiodarone and flecainide in particular can organize AF into more "coarse AF" or AFL. Antiarrhythmic drugs, which slow conduction velocity (eg, flecainide, amiodarone), can also slow AFL cycle lengths, sometimes dramatically. This has the potential to paradoxically increase the ventricular response rate to AFL if the slowed flutter rate can be conducted 1:1 to the ventricle, as opposed to 2:1 conduction which is the "best" a normal AV node can conduct with typically fast AFL cycle lengths. ECGs with 1:1 AFL with rate-dependent ventricular aberrancy can be difficult to distinguish from ventricular tachycardia (Chapter 17).

An important subgroup of patients is those who have had previous catheter or surgical ablation. These patients are increasingly common and likely to be encountered by general cardiologists and primary care physicians. Ablation procedures introduce regions of "scar" or tissue injury that can increase the likelihood of clinical atypical AFL. These arrhythmias tend to result in rapid ventricular responses that are difficult to control using hemodynamically tolerated doses of AV blockers (β-blocker or calcium blocker), and accordingly are often very symptomatic and refractory to drug therapy. Atypical AFL often requires early cardioversion and antiarrhythmic drug therapy or catheter ablation because the likelihood of recurrence is high given the demonstrated existence of the potential circuit to sustain atypical AFL in the first place.

In summary, clinical features which increase the likelihood of an individual patient developing atypical AFL include any pathophysiologic process producing an atrial myopathy such as hypertrophic cardiomyopathy, valvular heart disease with chronic pressure or volume overload of the atria, infiltrative cardiomyopathies, toxin exposure, or prior surgical or catheter-based procedures targeting atrial tissue. Importantly, any cardiac surgery involving a right atrial incision (eg, atrial septal defect repair, mitral valve surgery) produces a linear scar in the right atrium and can result in atypical right AFL. Similarly, surgical or catheter ablation for AF, or lung transplantation (which involves reimplantation of the pulmonary veins into the recipient left atrium) can result in atypical left AFL.

Twelve-Lead Electrocardiographic Characteristics of Atypical Atrial Flutter

The ECG characteristics of atypical AFLs include continuous or near continuous activation of the atrium represented by long-duration flutter waves in at least some surface ECG leads. The finding of "any" lead showing continuous atrial activation without an isoelectric atrial diastolic interval supports the diagnosis of macroreentrant AFL. Ultimately, the unequivocal definition of a given atrial arrhythmia mechanism such as atypical AFL requires an invasive electrophysiology study to define impulse propagation through the atria during the arrhythmia. In the last decade, studies have correlated ECG findings during organized atrial arrhythmias with mapping confirmed arrhythmia mechanisms. In general, atrial activation rates of less than 300 milliseconds are highly suggestive of macroreentrant AFL, especially when observed in patients with atrial enlargement and less than robust AV node conduction for whom common supraventricular tachycardias like orthodromic reciprocating tachycardia or AV node reentry would be unlikely to occur with short cycle lengths.[10,11]

As with peritricuspid annular (typical) AFL, perimitral annular AFL can propagate clockwise (up the atrial septum, over the left atrial roof, down the lateral left atrial wall, and from distal to proximal coronary sinus) or counterclockwise. Counterclockwise mitral annular flutter has positive F waves in the inferior and precordial leads with significant negative components in ECG leads I or aVL, unlike typical RA flutter (**Figure 16.11**). Negative atrial deflections in leads I and aVL occur because the activation is moving from left toward the right. Conversely, clockwise MA flutter demonstrated negative F waves in the inferior leads and positive F waves in the in leads I and aVL and can mimic typical cavotricuspid isthmus-dependent RA flutter. The finding of a positive F wave in lead I has been proposed to differentiate clockwise MA flutter from typical counterclockwise right AFL, which usually has a flat or negative F wave in lead I.[12] Nonetheless, it should be emphasized that the ECG appearance of atypical AFL is quite variable. **Figures 16.12** to **16.14** demonstrate additional macroreentrant atypical AFLs.

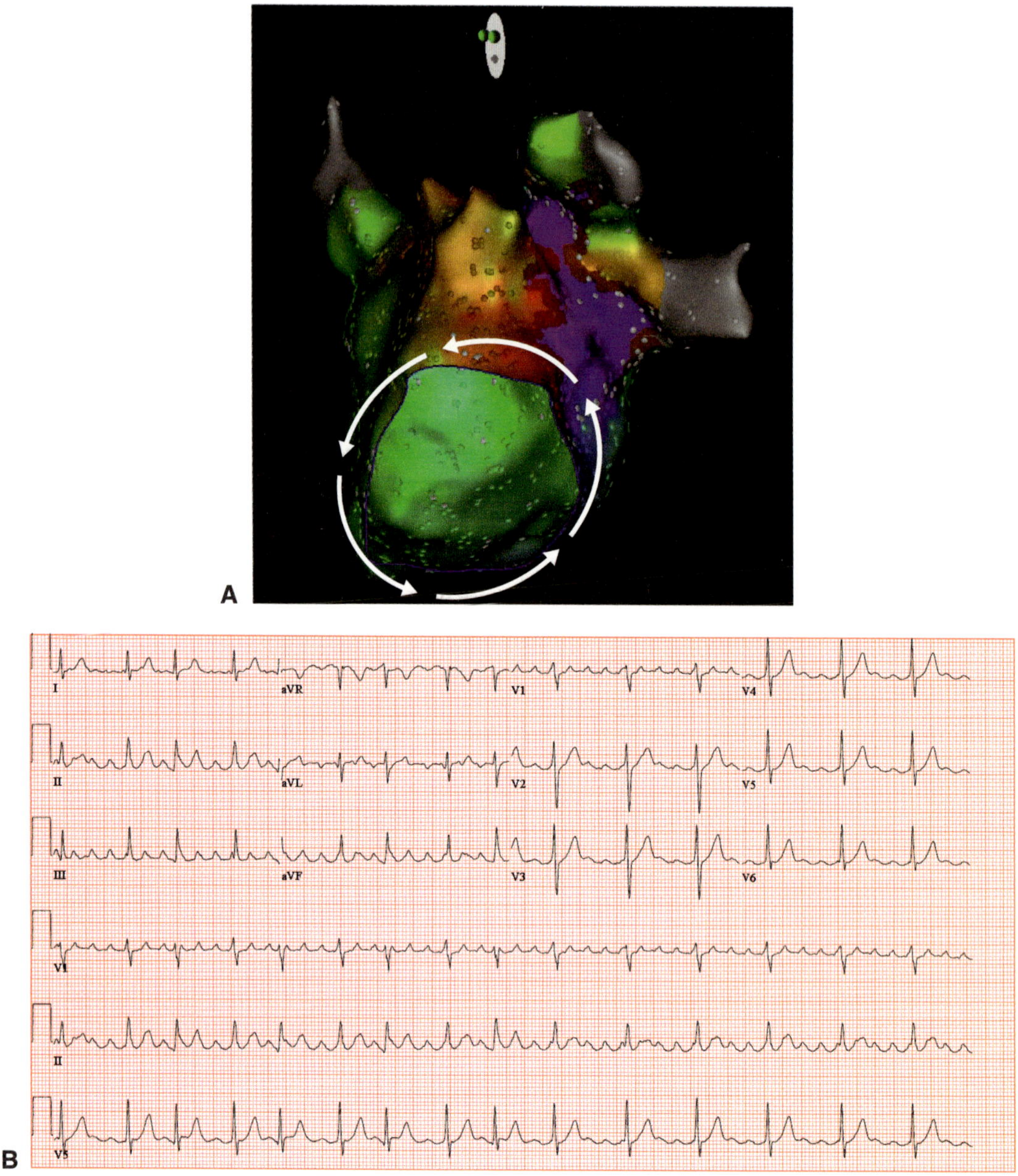

FIGURE 16.11. Counterclockwise perimitral annular atrial flutter. **A.** An atrial activation map obtained during an invasive electrophysiology (EP) study proving the mechanism of atrial flutter. Activation time relative to a fixed reference is depicted with color. Early activation is red with later activations represented by the color sequence: orange, yellow, green, and lavender. The red line between the lavender and orange areas represents that late activation meets early activation consistent with macroreentrant atrial flutter. The atrial flutter wavefront is seen to move around the mitral valve region in the counterclockwise direction (white arrows). **B.** The 12-lead electrocardiogram of this atypical flutter. The flutter CL is approximately 200 milliseconds as seen with the upright flutter waves in the inferior leads and across the precordium.

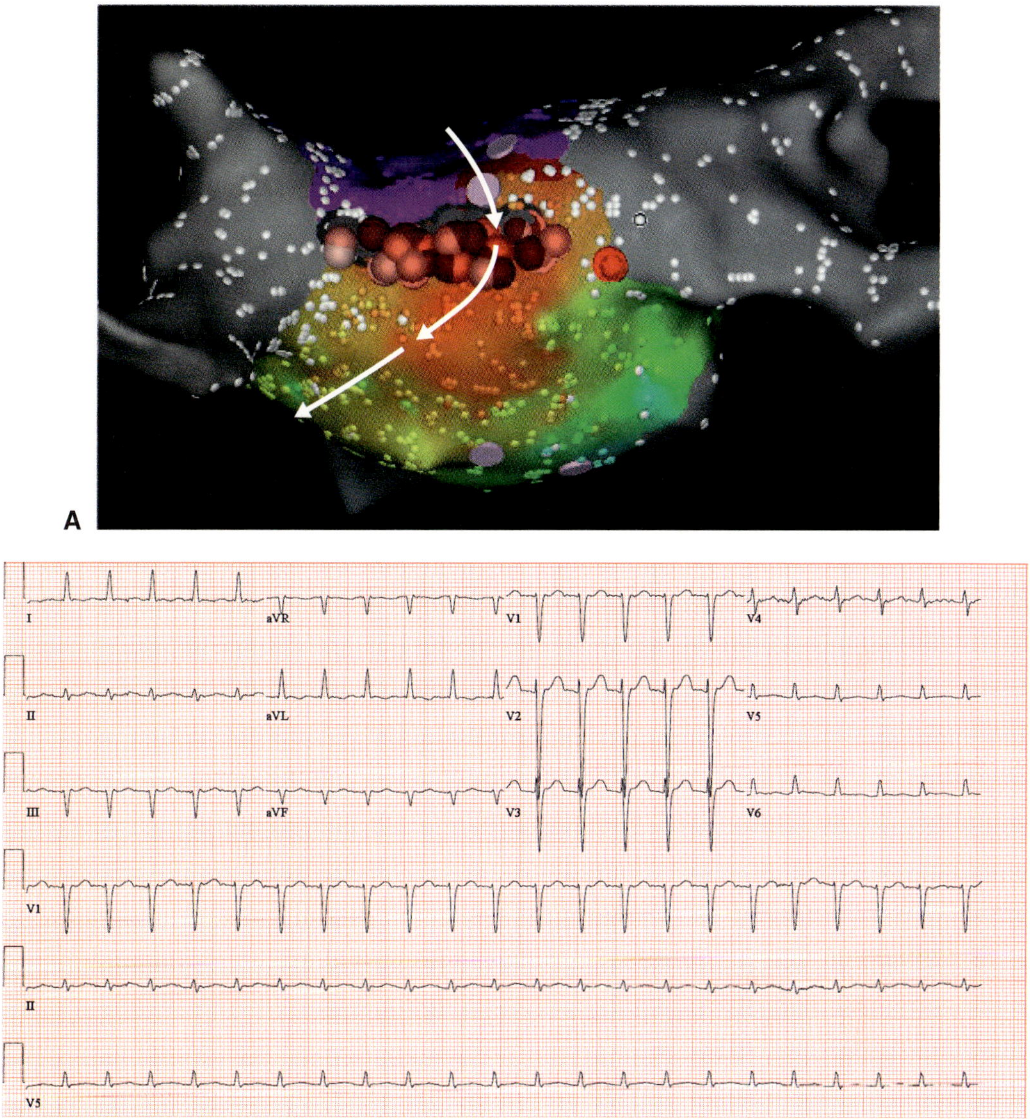

FIGURE 16.12. Left atrial roof-dependent atrial flutter. **A.** An activation map of atypical atrial flutter in the left atrium with a view "looking down at the heart from above" (see **Figure 16.11** legend for description of color scale). The mechanism of tachycardia was proven to be atypical atrial flutter by this activation map and by the fact that the atrial flutter was terminated with catheter ablation by creating a line of conduction block across the roof. Ablation lesions are depicted by the pink and red spheres and white arrows depict the activation path during flutter. **B.** Shows the electrocardiogram produced by this atrial flutter. It is difficult to discern flutter waves; however, the rhythm is regular, and the diastolic intervals contain repeating undulations without a clear appearance of P waves as would usually be seen with a focal atrial tachycardia. Given the proven mechanism, there must be 2:1 conduction and the flutter CL is about 235 milliseconds, one-half of the RR interval (~470 ms) with flutter waves concealed in the QRS and T waves. In this example, a maneuver to produce transient higher grade atrioventricular block (eg, carotid sinus massage or adenosine infusion) would be required to confirm the diagnosis by electrocardiogram alone.

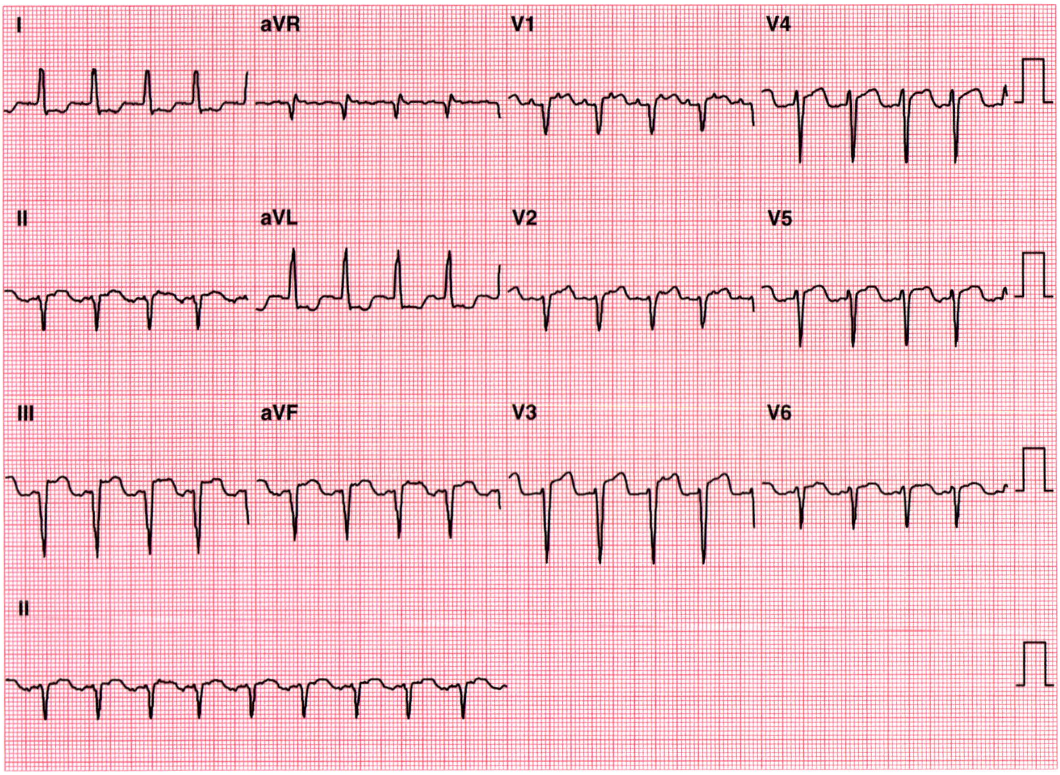

FIGURE 16.13. This patient had clockwise perimitral annular atrial flutter (atypical AFL) that was proven via electrophysiology study. Flutter waves are difficult to discern in this example and, if anything, appear to be negative in the inferior leads and upright in lead V_1 similar to that seen with typical atrial flutter (right atrial, counterclockwise cavotricuspid isthmus-dependent flutter). The regular rhythm together with organized atrial activity evident in leads V_1 and other leads such as lead II is consistent with macroreentrant atrial flutter. The atrial CL is about 260 milliseconds and the ventricular response rate is one-half of this, consistent with 2:1 conduction.

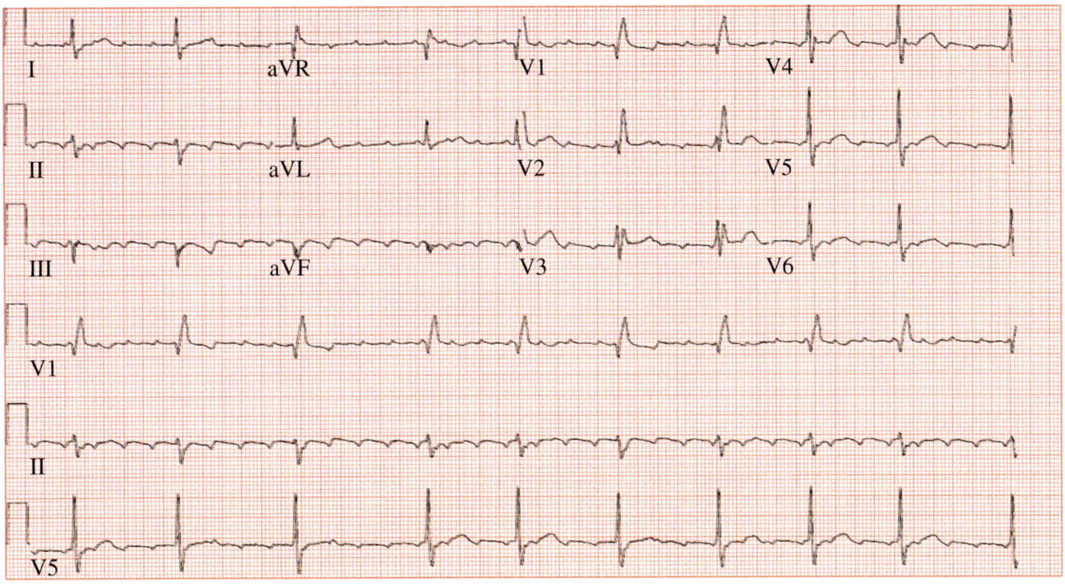

FIGURE 16.14. Right atriotomy-associated atypical atrial flutter. This patient had an EP study that proved atypical right atrial flutter. The circuit involved macroreentry around a high posterolateral atriotomy scar placed at the time of pulmonary endarterectomy. A critical area of slow conduction between the atriotomy scar and superior vena cava was demonstrated at EP study. The flutter CL is approximately 290 milliseconds and A:V conduction is variable. The flutter wave morphology could be confused with typical (counterclockwise cavotricuspid isthmus–dependent right atrial flutter). This flutter was terminated by ablation at the slowly conducting isthmus of tissue adjacent to the atriotomy scar near the superior vena cava. There is also evidence of a right-bundle-branch block pattern which is incidental.

Coarse AF can have features of AFL including discrete and regular F waves in lead V_1 which should not be mistaken for typical or atypical AFL and can be distinguished from AFL by noting that consistent atrial activation is not observed across all ECG leads (see **Figure 16.2**). Rhythm strips can also be helpful to diagnose pseudoflutter waves as the atrial deflection morphology varies over time as does the apparent cycle length. Importantly, AFL usually produces a regular ventricular response, and when the ventricular response is variable during AFL, some identical RR intervals can usually be identified on a rhythm strip recording representing multiples of the AFL cycle length. In distinction, the ventricular response during AF is "irregularly irregular" in the absence of complete heart block. When AFL conducts 2:1 to the ventricle, every other F wave is often buried in the QRS and may not be visible. Accordingly, regular tachycardias with rates between 130 and 160 beats/min (and rarely slower), especially with broad P waves, should prompt the ECG reader to consider the possibility that atrial tachycardia or AFL may be present with 2:1 conduction (**Figure 16.15**).

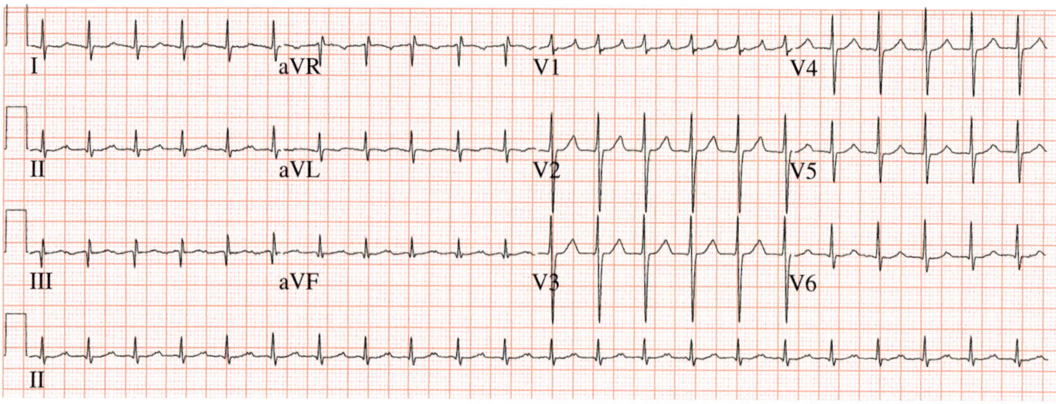

FIGURE 16.15. This figure illustrates a patient in atypical macroreentrant atrial flutter with 2:1 conduction and a heart rate in the 140s that could be falsely interpreted as sinus tachycardia. Carotid massage, vagal maneuvers, or the administration of adenosine in these cases can reveal the flutter waves and help make the diagnosis. In addition, significant discrepancy between the observed rate and the patient's prior sinus rates should raise a suspicion that sinus tachycardia might be an incorrect diagnosis.

As often performed with regular supraventricular tachycardias, maneuvers to produce transient higher grade atrioventricular block such as carotid sinus massage or adenosine administration can reveal underlying atypical AFL and "make the diagnosis." The correct diagnosis of atypical (or typical) AFL is important because adequate rate control with AV blockers is usually not possible, antiarrhythmic drug resistance is common, and an electrophysiology study with mapping and ablation may be required to prevent adverse outcomes such as tachycardia-mediated myopathy and heart failure.

Clinical Considerations of Atrial Fibrillation and Atrial Flutter

The symptoms of AF and AFL are diverse and vary widely between patients. The symptoms often include but are not limited to palpitations, fatigue, exercise intolerance, dyspnea on exertion, flushing, chest discomfort, diaphoresis, and syncope. Symptoms are typically more pronounced in younger and more active patients. Some patients are asymptomatic. The symptoms of AF and AFL and the impairment in cardiac performance are caused by several factors including the loss of effective atrial systole and atrial transport function, the irregularity of ventricular filling and contraction in the case of AF, and the tachycardia itself, which shortens diastole and ventricular filling. Some patients have symptoms limited to periods of rapid heart rates, whereas others experience symptoms despite rate control.

Thyrotoxicosis, obstructive sleep apnea, and alcohol intake are often missed in the evaluation of etiology of AF. A rare arrhythmia, dual atrioventricular nodal non-reentrant tachycardia can also cause an irregular rhythm that can often be misinterpreted as AF.[H] Here, every sinus beat conducts down through both fast and slow AV nodal pathways, and results in a fast and apparently irregular rhythm.

Treatment Goals

AF is associated with adverse outcomes, including reduced quality of life, stroke, heart failure, cognitive impairment, and an increased risk of mortality.[1] In particular, AF increases the risk of stroke by approximately 5-fold. Patients with AF who are at moderate or high risk of stroke are treated with oral anticoagulants to reduce the risk.[13] Similarly, patients with persistent tachycardia in AF are also at risk for developing left ventricular dysfunction and symptomatic heart failure. In general, most patients with AF are prescribed medications to control the heart rate. These atrioventricular nodal agents include β-blockers and nondihydropyridine calcium channel blockers. Before availability of β-blockers and calcium blockers for rate control of AF, digoxin was used for this purpose but has since fallen out of favor for several reasons: (1) digoxin's heart rate slowing effects are quite limited in ambulatory patients, and (2) digoxin shortens atrial refractory periods and interferes with normalization of AF-induced atrial refractory period shortening after cardioversion or AF termination (also called reverse remodeling) and increases abnormal automaticity and AF "triggers." All these factors are "proarrhythmic" for AF. Typically, clinicians aim for a resting heart rate in the 60 to 80 beats/min range, although some favor a more lenient approach and try and keep the resting heart rate less than 110 beats/min. Finally, some patients continue to have symptoms due to AF despite rate control. These patients should be treated with a rhythm control strategy to restore and maintain sinus rhythm.

Acutely, rhythm control may mean cardioverting the patient from AF back to sinus rhythm through the use of sedation and a direct current cardioversion (eg, a synchronized shock); however, sometimes, patients are cardioverted with medications like ibutilide. Patients with AF generally require anticoagulation before and after a cardioversion. Conversion to sinus rhythm with cardioversion is more frequent with coarse AF (commonly when the P wave amplitude is > 0.05 mV) rather than AF with fine fibrillatory waves.[I]

If adequate anticoagulation had not been achieved for 3 to 4 weeks prior to cardioversion, a transesophageal echocardiogram is often recommended to exclude the presence of a thrombus in the left atrial appendage or elsewhere in the left atrium.[13] Once a patient is back in normal sinus rhythm, maintaining sinus rhythm may require antiarrhythmic drug therapy. Antiarrhythmic drugs target ion channels to alter properties of myocardial conduction. Class IC medications, like flecainide and propafenone, block fast sodium channels and decrease myocardial conduction velocity. Class III antiarrhythmic medications, like sotalol and dofetilide, prolong refractoriness by blocking repolarizing potassium channel currents. Finally, the multichannel blockers (dronedarone and amiodarone) impact multiple cardiac ion channels including Na^+, K^+, and Ca^{2+} channels and adrenergic receptors. Catheter ablation is often performed to reduce or eliminate AF in patients who continue to experience recurrences of AF despite antiarrhythmic drugs or those who want to avoid the risks or side effects associated with these medications.

CHAPTER 16 SUMMARY ILLUSTRATION

Key Features of Atrial Fibrillation

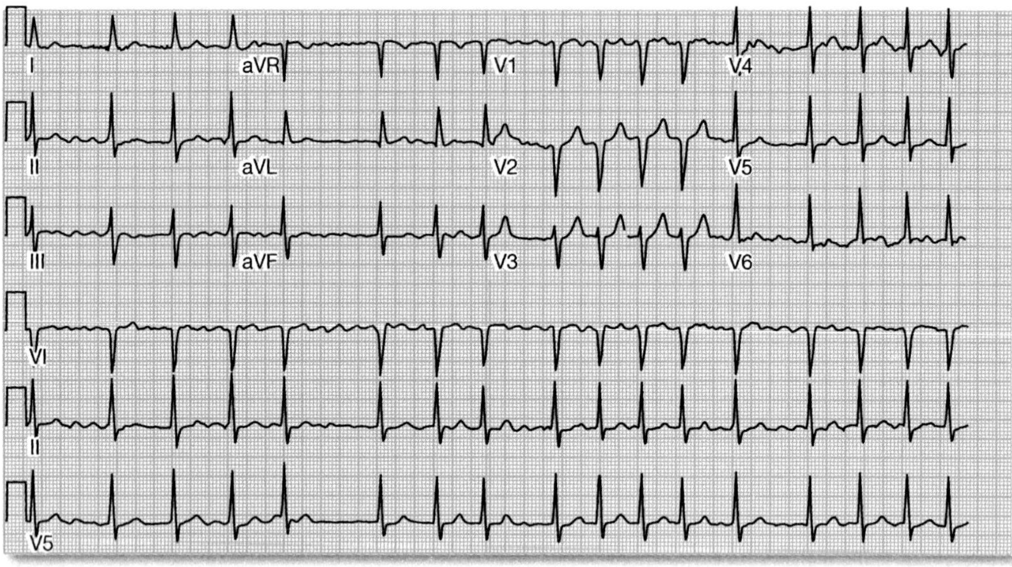

- No repetitive or organized atrial activity
- Irregularly irregular RR intervals

Key Features of Atrial Flutter

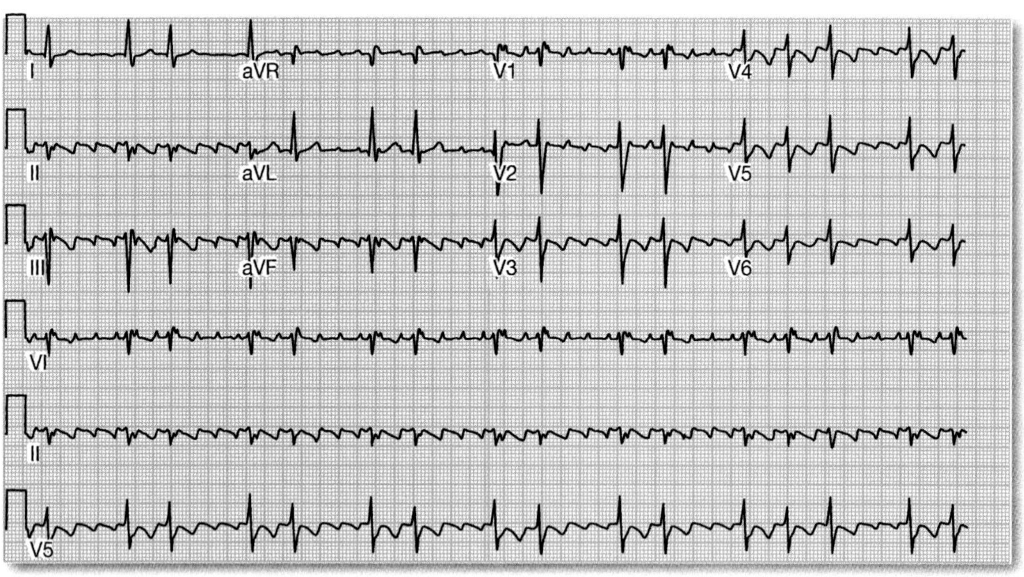

- Regular F-waves with no true isoelectric periods
- RR intervals are multiples of the FF intervals
- Not irregularly irregular

Atrial fibrillation and atrial flutter are distinct electrophysiology rhythms, although they share common risk factors, epidemiology, and pathophysiology.

Glossary

Atrial fibrillation: chaotic and disorganized electrical activation by multiple unstable "functional" wavelets of reentry in the atrial tissue with consequent irregularly irregular ventricular conduction. Often originates within the pulmonary veins or at their insertion sites with the posterior left atrial wall.

Atrial flutter: organized macroreentrant rhythm that results from a single stable activating wavefront traveling around a fixed nonconducting region of either atrium.

Atypical atrial flutter: may arise in either atrium. Often occurs in the setting of prior open-heart surgery or prior sites of arrhythmia ablation. Left atrial circuits for atypical flutter include reentry around the mitral annulus, and reentry around a pair of pulmonary veins (called roof dependent). Right atrial foci of atypical flutter include sites of atriotomy for surgical access or sites of prior arrhythmia ablation. The ECG characteristics of atypical flutter are highly variable can include isoelectric baseline in diastole, F waves that are variable in location by morphology but often positive in the inferior leads, and precordial leads. Invasive electrophysiologic study may be necessary to make a definitive diagnosis of atypical AFL and its site of origin.

F waves: waves characteristic of the underlying arrhythmia in the presence of typical AFL (sawtooth pattern), atypical AFL (small [sometimes very small]) deviations from the often isoelectric baseline, indicating continuous atrial macroreentry circuit. Sometimes may be confused with sinus P waves or P waves of ectopic atrial tachycardia. May be revealed by drugs that block the AV node, vagal maneuvers, or at the time of invasive electrophysiological study.

Typical atrial flutter: the circuit revolves in counterclockwise manner around the tricuspid valve and includes the inferior vena cava-tricuspid valve isthmus (cavotricuspid isthmus). The ECG features include sawtooth F waves and absence of isoelectric diastolic baseline, presence of negative F waves in the inferior leads, and positive F waves in leads V_1. Clockwise reentry around the same circuit is less common and is classified either as reverse (or clockwise) typical AFL or as an atypical flutter; notched positive F waves are present in inferior leads and mostly negative F wave in V_1.

Wavefront: Pattern of electrical activation of the myocardium as it spreads from initiating source (usually the sinoatrial node through normal conduction via the AV node and His-Purkinje system or via accessory pathways [see Chapter 19] or from other ectopic sites). This propagation of myocardial activation is often depicted by slow-motion tracking of simultaneous timed activation imaging (isochronic colored isobars). These imaging techniques are vital in localizing the source of arrhythmia initiation, thereby guiding arrhythmia ablation techniques.

Acknowledgment

We gratefully acknowledge the past contributions of the previous edition's author, Dr. Galen S. Wagner, as portions of that chapter were retained in this revision.

References

1. January CT, Wann LS, Alpert JS, et al. 2014 AHA/ACC/HRS guideline for the management of patients with atrial fibrillation: a report of the American College of Cardiology/American Heart Association Task Force on Practice Guidelines and the Heart Rhythm Society. *J Am Coll Cardiol*. 2014;64:e1-e76.
2. Waldo AL, Feld GK. Inter-relationships of atrial fibrillation and atrial flutter mechanisms and clinical implications. *J Am Coll Cardiol*. 2008;51:779-786.
3. Moore EN. Observations on concealed conduction in atrial fibrillation. *Circ Res*. 1967;21:201-208.
4. Kastor JA. Digitalis intoxication in patients with atrial fibrillation. *Circulation*. 1973;47:888-896.
5. Klein GJ, Bashore TM, Sellers TD, Pritchett EL, Smith WM , Gallagher JJ. Ventricular fibrillation in the Wolff-Parkinson-White syndrome. *N Engl J Med*. 1979;301:1080-1085.
6. Allessie MA, Boyden PA, Camm AJ, et al. Pathophysiology and prevention of atrial fibrillation. *Circulation*. 2001;103:769-777.
7. Haissaguerre M, Jais P, Shah DC, et al. Spontaneous initiation of atrial fibrillation

by ectopic beats originating in the pulmonary veins. *N Engl J Med.* 1998;339:659-666.
8. Philippon F, Plumb VJ, Epstein AE, Kay GN. The risk of atrial fibrillation following radiofrequency catheter ablation of atrial flutter. *Circulation.* 1995;92:430-435.
9. Gilligan DM, Zakaib JS, Fuller I, et al. Long-term outcome of patients after successful radiofrequency ablation for typical atrial flutter. *Pacing Clin Electrophysiol.* 2003;26(1, pt 1):53-58.
10. Jäis P, Matsuo S, Knecht S, et al. A deductive mapping strategy for atrial tachycardia following atrial fibrillation ablation: importance of localized reentry. *J Cardiovasc Electrophysiol.* 2009;20:480-491.
11. Chang SL, Tsao HM, Lin YJ, et al. Differentiating macroreentrant from focal atrial tachycardias occurred after circumferential pulmonary vein isolation. *J Cardiovasc Eletrophysiol.* 2011;22:748-755.
12. Gerstenfeld EP, Dixit S, Bala R, et al. Surface electrocardiogram characteristics of atrial tachycardias occurring after pulmonary vein isolation. *Heart Rhythm.* 2007;4:1136-1143.
13. January CT, Wann LS, Calkins H, et al. 2019 AHA/ACC/HRS focused update of the 2014 AHA/ACC/HRS Guideline for the Management of Patients with Atrial Fibrillation: a report of the American College of Cardiology/American Heart Association Task Force on Clinical Practice Guidelines and the Heart Rhythm Society in Collaboration with the Society of Thoracic Surgeons. *Circulation.* 2019;140:e125-e151.

References to the South Asian Edition

A. Cheniti G, Vlachos K, Pambrun T, Hooks D, et al. Atrial fibrillation mechanisms and implications for catheter ablation. *Front Physiol.* 2018; 9:1458.
B. Sauer WH, Alonso C, Zado E, et al. Atrioventricular nodal re-entrant tachycardia in patients referred for atrial fibrillation ablation: response to ablation that incorporates slow-pathway modification. *Circulation.* 2006; 114:191-195
C. Moorman JR, Pritchett EL. The arrhythmias of digitalis intoxication. *Arch Intern Med.* 1985; 145:1289-1292.
D. Wood P. Diseases of the heart and circulation. *Philadelphia, JB Lippincott Company;*1968. p. 625.
E. Selzer A, Cohn KE. Natural history of mitral stenosis: a review. *Circulation* 1972; 45: 878-890.
F. Bailey GWH, Braniff BA, Hancock EW, Cohn KE. Relation of left atrial pathology to atrial fibrillation in mitral valvular disease. *Ann Intern Med* 1968; 69:13-20.
G. Vaziri SM, Larson MG, Benjamin EJ, Levy D. Echocardiographic predictors of non-rheumatic atrial fibrillation. The Framingham heart study. *Circulation.*1994;89:724–730.
H. Peiker C, Pott C, Eckardt L, et al. Dual atrioventricular nodal non-re-entrant tachycardia. *Europace.* 2016; 18:332-339
I. Chou TC; Electrocardiography in clinical practice, 4thed. *Philadelphia, Saunders*, 1996; pp 351-370.

To view digital content associated with this chapter please access lww.co.in. Instructions are located on the inside front cover.

17 Ventricular Arrhythmias

ALBERT Y. SUN, JASON KOONTZ,
DEEPAK PADMANABHAN,
AND SAURABH DESHPANDE

Definitions of Ventricular Arrhythmias

Ventricular arrhythmias encompass a spectrum of rhythm disturbances from premature ventricular contractions (PVCs) to more persistent ventricular rhythms including *ventricular tachycardia* (VT), *ventricular flutter*, and *ventricular fibrillation*. PVCs are isolated depolarizations of a ventricular origin. VT is a ventricular arrhythmia with a rate over 100 beats/min and is considered sustained when it persists greater than 30 seconds; otherwise, it is classified as nonsustained. Ventricular flutter is a rapid ventricular arrhythmia without an easily identifiable onset to the QRS or electrical diastole. Ventricular fibrillation is a rapid and disorganized ventricular activity without identifiable QRS complexes.

Etiologies and Mechanisms

PVCs tend to arise from stereotypical locations within the ventricles; the electrocardiographic characteristics of the PVC point to the site of origin. PVCs typically are a result of triggered activity, reentry, or enhanced automaticity in ventricular myocardium and/or Purkinje fibers. PVCs can be seen in otherwise healthy individuals or in the context of structural heart disease.

VT is most often seen in the context of structural heart disease. Whereas an accelerated idioventricular rhythm (sometimes referred to as "slow VT"), a common reperfusion arrhythmia, is the result of enhanced automaticity, the majority of sustained ventricular arrhythmias are due to reentry. The substrate that typically leads to reentrant VT is scarring of the ventricular myocardium. Most often, reentrant VT occurs in the setting of ischemic heart disease and arises after myocardial infarction. The reentrant circuit may involve the diseased myocardium and/or specialized conduction system. For this reason, careful inspection of the individual's baseline electrocardiogram (ECG), if available, for evidence of prior myocardial infarction can provide significant insight when attempting to interpret the ECG of the tachycardia. Scarring is also seen in nonischemic cardiomyopathies including idiopathic dilated cardiomyopathy, hypertrophic cardiomyopathy, cardiac sarcoidosis, and arrhythmogenic (right) ventricular cardiomyopathy. In each of these conditions, the alteration of the underlying myocardium and replacement fibrosis provides the substrate to promote reentry.

The mechanism of macroreentry responsible for the majority of VT requires activation of a protected portion of the myocardium called the VT circuit throughout the tachycardia cycle. At first glance, this VT circuit would seem to be at odds with the typical electrocardiographic appearance of VT with a discrete QRS complex followed by electrical diastole (a T wave and an isoelectric period prior to the next QRS). This phenomenon is possible because circuit consists of surviving myocytes within scarred ventricular myocardium which owing to a combination of electrical, cellular, and geometrical reasons have low velocities of the cell-to-cell conduction. Depolarization of this "protected circuit" typically generates a very low voltage that is insufficient to be seen on the surface 12 lead ECG and results in the appearance of electrical diastole. Exit from this circuit results in the onset of the QRS owing to sufficient myocardial mass being activated. Therefore, the surface ECG provides only an estimate of this exit site from the circuit into the myocardium.

Acute ischemia can also cause ventricular arrhythmias, but in the absence of preexisting scar, these arrhythmias are likely to be polymorphic and perhaps have triggered activity as the mechanism of arrhythmia.

Two specific types of VT are typically seen in the context of individuals with otherwise normal hearts. The most common type is VT (or PVCs) arising from the right or left ventricular outflow tract. These arrhythmias result from triggered activity and as such are favored by conditions with high sympathetic stimulation such as exercise. They are classically catecholamine sensitive. and adenosine and/or beta-blocker responsive. The most common presentation of idiopathic ventricular arrhythmia (VA) is repetitive monomorphic VT (60-90%). The second type of "normal heart" VT involves the fascicles of the conduction system. These fascicular VT circuits are due to reentry or triggered activity between abnormally conducting peri-Purkinje tissue and the remaining conduction system, most frequently exiting at the terminal portion of the left posterior fascicle. ECG shows right bundle branch block (RBBB) with left axis in most of the cases. This type of VT is typically responsive to non-dihydropyridine calcium channel blockers (CCBs) like verapamil and diltiazem. In both outflow tract VT and fascicular VT, catheter ablation can be highly effective at eliminating the arrhythmia, and the patient does not need a defibrillator for secondary prevention of sudden cardiac arrest.

Conditions favoring sustained ventricular arrhythmias may paradoxically be promoted by antiarrhythmic medications. Antiarrhythmic drugs that prolong repolarization (eg, sotalol, dofetilide) may, in isolation or in combination with other medications that prolong repolarization, excessively prolong the QT interval and promote "torsade de pointes." Sodium channel blocking agents (eg, flecainide, propafenone) may slow conduction in diseased tissue and promote sustained reentry even in therapeutic concentrations (see Chapter 10).

Diagnosis

Various ECG algorithms have been developed to aid in the accurate diagnosis of VT from the 12-lead ECG. When evaluating the ECG of *wide complex tachycardia* (WCT), one must first consider the most common differential including VT, supraventricular tachycardia (SVT) with aberrancy in the His-Purkinje system, SVT via an antegrade conducting accessory pathway, ventricular pacing, electrogram artifact, as well as drug effect or electrolyte imbalances (see **Chapter 17 Summary Illustration**). The steps below focus on diagnosing VT when faced with a 12-lead ECG of WCT. Although these steps should be used as a guide only, many are widely practiced and well validated. This algorithm is summarized in **Figure 17.1**.

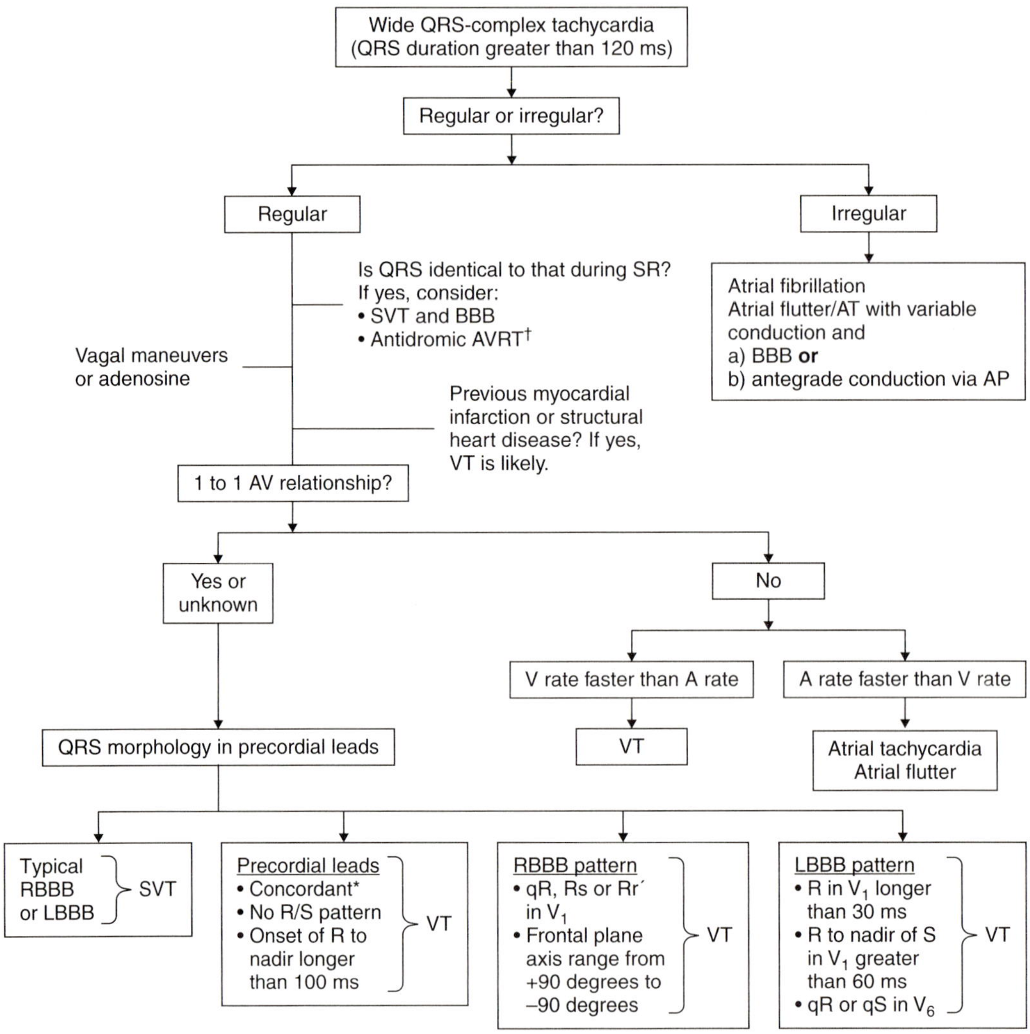

FIGURE 17.1. Differential diagnosis for wide QRS-complex tachycardia (more than 120 ms). *Concordant indicates that all precordial leads show either positive or negative deflections. Fusion complexes are diagnostic of VT. †In pre-excited tachycardias, the QRS is generally wider (ie, more pre-excited) compared with sinus rhythm. AP, accessory pathway; AT, atrial tachycardia; AV, atria-ventricles; AVRT, atrioventricular reentrant tachycardia; BBB, bundle branch block; LBBB, left bundle branch block; SR, sinus rhythm; SVT, supraventricular tachycardia; VT, ventricular tachycardia; RBBB, right bundle branch block. (Reprinted with permission from Blomström-Lundqvist C, Scheinman MM, Aliot EM, et al.)[1]

Step 1: Regular or Irregular

One's eye is often initially drawn to regularity of a rhythm even before detailed analysis of the various ECG characteristics. *Monomorphic VT* as opposed to ventricular fibrillation or *polymorphic VT* has a regular rhythm with a QRS morphology that is dissimilar to the native baseline morphology. Regular rhythms with identical QRS morphology to sinus rhythm are most likely SVT (see Chapter 15). Whereas VT can be somewhat irregular at the initiation, highly irregular, especially hemodynamically stable, irregular WCT is often atrial fibrillation or atrial flutter with variable conduction in the setting of concurrent bundle branch block, rate-related aberrancy, or preexcitation (**Figure 17.2**).

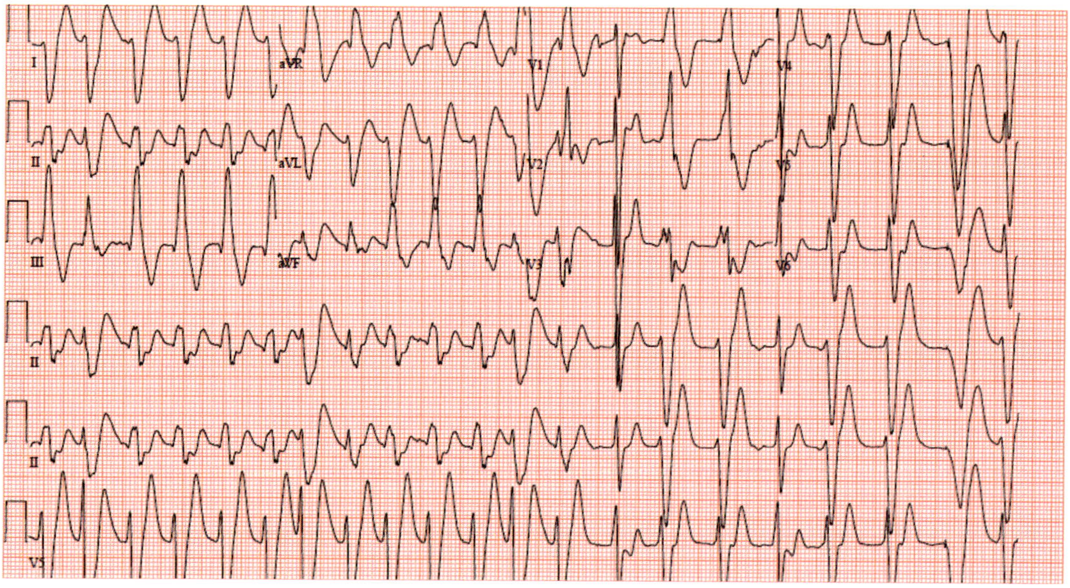

FIGURE 17.2. A 12-lead electrocardiogram from an elderly patient with atrial fibrillation with rapid ventricular response and intermittent left-bundle-branch block aberrancy.

Step 2: Understanding Clinical Substrate

Although ECG characteristics are extremely helpful in differentiating VT from other causes of WCT, the patient's clinical presentation is equally if not more predictive and should be the first step in the analysis of a regular wide complex rhythm. Without imposing any ECG criteria, WCT is VT over 80% of the time. In patients who present with abnormal cardiac substrate such as impaired ventricular function or known coronary artery disease, the likelihood of VT increases to over 90%.[2] Although the margin of error is small, it should be obvious that an accurate diagnosis is imperative. One study found that nearly all patients treated inaccurately for SVT while they were in VT suffered significant hemodynamic consequences, mostly from the use of calcium channel blockers and β blockers.[3] Baseline/old ECG with changes in the form of pathological q waves or loss of normal amplitude of R waves in precordial leads or presence of fractionation in the QRS complexes may direct one to VT being the cause of the WCT empirically.

Step 3: Identify P waves and Relationship to Ventricular Rhythm

AV Dissociation

By definition, VT arises from the ventricle, but activation of the atria can still occur via retrograde conduction. The atria, however, can be completely dissociated from the ventricles, with their own independent rhythm (usually sinus rhythm; **Figure 17.3**). When the ventricular rhythm is faster and dissociated from the atrial rhythm, then the rhythm is almost always VT.

Because wide QRS complexes or T waves are occurring constantly in both of these situations, the P waves are often lost during the rapid ventricular cycles. Sometimes, however, the P waves may be recognized as bumps or notches in the vicinity of T waves.

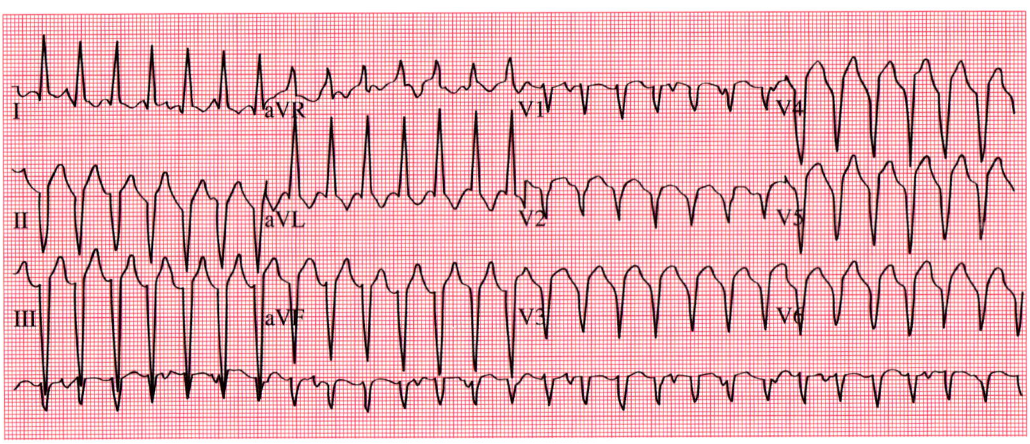

FIGURE 17.3. A 12-lead electrocardiogram from a young patient with a previous myocardial infarction and resultant ventricular aneurysm. Note the QRS duration is slightly <0.12 second because of the patient's age. Arrows indicate the P waves occurring without a fixed relationship to the QRS complexes. The P waves are clearly visible only in leads II, III, and V_1 to V_4.

One may look in lead V_1, where atrial activity tends to be most prominent, or in any lead with low amplitude or isoelectric QRS to improve accuracy.

Figure 17.4 is an example in which the low QRS amplitude in lead II facilitates observation of P waves. Presence of AV dissociation (defined above) is entirely specific for the diagnosis of VT but minimally sensitive because of difficulty in finding definitive P waves among the wide QRS complexes and T waves.[4]

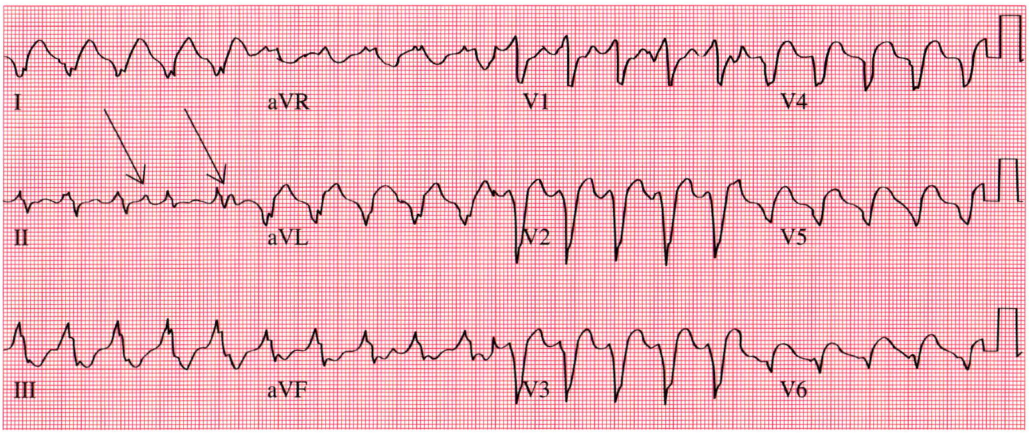

FIGURE 17.4. A 12-lead electrocardiogram from an elderly patient with a dilated cardiomyopathy. Arrows indicate consecutive P waves in lead II.

Intermittent Irregularity—Fusion and Capture Beats

When the ECG waveform morphology of VT is consistent from beat to beat, the term *monomorphic* is applied. When an intermittent on-time narrowing of the QRS complex occurs, the most likely cause is a breakthrough of conduction of the atrial rhythm to the ventricles. If the atrial breakthrough occurs during a QRS complex of the VT, the result is a "fusion beat" (Dressler beat). If the atrial breakthrough occurs before a QRS complex has begun, the result is a "capture beat," as in beats 5 and 18 in **Figure 17.5**. Fusion describes a hybrid QRS morphology, in which a portion of the QRS complex represents the areas of the ventricles activated by the VT, whereas the other portion represents the areas activated by a competing atrial impulse, as in **Figure 17.5**, beats 10 and 15. "Capture" means that the entire QRS complex represents activation of the ventricles by a competing atrial impulse. If either fusion or capture beats are proven to be present, the diagnosis is almost certainly VT. Fusion and/or capture beats are, however, seldom seen in VT and usually at the less rapid rates (<160 beats/min). Indeed, they appeared in only 4 of a series of 33 reported patients with *sustained VT*.[5]

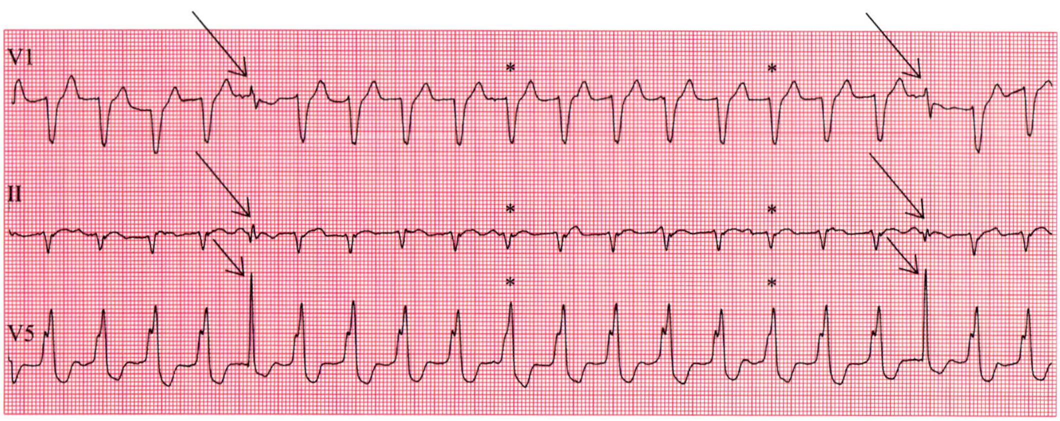

FIGURE 17.5. A three-lead rhythm strip from a 62-year-old man who presented with acute shortness of breath 2 months after an inferior-lateral (posterior) myocardial infarction. Arrows indicate capture beats and asterisks indicate fusion beats.

Atrioventricular Association

When atrial and ventricular activations are associated, there is a particular ventricular-to-atrial ratio, such as 1:1, 2:1, or 3:2. In **Figure 17.6A**, the VT with retrograde 1:1 conduction is terminated by the premature ventricular activation (arrow), either a ventricular premature beat or an atrial capture with aberrancy. The termination of the VT is followed by a sinus capture beat with normal QRS morphology (asterisk). In **Figure 17.6B**, there is initially variable retrograde conduction during *nonsustained VT*. Then, after the VT resumes, there is 1:1 retrograde conduction.

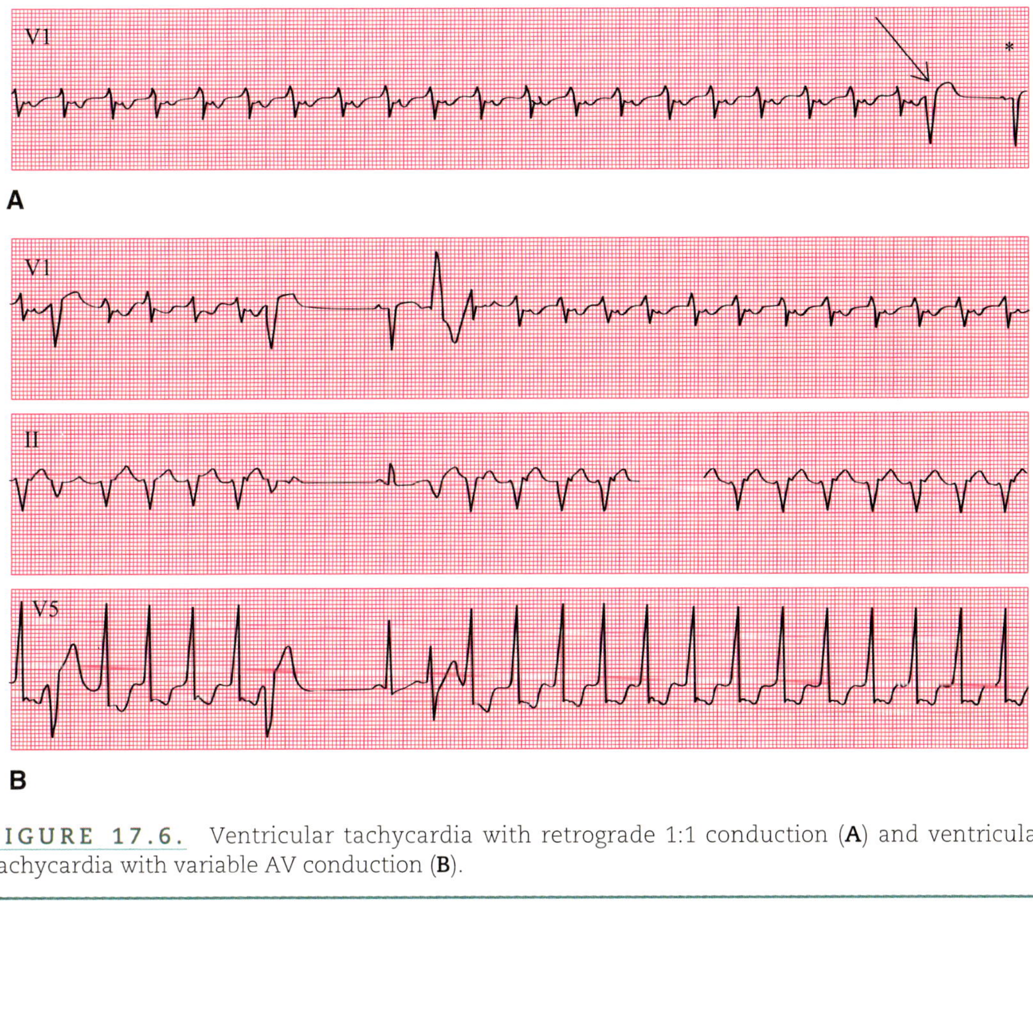

FIGURE 17.6. Ventricular tachycardia with retrograde 1:1 conduction (**A**) and ventricular tachycardia with variable AV conduction (**B**).

Step 4: RS Morphology

No RS Pattern

Typically, right- or left-bundle-branch block has an RS pattern in at least one of the precordial leads (V_1-V_6), and the time from the beginning of the R wave to the nadir of the S is <100 milliseconds ("steep downslope") (see Chapter 5).

When there is no RS morphology in any of the precordial leads, VT is strongly suggested, but this finding has low sensitivity (21%) as documented by Brugada et al.[6] Scanning all the precordial leads reveals R, qR, or qS QRS complex morphologies (**Figure 17.7**). The presence of QS in all precordial leads (negative concordance) is suggestive of VT on most occasions. The presence of R in all precordial leads (positive concordance) is likely to be either VT or an antidromic atrioventricular reentrant tachycardia (AVRT).

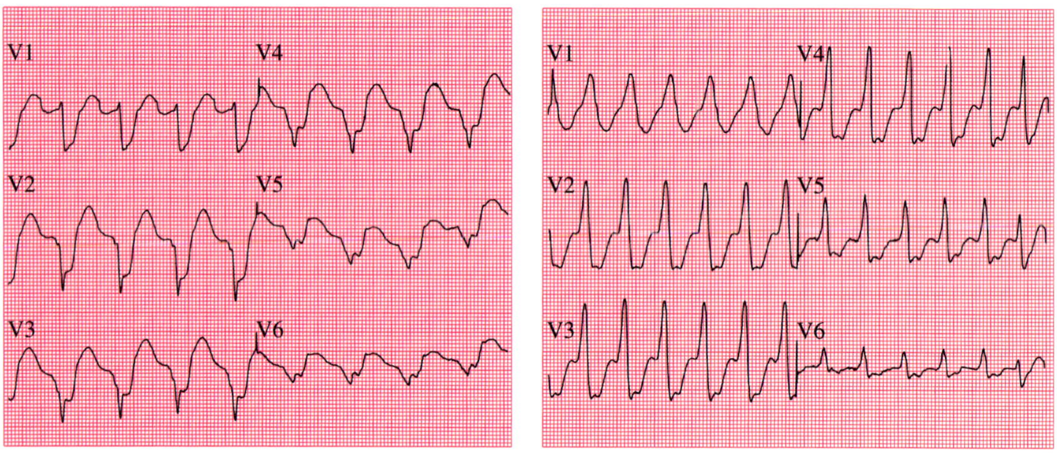

A B

FIGURE 17.7. The electrocardiogram recordings in the six precordial leads from a patient with recurrent ventricular tachycardia and heart failure (**A**) are contrasted with those of a patient who returned with acute chest pain 1 month after a posterolateral myocardial infarction (**B**).

RS Is Present

An interval >100 milliseconds from the beginning of the R wave to the nadir of the S wave ("slurred downslope") in one precordial lead had a specificity of 0.98 and sensitivity of 0.66.[6] An RS interval >100 milliseconds is difficult to calculate when the QRS merges with the previous T wave, masking the QRS onset during rapid tachycardia. Moreover, an increased RS interval occurs in SVT with conduction over an accessory pathway and with drugs that prolong QRS duration (**Figure 17.8**).

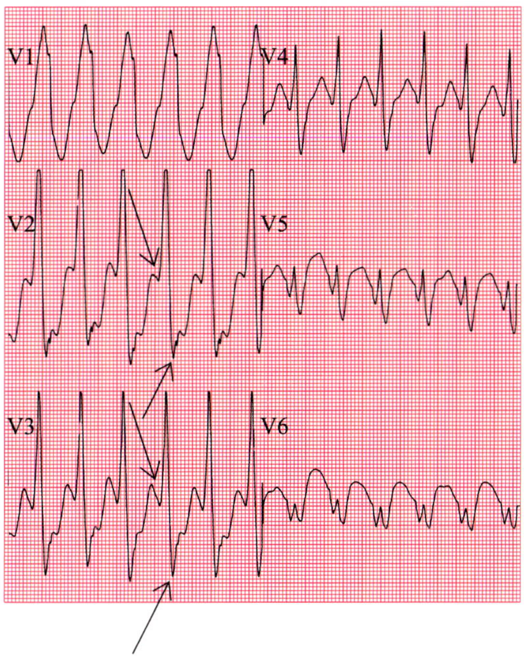

FIGURE 17.8. The six precordial leads of the electrocardiogram from a patient illustrating ventricular tachycardia with a prolonged interval from onset of the QRS complex to the nadir of the S wave. Arrows indicate the period of 0.12 second from QRS onset to S nadir in leads V_2 and V_3.

Step 5: QRS Morphology

Right-Bundle-Branch Block Pattern

EXAMINE LEAD V_1 Just as the presence of the terminal positive (R or R′) morphology in lead V_1 of conducted beats indicates a right-bundle-branch block, this morphology during VT indicates that the right ventricle is activated after the left ventricle. Therefore, the term *right-bundle-branch block pattern* is used to classify VT as left ventricular in origin (**Figure 17.9**). The terminal positive wave is preceded in **Figure 17.9A,B** by a smooth or notched R wave but by a Q wave in **Figure 17.9C**. The most commonly occurring variety of the right-bundle-branch block is the notched downslope R.

Wellens and colleagues[7] and Drew and Scheinman[4] analyzed the morphologic features of the ECGs of 122 and 121 patients, respectively, with proven SVT or SVT with aberration established by electrophysiologic studies. These three QRS morphologies were strongly suggestive of VT.

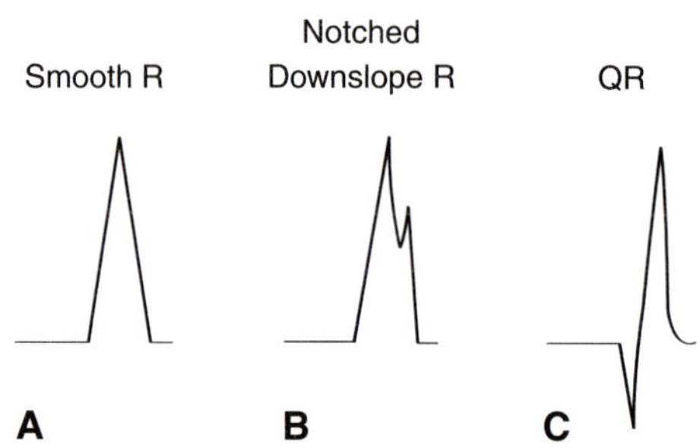

FIGURE 17.9. The three variations in QRS complex morphology in lead V, during "left-bundle-branch block pattern ventricular tachycardia." See text above.

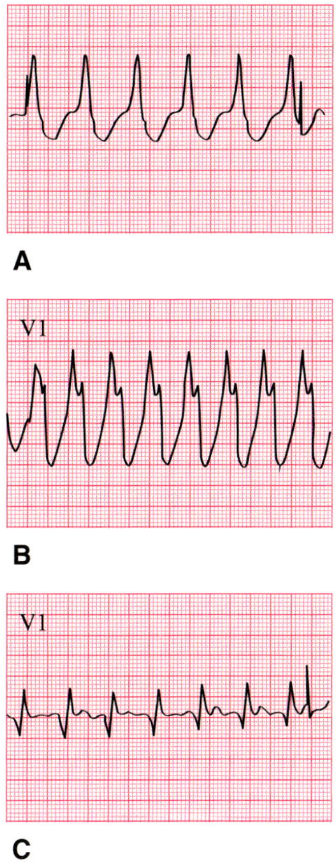

FIGURE 17.10. Signs of ventricular tachycardia **A.** Smooth R. **B.** Notched downslope R. **C.** QR pattern.

QRS Morphologies Strongly Suggestive of VT

1. Monophasic R waves (**Figure 17.10A**)
2. Biphasic RR′ with the taller first rabbit ear (Marriott sign; **Figure 19.10B**) is by far the most specific criteria for VT, but the sensitivity is low.
3. A qR pattern (**Figure 17.10C**) can also be associated with SVT with right-bundle-branch block and myocardial infarction.

"Left rabbit ear taller than right in V_1 with RBBB morphology has high specificity for VT."

HJL Marriott

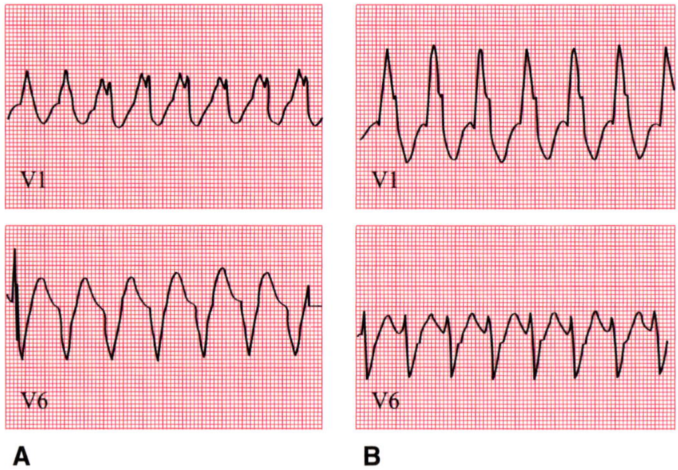

FIGURE 17.11. The QS (**A**) and RS (**B**) morphologies of the QRS complex in lead V_6 during "right-bundle-branch block pattern ventricular tachycardia" are illustrated.

EXAMINE LEAD V_6 Observation of a QS morphology in lead V_6, illustrated in **Figure 17.11A**, is valuable in either left- or right-bundle-branch block pattern VTs. The R/S <1 pattern in lead V_6 in **Figure 17.11B** should only be considered indicative of VT when there is left-axis deviation evident in the limb leads.

Left-Bundle-Branch Block Pattern

EXAMINE LEADS V_1 AND V_2 Just as the presence of the terminal negative morphology in lead V_1 of conducted beats indicates a left-bundle-branch block, this morphology during VT indicates that the right ventricle is activated after the left ventricle. Therefore, the term *left-bundle-branch block pattern* is used to classify VT as right ventricular or septal in origin.

The ECG criteria illustrated in the diagram and presented in the box in **Figure 17.12** were proposed by Kindwall et al.[8] They evaluated 118 patients with VT or SVT with aberration who underwent intracavitary recording. Predictive accuracy was 96%.

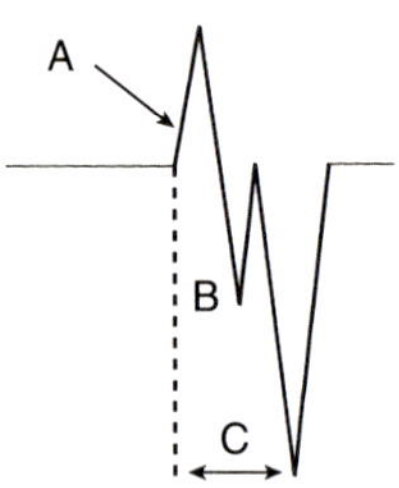

A = broad R wave (≥.04 s)
B = notched downslope in S wave
C = onset of R wave to the nadir of S wave (≥.06 s)

FIGURE 17.12. The three characteristics of the QRS morphology of "left-bundle-branch block pattern ventricular tachycardia" in leads V_1 and V_2 are illustrated.

Examining leads V_1 and V_2 for the three ECG examples provides observation of the criteria of Kindwall et al[8] for VT with the left-bundle-branch block pattern, as indicated by the arrows:

- **Figure 17.13A**: the broad R wave in V_1
- **Figure 17.13B**: the notched S wave downslope in V_2
- **Figure 17.13C**: the prolonged R onset to the S nadir in V_2

Note that the latter two criteria are not present in lead V_1 in either **Figure 17.13B** or **17.13C**.

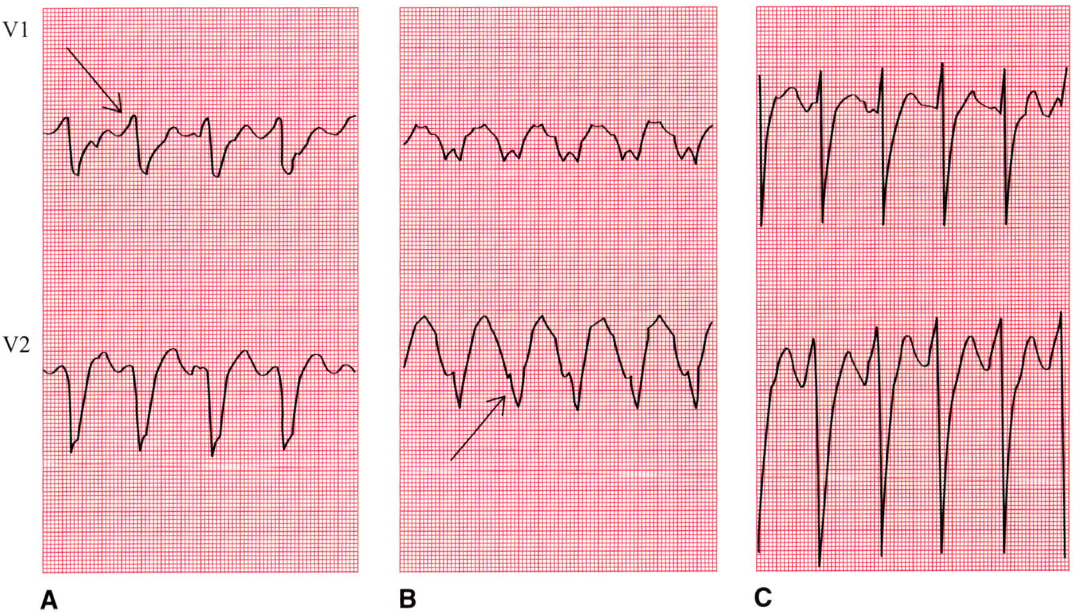

FIGURE 17.13. **A-C.** Each of the three characteristics of "left-bundle-branch block pattern ventricular tachycardia" in leads V_1 and V_2 are illustrated. See text above.

EXAMINE LEAD V_6 QRS (**Figure 17.14A**) and qR (**Figure 17.14B**) in V_6 are diagnostic of VT but are seldom seen.

In conclusion, there are limitations with this approach. The usefulness of so many criteria is related to a low sensitivity yield (20%-50%) of each criterion, even though they are associated with a high probability in favor of VT.

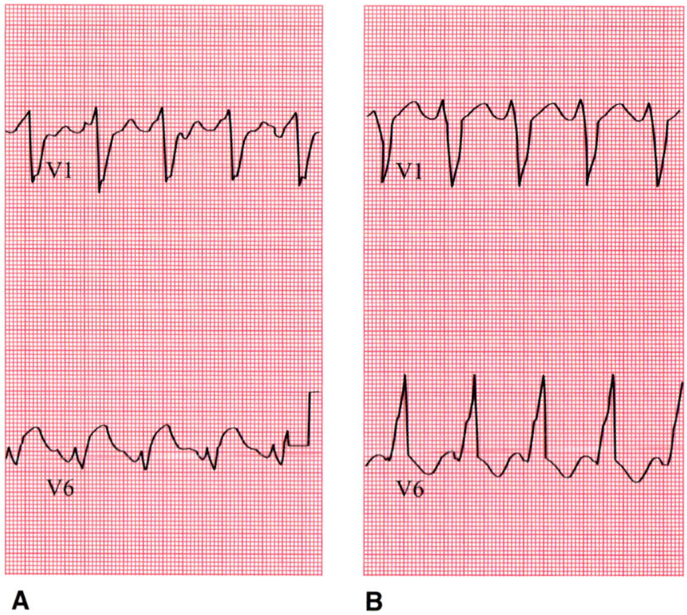

FIGURE 17.14. The QRS (**A**) and qR (**B**) morphologies of the QRS complex in lead V_6 during "left-bundle-branch block pattern ventricular tachycardia" are illustrated.

Variations in the Electrocardiographic Appearance of Ventricular Tachycardia: Torsades de Pointes

All of the examples provided in the previous sections have been of monomorphic VT with consistency of their QRS complex morphologies. However, *torsades de pointes* represents a commonly occurring VT with variations in morphology (polymorphic VT; see **Figure 17.1**). This French term translates as "twistings of the points."[9,10] Torsades de pointes VT is characterized by undulations of continually varying amplitudes that appear alternately above and below the baseline. The wide ventricular waveforms are not characteristic of either QRS complexes or T waves, and the rate varies from 180 to 250 beats per minute (**Figure 17.15**).[11] Torsades de pointes VT is usually nonsustained; however, it may persist for >30 seconds, satisfying the definition of a sustained tachyarrhythmia. It may also at times evolve into ventricular fibrillation.

Torsades de pointes always occurs in the presence of QTc-interval prolongation.[12-14] This prolonged QTc may be caused by the proarrhythmic effect of drugs that prolong ventricular recovery time, such as sotalol, phenothiazines, some antibiotics, some antihistamines, and tricyclic antidepressants.[15,16] It also occurs with electrolyte abnormalities such as hypokalemia and hypomagnesemia, insecticide poisoning,[17] subarachnoid hemorrhage,[18] congenital prolongation of the QTc interval,[19] ischemic heart disease,[20] and bradyarrhythmias.[21]

Intravenous magnesium is effective in the treatment of Torsades. In this situation, magnesium may suppress the arrhythmia even before normalization of the QT interval and this is thought to be related to its calcium channel blocking effect.

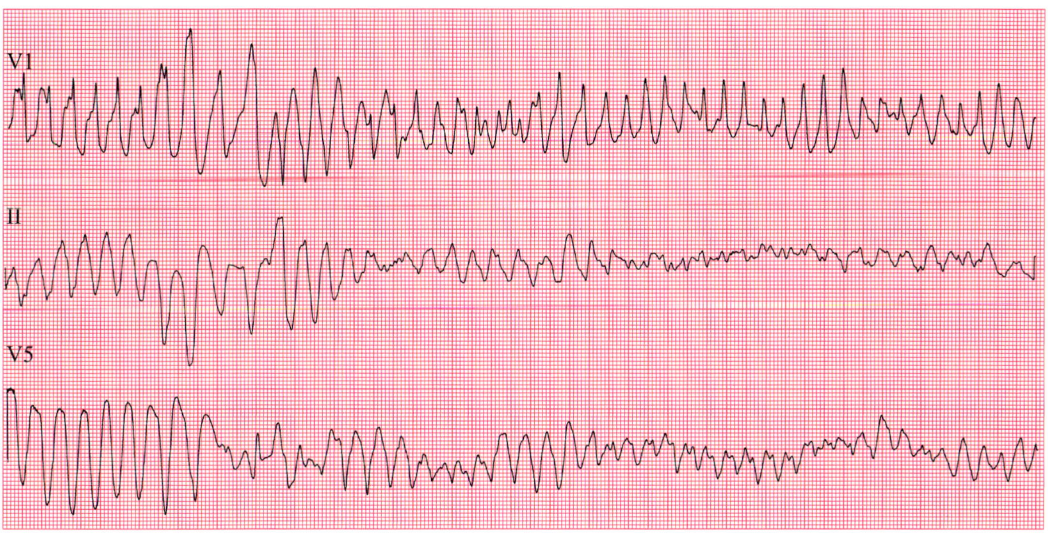

FIGURE 17.15. Simultaneous recordings of leads V_1, II, and V_5 from a 62-year-old woman receiving diuretic therapy who presented after experiencing a syncopal episode at home. Syncope recurred in the emergency department during this electrocardiogram recording. The patient's serum potassium concentration was 2.3 mEq/L.

Ventricular Flutter/Fibrillation

Ventricular flutter/fibrillation is a macroreentrant tachyarrhythmia within the ventricular muscle that is analogous to the atrial flutter/fibrillation spectrum discussed in Chapter 16 (**Figure 17.16A**). Neither QRS complexes nor T waves are clearly formed, and the rhythm looks similar when viewed right side up or upside down. Immediately after the onset of reentry, a regularly undulating baseline is present (**Figure 17.16B**, top). This ventricular flutter looks like a larger version of atrial flutter, but it remains regular and orderly only transiently because the rapid, weak myocardial contractions produce insufficient coronary blood flow (**Figure 17.16B**, middle). As a result, there is prompt deterioration toward the irregular appearance of ventricular fibrillation (**Figure 17.16B**, bottom). See also **Animation 17.1**.

To view the animation(s) and video(s) associated with this chapter please access lww.co.in. Instructions are located on the inside front cover.

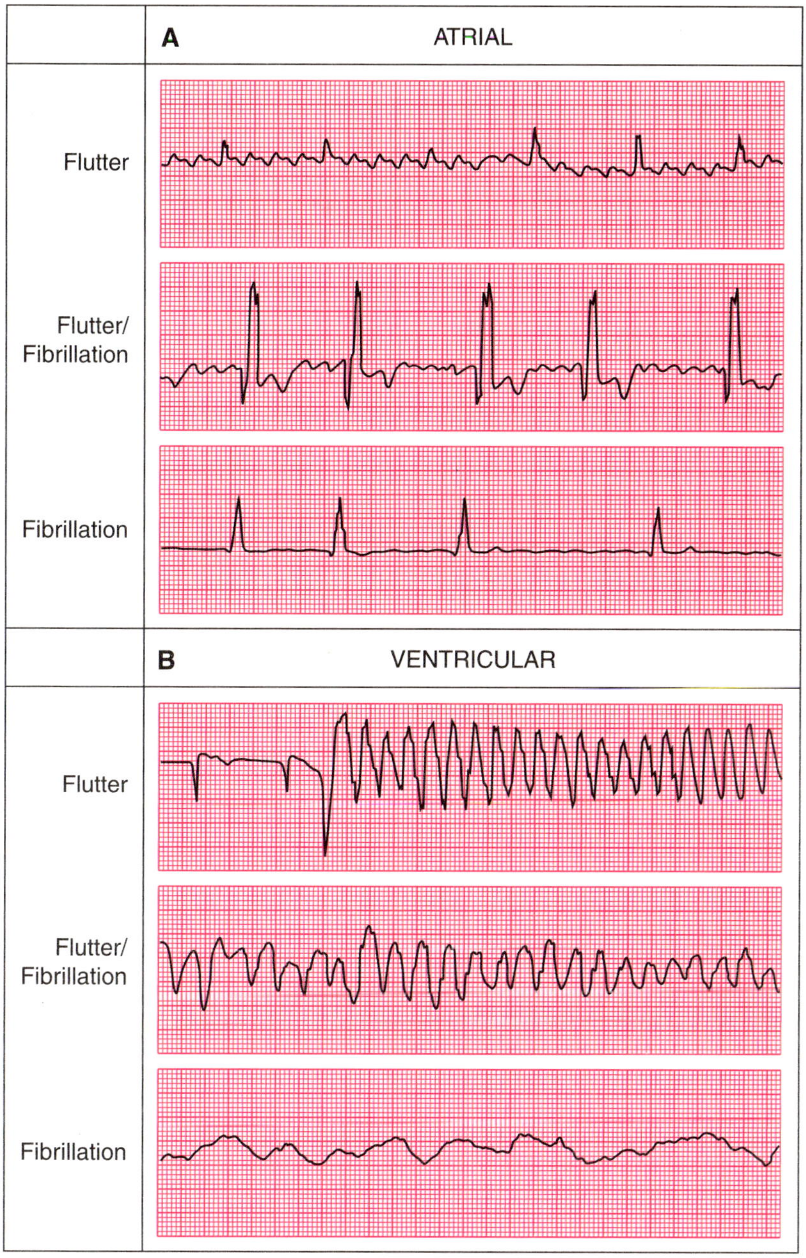

FIGURE 17.16. The atrial flutter/fibrillation spectrum (**A**) is compared with its ventricular counterpart (**B**). (Reprinted from Wagner GS, Waugh RA, Ramo BW. *Cardiac Arrhythmias*. New York, NY: Churchill Livingstone; 1983:22. Copyright © 1983 Elsevier. With permission.)

CHAPTER 17 SUMMARY ILLUSTRATION

Ventricular Tachycardia - Ischemic Cardiomyopathy

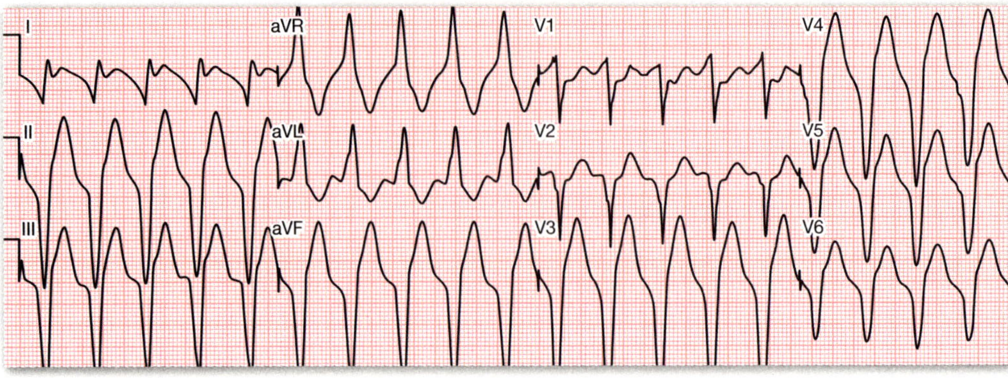

Note the atrial ventricular (AV) dissociation as well as bizarre QRS pattern and bizarre axis as some of the key features suggesting VT

SVT (Atrial Flutter) with 1:1 Conduction and Right Bundle Branch Block Aberrancy

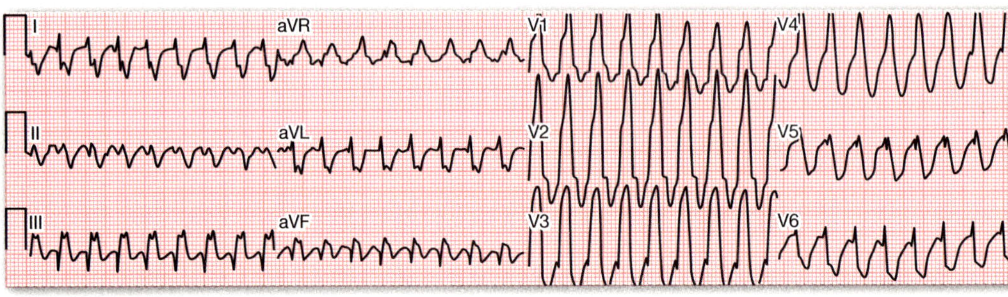

Atrial Fibrillation with Intermittent Preexcitation and Antegrade Conduction via Accessory Pathway

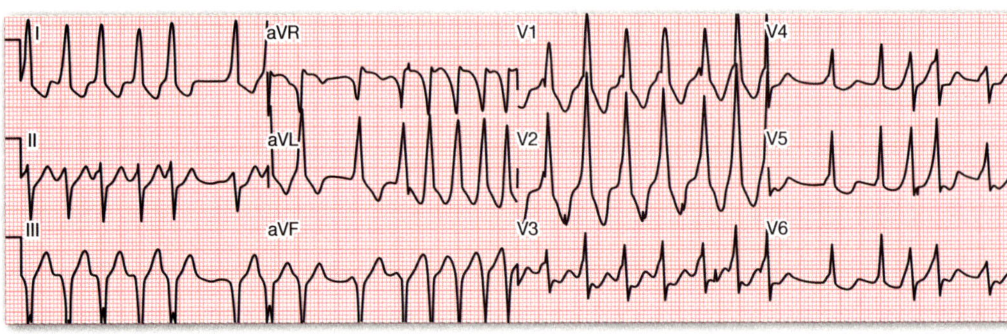

(continued)

CHAPTER 17 SUMMARY ILLUSTRATION (continued)

Permanent Atrial Fibrillation with Complete Heart Block and Single Chamber Ventricular Pacing

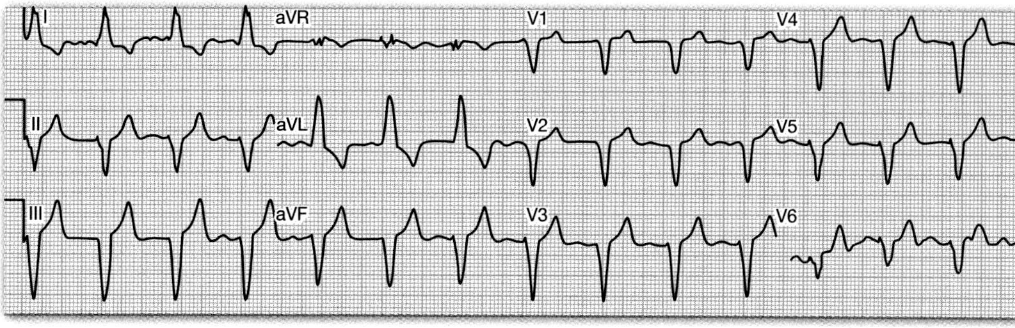

Drug Effects - Junctional Tachycardia with Intraventricular Conduction Delay and Underlying Ischemic Cardiomyopathy

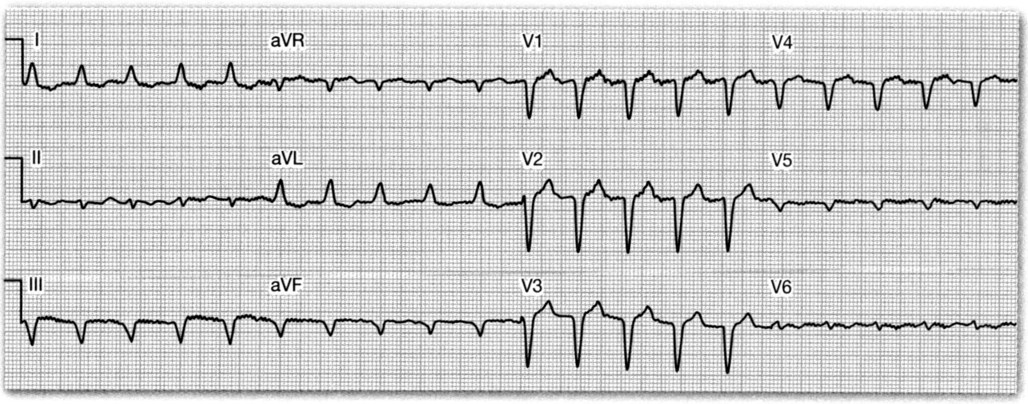

Electrolyte Abnormalities – Renal Failure with Hyperkalemia

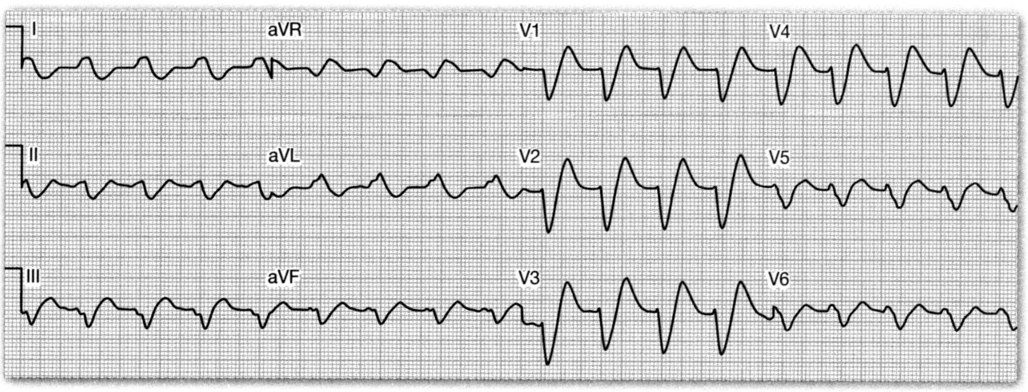

Abbreviations: SVT, supraventricular tachycardia; VT, ventricular tachycardia.

(Reprinted with permission from Kummer JL, Nair R, Krishnan SC. Images in cardiovascular medicine. Bidirectional ventricular tachycardia caused by digitalis toxicity. *Circulation*. 2006;113(7):e156-e157.)

Glossary

Monomorphic: a single appearance of all QRS complexes.

Monomorphic VT: VT with a regular rate and consistent QRS complex morphology.

Nonsustained VT: VT of <30-second duration.

Polymorphic VT: VT with a regular rate but frequent changes in QRS complex morphology.

Sustained VT: VT of ≥30-second duration or requiring an intervention for its termination.

Torsades de pointes: a polymorphic ventricular tachyarrhythmia with the appearance of slow polymorphic ventricular flutter without discernible QRS complexes or T waves. The ventricular activity has constantly changing amplitudes and seems to revolve around the isoelectric line.

Ventricular fibrillation: rapid and totally disorganized ventricular activity without discernible QRS complexes or T waves in the ECG.

Ventricular flutter: rapid, organized ventricular activity without discernible QRS complexes or T waves in the ECG.

Ventricular tachycardia: a rhythm originating distal to the branching of the common bundle, with a ventricular contraction

Acknowledgment

We gratefully acknowledge the past contributions of the previous edition's authors, Marcel Gilbert, Galen S. Wagner, and David G. Strauss, as portions of that chapter were retained in this revision.

References

1. Blomström-Lundqvist C, Scheinman MM, Aliot EM, et al. ACC/AHA/ESC guidelines for the management of patients with supraventricular arrhythmias—executive summary: a report of the American College of Cardiology/American Heart Association Task Force on Practice Guidelines and the European Society of Cardiology Committee for Practice Guidelines (Writing Committee to Develop Guidelines for the Management of Patients With Supraventricular Arrhythmias). *Circulation.* 2003;108[15]:1871-1909.
2. Baerman JM, Morady F, DiCarlo LA Jr, de Buitleir M. Differentiation of ventricular tachycardia from supraventricular tachycardia with aberration: value of the clinical history. *Ann Emerg Med.* 1987;16(1):40-43.
3. Stewart RB, Bardy GH, Greene HL. Wide complex tachycardia: misdiagnosis and outcome after emergent therapy. *Ann Intern Med.* 1986;104(6):766-771.
4. Drew BJ, Scheinman MM. Value of electrocardiographic leads MCL_1, MCL_6, and other selected leads in the diagnosis of wide QRS complex tachycardia. *J Am Coll Cardiol.* 1991;18:1025-1033.
5. Gozensky C, Thorne D. Rabbit ears: an aid in distinguishing ventricular ectopy from aberration. *Heart Lung.* 1974;3:634-636.
6. Brugada P, Brugada J, Mont L, Smeets J, Andries EW. A new approach to the differential diagnosis of a regular tachycardia with a wide QRS complex. *Circulation.* 1991;83:1649-1659.
7. Wellens HJJ, Bär FW, Lie KI. The value of the electrocardiogram in the differential diagnosis of a tachycardia with a widened QRS complex. *Am J Med.* 1978;64:27-33.
8. Kindwall E, Brown JP, Josephson ME. ECG criteria for ventricular and supraventricular tachycardia in wide complex tachycardias with left bundle branch morphology. *J Am Coll Cardiol.* 1987;9:206A.
9. Kossmann CE. Torsade de pointes: an addition to the nosography of ventricular tachycardia. *Am J Cardiol.* 1978;42:1054-1056.
10. Smith WM, Gallagher JJ. "Les torsades de pointes": an unusual ventricular arrhythmia. *Ann Intern Med.* 1980;93:578-584.
11. Kay GN, Plumb VJ, Arciniegas JG, Henthorn RW, Waldo AL. Torsade de pointes: the long-short initiating sequence and other clinical features: observations in 32 patients. *J Am Coll Cardiol.* 1983;2:806-817.
12. Soffer J, Dreifus LS, Michelson EL. Polymorphous ventricular tachycardia associated with normal and long Q-T intervals. *Am J Cardiol.* 1982;49:2021-2029.
13. Reynolds EW, Vander Ark CR. Quinidine syncope and the delayed repolarization syndromes. *Mod Concepts Cardiovasc Dis.* 1976;45:117-122.
14. Roden DM, Thompson KA, Hoffman BF, Woosley RL. Clinical features and basic mechanisms of quinidine-induced arrhythmias. *J Am Coll Cardiol.* 1986;8(1 suppl A):73A-78A.

15. Nicholson WJ, Martin CE, Gracey JG, Knoch HR. Disopyramide-induced ventricular fibrillation. *Am J Cardiol.* 1979;43:1053-1055.
16. Wald RW, Waxman MB, Colman JM. Torsade de pointes ventricular tachycardia. A complication of disopyramide shared with quinidine. *J Electrocardiol.* 1981;14:301-307.
17. Ludomirsky A, Klein HO, Sarelli P, et al. Q-T prolongation and polymorphous ("torsades de pointes") ventricular arrhythmias associated with organic insecticide poisoning. *Am J Cardiol.* 1982;49:1654-1658.
18. Carruth JE, Silverman ME. Torsade de pointe atypical ventricular tachycardia complicating subarachnoid hemorrhage. *Chest.* 1980;78:886-888.
19. Jervell A, Lange-Nielsen F. Congenital deaf-mutism, functional heart disease with prolongation of the Q-T interval and sudden death. *Am Heart J.* 1957;54:59-68.
20. Krikler DM, Curry PVL. Torsade de pointes, an atypical ventricular tachycardia. *Br Heart J.* 1976;38:117-120.
21. Ben-David J, Zipes DP. Torsades de pointes and proarrhythmia. *Lancet.* 1993;341:1578-1582.

To view digital content associated with this chapter please access lww.co.in.
Instructions are located on the inside front cover.

18 Bradyarrhythmias

LARRY R. JACKSON II,
CAMILLE GENISE FRAZIER-MILLS,
FRANCIS E. UGOWE,
JAMES P. DAUBERT, AND
AMEYA UDYAVAR

Introduction

The bradyarrhythmias can be summed up as being the result of either a failure of electrical impulse generation or a failure of effective conduction. Sinoatrial (SA or sinus) node dysfunction and atrioventricular (AV) conduction block are the most common causes of pathologic bradycardia. Cardiac electrical activation normally originates in the sinus node, the predominant pacemaker in the heart. Auxiliary pacemakers exist within the cardiac muscle, the AV node, and His-Purkinje system that can elicit automaticity if the sinus node is suppressed or otherwise fails to function appropriately. When the automaticity of the sinus node is decreased, the result is a bradyarrhythmia originating either from the sinus node itself or from subsidiary pacemakers that spontaneously depolarize to maintain a cardiac rhythm.

When the decelerated rhythm originates from the sinus node, the term sinus bradycardia is used. When it originates from a lower site, the terms *atrial rhythm*, *junctional rhythm*, or *ventricular rhythm* are used. These subsidiary rhythms are not true primary arrhythmias but rather *escape rhythms* that attempt to compensate for decreased sinus node automaticity. **Figure 18.1** illustrates the various consequences of the slowing of sinus automaticity to <60 beats/min. The automaticity of the distal sites is suppressed if the sinus node has normal pacemaker function, but their automaticity returns (escapes) at its own, slower rate when the sinus node fails. Escape beats emerge from an atrial (**Figure 18.1A**), His bundle (**Figure 18.1B**), or ventricular (**Figure 18.1C**) site after the sinus impulses fail to appear.

Causes of Decreased Automaticity

1. Physiologic slowing of the sinus rate
2. Physiologic or pathologic enhancement of parasympathetic nervous activity
3. Pathologic pacemaker failure

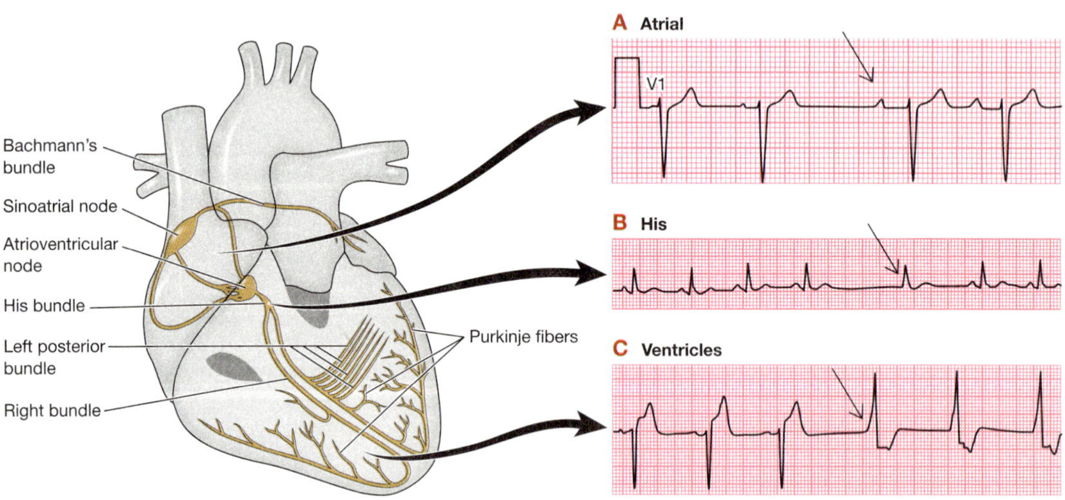

FIGURE 18.1. Schematic diagram of the cardiac conduction system depicting the sinoatrial and atrioventricular nodes and the common bundle (His) and bundle branches that lead toward the ventricles from the atrioventricular node. Arrows indicate the atrial (**A**), His-bundle (**B**), and ventricular escape (**C**) beats that terminate the pauses after the sinus node has failed to maintain its dominant rhythmicity.

Mechanisms of Bradyarrhythmias: Decreased Automaticity

Physiologic Slowing of the Sinus Rate

Although a rate of <60 beats/min is technically termed a bradyarrhythmia, sinus bradycardia is often a normal variation of cardiac rhythm (especially in trained athletes, whose heart rates may be as low as 30-40 beats per min at rest). With slowing of the sinus rate, the emerging rhythm may be either sinus bradycardia or, as shown in **Figure 18.2**, a junctional (see **Figure 18.2A**) or ventricular (see **Figure 18.2B**) escape rhythm. Bradycardia is a physiologic response to relaxation or sleep, when the parasympathetic effect on cardiac automaticity dominates over the sympathetic effect. Even during the expiratory phase of the respiratory cycle, there is slowing of the sinus rate, often into the bradycardic range.

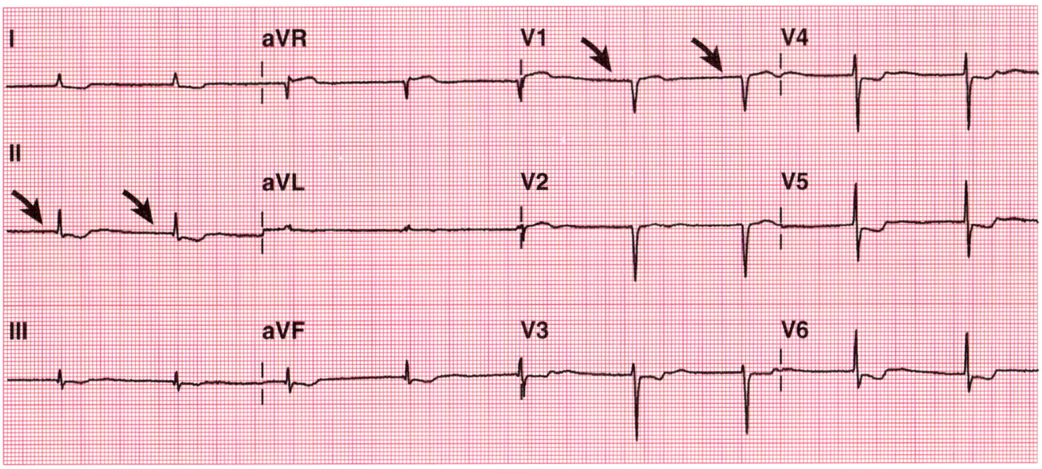

A

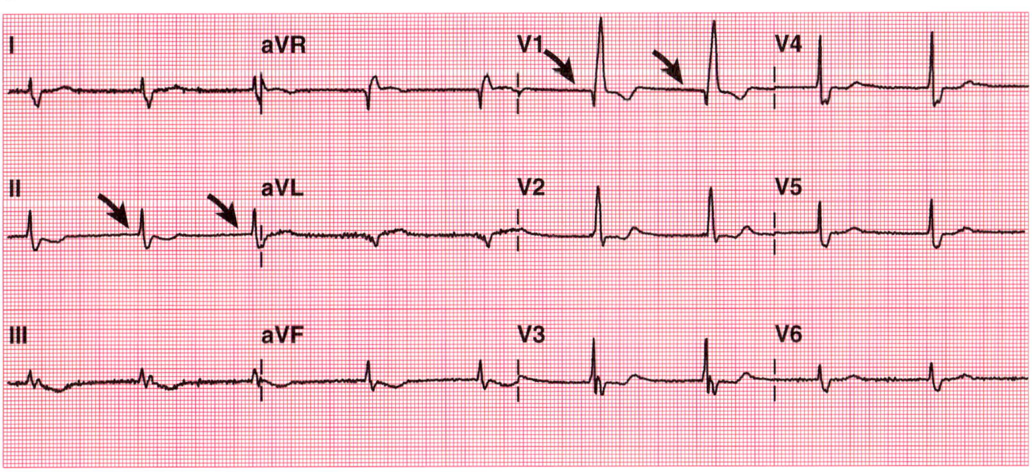

B

FIGURE 18.2. Twelve-lead electrocardiograms from a woman receiving β-adrenergic–blocking therapy for ischemic heart disease (**A**) and an otherwise healthy man on the day after prostate surgery (**B**). Arrows indicate complete absence of P waves preceding the normal (**A**) and abnormally wide QRS complexes (**B**). The lead V_1–positive QRS complexes in **B** indicate that the escape site is in the left bundle.

Physiologic or Pathologic Enhancement of Parasympathetic Activity

All cells with pacemaking capability are under some influence of both the sympathetic and parasympathetic divisions of the autonomic nervous system. This influence is greatest in the sinus node and diminishes in the lower sites with pacemaker function. Usually, the shifting autonomic balance causes a gradual increase or decrease in the pacing rate. Many factors, however, can induce autonomic imbalance and parasympathetic dominance including the following:

Factors Producing Autonomic Imbalance and Parasympathetic Dominance

1. Carotid sinus massage
2. Hypersensitivity of the carotid sinus
3. Straining (ie, a Valsalva maneuver)
4. Ocular pressure
5. Increased intracranial pressure
6. Sudden movement from a recumbent to an upright position
7. Drugs that cause pooling of blood by dilating the veins
8. Drugs with primary parasympathomimetic activity (eg, pilocarpine, bethanechol, neostigmine, donepezil)

This increase in parasympathetic tone called a *vasovagal reaction* (vasovagal reflex) has a prominent component of vascular relaxation, in addition to cardiac slowing, and is mediated by the vagus nerve. Typical bradyarrhythmias that occur suddenly during a vasovagal reaction are presented in **Figure 18.3**. A sudden increase in parasympathetic activity is manifested by both slowing of the sinus rate and slowing/failure of AV conduction (note the nonconducted P wave in the electrocardiogram [ECG] shown in **Figure 18.3**). The increase in parasympathetic tone also suppresses escape pacemakers, and the resulting pause is interrupted only by the return of sinus rhythm. The combination of vascular relaxation and cardiac slowing may result in a fall in cardiac output so severe that dizziness or even loss of consciousness may occur, also known as *vasovagal syncope*. This type of syncope is one of a family of neurally mediated syncope events including vasovagal and *neurocardiogenic syncope*.[1-3]

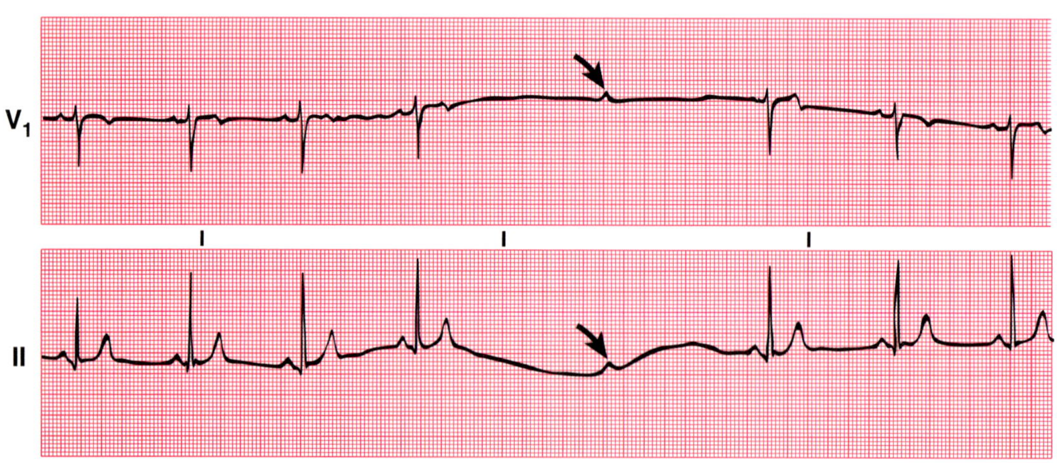

FIGURE 18.3. Simultaneous recording of leads V_1 and II from a patient soon after cholecystectomy. Arrows indicate a nonconducted P wave. (Reprinted from Wagner GS, Waugh RA, Ramo BW. *Cardiac Arrhythmias*. New York, NY: Churchill Livingstone; 1983:208. Copyright © 1983 Elsevier. With permission.)

Vasovagal syncope is typically reversed when the individual falls into a recumbent position, thereby increasing venous return to the heart. When a person who has fainted due to vasovagal syncope is encountered, consciousness can usually be restored by lowering the head and chest and elevating the legs.

A physiologic vasovagal reaction, although appearing benign in isolation, can have severe pathologic consequences if the individual is injured during a consequent fall or if the change in body position required to restore venous return to the heart is not possible. Repeated, severe, and sudden episodes of bradyarrhythmia with vasodilation require medical intervention to prevent serious injury or death.

Pathologic Pacemaker Failure

When a sudden period of complete absence of P waves appears in the ECG, the name *asystole* (or sinus arrest) is used. A prolonged atrial pause may be caused by either enhanced parasympathetic activity or impairment of all cells with impulse formation capability. Often, failure in impulse generation is attributed to sinus node dysfunction. If the problem was limited to the sinus node, however, it would not be expected to produce any serious bradyarrhythmia as a 1- to 2-second sinus pause would be interrupted by escape from a lower site with the capacity for impulse formation (**Figure 18.4**).

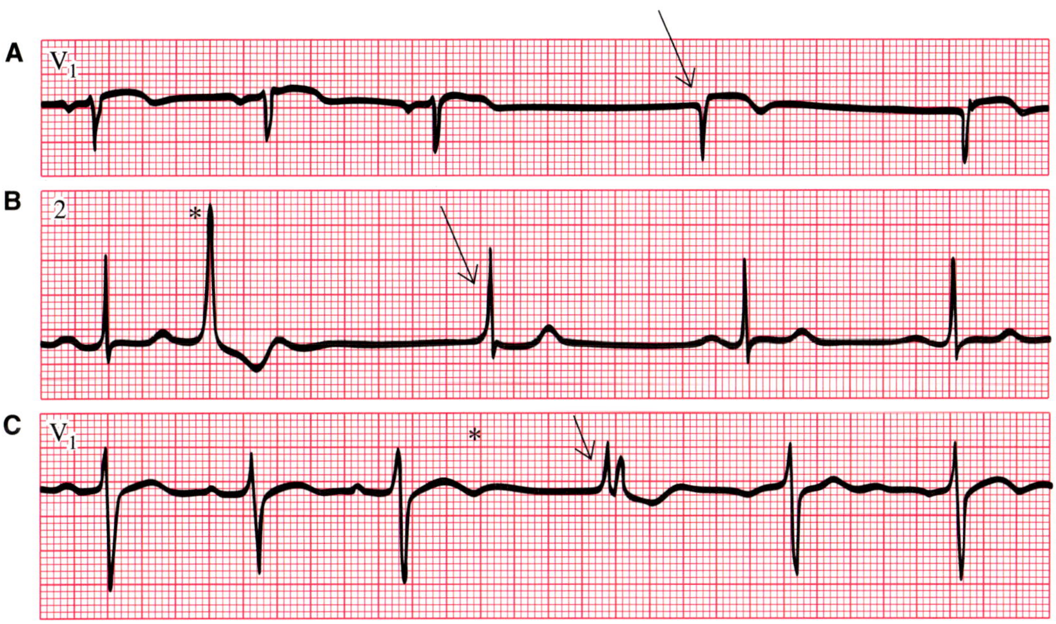

FIGURE 18.4. Rhythm strips from three individuals during postoperative monitoring: lead V_1 (**A**,**C**) and lead II (**B**). Arrows indicate junctional escape beats in **A** and **B** and the ventricular escape beat in **C**. Asterisks indicate the ventricular premature beat in **B** and nonconducted atrial premature beat in **C**. After three sinus beats (see **Figure 18.4A**), there is no further evidence of atrial activity, but then two junctional escape beats result. The pause following a ventricular premature beat (see **Figure 18.4B**) ends with a junctional escape beat. After three sinus beats (see **Figure 18.4C**), a nonconducted atrial premature beat provides a cycle long enough for the ventricular Purkinje system to provide an escape beat. (Reprinted from Marriott HJL. *ECG/PDQ*. Baltimore, MD: Williams & Wilkins; 1987:171. Copyright © 1987 Elsevier. With permission.)

The term *sick sinus syndrome* (SSS) is often applied to this situation. Although sick pacemaker syndrome would be a more accurate term, *sick sinus syndrome* is used here because of its general acceptance.

In the example of atrial flutter/fibrillation shown in **Figure 18.5**, the arrhythmia terminated abruptly and was followed by a 2.5-second pause. All potential atrial, junctional, and ventricular pacemakers were suppressed during the atrial tachyarrhythmia. An escape junctional pacemaker eventually emerged. After three beats, atrial reentry recurred, and atrial flutter/fibrillation reappeared.

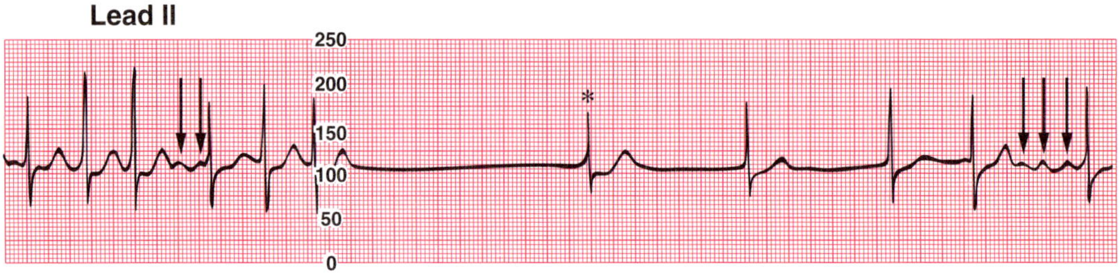

FIGURE 18.5. A lead II rhythm strip from a patient with paroxysmal atrial fibrillation. Arrows indicate the F waves, and an asterisk indicates the junctional escape after a 2.5-second pause. (Reprinted from Wagner GS, Waugh RA, Ramo BW. *Cardiac Arrhythmias*. New York, NY: Churchill Livingstone; 1983:210. Copyright © 1983 Elsevier. With permission.)

Sick Sinus Syndrome

The SSS is a part of the *tachycardia-bradycardia syndrome*[4-6] in which bursts of an atrial tachyarrhythmia, often atrial fibrillation, alternate with prolonged pauses. Its characteristics are

Characteristics of Sick Sinus Syndrome[7]

1. Bradyarrhythmia at rest
2. Inability to appropriately increase the pacemaking rate with increased sympathetic nervous activity
3. Absence of escape rhythms when the sinus rate slows
4. Increased sensitivity to suppression of impulse formation by various drugs
5. Increased sensitivity to suppression of impulse formation during a reentrant tachyarrhythmia (see **Figure 18.5**)
6. Tachy-brady syndrome

In **Figure 18.6**, an irregular atrial tachyarrhythmia (probably atrial fibrillation) stops abruptly and is followed by a 4-second pause. Because the sinus node fails to establish a rhythm, there is only slow junctional escape followed by the return of an atrial tachyarrhythmia.

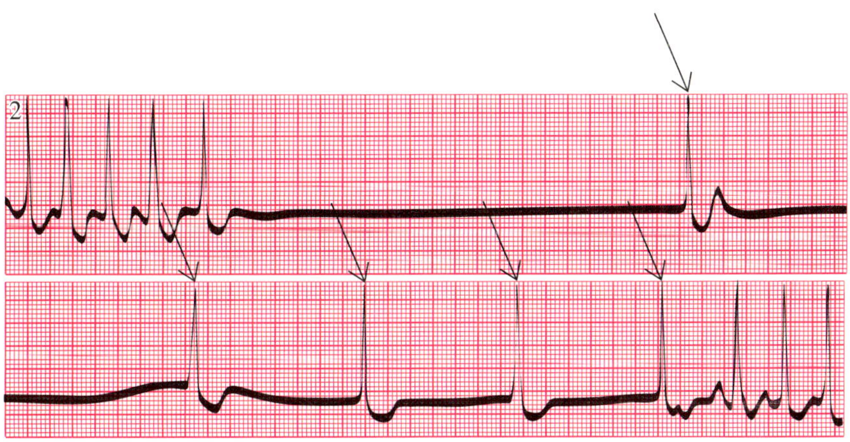

FIGURE 18.6. A lead II rhythm strip from a patient with history of recurrent syncopal episodes. Arrows indicate the junctional escape rhythm following the initial failure of emergence of an adequate escape rhythm.

Tachycardia-Bradycardia Syndrome (Tachy-Brady)

Although SSS predominantly affects the elderly, it has been recognized as early as the first day of life.[8] Temporary and reversible manifestations of the syndrome can be caused by pharmacologic agents (digitalis, antiarrhythmic drugs, β-blockers, lithium), metabolic disturbances, obstructive sleep apnea, and toxins. The chronically progressive SSS was formerly believed to be due to ischemia, but a postmortem angiographic study of the sinus nodal artery confirmed vascular involvement in fewer than one-third of 25 subjects with the chronic syndrome.[9]

The SSS may result from inflammatory and autoimmune diseases, cardiomyopathy, amyloidosis,[10] collagen vascular disease, metastatic disease, or surgical injury. In many patients, no cause is evident, and the syndrome is, therefore, classified as idiopathic. In these patients, it may be part of a sclerodegenerative process also affecting the lower parts of the cardiac pacemaking and conduction systems. Two complications that affect the prognosis of patients with SSS are atrial fibrillation and AV block. During a 3-year follow-up study, atrial fibrillation developed in 16% and AV block developed in 8% of patients with SSS.[11]

The diagnosis of SSS can usually be made from the standard ECG or from a 24-hour Holter recording carefully correlated with the patient's clinical history. Pauses of ≥3 seconds in sinus rhythm, although uncommon, do not necessarily indicate a poorer prognosis, cause symptoms, or require permanent pacemaker implantation, if the patient is asymptomatic.[12] In some patients, definitive diagnostic tests may be required. One of the best of these diagnostic tests is measurement of sinus node recovery time after rapid atrial pacing. Sinus node recovery time testing is useful in recognizing SA block or other mechanisms for SSS.[13,14] Disorders of cardiac impulse formation probably account for half of all implantations of permanent pacemakers.

In some patients, the tachyarrhythmia is the primary abnormality and ablation of the arrhythmia can abolish episodes of bradycardia that occur after termination of tachycardia episodes.

Sinus Pause or Arrest

Sudden pauses in sinus rhythm are common and rarely associated with hemodynamic changes or clinical symptoms. However, it is often impossible to determine their etiology with the standard ECG or any other clinical test. When the sinus pauses are brief, the differential diagnosis includes sinus node failure, SA block, and an atrial premature beat (APB) that fails to conduct to the ventricles. When sinus node dysfunction or SA block results in prolonged periods of asystole, this situation is termed sinus arrest. It is often impossible to establish the etiology of a sudden sinus pause because underlying sinus arrhythmia makes it difficult to determine whether the pause is a precise multiple of the P-P interval (**Figure 18.7**). Also, when a nonconducted APB is present, the premature P wave is often obscured by a T wave.

> "The most common cause of a sinus pause is a non-conducted premature atrial contraction."
>
> HJL Marriott

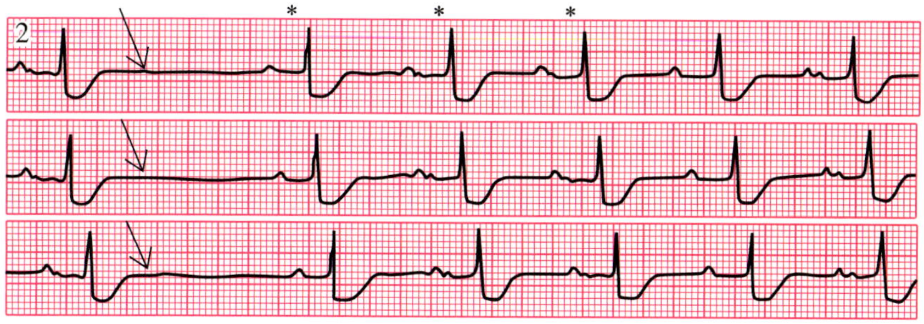

FIGURE 18.7. A continuous lead II rhythm strip from an elderly patient receiving digitalis therapy for chronic congestive heart failure. Arrows indicate the times when P waves should have emerged from the sinus node pacemaker, and asterisks indicate the accompanying first-degree atrioventricular block (PR interval = 0.28 s).

When sudden pauses in sinus rhythm are prolonged, however, nonconducted APBs are less of a consideration. Instead, failure of all pacemaking cells, rather than of only the sinus node, must be considered. The distinction between an abnormality within the pacemaking cells and aberrant control of these pacemakers by the autonomic nervous system is often difficult to determine.

When pauses in sinus rhythm are brief, no clinical intervention is required, and the patient may not actually be at increased future risk for either the generalized pacemaker failure or autonomic abnormality that produces prolonged pauses. Sometimes when sinus pauses are prolonged, it may be necessary to proceed with treatment without differentiating between a neurologic and cardiologic etiology.

Sinoatrial Block

The SA block is characterized by the intermittent failure of an impulse to emerge from the SA node and stimulate activation of the surrounding atria, resulting in the occasional complete absence of beats (see **Figure 18.7**). The long cycle at the beginning of each strip is due to an absent sinus beat, in which an entire P-QRS-T sequence is missing. Note that the pauses are approximately equal to twice the observed sinus cycle length. When no such pattern can be established, **sinus pause** is a useful and appropriate term for the abnormally long cycle, accompanied by indication of its duration in seconds.

The SA block should be diagnosed only when an arithmetical relationship (ie, equals two or more P-P intervals) between the longer and shorter sinus cycles can be demonstrated or when the sinus cycles show the characteristic classical *Wenckebach sequence* of Mobitz type I block.

Atrioventricular Conduction Disease

An AV block refers to an abnormality in electrical conduction between the atria and ventricles. The term *heart block* has also been used to describe this abnormality. Normal AV conduction was discussed in Chapter 3, and the parts of the cardiac pacemaking and conduction system that electrically connect the atrial and ventricular myocardia are illustrated in **Figure 18.1**. The term *degree* is used to indicate the severity of AV block. This severity varies from minor (first degree), in which all impulses are conducted with a slight delay; through moderate (second degree), in which some impulses are not conducted; to complete (third degree), in which no impulses are conducted. Any of these three levels of severity of AV block can be caused by conduction abnormality in the AV node, His bundle, or both the right bundle branch (RBB) and left bundle branch (LBB).[7]

Severity of Atrioventricular Block

First-Degree Atrioventricular Block

The "normal" PR interval has a duration of 0.12 to 0.20 second. *First-degree* AV *block* is generally defined as a prolongation of AV conduction time (PR interval) to >0.20 seconds. In analyses of records from normal young persons, the prevalence of first-degree block by this definition ranged from 0.5%[14] to 2%.[15] In healthy middle-aged men, a prolonged PR interval in the presence of a normal QRS complex was found not to affect prognosis and to be unrelated to ischemic heart disease.[16] Rhematic carditis is one of the causes of prolonged PR interval in the South Asian continent due to higher prevalence of rheumatic fever. **Figure 18.8** illustrates two examples of first-degree AV block. The first of these (**Figure 18.8A**) is minor, with a PR interval of 0.24 second, and the second (**Figure 18.8B**) shows extreme PR lengthening. Note that in **Figure 18.8B**, the P wave is superimposed on the T wave of the preceding cycle.

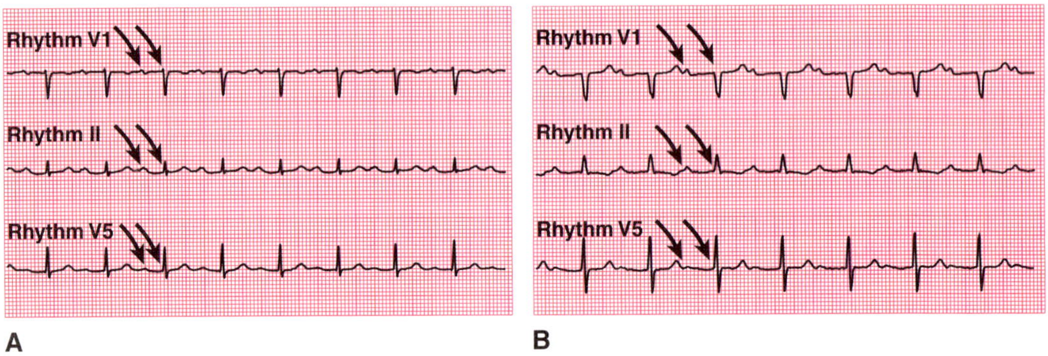

FIGURE 18.8. Simultaneous three-lead (V_1, II, and V_5) rhythm strips showing examples of first-degree AV block from healthy patient (**A**) and a woman receiving no medications (**B**). Arrows indicate PR intervals of 0.25 (**A**) and 0.35 second (**B**).

Second-Degree Atrioventricular Block

By definition, *second-degree AV block* is present when one or more, but not all, atrial impulses fail to reach the ventricles. **Figure 18.9** presents an example of both first- and second-degree AV block in which on-time P waves either have delayed AV conduction (first and second cycles of the series) or no AV conduction (third cycle).

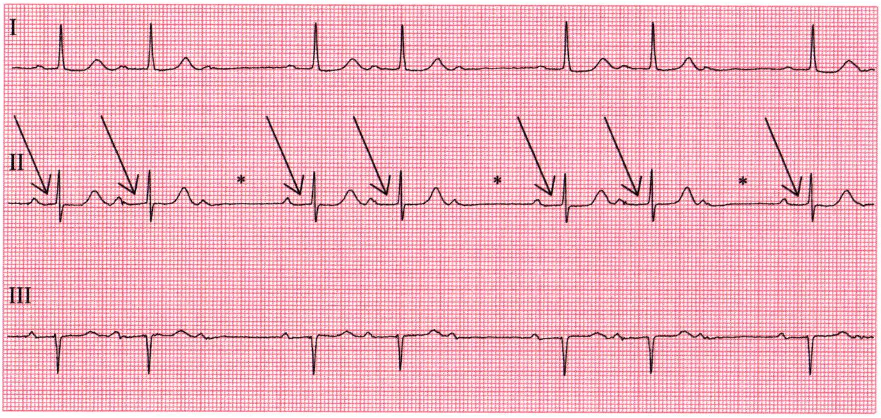

FIGURE 18.9. Leads I, II, and III rhythm strips from an elderly patient receiving digitalis therapy for chronic heart failure. Arrows indicate first-degree AV block and asterisks indicate second-degree AV block with 3:2 conduction with Wenckebach periodicity.

Second-degree AV block may be intermittent (**Figure 18.10A**) or continuous (**Figure 18.10B**). Note that in **Figure 18.10A**, the second-degree block occurs only after a sequence of six conducted beats, of which the first shows no AV block and the latter five show first-degree block (7:6 block). In **Figure 18.10B**, there is continually alternating first- and second-degree AV block with a 2:1 AV ratio. This finding is termed **2:1 (AV) block**.

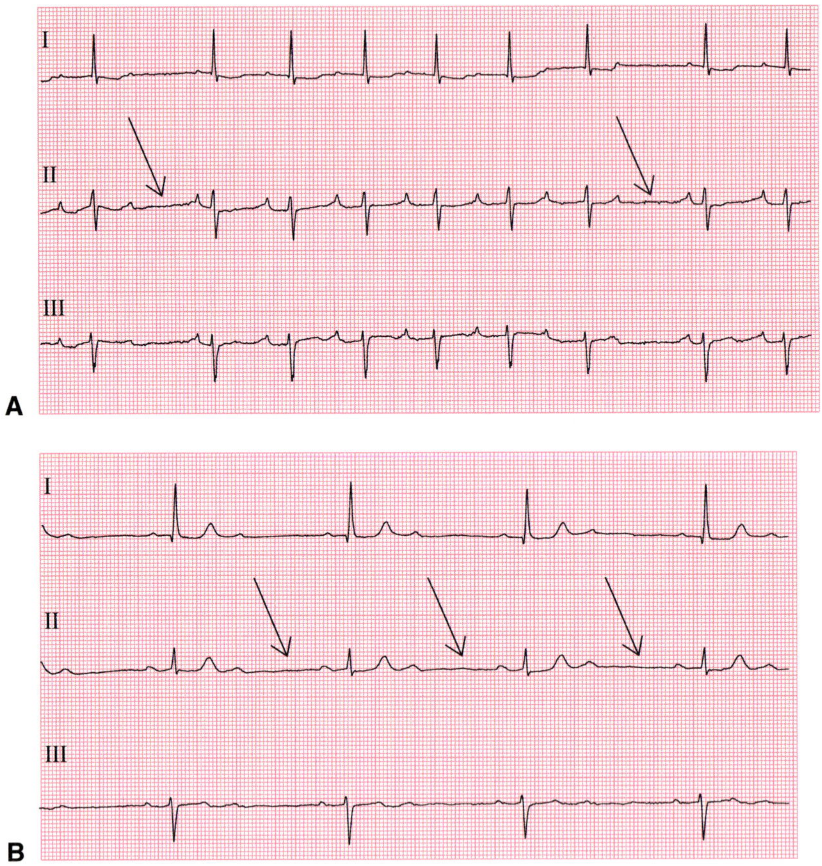

FIGURE 18.10. Leads I, II, and III rhythm strips from a patient with chronic pulmonary disease and receiving digitalis therapy (**A**) and a woman with hypertension and receiving both β-adrenergic and calcium antagonist therapy (**B**). Arrows indicate failure of atrioventricular conduction and therefore the presence of second-degree atrioventricular block.

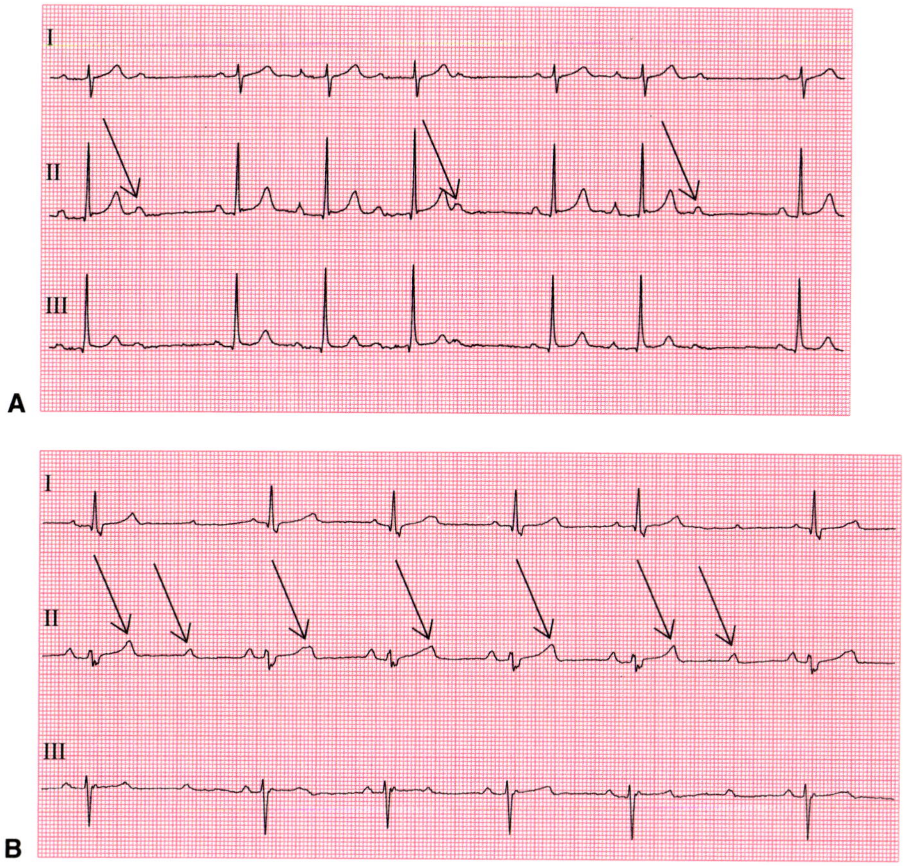

FIGURE 18.11. Leads I, II, and III rhythm strips from a patient with chronic bronchitis and cor pulmonale (**A**) and a 79-year-old woman with acute pulmonary edema (**B**), both of whom were receiving long-term digitalis therapy for heart failure. Arrows indicate P waves that completely fail to conduct to the ventricles.

Second-degree AV block may have any ratio of P waves to QRS complexes (**Figure 18.11**). In **Figure 18.11A**, there are the commonly appearing 3:2 and 4:3 AV conduction ratios. In **Figure 18.11B**, however, the sinus rate is in the tachycardia range, and the more rapid "bombardment" of the AV node causes the 2:1 ratio to be intermittently increased to 3:1. When 2 or more consecutive P waves are blocked from conducting to the ventricle, i.e., ratios like 3:1 or 4:1 AV conduction, it is called advanced AV block. When "AV block" occurs in the presence of an atrial tachyarrhythmia, the block itself is considered a normal occurrence due to the normal conduction properties of the AV node and not an additional arrhythmia (**Figure 18.12A**) unless the ventricular rate is reduced into the bradycardic range (**Figure 18.12B**).

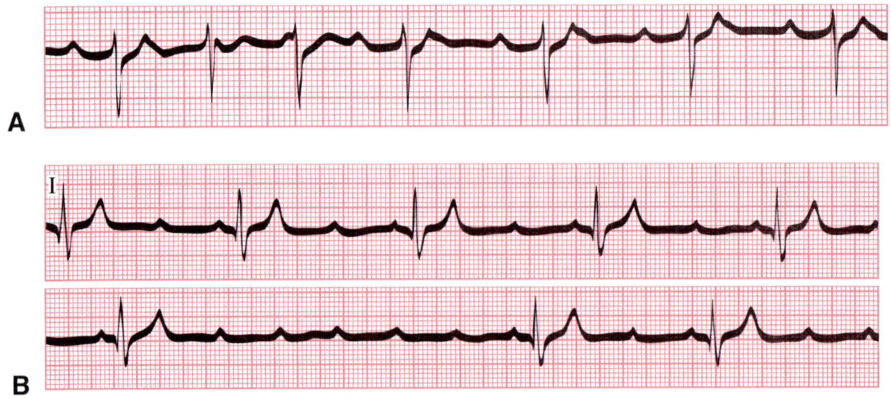

FIGURE 18.12. Lead II rhythm strips from elderly patients receiving digitalis therapy. The ventricular rates are in the normal (60-100 beats/min) (**A**) and bradycardic (15-40 beats/min) (**B**) ranges. Note the prolonged pause in the ventricular rhythm (3.5 s) in **B**.

When both second-degree AV block and sinus pauses are present, the cause is most likely not within the heart itself but rather due to the influences of the autonomic nervous system, specifically conditions that promote parasympathetic dominance via increased vagal tone. Second-degree AV block usually occurs in the AV node[17,18] and is associated with reversible conditions such as the acute phase of an inferior myocardial infarction or treatment with digitalis, a β-adrenergic blocker, or a calcium channel–blocking drug. Because second-degree AV block is generally a transient disturbance in rhythm, it seldom progresses to complete AV block. However, in one study of 16 children manifesting second-degree AV block, 7 developed complete block.[19] Chronic second-degree AV block may occasionally occur in many conditions, including aortic valve disease, atrial septal defect, heavy physical training, amyloidosis, Reiter syndrome (reactive arthritis), and (rarely) tumor of the AV node.[20]

Third-Degree Atrioventricular Block

When no atrial impulses are conducted to the ventricles, the cardiac rhythm is termed *third-degree AV block* and the clinical status is determined by the automaticity and "escape" capability of the more distal Purkinje cells. The junctional or ventricular escape rhythm in the presence of third-degree AV block is almost always precisely regular because these sites are not as influenced by the autonomic influences as is the sinus node. **Figure 18.13A** shows junctional escape in a case of third-degree AV block. **Figure 18.13B**, however, illustrates ventricular escape. Note the slower intrinsic rate and wider QRS, which suggest a lower or more distal origin of the escape rhythm.

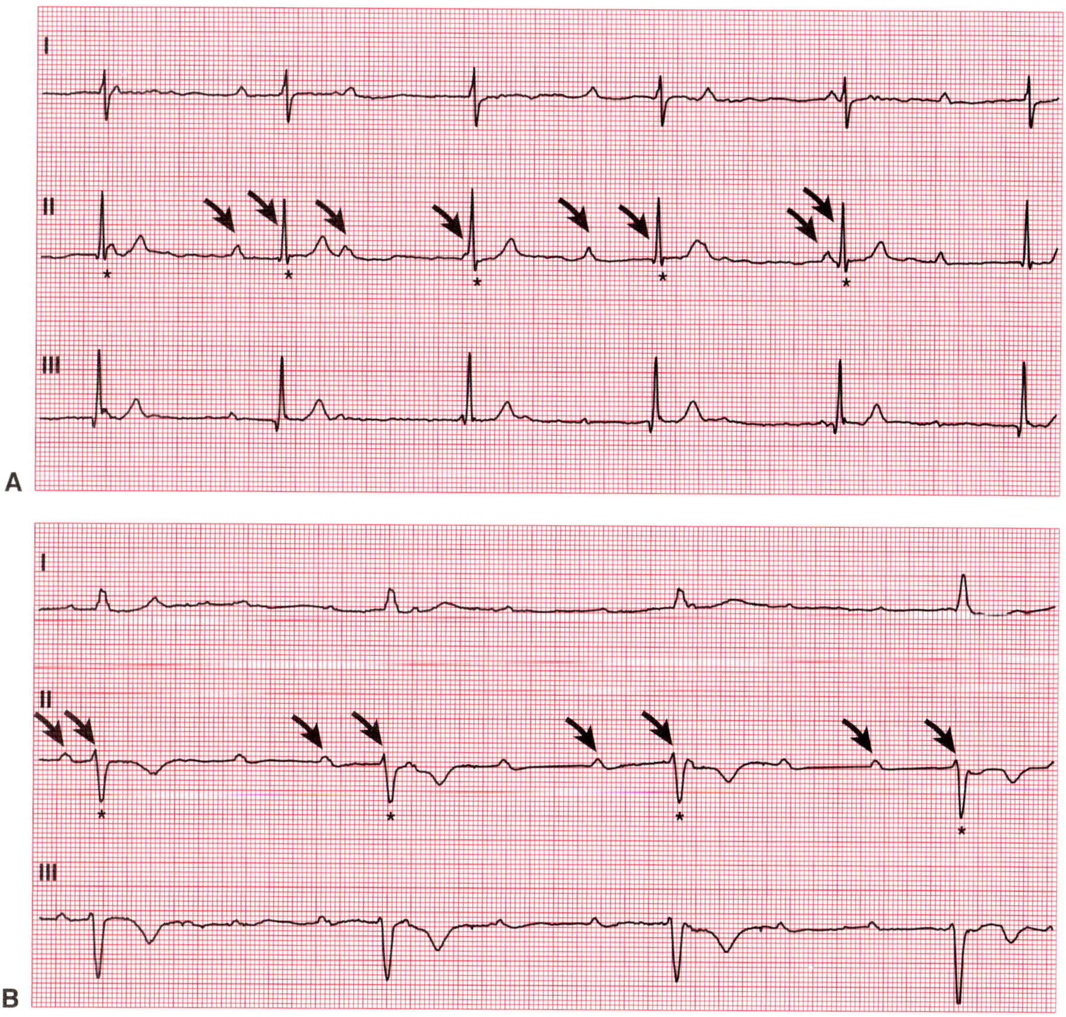

FIGURE 18.13. Leads I, II, and III rhythm strips from two patients presenting with complaints of dyspnea on exertion. Arrows indicate the varying PR-interval relationships and asterisks indicate the regular junctional (**A**) and ventricular (**B**) escape rates.

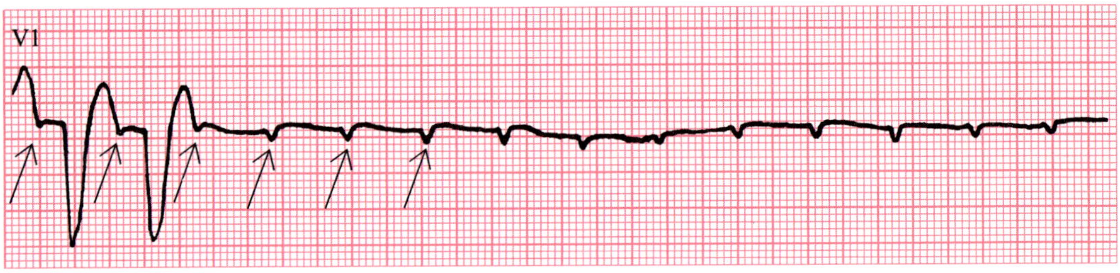

FIGURE 18.14. A lead V_1 rhythm strip from elderly patient on telemetry monitoring during hospitalization following an episode of syncope. Arrows indicate the continuing sinus tachycardia before and after the onset of complete atrioventricular block.

In most clinical instances, complete AV block is at least partly compensated by an escape rhythm originating from an area distal to the site of the block. Complete AV block of sudden onset may, however, cause syncope with catastrophic consequences, or even sudden death, when there is no escape rhythm (**Figure 18.14**). As seen in the figure, P waves occur immediately after the T waves, and the first two P waves are conducted without even first-degree block, but the third and all subsequent P waves are not conducted at all. Thus, third-degree AV block need not be preceded by first- or second-degree AV block.Third-degree AV block always produces AV dissociation with its independent atrial and ventricular rhythms. An AV dissociation may, however, result from sources other than third-degree AV block. Decreased sinus automaticity (sinus slowing), increased junctional and ventricular automaticity (junctional or ventricular speeding), and reentrant ventricular tachycardia can all produce AV dissociation by creating the condition in which anterograde impulses fail to traverse the AV node. More cranial atrial impulses encounter refractoriness that follows AV nodal activation by retrograde impulses. Therefore, AV dissociation caused solely by impaired function of the AV conduction system should actually be termed AV dissociation due to AV block (**Figure 18.15A,B**) and AV dissociation caused solely by an accelerated distal pacing site should be termed functional AV dissociation (see **Figure 18.15A**). Both causes can coexist, producing "AV dissociation due to a combination of AV block and increased refractoriness," when there are P waves that are obviously not conducted to the ventricles, but the ventricular rate is slightly above the upper limit of the bradycardic range of 60 beats/min (see **Figure 18.15B**). The term interference is often used to describe the condition of refractoriness that either causes or contributes to the two types of AV dissociation described here.

Causes of Atrioventricular Dissociation

1. Atrioventricular block
2. Increased automaticity of subsidiary pacemakers (atrioventricular nodal, junctional, ventricular)
3. Decreased automaticity of the sinoatrial node
4. Combination of the abovementioned factors
5. Reentrant arrhythmias including ventricular tachyarrhythmias

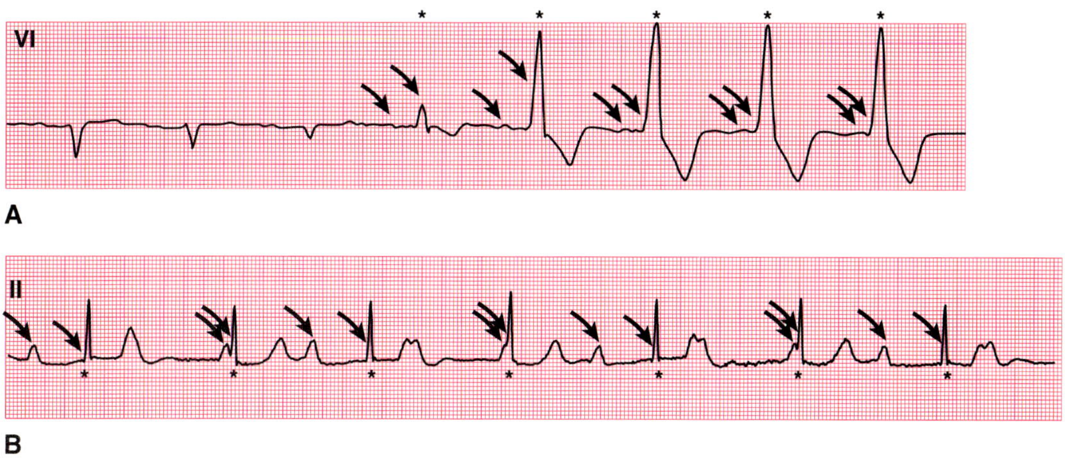

FIGURE 18.15. Rhythm strips from two patients receiving digitalis therapy for congestive heart failure. **A.** Lead V_1. **B.** Lead II. Note in **A** that the initial independent ventricular beat is a "fusion beat" produced partly by conduction from the atria and partly from the ventricular pacing site. Arrows indicate the varying relationships between adjacent P waves and QRS complexes, and asterisks indicate the regular ventricular rates. Note that the P waves are unusually small in **A** and unusually large in **B**.

Often, the AV dissociation produced by third-degree AV block is "isoarrhythmic," with similar atrial and ventricular rates and with P waves and QRS complexes occurring almost simultaneously. Insight into the presence or absence of AV block can be attained only when a P wave appears at a time sufficiently remote from a QRS complex that the ventricular refractory period would be expected to have been completed. In **Figure 18.16**, there is AV dissociation during the first three cycles, in which the independent sinus and ventricular rhythms are similar. Then, when variation in rate caused by respiration (sinus arrhythmia) accelerates the sinus rate but does not affect the ventricular escape focus during the fourth cycle, atrial capture occurs. This event proves AV conduction to be possible and eliminates complete AV block as a contributor to the AV dissociation seen here. Block in both the RBB and

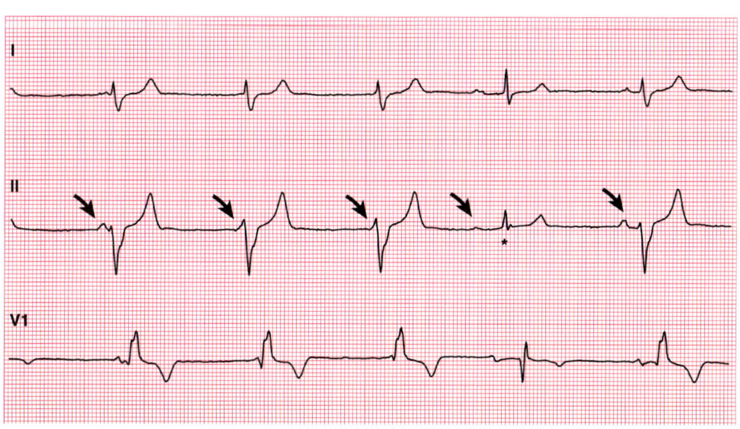

FIGURE 18.16. Leads I, II, and V_1 rhythm strips from a patient receiving digitalis therapy for congestive heart failure. Arrows indicate P-wave locations (the irregularity is due to sinus arrhythmia), and an asterisk indicates a QRS complex produced by atrial capture.

LBB, rather than block at the AV node or in the His bundle, is usually the cause of chronic complete AV block.[21] Idiopathic fibrosis, called either Lev disease or Lenègre disease, is the most common pathologic cause of chronic complete AV block.[22,23] Acute complete AV block within the AV node may result from inferior myocardial infarction, digitalis intoxication, and hypertrophic cardiomyopathy.[24] Acute complete AV block within the bundle branches results from extensive septal myocardial infarction.[25,26] Complete AV block may also be congenital, as when it results from maternal anti-Ro antibodies affecting the AV node.[27]

Differential Diagnosis for Atrioventricular Block

1. Idiopathic fibrosis and sclerosis of the conduction system
2. Hypertrophic cardiomyopathy
3. Ischemic heart disease (atrioventricular nodal block from inferior wall myocardial infarction, atrioventricular block arising in bundle branches from extensive septal myocardial infarction)
4. Idiopathic dilated cardiomyopathy
5. Infiltrative cardiomyopathies (amyloidosis, sarcoidosis, hemochromatosis, etc.)
6. Drugs (antiarrhythmic drugs, digoxin, calcium channel blockers, β-adrenergic blockers)
7. Valvulopathies
8. Congenital, genetic, or other disorders

In the presence of chronic LBB or RBB block, the individual is at risk for suddenly developing complete AV block. In the event of complete AV block in the setting of BBB, the ventricles either remain inactive (ventricular asystole; see **Figure 18.14**) and the patient experiences syncope or even sudden death or a more distal pacing site takes over (see **Figure 18.13B**) and controls the ventricles (ventricular escape). In this event, the atria continue to beat at their own rate and the ventricles beat at a slower rhythm. This independence (AV dissociation due to AV block) is readily recognized in the ECG recording from the lack of relationship between the infrequent QRS complexes and the more frequent P waves. Each maintains its own rhythm.

Differentiation between second- and third-degree AV block is accomplished by considering the relationship among the ventricular waveforms in a series of cycles (R-R intervals) and the relationship between the atrial and ventricular waveforms in each of these cycles (PR or flutter-R intervals). If the R-R interval is irregular, some AV conduction can be assumed, and second-degree block is present. If the R-R interval is regular, a constant PR or flutter-R interval indicates second-degree AV block. In contrast, a varying PR or flutter-R interval indicates third-degree block, with an escape rhythm generated by a lower site. **Figure 18.17** presents examples of AV block occurring in the presence of three different atrial tachyarrhythmias: sinus tachycardia (**Figure 18.17A**), atrial flutter (**Figure 18.17B**), and atrial fibrillation (**Figure 18.17C**). Consecutive R-R intervals are constant in all of the examples, at 2.84, 1.40, and 1.96 seconds, respectively. In **Figure 18.17A,B**, it is obvious that there is third-degree AV block because the adjacent PR relationships in **Figure 18.17A** and flutter wave-R relationships in **Figure 18.17B** are quite variable. In **Figure 18.17C**, third-degree AV block can be assumed because the absence of regular atrial activity in atrial fibrillation prohibits any constancy in AV conduction relationships.

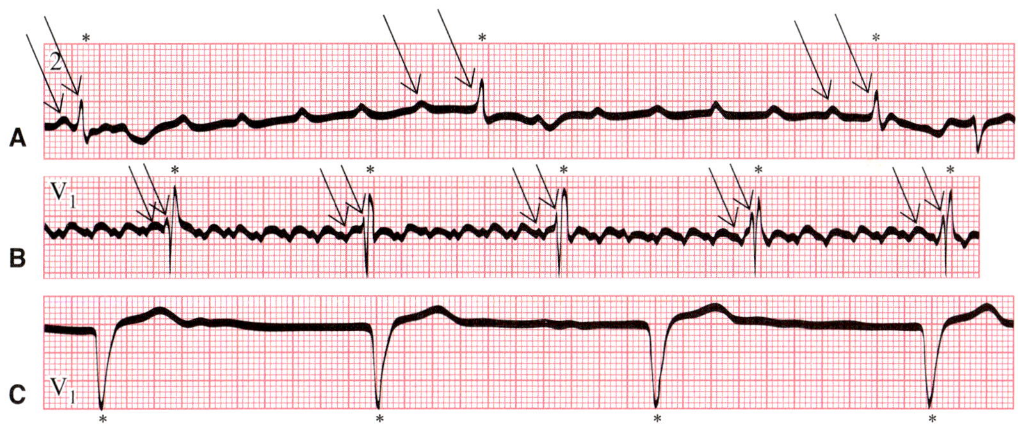

FIGURE 18.17. Three examples of atrial tachyarrhythmias with third-degree atrioventricular block and lower escape rhythms. In **A** and **B**, the QRS duration of <0.12 second indicates escape from the common bundle, but in **C**, the QRS duration of 0.16 second indicates either escape from the common bundle accompanied by left-bundle-branch block or escape from the right bundle branch. Arrows indicate the varying P-QRS (**A**) and F-QRS (**B**) intervals, and asterisks indicate the constant ventricular rates in all three examples.

Location of Atrioventricular Block

AV block can be located in the AV node, the common bundle, or the bundle branches (**Figure 18.1**). This distinction is important because both the etiology and prognosis are quite different with proximal (AV nodal) versus distal (infranodal) block. Fortunately, block within the common bundle is so rare that the clinical decision about the location of an AV block is essentially limited to the AV node versus the bundle branches.

Two aspects of the electrocardiographic appearance of rhythm may help in differentiating AV block at the AV node versus AV block in a bundle branch.

Factors Determining the Site of AV Block Within AV Node Versus Bundle Branches

1. The consistency of the PR intervals of conducted impulses
2. The width of the QRS complexes of either conducted or escape impulses

Because only the AV node has the ability to vary its conduction time, the Purkinje cells of the common bundle and bundle branches must conduct at a particular speed or not at all. Therefore, when a varying PR interval is present, the AV block is most likely within the AV node.

A QRS complex of normal duration (<0.12 s) can occur only when the impulse producing the complex has equal access to both the RBB and LBB. Therefore, when AV block is located at the bundle-branch level, the conducted or escape QRS complexes must be ≥0.12 second. The diagnosis is complicated by the possibility of either a fixed bundle-branch block accompanying AV nodal block or an aberrancy of intraventricular conduction. Consequently, a QRS complex of normal duration confirms that a block has an AV nodal location, whereas a QRS complex of prolonged duration is not helpful in locating the site of an AV block.

The AV node has this ability to vary its conduction time because its cells have uniquely prolonged periods of partial refractoriness as they return from their depolarized to their repolarized states. Therefore, in less than complete AV block, a nodal versus an infranodal (bilateral bundle) location can be determined by observing whether the PR interval is variable, as in the first case, or constant, as in the second.

The AV conduction patterns can be considered only when some conduction is present (first- or second-degree AV block). No differentiation between an AV nodal and an infranodal location is possible in *complete (third-degree)* block with wide escape QRS complexes (see **Figure 18.13B**).

Tips for Identifying Location of AV Block Within AV Node Versus Bundle Branches

1. Varying PR interval indicates that the atrioventricular (AV) block is located in the AV node. Prolonged PR of conducted beat indicates that the AV block is located in the AV node.
2. QRS of normal duration (<0.12 s) indicates that the AV block is located in the AV node.
3. A prolonged QRS (≥0.12 s) is not helpful in determining the location of AV block.

Atrioventricular Nodal Block

The classic form of AV nodal block is reflected by the Wenckebach sequence, in which the PR interval may begin within normal limits but is usually somewhat prolonged. With each successive beat, the PR interval gradually lengthens until there is failure to conduct an impulse to the ventricles. Examples are presented in **Figures 18.9**, **18.10A**, and **18.11A**. Following the nonconducted P wave, the PR interval reverts to normal (or near normal) and the sequence is repeated. At times, the PR interval may increase to surprising lengths.

Progressive lengthening of the PR interval occurs in the Wenckebach sequence because each successive atrial impulse arrives progressively earlier in the relative refractory period of the AV node and, therefore, takes progressively longer to penetrate the node and reach the ventricles. This lengthening PR is a physiologic mechanism during atrial fibrillation/flutter, but its occurrence at normal heart rates implies impairment of AV conduction. The progressive lengthening of the PR interval usually follows a predictable pattern: The maximal increase in the PR interval occurs between the first and second cardiac cycles, and the increase between subsequent cycles then becomes progressively smaller. Three characteristic features of the cardiac cycle, which were figuratively referred to by Dr. Marriott as the *"footprints" of the Wenckebach* AV nodal block follow:

"Footprints" of Wenckebach Atrioventricular Nodal Block

1. The beats tend to cluster in small groups, particularly in pairs, because 3:2 P-to-QRS ratios are more common than 4:3 ratios, which are more common than 5:4 ratios, and so forth.
2. In each group of ventricular beats, the first cycle is longer than the second cycle, and there is a tendency for progressive shortening to occur in successive cycles.
3. The longest cycle (the one containing the dropped ventricular beat) is less than twice the length of the shortest cycle (**Figure 18.18**).

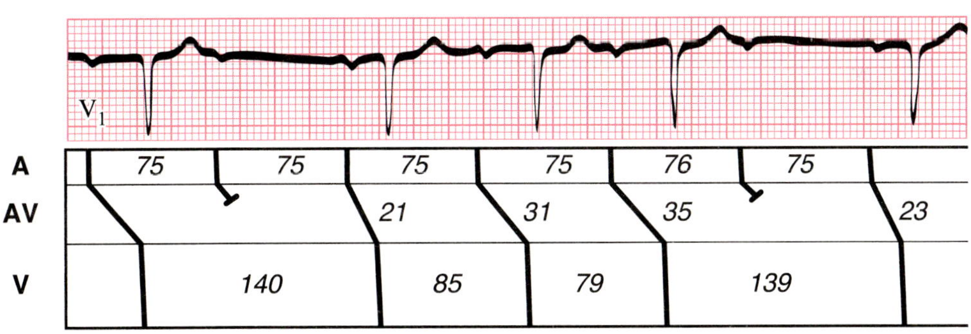

FIGURE 18.18. A lead V_1 rhythm strip accompanied by a ladder diagram with atrial (A), AV nodal (AV), and ventricular (V) levels. The various intervals are indicated in hundredths of a second.

This phenomenon influences the rhythm of the ventricles. After the pause produced by complete failure of AV conduction, the R-R intervals in the ECG tend to decrease progressively, and the long cycle (the one containing the nonconducted beat) is of shorter duration than two of the shorter cycles because it contains the shortest PR interval. This pattern of progressively decreasing R-R intervals preceding a pause in AV conduction that lasts for less than twice the duration of the shortest R-R interval is of only academic interest in the presence of AV nodal block, but a similar pattern of P-P intervals may provide the only clue to the presence of sinus nodal exit block.

"Decremental conduction delay may occur in any cardiac conduction pathway. Group beating is the hallmark of such activity."

HJL Marriott

When second-degree AV block appears during an acute inferior myocardial infarction, the elevation of the ST segment in the ECG may obscure many of the P waves, as seen in **Figure 18.19**. The visible P waves with prolonged PR intervals during the pauses allow diagnosis of first-degree block, but only the typical R-R interval pattern allows a diagnosis of second-degree AV nodal block.The features described are typical of a classic Wenckebach period, but AV nodal block rarely fits this pattern because both the sinus rate and the AV conduction are under the constant influence of the autonomic nervous system. Among common variations from the classic pattern are (1) the first incremental increase in PR interval may not be the greatest, (2) the PR intervals may not lengthen progressively, (3) the last PR increment may be the longest of all, and (4) a nonconducted atrial beat may not occur. The only criterion needed to identify the form of AV block that typically occurs in the AV node is a variation in the PR intervals. The term *Mobitz type I* or simply *type I AV block* is used when variation of the PR intervals is virtually diagnostic of block in the AV node.

The Common Variants of "Footprints" of Wenckebach

1. The first incremental increase in PR interval may not be the greatest.
2. The PR intervals may not lengthen progressively.
3. The last PR increment may be the longest of all.
4. A nonconducted atrial beat may not occur.

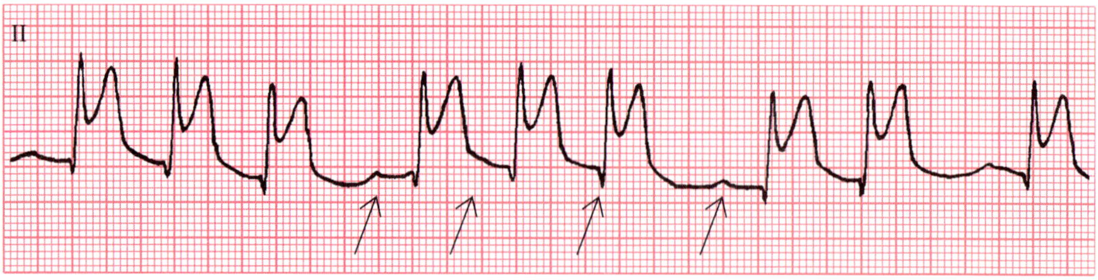

FIGURE 18.19. A continuous recording of lead II from a patient with acute inferior myocardial infarction. Arrows indicate both the obvious and the assumed locations of sinus-originated P waves.

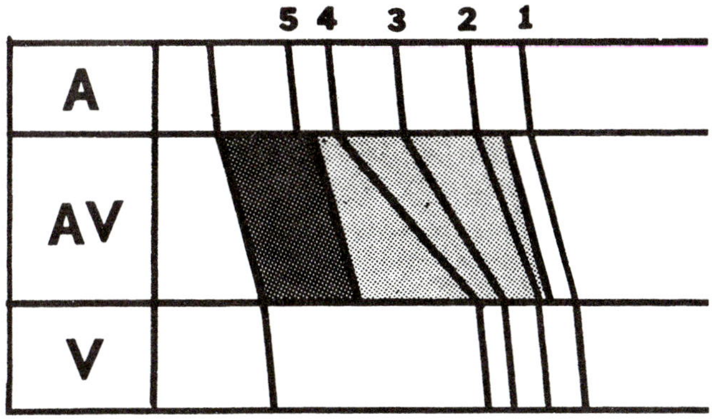

FIGURE 18.20. A ladder diagram illustrating the effect of progressively earlier entry of atrial impulses 1 to 5 into the atrioventricular (AV) node. The light stippled area indicates the atrioventricular node's relative refractory period, during which impulses 2, 3, and 4 encounter progressively slower conduction. The dark stippled area indicates the node's absolute refractory period, during which impulse 5 cannot be conducted to the ventricles.

The earlier an impulse arrives during the prolonged partial refractory period of the AV node, the longer the time required for conduction of the impulse through to the ventricles. Therefore, when the AV node remains in its refractory period, the shorter the interval between a conducted QRS complex and the next conducted P wave (*RP interval*), the longer is the following conduction time (PR interval). This inverse or reciprocal relationship between RP and PR intervals is illustrated schematically in **Figure 18.20**.

The need to consider the variability in AV conduction times to determine the location of an AV block is illustrated in **Figure 18.21**. There is normal sinus rhythm with second-degree AV block and RBB block. For the initial complete cardiac cycles, the RP intervals are constant (1.36 s) and the PR intervals are also constant (0.24 s). It is tempting to locate the AV block below the AV node because the PR intervals do not vary and there is an obvious intraventricular conduction problem. The possibility of AV nodal block has, however, not been eliminated because with a constant RP interval the AV node would be expected to conduct with a constant PR interval. Only when the conduction ratio changes from 2:1 (P waves 1-4) to 3:2 (P waves 5-7) is a change produced in the RP interval (from 1.36 to 0.56 s). This shorter RP interval is accompanied by a reciprocally greater PR interval (from 0.24 to 0.36 s), identifying the AV node rather than the ventricular Purkinje system as the location of the AV block.

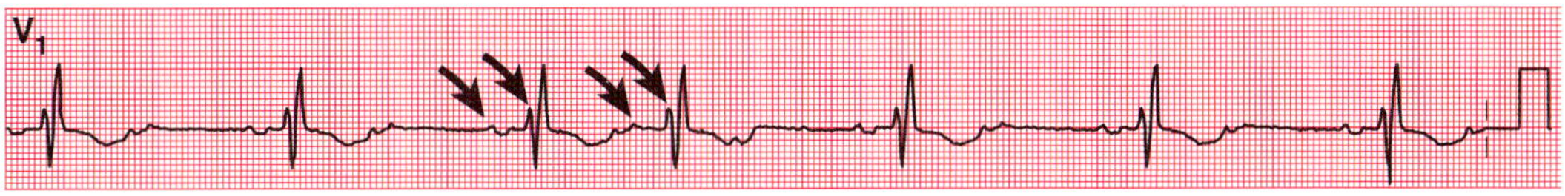

FIGURE 18.21. A lead V_1 rhythm strip from an elderly patient on digitalis therapy for congestive heart failure. Arrows indicate the varying PR intervals during the third and fourth cycles that prove the capacity for variable conduction times.

Infranodal (Purkinje) Block

Although infranodal (ie, occurring in the Purkinje system) block is much less common than AV nodal block, it is a much more serious condition. *Infranodal block* is almost always preceded by a bundle-branch block pattern for the conducted beats, with the nonconducted beats resulting from intermittent block in the other bundle branch.[17,18] Continuous block in the other bundle branch results in syncope or heart failure if ventricular escape occurs and sudden death if there is no ventricular escape. Infranodal block is almost always due to bilateral bundle-branch block rather than His-bundle block. First-degree AV block may or may not accompany the bundle-branch block, but there is usually no stable period of second-degree AV block. Infranodal block is typically characterized by a sudden progression from no AV block to third-degree (complete) AV block. Because it occurs in the distal part of the pacemaking and conduction system, the escape rhythm may be too slow or too unreliable to support adequate circulation of blood, thereby causing serious and even fatal clinical events.

Unlike the cells in the AV node, those in the Purkinje system have an extremely short relative refractory period. Therefore, they either conduct at a particular speed or not at all. Infranodal block is characterized by a lack of lengthening of the PR interval preceding the nonconducted P wave and a lack of shortening of the PR interval in the following cycle. This pattern is termed *Mobitz type II* or simply *type II AV block* and should be diagnosed whenever there is second-degree AV block with a constant PR interval despite a change in the RP interval.

The cardiac rhythm shown in **Figure 18.22A** should be compared with that in **Figure 18.22B**. The consistent 3:2 AV ratio provides varying RP intervals. However, in **Figure 18.22A**, the PR intervals remain constant at 0.20 second, in contrast with **Figure 18.22B** in which the varying P-P intervals result in varying PR intervals. Therefore, the AV block producing the rhythm shown in **Figure 18.22A** is in a location that is incapable of varying its conduction time even when it receives impulses at varying intervals. The PR intervals are independent of, rather than reciprocal to, their associated RP intervals. This type II block in **Figure 18.22A** is indicative of an infranodal (Purkinje) site of failure of AV conduction, in contrast to type I block in **Figure 18.22B**, which is indicative of an AV nodal site. **Figure 18.23** presents another example of type II block. Note that the PR

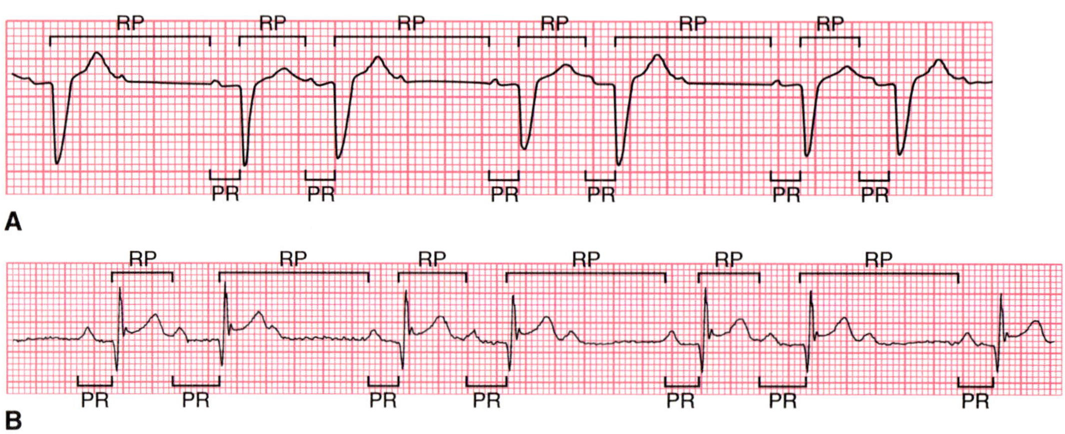

FIGURE 18.22. Lead II rhythm strips from a woman with recurrent presyncopal episodes (**A**) and another patient with an acute inferior myocardial infarction (**B**). Brackets indicate the variable RP/constant PR pattern typical of type II atrioventricular block in **A** and the variable RP/variable PR pattern typical of type I AV block in **B**.

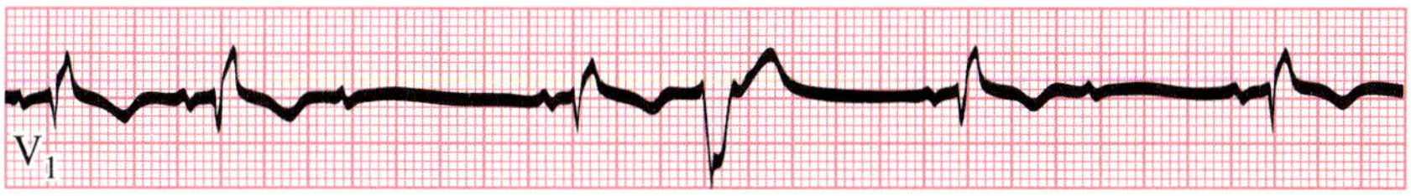

FIGURE 18.23. A lead V_1 rhythm strip from a patient with chronic congestive heart failure. There is a lack of increase in the PR interval when a decrease occurs in the RP interval.

intervals remain unchanged despite longer and shorter RP intervals (ie, there is no *RP/PR reciprocity*). The recording illustrates the two sources of variation in RP intervals: a change in the AV conduction ratio (from 1:1 to 2:1) and the presence of a ventricular premature beat.

A stepwise method for determining the location of AV block is illustrated in **Figure 18.24**. This algorithm does not consider the localization of AV block within the common bundle because of the rarity of AV block in this location. (Such a location should be considered only when a QRS complex of normal duration [step 1] is accompanied by a pattern characteristic of type II block [step 4].) Note that both steps 2 and 4 may lead to situations in which it is impossible to determine the location of a block from a particular ECG recording. In this case, additional recordings should be obtained. If these are also nondiagnostic, the patient should be managed as though the block were located in the bundle branches because such a location has the most serious clinical consequences. This management usually requires insertion of a temporary pacemaker, which provides time for further studies to determine the location of the AV block. *His-bundle electrograms* can be obtained via intracardiac recordings. A prolonged atrial-to-His interval (from the onset of the atrial signal to the time of the His-bundle signal), or the absence of a signal from the His bundle, indicates block in an AV nodal location, whereas a prolonged His-to-ventricle interval (from the His-bundle signal to the onset of the ventricular signal), or absence of a signal from the ventricles after a His signal, indicates block in a bilateral bundle branch location.

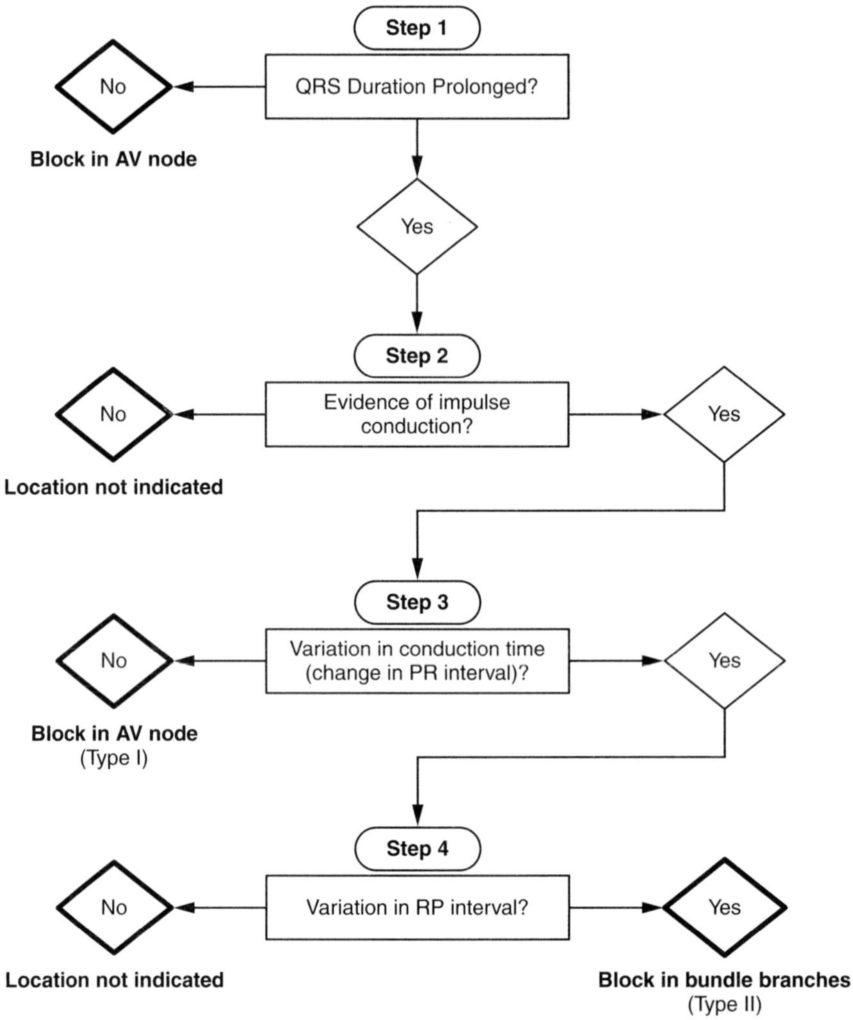

FIGURE 18.24. The four-step algorithm for identifying the location of atrioventricular (AV) block from an electrocardiogram recording. Step 1: Consider the duration of the QRS complex. Step 2: Consider whether conducted beats are present. Step 3: Consider whether there is variation in the conduction times. Step 4: Consider whether there are constant PR intervals with changing RP intervals. Situations that indicate an end point in the algorithm are indicated by boxes with accentuated borders.

CHAPTER 18 SUMMARY ILLUSTRATION

Location	ECG	Summary
Sinus Pause/ Arrest	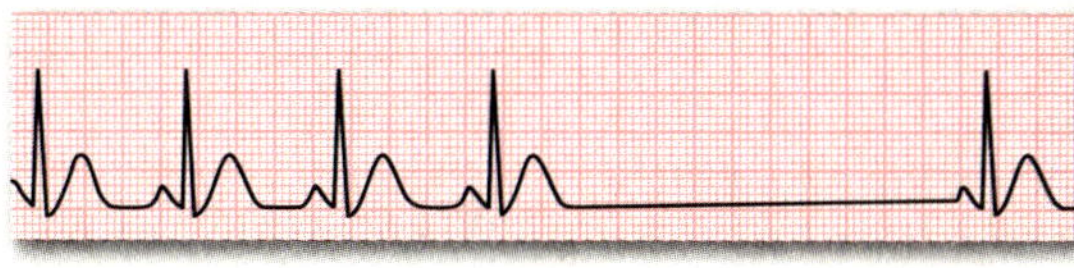	• Intermittent failure of SA node discharge resulting in absence of P wave and no recorded rhythm until SA node eventually fires or lower pacemaker initiates escape rhythm
Sinoatrial Exit Block	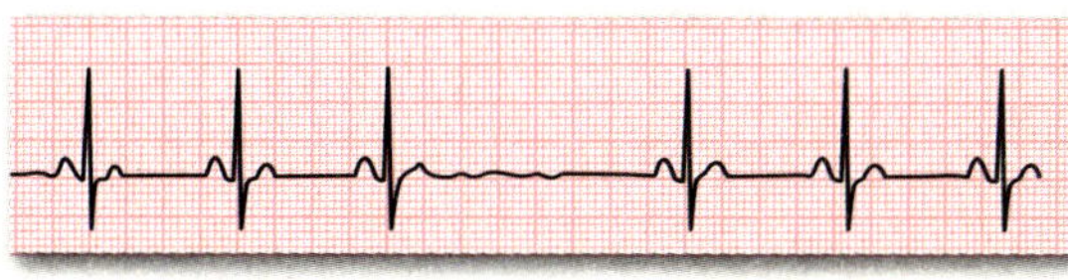	• Intermittent block at level of SA node from delivering impulse • Can be diagnosed only when cycle length of pause is a multiple of the basic sinus cycle length • Follows convention of AV block with 1st, 2nd type I/II, and 3rd degree classifications
1st Degree AV Block	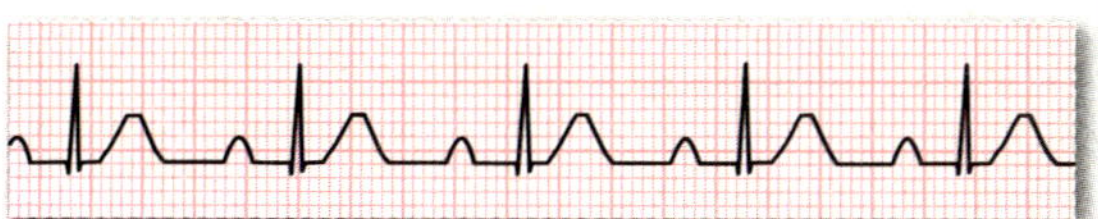	• Stable prolongation of AV conduction time (PR interval) to >0.20 seconds • Every impulse conducted (every P wave followed by QRS)
2nd Degree AV Block: Mobitz Type I "Wenckebach"	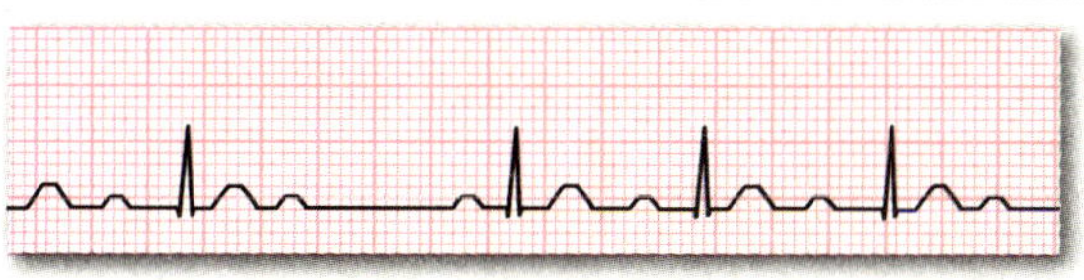	• Intermittent block at level of AV node • PR interval gets progressively longer until QRS is dropped
2nd Degree AV Block: Mobitz Type II	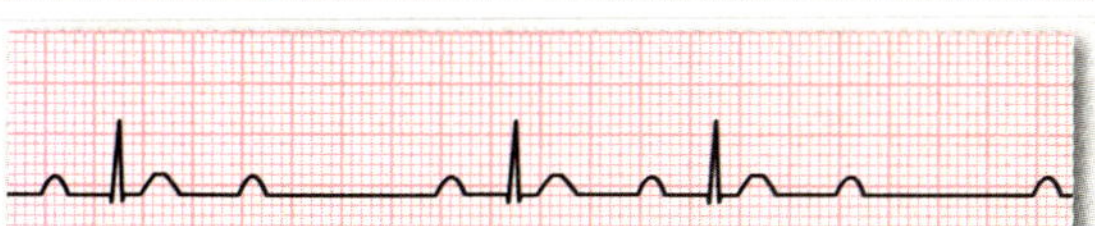	• Intermittent infranodal block (level of His or at bundle branches) • Stable prolongation of PR interval • Not all impulses conducted (not every P wave followed by QRS)
3rd Degree AV Block "Complete Heart Block"	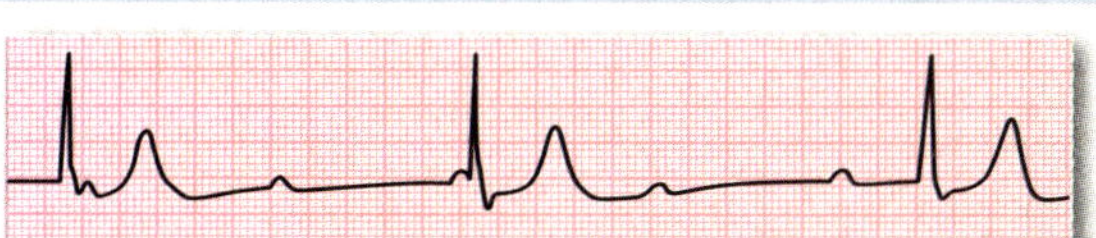	• Complete block at level of AV node or lower • Lack of concordance between P wave and QRS

Examples of sinus node and conduction system pathology that can lead to various bradyarrhythmias. At the sinus node, the heart's primary pacemaker, associated dysfunction in impulse generation, or its exit from the node can result in a pause/arrest or sinoatrial exit block, respectively. Dysfunction at the atrioventricular node or lower conduction sites can result in atrioventricular nodal block of varying degrees depending on location. Although the mechanisms vary at different anatomic sites, the result is an alteration in the efficient impulse generation and conduction and slowing of the cardiac rhythm. Abbreviations: AV, atrioventricular; SA, sinoatrial.

Glossary

Asystole: a pause in the cardiac electrical activity with neither atrial nor ventricular waveforms present on the ECG.

Atrial rhythm: a rhythm with a rate of <100 beats/min and with abnormally directed P waves (indicating origination from a site in the atria other than the sinus node) preceding each QRS complex.

Atrioventricular (AV) block: a conduction abnormality located between the atria and the ventricles. Both the severity and the location of the abnormality should be considered.

Degree: a measure of the severity of AV block.

Escape rhythms: rhythms that originate from sites in the pacemaking and conduction system other than the sinus node after a pause created by the failure of either normal sinus impulse formation or AV impulse conduction.

First-degree AV block: conduction of atrial impulses to the ventricles with PR intervals of >0.21 second.

Footprints of the Wenckebach sequence: the pattern of clusters of beats in small groups (group beating), with gradually decreasing intervals between beats, preceding a pause that is less than twice the duration of the shortest interval.

Heart block: another term used for AV block.

His-bundle electrograms: intracardiac recordings obtained via a catheter positioned across the tricuspid valve adjacent to the common or His bundle. These recordings are used clinically to determine the location of AV block when this is not apparent from the surface ECG recordings.

Infranodal block: AV block that occurs distal to or below the AV node and therefore within either the common bundle or in both the RBB and LBB.

Junctional rhythm: a rhythm with a rate of 45 to 60 beats/min with an inverted P-wave direction visible in the frontal plane leads and normally appearing QRS complexes. The P waves may precede or follow the QRS complexes or may be obscured because they occur during the QRS complexes. Slower junctional rhythms are termed *junctional bradycardia*. Faster junctional rhythms in the range 60 to 100 beats/min are termed *accelerated junctional rhythms*, whereas those junctional rhythms faster than 100 beats/min are designated junctional tachycardias.

Mobitz type I (type I): a pattern of AV block in which there are varying PR intervals. This pattern is typical of block within the AV node, which has the capacity for wide variations in conduction time. Wenckebach sequences are the classic form of type I block.

Mobitz type II (type II): a pattern of AV block in which there are constant PR intervals despite varying RP intervals. This pattern is typical of block in the ventricular Purkinje system, which is incapable of significant variations in conduction time.

RP interval: the time between the beginning of the previously conducted QRS complex and the beginning of the next conducted P wave.

RP/PR reciprocity: the inverse relationship between the interval of the last previously conducted beat (RP interval) and the time required for AV conduction (PR interval). This occurs in type I AV block.

Second-degree AV block: the conduction of some atrial impulses to the ventricles, with the failure to conduct other atrial impulses.

Sick sinus syndrome: inadequate function of cardiac cells with pacemaking capability, resulting in continuous or intermittent slowing of the heart rate at rest and an inability to appropriately increase the rate with exercise.

Tachycardia-bradycardia syndrome: a condition in which both rapid and slow cardiac rhythms are present. The rapid rhythms tend to appear when the rate slows abnormally, whereas the slow rhythms are prominent immediately after the sudden cessation of a rapid rhythm.

Third-degree AV block: failure of conduction of any atrial impulses to the ventricles. This is often referred to as "complete AV block."

Vasovagal reaction (vasovagal reflex): sudden slowing of the heart rate either from decreased impulse formation (sinus pause) or decreased impulse conduction (AV block) resulting from increased activity of the parasympathetic or decreased activity of the sympathetic nervous system. The slowing of the cardiac rhythm is accompanied by peripheral vascular dilation.

Vasovagal syncope: loss of consciousness caused by a vasovagal reaction. Consciousness is almost always regained when the individual falls into a recumbent position because this results in increased venous return to the heart. See also Neurocardiogenic syncope.

Ventricular rhythm: a rhythm with a rate of <100 beats/min with abnormally wide QRS complexes. There may be either retrograde association or AV dissociation.

Wenckebach sequence: the classic form of type I AV block, which would be expected to occur in the absence of autonomic influences on either the SA or AV nodes.

Acknowledgment

We gratefully acknowledge the past contributions of the previous edition's author, Dr. Galen S. Wagner, as portions of that chapter were retained in this revision.

References

1. Abboud FM. Neurocardiogenic syncope. *N Engl J Med.* 1993;328:1117-1120.
2. Fouad FM, Siitthisook S, Vanerio G, et al. Sensitivity and specificity of the tilt table test in young patients with unexplained syncope. *Pacing Clin Electrophysiol.* 1993;16:394-400.
3. Thilenius OG, Ryd KJ, Husayni J. Variations in expression and treatment of transient neurocardiogenic instability. *Am J Cardiol.* 1992;69:1193-1195.
4. Kaplan BM, Langendorf R, Lev M, Pick A. Tachycardia-bradycardia syndrome (so-called "sick sinus syndrome"). Pathology, mechanisms and treatment. *Am J Cardiol.* 1973;31:497-508.
5. Moss AJ, Davis RJ. Brady-tachy syndrome. *Prog Cardiovasc Dis.* 1974;16:439-454.
6. Ferrer MI. *The Sick Sinus Syndrome.* Mt. Kisco, NY: Futura Publishing; 1974.
7. Kusumoto FM, Schoenfeld MH, Barrett C, et al. 2018 ACC/AHA/HRS guideline on the evaluation and management of patients with bradycardia and cardiac conduction delay: executive summary. A report of the American College of Cardiology/American Heart Association Task Force on Clinical Practice Guidelines, and the Heart Rhythm Society. *J Am Coll Cardiol.* 2019;74:c51.
8. Ector H, Van der Hauwaert LG. Sick sinus syndrome in childhood. *Br Heart J.* 1980;44:684-691.
9. Shaw DB, Linker NJ, Heaver PA, Evans R. Chronic sinoatrial disorder (sick sinus syndrome): a possible result of cardiac ischaemia. *Br Heart J.* 1987;58:598-607.
10. Evans R, Shaw DB. Pathological studies in sinoatrial disorder (sick sinus syndrome). *Br Heart J.* 1977;39:778-786.
11. Sutton R, Kenny RA. The natural history of sick sinus syndrome. *Pacing Clin Electrophysiol.* 1986;9:1110-1114.
12. Hilgard J, Ezri MD, Denes P. Significance of ventricular pauses of three seconds or more detected on twenty-four-hour Holter recordings. *Am J Cardiol.* 1984;55:1005-1008.
13. Chung EK. Sick sinus syndrome: current views. Part II. *Mod Concepts Cardiovasc Dis.* 1980;49:67-70.
14. Gann D, Tolentino A, Samet P. Electrophysiologic evaluation of elderly patients with sinus bradycardia: a long-term follow-up study. *Ann Intern Med.* 1979;90:24-29.
15. Johnson RL, Averill KH, Lamb LE. Electrocardiographic findings in 67,375 asymptomatic individuals. VII. Atrioventricular block. *Am J Cardiol.* 1960;6:153-157.
16. Eriksen J, Otterstad JE. Natural course of a prolonged PR interval and the relation between PR and incidence of coronary heart disease. A 7-year follow-up study of 1832 apparently healthy men aged 40-59 years. *Clin Cardiol.* 1984;7:6-13.
17. Damato AN, Lau SH. Clinical value of the electrogram of the conduction system. *Prog Cardiovasc Dis.* 1970;13:119-140.
18. Narula OS. Wenckebach type I and type II atrioventricular block (revisited). *Cardiovasc Clin.* 1974;6:137-167.
19. Young D, Eisenberg R, Fish B, Fisher JD. Wenckebach atrioventricular block (Mobitz type I) in children and adolescents. *Am J Cardiol.* 1977;40:393-399.
20. Strasberg B, Amat-Y-Leon F, Dhingra RC, et al. Natural history of chronic second-degree atrioventricular nodal block. *Circulation.* 1981;63:1043-1049.
21. Lepeschkin E. The electrocardiographic diagnosis of bilateral bundle branch block in relation to heart block. *Prog Cardiovasc Dis.* 1964;6:445-471.
22. Rosenbaum MB, Elizari MV, Kretz A, Taratuto AL. Anatomical basis of AV conduction disturbances. *Geriatrics.* 1970;25:132-144.
23. Steiner C, Lau SH, Stein E, et al. Electrophysiologic documentation of trifascicular block as the common cause of complete heart block. *Am J Cardiol.* 1971;28:436-441.

24. Louie EK, Maron BJ. Familial spontaneous complete heart block in hypertrophic cardiomyopathy. *Br Heart J.* 1986;55: 469-474.
25. Hindman MC, Wagner GS, JaRo M, et al. The clinical significance of bundle branch block complicating acute myocardial infarction. 1. Clinical characteristics, hospital mortality, and one-year follow-up. *Circulation.* 1978;58:679-688.
26. Hindman MC, Wagner GS, JaRo M, et al. The clinical significance of bundle branch block complicating acute myocardial infarction. 2. Indications for temporary and permanent pacemaker insertion. *Circulation.* 1978;58:689-699.
27. Ho SY, Esscher E, Anderson RH, Michaëlsson M. Anatomy of congenital complete heart block and relation to maternal anti-Ro antibodies. *Am J Cardiol.* 1986;58:291-294.

19

Ventricular Preexcitation

DONALD D. HEGLAND, STEPHEN GAETA, JAMES P. DAUBERT, AND SHOMU BOHORA

Introduction

In the normal heart, electrical signals can only pass between the atria and the ventricles through the atrioventricular (AV) node (AVN). In 1893, however, Kent[1] described the rare occurrence of extranodal, electrically active tissue between the atria and the ventricles. Mines suggested in 1914 that this AV tissue (*accessory pathway*) may create a circuit that can allow for the creation of a tachyarrhythmia circuit. Wolff and White in Boston and Parkinson in London reported in 1930 their combined series of 11 patients with slurred upstroke to their QRS complexes and short PR intervals.[2] In 1944, Segers then introduced the triad of short PR interval, preexcitation of the ventricles characterized by an early slurred upstroke of the QRS complex (*delta wave*), and tachyarrhythmia that constitute the *Wolff-Parkinson-White (WPW) syndrome*. Its history has been reviewed.[3] The prevalence of preexcitation is approximately 0.1% to 0.2% in the population.[4,5] Most of the patients are asymptomatic. Only a few patients who have pathological tachycardia present with history of palpitations, presyncope, and syncope. Sudden cardiac death can rarely be a presentation of preexcitation syndrome.

Clinical Perspective

Ventricular preexcitation refers to a congenital cardiac abnormality where part of the ventricular myocardium receives electrical activation from the atria before the impulse arrives via the normal AV conduction system. A schematic illustration of the anatomic relationship between the normal AV conduction system and the accessory AV conduction pathway provided by the accessory pathway is displayed in **Figure 19.1**. Nonconducting structures, which include the coronary arteries and veins, valves, and fibrous and fatty connective tissues, prevent conduction of electrical impulses from the atrial myocardium to the ventricular myocardium. The AV myocardial bundles commonly exist during fetal life but then disappear by the time of birth.[6] When even a single myocardial connection persists, there is the potential for ventricular preexcitation. In some individuals, evidence of preexcitation and/or the WPW syndrome may not appear until later in life. Conversely, WPW syndrome may present in infants and require treatment. In some such patients, the accessory pathway conduction may decrease over time or even cease all together.[7] WPW syndrome is not associated with congenital structural abnormalities in most patients, but is seen with increased frequency in patients with Ebsteins anomaly, hypertrophic cardiomyopathy, and transposition physiology.

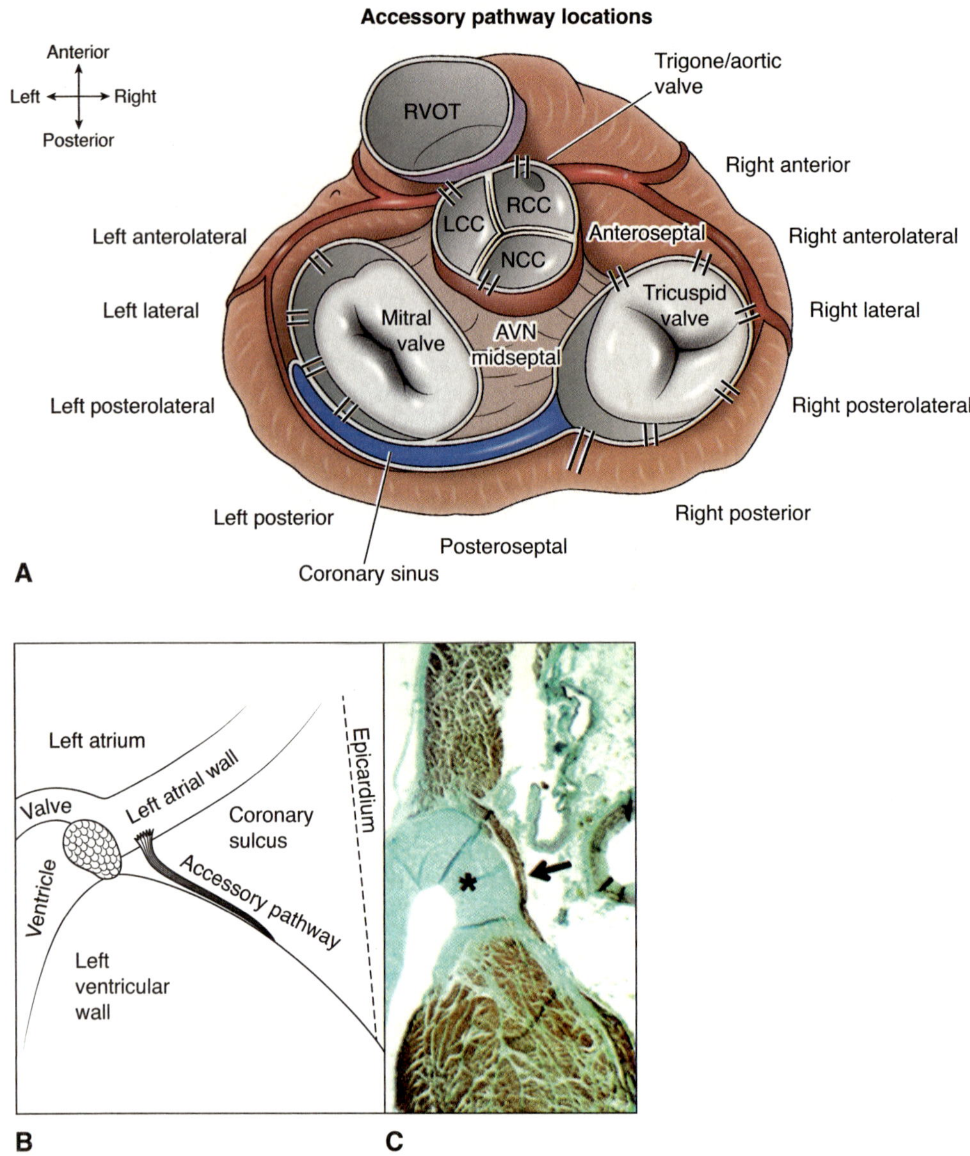

FIGURE 19.1. Normal atrioventricular (AV) conduction system (AV node [AVN]) is located in the mid-superior aspect of the interatrial septum separating the right atrium from the left atrium and communicates electrical signals to the ventricles via the His-Purkinje system. **A.** The AV aspect of the heart in short axis. Accessory pathways may exist at any location around the tricuspid and/or mitral valve annulus where there is atrial myocardium on the atrial side of the AV groove and ventricular myocardium on the ventricular side of the AV groove (including within the coronary sinus and cardiac venous system). LCC, left-coronary cusps of aortic valve; NCC, non-coronary cusps of aortic valve; RCC, right-coronary cusps of aortic valve; RVOT, right ventricular outflow tract. **B,C.** Histologic section perpendicular to the AV groove demonstrating an accessory pathway, a small band of muscular tissue crossing the AV groove from atrium to ventricle.

Figure 19.2 illustrates the two types of altered conduction from the atria (PR interval) to the ventricles (QRS interval) that result in a wide QRS, due to either delayed ventricular activation from aberrancy in the His-Purkinje system (eg, bundle-branch block) and/or fascicular block or earlier ventricular activation (ie, ventricular preexcitation) due to presence of an accessory pathway. Normally, the QRS is narrow because of synchronous activation of both the ventricles through the bundle branches (**Figure 19.2A**). Right- or left-bundle-branch block (LBBB) does not alter the PR interval but prolongs the QRS complex by delaying activation of one of the ventricles (**Figure 19.2B**). Ventricular preexcitation, due to a connection of the ventricle to the atria via an accessory muscle bundle, shortens the PR interval and produces a "delta wave" in the initial part of the QRS complex (**Figure 19.2C**). The total time from the beginning of the P wave to the end of the QRS complex remains the same as in the normal condition because conduction via the accessory pathway does not interfere with conduction via the normal AV conduction system. Therefore, before the entire ventricular myocardium can be activated by progression of the preexcitation wavefront, electrical impulses from the more rapidly conducting His-Purkinje system arrive to activate the remainder of the ventricular myocardium.[8]

Because the accessory pathway and His-Purkinje compete to activate ventricular myocardium, more rightward accessory pathways (closer to the impulse initiating sinus node) that conduct rapidly will create more ventricular preexcitation (larger, more prominent delta waves and a wider QRS complex). On the other hand, patients with a relatively shorter native PR interval (due to more rapid AV nodal conduction) and/or patients with left free wall accessory pathways (further away from the impulse initiating sinus node) will exhibit less ventricular preexcitation (a relatively longer PR interval; smaller, less prominent delta waves; and a less wide QRS).

In some cases, if AV nodal conduction is fast, then findings of ventricular preexcitation from a left-sided pathway may be subtle or even inapparent. The most common location for an accessory pathway is "left lateral," far away from the sinus node. As a result, if a patient with documented tachyarrhythmia has a baseline electrocardiogram (ECG) with a short PR, especially if there is lack of an isoelectric segment between the P wave and the onset of the QRS, there should be a high level of suspicion that an accessory pathway may be present.

Pathophysiology

Wolff-Parkinson-White Syndrome

The combination of the following has been termed the WPW syndrome:

1. PR interval duration of <0.12 second
2. A delta wave at the beginning of the QRS complex
3. Tachyarrhythmia with mechanism dependent on accessory pathway conduction

The PR interval is short because the electrical impulse bypasses the normal AV nodal conduction delay. The delta wave is produced by early but relatively slow intramyocardial conduction that results when the impulse, instead of being delivered to the ventricular myocardium via the His-Purkinje system, is delivered directly into the ventricular myocardium via an abnormal or "anomalous" muscle bundle. The duration of the QRS complex

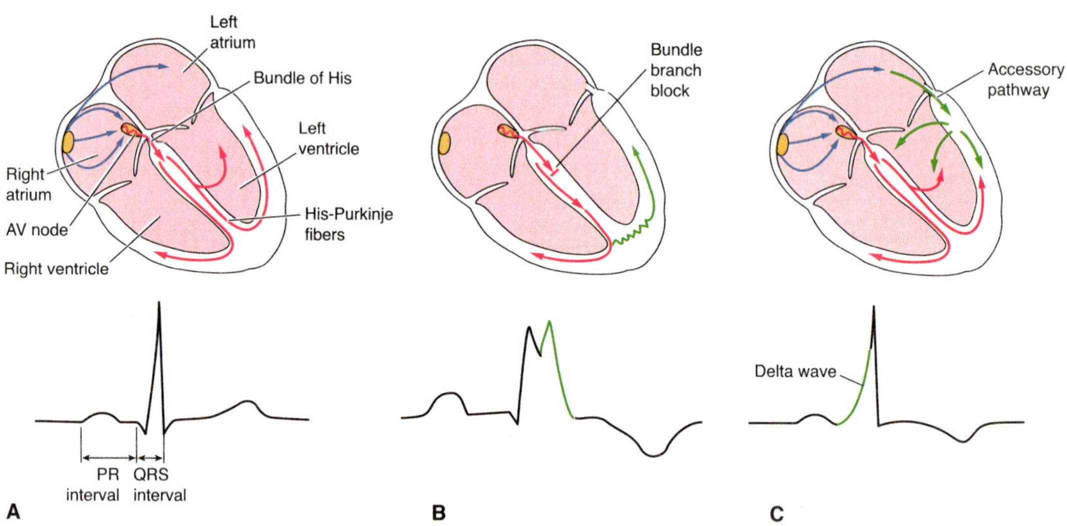

FIGURE 19.2. Basis for wide QRS due to bundle branch block or preexcitation. Normal atrioventricular (AV) conduction with-out bundle branch block or an accessory pathway (**A**). Wide QRS with a normal or prolonged PR interval due to bundle branch block. Delayed activation of the ventricle on the side of the blocked bundle produces widening of the QRS (**B**). Short PR interval with ventricular preexcitation due to the presence of an accessory pathway (**C**). Accessory pathway conduction to the ventricle activates the ventricle early because it does not need to pass through the slower conducting fibers of the AV node (short PR) but propagates more slowly through the ventricular myocardium because of lack of immediate access to the His-Purkinje fibers producing a slurred onset to the QRS (delta wave).

is prolonged because it begins "too early," in contrast with the situations presented in Chapter 5, in which the duration of the QRS complex is prolonged because it ends too late. The preexcited ventricular myocardium is activated initially from the accessory pathway, and then from the His-Purkinje system, rather than just from the His-Purkinje system (**Figure 19.2**). For additional instruction, see **Animation 19.1**, which illustrates the initiation of AV bypass SVT by competing conduction pathways through the accessory pathway (Kent bundle) and through the AV node to the His-Purkinje system.

The relationship between an accessory pathway conduction resulting in preexcitation of the ventricular myocardium and the typical ECG changes of ventricular preexcitation are illustrated on top and on bottom, respectively (see **Figure 19.2C**). **Figure 19.2A** illustrates the normal cardiac anatomy that permits AV conduction only via the AVN. Thus, there is normally a delay in the activation of the ventricular myocardium (PR segment), as noted in the ECG recording shown in the figure. When the congenital abnormality responsible for the WPW syndrome is present, the ventricular myocardium is activated from two sources via (1) the accessory pathway and (2) the His-Purkinje system. The initial part of the QRS complex is formed by the delta wave (slurred upstroke of the QRS complex), which is due to an abnormal preexcitation wave, and the mid and terminal portions of the QRS are formed due to activation by a normal His-Purkinje conduction. Right-sided pathways and patients with AV nodal disease demonstrate wider QRS complex as activation predominantly occurs due to abnormal preexcitation wave.

Arrhythmias associated with accessory pathways

A. Accessory pathway is integral in causing the tachycardia. (Treatment of pathway by ablation will result in abolishing the tachycardia.)

1. Orthodromic reciprocating tachycardia. (Narrow complex regular tachycardia, most common.)
2. Antidromic reciprocating tachycardia. (Broad complex regular tachycardia, commonly associated with multiple pathways, differentiating from VT sometimes is difficult.)
3. Duodromic tachycardia. (Involving more than one accessory pathway where both antegrade and retrograde conduction occur from pathways resulting in a broad QRS tachycardia.)
4. Atrial fibrillation (AF) causes a fast, irregularly irregular rhythm of broad QRS morphology and has varying QRS width due to varying preexcitation. Accessory pathway is considered essential for AF to occur, and treatment of pathway causes no further episodes of atrial fibrillation.
5. Spontaneous automaticity from accessory pathways.

B. Innocent bystander where accessory pathway is not necessary for causing the tachycardia, but merely results in preexcitation, resulting in a broad QRS preexcited rhythm. (Treatment of pathway by ablation will not result in the treatment of tachycardia but will only result in loss of preexcitation.) Primary tachycardia (atrio-ventricular nodal reentrant tachycardia [AVNRT], atrial tachycardia, atrial flutter, or atrial fibrillation) needs additional treatment along with pathway during ablation.

To view the animation(s) and video(s) associated with this chapter please access lww.co.in. Instructions are located on the inside front cover.

The abnormal AV muscular connection (accessory pathway) produces ventricular preexcitation. This abnormal connection may have the ability to conduct retrogradely as well as anterogradely. Under certain circumstances, an atrial premature beat may come too soon after the prior sinus beat to conduct anterogradely down the accessory pathway. Provided that retrograde accessory pathway conduction is present, that beat which had blocked in the accessory pathway in the anterograde direction may conduct via the AVN and His-Purkinje fibers to activate the ventricles. By the time this signal reaches the ventricular end of the accessory pathway, it may be able to conduct retrogradely to the atrium. This atrial activation is termed an "echo beat" (a beat that returns to the chamber of origin, in this case the atrium, making it an "atrial echo"). If this atrial echo beat reaches the AVN and finds the AVN able to conduct it to the ventricles, then this cycle may repeat, establishing a tachycardia circuit known as *atrioventricular reentrant* (or "reciprocating") *tachycardia* (AVRT). This type of tachycardia is specifically referred to as *orthodromic reciprocating tachycardia* (ORT) because the anterograde limb is using the His-Purkinje system, creating a narrow (normal) QRS complex in tachycardia, as opposed to *antidromic reciprocating tachycardia* (ART) that uses the accessory pathway as the anterograde limb of the tachycardia (producing a wide, preexcited QRS).

The ORT and ART are the two most common forms of AVRT. The ORT is more common than ART. The ORT could also be induced by a premature ventricular complex that happens to find the AVN–His-Purkinje system refractory. That premature ventricular complex may instead conduct to the atrium retrogradely up the accessory pathway and then anterogradely back the AVN–His-Purkinje system (if it has electrically recovered) (**Figure 19.3**). **Animation 19.2** provides additional information comparing micro reentry circuits that lead to AV nodal reentry tachycardia (see Chapter 15) vs. macro reentry circuits with WPW syndrome that cause supraventricular tachyarrhythmias. **Animation 19.3** then further explains the two mechanisms of ORT.

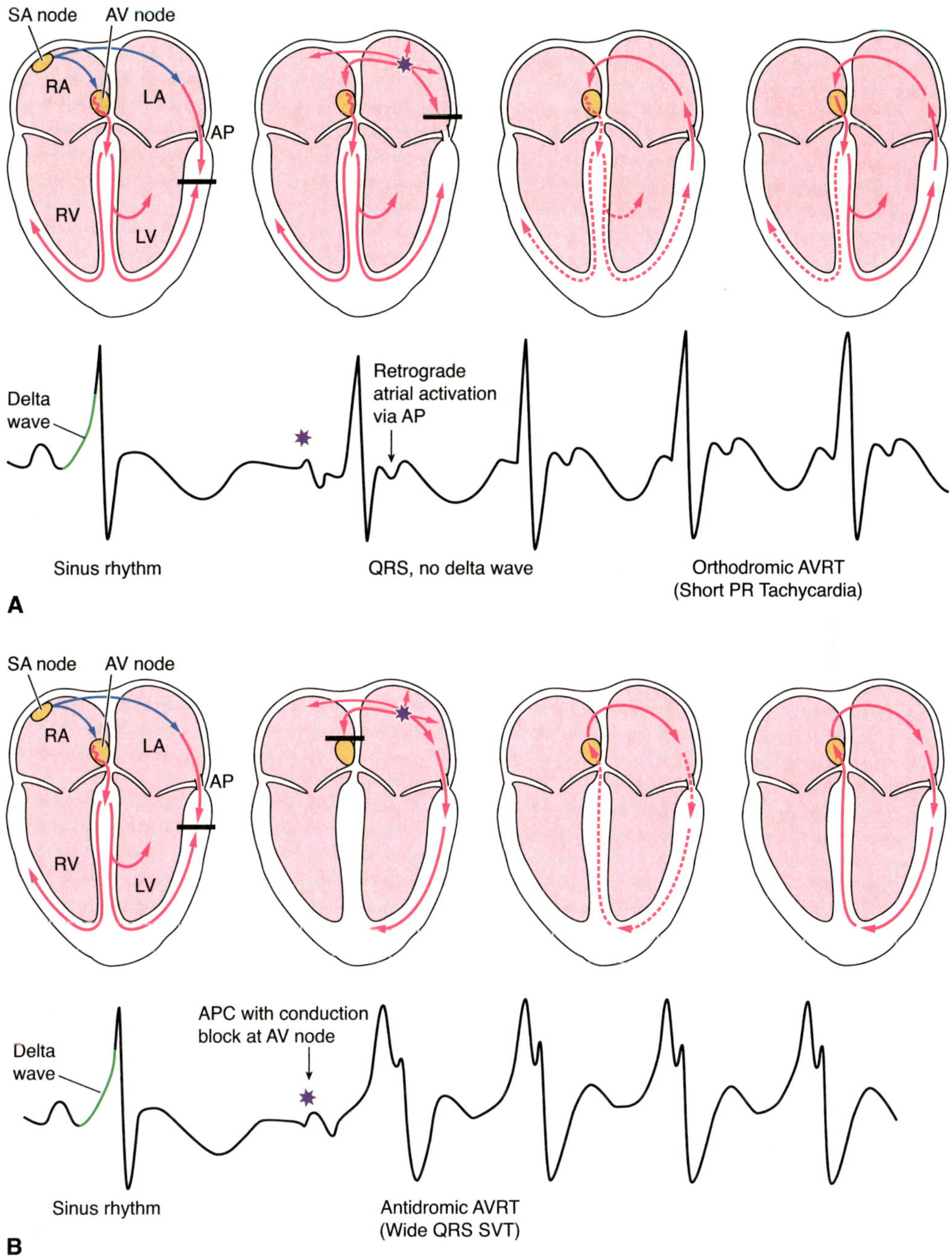

FIGURE 19.3. Induction of atrioventricular (AV) reentrant tachycardia from a premature atrial contraction (PAC). **A.** The PAC (*) blocks in the accessory pathway (AP) but after delay in the AV node is able to conduct down the His-Purkinje system producing a narrow QRS, "short RP" ("short RP" = RP interval < PR interval) tachycardia known as orthodromic reciprocating tachycardia (orthodromic because it conducts from the atrium to the ventricle anterograde down the His-Purkinje system). **B.** The PAC (*) blocks in the AV node but is able to conduct anterograde down the AP producing a wide QRS, "maximally preexcited" tachycardia ("maximally preexcited" = the majority or all of the ventricular myocardium is being activated by the AP, and minimal or none of the ventricular myocardium is being activated by His-Purkinje system). APC, atrial premature complexes; AVRT, antidromic reciprocating tachycardia; LA, left atrium; LV, left ventricle; RA, right atrium; RV, right ventricle; SA, sinoatrial.

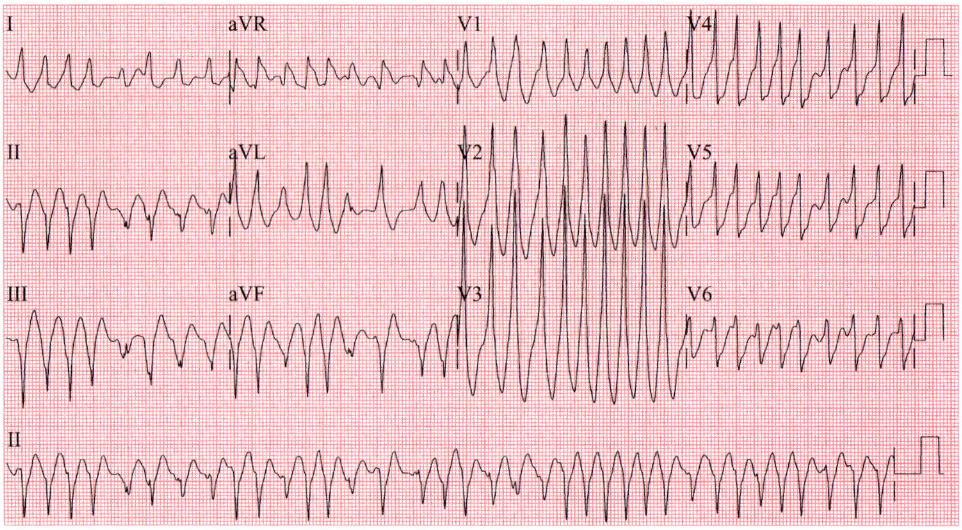

FIGURE 19.4. Ventricular preexcitation during atrial fibrillation.

Ventricular preexcitation, induced by an accessory pathway, influences the ventricular rate to become rapid in the presence of an atrial tachyarrhythmia such as atrial flutter/fibrillation (see Chapter 15). During such an episode, the ventricles are no longer "protected" by the delay in the AVN. A 12-lead ECG recording with a lead II rhythm strip of a 24-year-old woman with ventricular preexcitation during atrial fibrillation is displayed in **Figure 19.4**. The irregularities of both the ventricular rate and QRS complex morphology are apparent, especially on the 10-second lead II rhythm strip at the bottom of the figure. Although ECGs of preexcited atrial fibrillation may in some cases look so bizarre that it may be difficult to tell exactly what is going on, the "irregularly irregular" heart rhythm should be a clue that atrial fibrillation is present. Likewise, the variability in QRS complexes when reviewed closely demonstrate consistency among the widest QRS complexes ("maximally preexcited") and the narrowest ("minimally preexcited") with the intermediate width QRS complexes in between representing variable degrees of fusion of these two extremes.

Preexcited atrial fibrillation is a life-threatening arrhythmia and therefore is important to recognize and treat appropriately. Unlike rapid conduction of atrial fibrillation in the absence of ventricular preexcitation, it is important to avoid administering medications that may slow conduction through the AVN (eg, β-blockers, digitalis preparations, nondihydropyridine calcium channel blockers, and/or adenosine). By blocking conduction through the AVN, these agents force all atrial fibrillation to travel over the more rapidly conducting accessory pathway, potentially causing atrial fibrillation to become ventricular fibrillation.[9] Direct current cardioversion is a safe and effective treatment of preexcited atrial fibrillation if the rhythm is hemodynamically unstable. Antiarrhythmic drug suppression with procainamide, which will likely slow conduction over the accessory pathway and may terminate the atrial fibrillation, may also be effective. Amiodarone, although potentially effective, can cause hypotension and worsening, due to its acute beta-blocker action, and therefore, it should always be administered only when direct current cardioversion backup is available.

Electrocardiographic Diagnosis of Ventricular Preexcitation

Typically, with ventricular preexcitation, the PR interval is <0.12 second in duration, and the QRS complex is >0.10 second. Ventricular preexcitation produces a slurred onset to the QRS, which has been termed a "delta wave." The delta wave polarity should be based on the first 20 milliseconds of ventricular preexcitation. The timing of onset of ventricular preexcitation is best determined by identifying the earliest point of QRS onset/slurring in the most preexcited QRS complex in the frontal leads (ie, the QRS that is most slurred, earliest onset, broadest delta wave). The delta wave may be positive, negative, or isoelectric as illustrated in **Figure 19.5**.

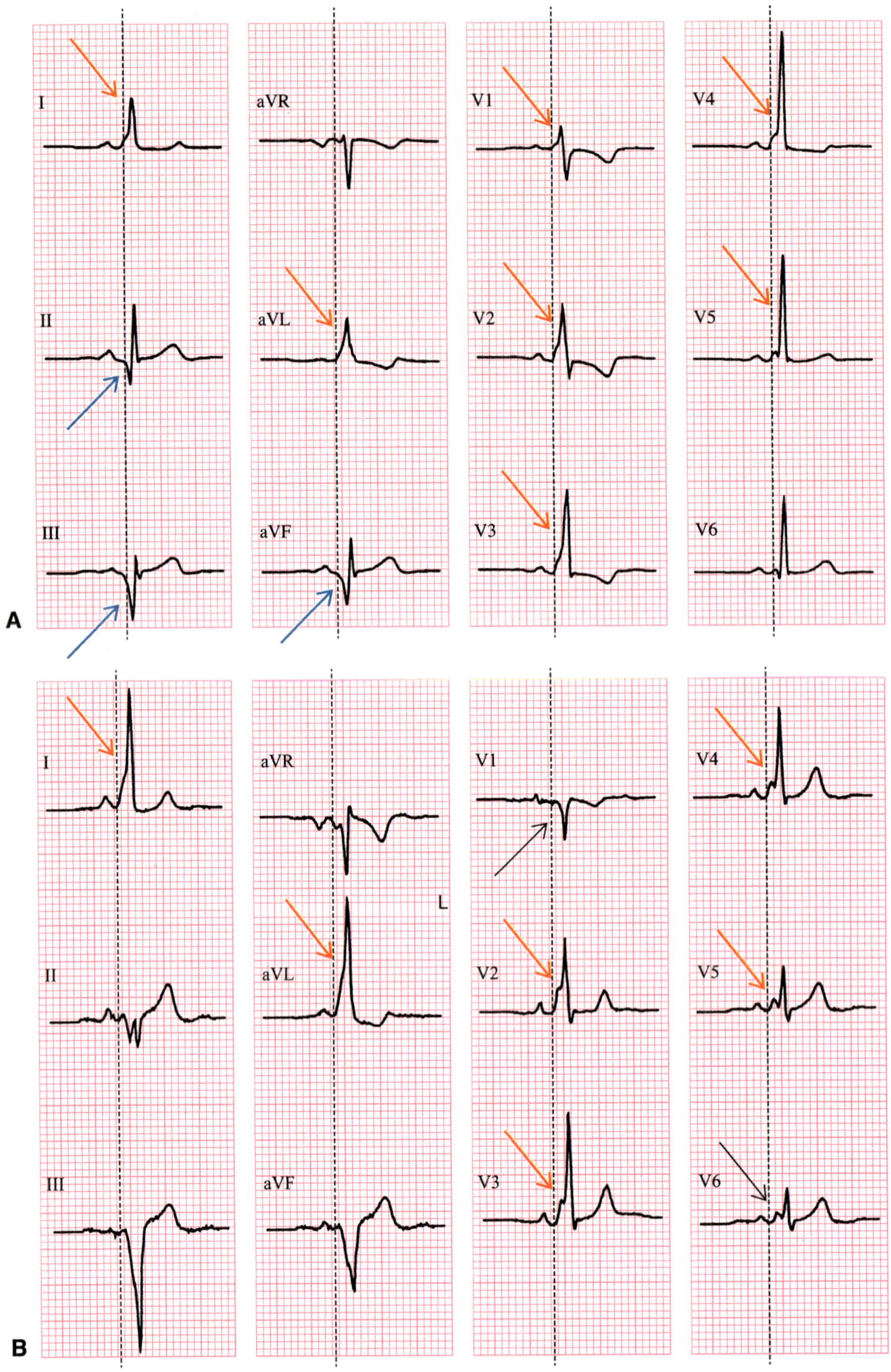

FIGURE 19.5. Positive and negative delta waves (arrows) in two patients. Both electrocardiograms (**A**,**B**) have negative delta waves in III and aVF indicating a posteroseptal or posterior accessory pathway position (ventricular activation directed superiorly) with V_1 delta wave positive in **A** indicating a more leftward origin (activation traveling toward the right-sided V_1 lead) consistent with a left posteroseptal (or left posterior) accessory pathway and V_1 delta negative in **B** indicating a more rightward origin (activation traveling away from the right-sided V_1 lead) consistent with a right posteroseptal accessory pathway.

The PR interval, however, is not always abnormally short, and the QRS complex is not always abnormally prolonged. **Figure 19.6A** illustrates an abnormally slow onset of the QRS complex following a normal PR interval (0.16 s). **Figure 19.6B** illustrates an abnormally short PR interval preceding a QRS complex of normal duration (0.08 s) but with no delta wave. When the PR is short but with no delta wave, ECG is classified as having Lown-Ganong-Levine (LGL) syndrome and is likely due to faster AV nodal conduction or due to accessory pathways inserting in the conduction system. P-wave morphology should be looked in these cases to see for ectopic low atrial rhythms. Conduction through an accessory pathway is usually fast and nondecremental. Less commonly, accessory pathways could, conduct slowly, be decremental, or even insert into the His-Purkinje system. Among almost 600 patients with documented ventricular preexcitation, 25% had PR intervals of ≥0.12 second, and 25% had a QRS complex duration of ≤0.10 second.[10] As if that were not confusing

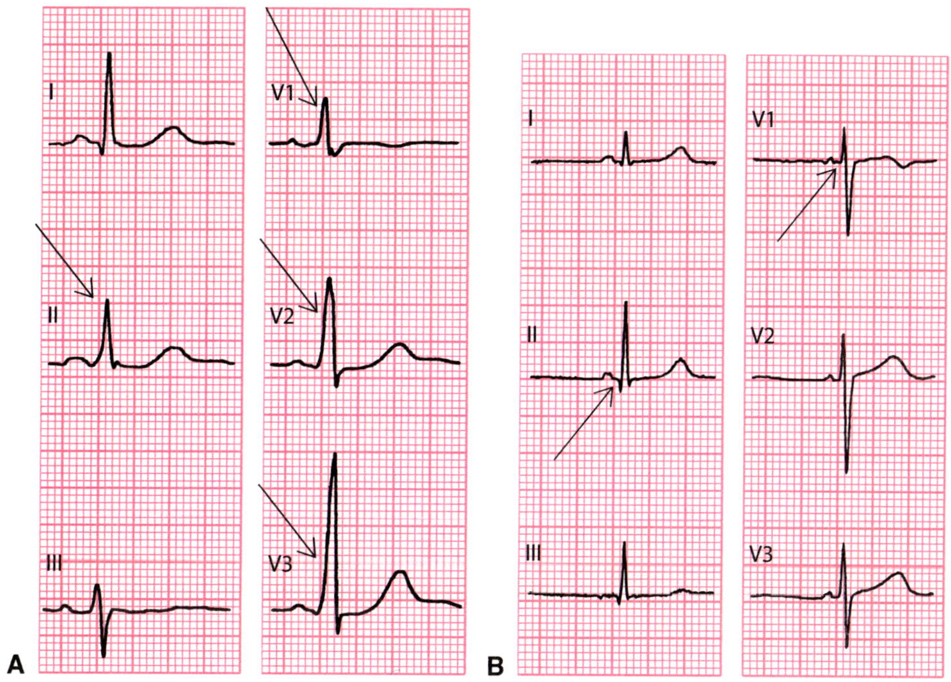

FIGURE 19.6. **A.** Slurred onset of the QRS complex following a normal PR interval (arrows); that is, there is a delta wave and preexcitation even though the PR is not short. **B.** Short PR interval preceding a normal QRS complex duration (arrows); that is, there is no delta wave or preexcitation even though the PR is short.

enough, accessory pathways may conduct retrograde only (referred to as a "concealed accessory pathway"). A "retrograde conducting only" pathway, by definition, cannot produce ventricular preexcitation and therefore cannot be seen on a sinus rhythm 12-lead ECG. Such a "retrograde conducting only" pathway could, however, participate in an AVRT (ie, ORT).

When evidence of ventricular preexcitation is subtle in a patient with tachyarrhythmia or suspected ventricular preexcitation, the following diagnostic procedures may be helpful:

Potentially Helpful Diagnostic Procedures for Identifying Ventricular Preexcitation

1. Perform a Holter monitor and look for electrocardiograms at times of varying autonomic tone (eg, higher vagal tone), or look for heart rate changes or premature atrial contractions that might slow in the atrioventricular (AV) node and make ventricular preexcitation more clear.
2. Perform maneuvers to increase vagal tone to create decrement in the AV node to make changes of ventricular preexcitation more apparent.
3. Perform an ECG while giving intravenous adenosine to block the AV node and increase conduction through the accessory pathway bringing out preexcitation.
4. Perform an electrophysiology study to look for retrograde and/or anterograde conduction external to the AV node.

Ventricular Preexcitation as a "Great Mimic" of Other Cardiac Problems

Ventricular preexcitation may mimic a number of other cardiac abnormalities. When there is a wide, positive QRS complex in leads V_1 and V_2, it may simulate right-bundle-branch block, right-ventricular hypertrophy, or a posterior myocardial infarction. When there is a wide, negative QRS complex in lead V_1 or V_2, preexcitation may be mistaken for LBBB (**Figure 19.7A**) or left-ventricular hypertrophy. A negative delta wave, producing Q waves in the appropriate leads, may imitate anterior, lateral, or inferior infarction. The prominent Q waves in leads aVF and V_1 in **Figure 19.7B** could be mistaken for inferior or anterior infarction, respectively (see Chapter 9). Similarly, the deep, wide Q wave in lead aVF and broad initial R wave in lead V_1 in **Figure 19.7C** could be mistaken for inferior or posterior infarction, respectively.

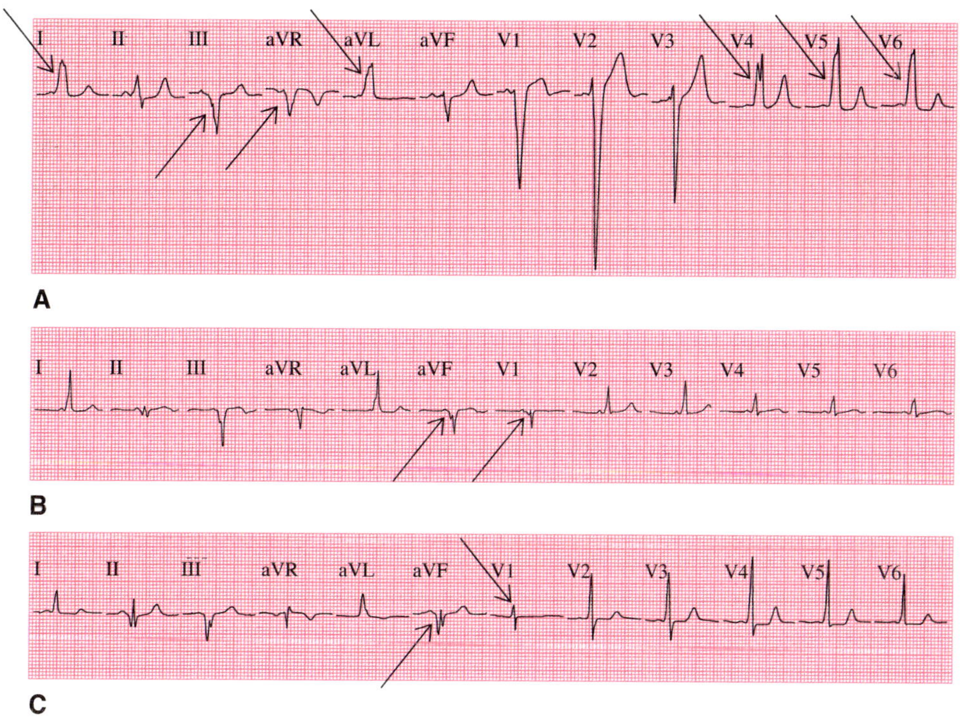

FIGURE 19.7. **A.** Delta waves (arrows). **B,C.** Delta waves mimicking myocardial infarction (arrows).

Although accessory pathways may be found anywhere in the connective tissue between the atria and ventricles, nearly all are found in three general locations, as follows:

Common Locations for Accessory Pathways Producing Ventricular Preexcitation

1. Left laterally, between the left-atrial and left-ventricular free walls (50%)
2. Posteriorly, between the atrial and ventricular (30%) (right AV valve, left AV valve, and the coronary sinus [CS]; CS sinus ostium, CS body, middle cardiac vein [MCV]-CS junction, and coronary sinus diverticulum)
3. Right laterally or anteriorly, between the right-atrial and right-ventricular free walls (20%)

The three general locations are illustrated as a schematic view (from above) of a cross-section of the heart at the junction between the atria and the ventricles in **Figure 19.1**. The ventricular outflow aortic and pulmonary valves are located anteriorly, and the ventricular inflow mitral (bicuspid) and tricuspid valves are located posteriorly.

Parahisian (antero-septal and mid-septal) location and epicardial (CS and appendage to ventricular connections) location of pathways are uncommon.

Electrocardiographic Localization of the Pathway of Ventricular Preexcitation

Many attempts have been made to determine the myocardial location of ventricular preexcitation according to the direction of the delta waves in the various ECG leads.[11-16] All the available algorithms to localize the pathway are based on preexcitation (delta wave) axis and/or QRS axis and/or QRS morphology, and they provide a rough guide to limit the area of mapping during treatment by ablation.[11-20] Precise localization of an accessory AV pathway is made difficult by several factors. These factors include minor degrees of preexcitation, the presence of more than one accessory pathway, obliquity of pathways, and distortions of the QRS complex caused by structural heart disease (congenital abnormalities, myocardial infarction, ventricular hypertrophy, etc.).

Rosenbaum and colleagues[11] divided patients into two groups (groups A and B) on the basis of the direction of the "main deflection of the QRS complex" in transverse plane leads V_1 and V_2 (**Table 19.1**).

Table 19.1.

Relationship Between Accessory Pathway Location and Electrocardiographic (ECG) Changes

ECG Appearance	Location of Abnormal Pathway
Group A: QRS mainly positive in leads V_1 and V_2	LA-LV
Group B: QRS mainly negative in leads V_1 and V_2	RA-RV

Abbreviations: LA, left atrium; LV, left ventricle; RA, right atrium; RV, right ventricle.

Other classification systems consider predominantly the direction of the delta wave in attempting to better localize the pathway of ventricular preexcitation. Milstein and associates[12] devised an algorithm that enabled them to correctly identify the location of 90% of >140 accessory pathways. Arruda algorithm is commonly used in electrophysiology (EP) laboratories.[14] **(Figure 19.8)** A negative or positive-negative delta in lead I and/or R/S ratio of more than 1 in lead V_1 suggests a left-sided pathway location. A negative delta in lead II suggests the pathway location to be in the CS/MCV region. When delta wave in V_1 is positive-negative or predominantly negative with positive delta/QRS in V_2, septal location of the pathway is considered, of which anteroseptal and midseptal pathway location can be recognized if there is positive in lead aVF, while if delta wave is positive-negative or negative in aVF, then the location of the pathway is considered to be posteroseptal.[14] A negative delta in V_1 and V_2 suggests the pathway location to be right sided.

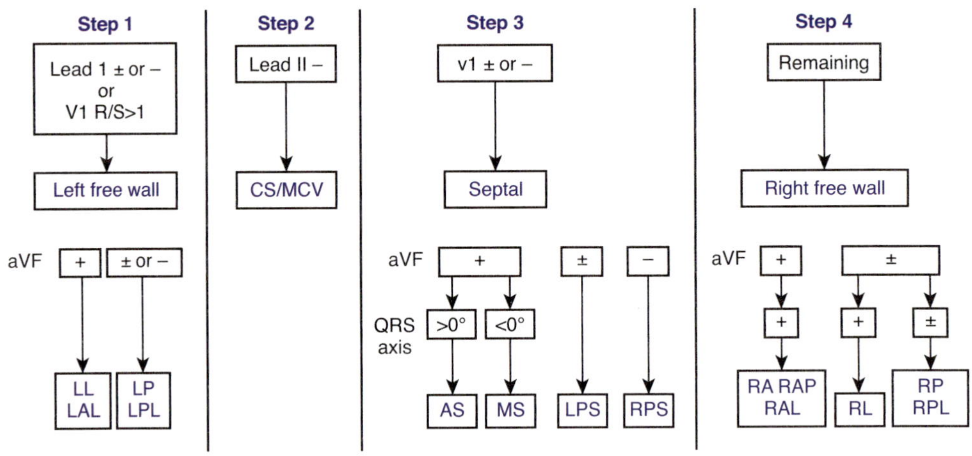

FIGURE 19.8. Mapping algorithm described by Arruda et al. to localize a pathway location using morphology of delta wave and QRS morphology on electrocardiogram. Reused with permission from Arruda et al, *Pacing Clin Electrophysiol* 1993; 16:865.

Tonkin and associates[13] presented a simple method for localizing accessory pathways to one of the foregoing areas on the basis of the direction of the delta wave (**Table 19.2**). They considered a point 20 milliseconds after the onset of the delta wave in the QRS complex as their reference.

Table 19.2.

Consideration of Delta Wave at QRS Onset + 0.02 s[a]

Direction of Preexcitation	Location of Pathway	Incidence Correct
Rightward	LA-LV free wall	10 of 10
Leftward and superior	Posterior septal	9 of 10
Leftward and inferior	RA-RV free wall	6 of 7

Abbreviations: LA, left atrial; LV, left ventricular; RA, right atrial; RV, right ventricular.

[a]From Sano S, Komori S, Amano T, et al. Prevalence of ventricular preexcitation in Japanese schoolchildren. *Heart*. 1998;79:374-378.

Ablation of Accessory Pathways

Although the first accessory pathway ablation procedures were performed with surgical dissection, virtually all accessory pathway ablations now are performed by catheter-based ablation techniques, in conjunction with a diagnostic electrophysiology testing and often three-dimensional electroanatomic mapping to localize and eliminate accessory pathway conduction. **Figures 19.9A** and **19.10A** illustrate the typical ECG appearances of preexcitation of the right ventricular free wall and the interventricular septum, respectively. Successful ablation of the accessory pathways (**Figures 19.9B** and **19.10B**) revealed the underlying presence of normal QRS complexes. The guidelines for electrophysiologic study and catheter ablation have been described.[20]

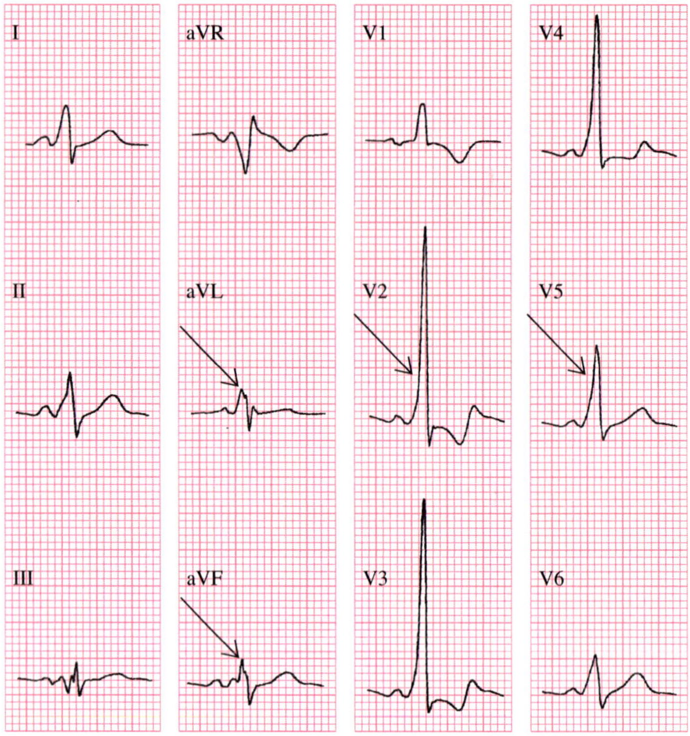

A

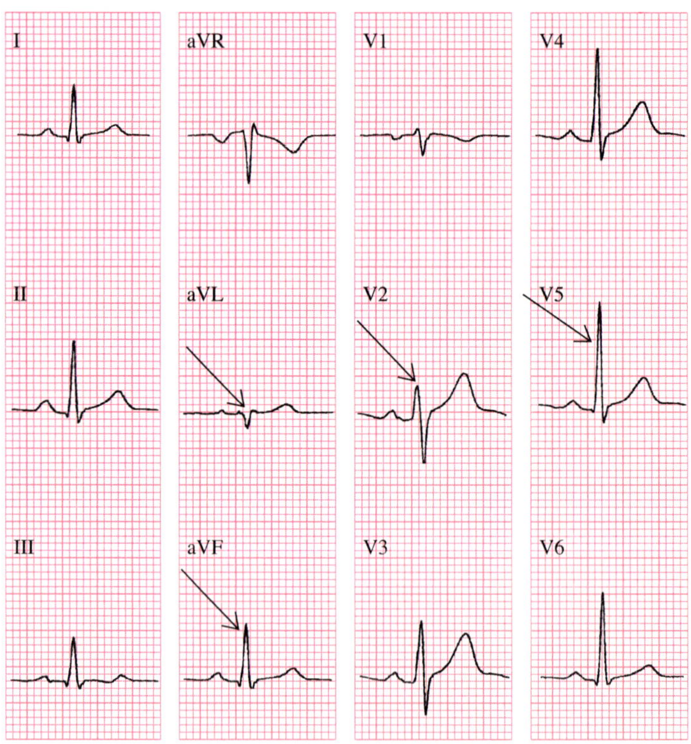

B

FIGURE 19.9. Radiofrequency ablation of a left ventricular free wall accessory pathway. **A.** Before the procedure. Delta waves are seen as shown by arrows. **B.** After the procedure. Arrows, Normal QRS complex is seen with disappearance of delta waves (arrows).

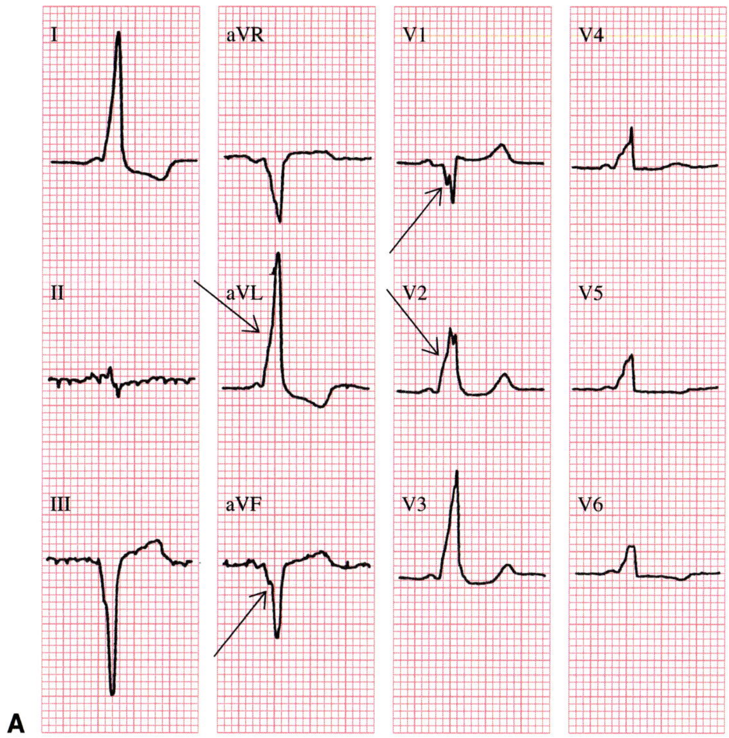

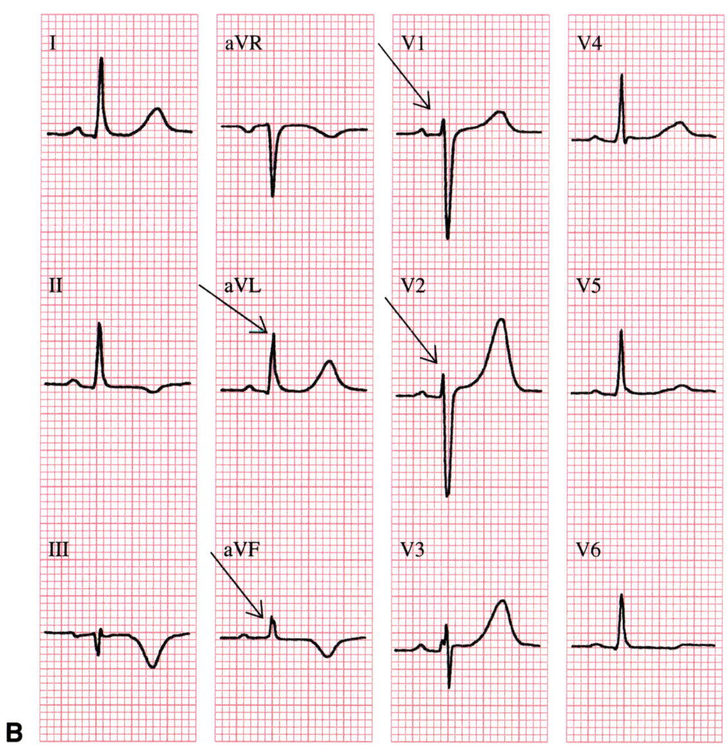

FIGURE 19.10. Radiofrequency ablation of a posteroseptal accessory pathway. **A.** Before the procedure. Arrows, delta waves. **B.** After the procedure. Arrows, normal QRS complex.

CHAPTER 19 SUMMARY ILLUSTRATION

ECG

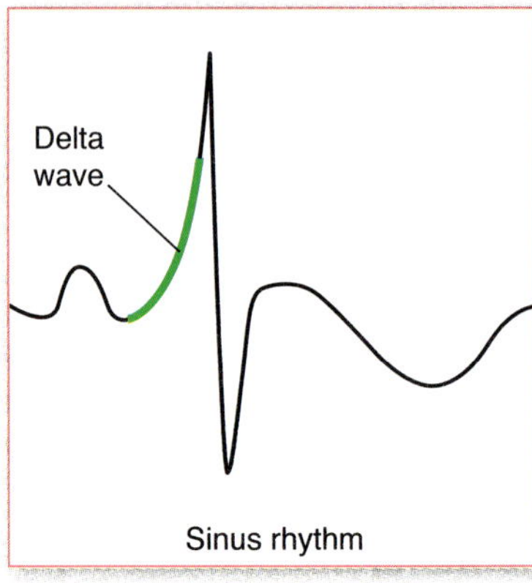

Schematic

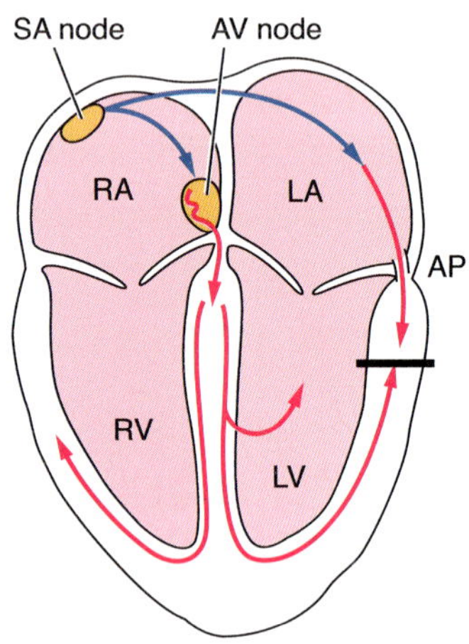

Arrhythmias

Orthodromic AVRT
Antidromic AVRT
Preexcited atrial fibrillation

Abbreviations: AP, accessory pathway; AV, atrioventricular; AVRT, atrioventricular reentrant (or "reciprocating") tachycardia; LA, left atrium; LV, left ventricle; RA, right atrium; RV, right ventricle; SA, sinoatrial.

Glossary

Accessory pathway: ectopic myocardial muscle bundles capable of conducting electrical signals between the atria and ventricles more rapidly than the slower conduction speeds of the AVN and His-Purkinje system. These accessory pathways may facilitate reentrant tachycardias by conduction in antegrade (atria to ventricles) and/or retrograde (ventricles to atria) direction.

Wolff-Parkinson-White (WPW) syndrome: combination of delta wave, short PR interval, and tachyarrhythmia.

Ventricular preexcitation: activation of the ventricles via an accessory pathway that conducts impulses at a faster conduction velocity than the AVN, thereby reaching the ventricles sooner than expected (eg, preexcited).

Delta wave: "slurred" initial portion of a QRS indicating evidence of early activation (preexcitation) of ventricles via an accessory pathway.

Atrioventricular reentrant tachycardia (also referred to as reciprocating tachycardia): tachyarrhythmia requiring both atrium and ventricles to be part of the circuit.

Antidromic reciprocating tachycardia: involves a continuous electrical circuit where the impulse travels from the atria to the ventricles via an accessory pathway and is sustained by retrograde conduction up the His-Purkinje system and the AVN to reach the atria and then return back down to the ventricles again via the accessory pathway.

Orthodromic reciprocating tachycardia: involves a continuous circuit where the impulse travels from the atria to the ventricles via the usual pathway of the AVN and His-Purkinje system but is sustained by retrograde conduction from the ventricles to the atria by an accessory pathway and then down again to the ventricles via the AVN and His-Purkinje system.

Acknowledgment

We gratefully acknowledge the past contributions of the previous edition's author, Dr. Galen S. Wagner, as portions of that chapter were retained in this revision.

References

1. Kent AFS. Research on the structure and function of the mammalian heart. *J Physiol.* 1893;14:i2-254.
2. Wolff L. Syndrome of short P-R interval with abnormal QRS complexes and paroxysmal tachycardia (Wolff-Parkinson-White syndrome). *Circulation.* 1954;10:282-291.
3. Scheinman MM. The history of the Wolff-Parkinson-White syndrome. *Rambam Maimonides Med J.* 2012;3:e0019.
4. Pelliccia A, Culasso F, Di Paolo FM, et al. Prevalence of abnormal electrocardiograms in a large, unselected population undergoing pre-participation cardiovascular screening. *Eur Heart J.* 2007;28:2006-2010.
5. Sano S, Komori S, Amano T, et al. Prevalence of ventricular preexcitation in Japanese schoolchildren. *Heart.* 1998;79:374-378.
6. Becker AE, Anderson RH, Durrer D, Wellens HJ. The anatomical substrates of Wolff-Parkinson-White syndrome. A clinicopathologic correlation in seven patients. *Circulation.* 1978;57:870-879.
7. Giardina ACV, Ehlers KH, Engle MA. Wolff-Parkinson-White syndrome in infants and children. A long-term follow-up study. *Br Heart J.* 1972;34:839-846.
8. Gallagher JJ, Gilbert M, Svenson RH, Sealy WC, Kasell J, Wallace AG. Wolff-Parkinson-White syndrome. The problem, evaluation, and surgical correction. *Circulation.* 1975;51:767-785.
9. Obeyesekere MN, Leong-Sit P, Massel D, et al. Risk of arrhythmia and sudden death in patients with asymptomatic preexcitation: a meta-analysis. *Circulation.* 2012;125:2308-2315.
10. Goudevenos JA, Katsouras CS, Graekas G, Argiri O, Giogiakas V, Sideris DA. Ventricular pre-excitation in the general population: a study on the mode of presentation and clinical course. *Heart.* 2000;83:29-34.
11. Rosenbaum FF, Hecht HH, Wilson FN, Johnston FD. Potential variations of thorax and esophagus in anomalous atrioventricular excitation (Wolff-Parkinson-White syndrome). *Am Heart J.* 1945;29:281-326.
12. Milstein S, Sharma AD, Guiraudon GM, Klein GJ. An algorithm for the electrocardiographic localization of accessory pathways in the Wolff-Parkinson-White syndrome. *Pacing Clin Electrophysiol.* 1987;10(3, pt 1):555-563.
13. Tonkin AM, Wagner GS, Gallagher JJ, Cope GD, Kasell J, Wallace AG. Initial forces of

ventricular depolarization in the Wolff-Parkinson-White syndrome. Analysis based upon localization of the accessory pathway by epicardial mapping. *Circulation*. 1975;52:1030-1036.
14. Arruda MS, McClelland JH, Wang X, et al. Development and validation of an ECG algorithm for identifying accessory pathway ablation site in Wolff-Parkinson-White syndrome. *J Cardiovasc Electrophysiol*. 1998;9:2-12.
15. Teixeira CM, Pereira TA, Lebreiro AM, Carvalho SA. Accuracy of the electrocardiogram in localizing the accessory pathway in patients with Wolff-Parkinson-White Pattern. *Arq Bras Cardiol*. 2016;107:331-338.
16. Maden O, Balci KG, Selcuk MT, et al. Comparison of the accuracy of three algorithms in predicting accessory pathways among adult Wolff-Parkinson-White syndrome patients. *J Interv Card Electrophysiol*. 2015;44:213-219.
17. Cobb FR, Blumenschein SD, Sealy WC, Boineau JP, Wagner GS, Wallace AG. Successful surgical interruption of the bundle of Kent in a patient with Wolff-Parkinson-White syndrome. *Circulation*. 1968;38:1018-1029.
18. Gallagher JJ, Pritchett EL, Sealy WC, Kasell J, Wallace AG. The preexcitation syndromes. *Prog Cardiovasc Dis*. 1978;20:285-327.
19. Jackman WM, Beckman KJ, McClelland JH, et al. Treatment of supraventricular tachycardia due to atrioventricular nodal reentry by radiofrequency catheter ablation of slow-pathway conduction. *N Engl J Med*. 1992;327:313-318.
20. Page RL, Joglar JA, Caldwell MA, et al. 2015 ACC/AHA/HRS Guideline for the Management of Adult Patients With Supraventricular Tachycardia: A Report of the American College of Cardiology/American Heart Association Task Force on Clinical Practice Guidelines and the Heart Rhythm Society. *J Am Coll Cardiol*. 2016;67:e27-e115.

To view digital content associated with this chapter please access lww.co.in. Instructions are located on the inside front cover.

20 Inherited Arrhythmia Disorders

JOHN SYMONS, ALBERT Y. SUN,
AND BHIMA SHANKAR P R

Introduction

Subtle differences in QRS-, ST-, or T-wave morphologies on electrocardiogram (ECG) most commonly represent benign variations on a population basis; however, in some instances, these changes represent diagnostic clues to identify rare, inherited disorders associated with an increased risk of sudden cardiac death (SCD). This group of inherited arrhythmia disorders is heterogeneous in regard to underlying mechanism and presentation. They do, however, share some important characteristics: (1) an increased risk of SCD; (2) result from functional mutations in ion channel, ion channel accessory proteins, or myocardial structural genes; (3) mostly appear in the absence of overt structural heart disease; and (4) have characteristic ECG patterns. The identification of these ECG patterns that include prolonged or shortened QT intervals, low amplitude notching in QRS complexes, or unusual-appearing bundle branch patterns is extremely important in the proper identification of these rare syndromes. This chapter explores this group of inherited arrhythmia disorders, their accompanying ECG patterns, and some of their defining clinical features.

The Long QT Syndrome (LQTS)

The *long QT syndrome* (LQTS) is a disorder of abnormal myocardial repolarization characterized by a prolonged QT interval (see Chapter 3) on ECG and an increased risk of SCD.[1] This abnormal repolarization can lead to the development of fatal ventricular arrhythmias such as torsades de pointes (see Chapter 17). The LQTS can either be an inherited condition, often involving a mutation in an ion channel-associated gene, or an acquired condition resulting from medication exposure, electrolyte derangements, or myocardial ischemia.[2]

LQTS Electrocardiographic Characteristics

QT Interval

A prolonged QTc interval (see Chapter 3) is the hallmark of LQTS. However, prolonged QTc should not be used as the sole diagnostic criteria because up to a quarter of genotype-positive LQTS patients may have a normal QTc. In addition, as QT intervals in a population follow a normal distribution, at least 2.5% of the general population will have a "prolonged QTc" (≥450 ms in men and ≥460 ms in women) as per the guidelines.[3] See the "Electrocardiogram as Used in Diagnosis" section.

In general, QTc intervals >500 milliseconds are associated with an increased risk of sudden death. Because the QTc interval is dynamic and changes under different physiologic conditions, the longest QTc interval should be used for risk stratification.[4]

T-wave Morphology

Currently, there have been at least 15 genes identified as loci for congenital LQTS; however, three major genes (*KCNQ1*, *KCNH2*, and *SCN5A*) represent the majority of cases.[5] These three main subtypes of LQTS often have subtle characteristic differences in T-wave morphology that should be noted.[6]

LQT1 represents the most common loci of LQTS (30%-25%) and results from a loss-of-function mutation in the *KCNQ1* gene that encodes the α-subunit of Kv7.1, the slow-activating potassium channel responsible for the IKs current. The ECG in LQT1 is characterized by an early-onset broad-based T wave (**Figure 20.1A**).

LQT2 is the second most common loci for LQTS (35%-40%) and stems from mutations in the *KCNH2* gene encoding the alpha (HERG) subunit of the potassium channel responsible for the IKr current. The T waves in LQT2 are usually low amplitude and bifid (**Figure 20.1B**).

LQT3 arises from gain of function mutations in the SCN5A that encodes for the rapidly inactivating sodium channels NaV1.5. The ECG in LQT3 shows long isoelectric ST segments with a late-appearing T wave (**Figure 20.1C**).

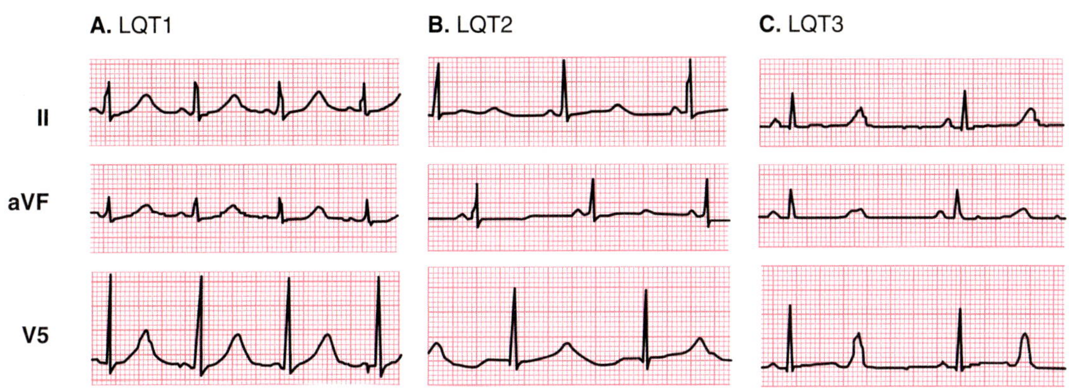

FIGURE 20.1. Genotype specific electrocardiogram patterns in long QT syndrome. **A.** LQT1—early onset broad-based T wave. **B.** LQT2 low amplitude and bifid T wave. **C.** LQT3 long isoelectric ST segment with a late-appearing T wave.[7]

Electrocardiogram as Used in Diagnosis for LQTS

It is important to remember that a prolonged QT interval alone is not sufficient to make the diagnosis of LQTS; an increased risk of SCD is necessary. To assist with the diagnosis of LQTS, a diagnostic score has been created, known as the International Long QT Score or "Schwartz score" (**Table 20.1**). Although a score ≥3.5 makes the diagnosis of LQTS more likely, it also is not diagnostic.[8]

Table 20.1.

Schwartz Score[a]

Characteristics	Points
Electrocardiographic findings	
• QTc (calculated with Bazett formula)	
≥480 ms	3
460-470 ms	2
450 ms and male gender	1
• QTc fourth minute of recovery from exercise stress test ≥480 ms	1
• Torsades de pointes	2
• T-wave alternans	1
• Notched T wave in three leads	1
• Low heart rate for age (children), resting heart rate below second percentile for age	0.5
Clinical history	
• Syncope (one cannot receive points both for syncope and torsades de pointes)	
With stress	2
Without stress	1
• Congenital deafness	0.5
Family history	
• Other family members with definite LQTS	1
• Sudden death in immediate family members (before age 30 years)	0.5

Abbreviation: LQTS, long QT syndrome.

[a]Score: ≤1 point, low probability of LQTS; 1.5 to 3 points, intermediate probability of LQTS; ≥3.5 points, high probability.

The Short QT Syndrome (SQTS)

As with LQTS, *short QT syndrome* (SQTS) is a disorder of repolarization in this case associated with more rapid repolarization and therefore a short QT interval. Again, like LQTS, this condition can be congenital or acquired. Acquired causes of short QT include hyperthermia, hyperkalemia, hypercalcemia, acidosis, and changes in autonomic tone. Congenital SQTS is much more rare than LQTS, with <100 cases reported worldwide. The SQTS is defined by the presence of an abnormal QT interval (<300 ms) and an increased risk of ventricular arrhythmias and SCD. Not surprisingly, the genes currently associated with SQTS are involved in the repolarization phase of the cardiac action potential. These functional mutations lead to a gain-of-function in the three voltage-gated potassium channel genes: *KCNH2*, *KCNQ1*, and *KCNJ2*. This gain of function results in an increased efflux of potassium from the cell during the repolarization phase and a shortening of the action potential.[9]

SQTS Electrocardiographic Characteristics

QT Interval

Similar to LQTS, the QT interval in a population follows a normal distribution; thus, there will be many "normal" patients in the general population with a short QT interval <360 milliseconds. Regardless, patients with very short QT intervals (QTc <330 ms in males and QTc <340 ms in females) should be considered for SQTS even if they are asymptomatic because QT intervals this short are quite rare.

T-wave Morphology

Most SQTS patients have an absent ST segment, with the T wave beginning immediately after the S wave. The T wave also often appears peaked and narrow (**Figure 20.2**).

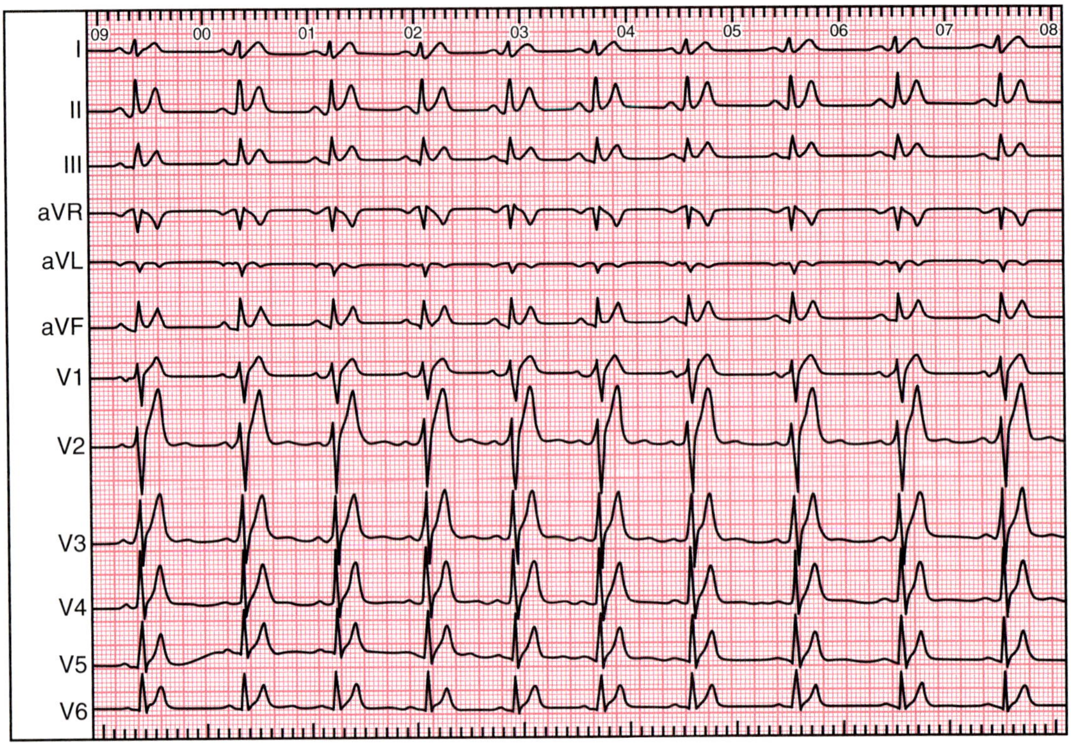

FIGURE 20.2. Short QT syndrome. (From Moreno-Reviriego S, Merino JL. Short QT syndrome. *E-J ESC Counc Cardiol Prac.* 2010;9:2-17, with permission.)

Electrocardiogram as Used in Diagnosis for SQTS

Similar to LQTS, a short QT interval alone is not sufficient to make the diagnosis of SQTS; an increased risk of SCD is necessary. To assist with the diagnosis of SQTS, a diagnostic score has been created (**Table 20.2**).[9] Although a score ≥4 makes the diagnosis of SQTS more likely, it is not sufficient to make the diagnosis.

Table 20.2.

Short QT Syndrome Diagnostic Criteria[a]

Characteristic	Points
Electrocardiographic findings	
• QTc (calculated with Bazett formula)	
<370 ms	1
<350 ms	2
<330 ms	3
• J-point–T-peak interval <120 ms	1
Clinical history	
• History of sudden cardiac arrest	2
• Documented polymorphic VT or VF	2
• Unexplained syncope	1
• Atrial fibrillation	1
Family history	
• First- or second-degree relative with high-probability SQTS	2
• First- or second-degree relative with autopsy-negative SCD	1
• Sudden infant death syndrome	1
Genotype	
• Genotype positive	2
• Mutation of undetermined significance in a culprit gene	1

Abbreviations: SCD, sudden cardiac death; SQTS, short QT syndrome; VF, ventricular fibrillation; VT, ventricular tachycardia.

[a]Score: ≤2 points, low probability; 3 points, intermediate probability; ≥4 points, high probability of SQTS.

The Brugada Syndrome

The *Brugada pattern* was first reported in 1953, but it was not until the ECG pattern was associated with SCD in 1992 that it became a recognized clinical syndrome.

The Brugada pattern is the hallmark of the *Brugada syndrome* and has a characteristic pattern on the ECG consisting of a pseudo–right-bundle-branch block (RBBB) and persistent ST-segment elevation in leads V_1 to V_3.[10]

Since the original description by Brugada and Brugada,[11] there have been three main patterns described (**Table 20.3**; **Figure 20.3**):

Brugada Patterns

1. Type 1: prominent high takeoff J-point elevation with a "coved-type" ST-segment elevation with amplitude of ≥2 mm leading to a negative T wave (**Figure 20.4**)
2. Type 2: high takeoff J-point elevation ≥2 mm with a gradually descending ST segment that remains ≥1 mm above the baseline leading to a positive or biphasic T wave; a "saddleback configuration"
3. Type 3: right precordial ST-segment elevation of <1 mm with either coved- or saddleback-type morphology

It is important to recognize that this pattern is often dynamic, and all three patterns can be observed in a single individual or even be completely concealed. Intravenous administration of certain drugs (mostly sodium channel blockers—Class I antiarrhythmic drugs) may exaggerate the ST-segment elevation or unmask it if it is initially absent.

A diagnosis of Brugada syndrome is made in patients with type 1 morphology that occurs either spontaneously or after provocative drug test and in patients with type 2 or type 3 patterns, when a provocative drug test induces a type I ECG morphology.[A]

Table 20.3.

ST-segment Abnormalities in Leads V_1 to V_3[a]

	Type 1	Type 2	Type 3
J-wave amplitude	≥2 mm	≥2 mm	≥2 mm
T wave	Negative	Positive or biphasic	Positive
ST-T configuration	Coved type	Saddleback	Saddleback
ST segment (terminal portion)	Gradually descending	Elevated ≥1 mm	Elevated <1 mm

[a]From Wilde AA, Antzelevitch C, Borggrefe M, et al. Proposed diagnostic criteria for the Brugada syndrome. *Eur Heart J*. 2002;23:1648-1654.

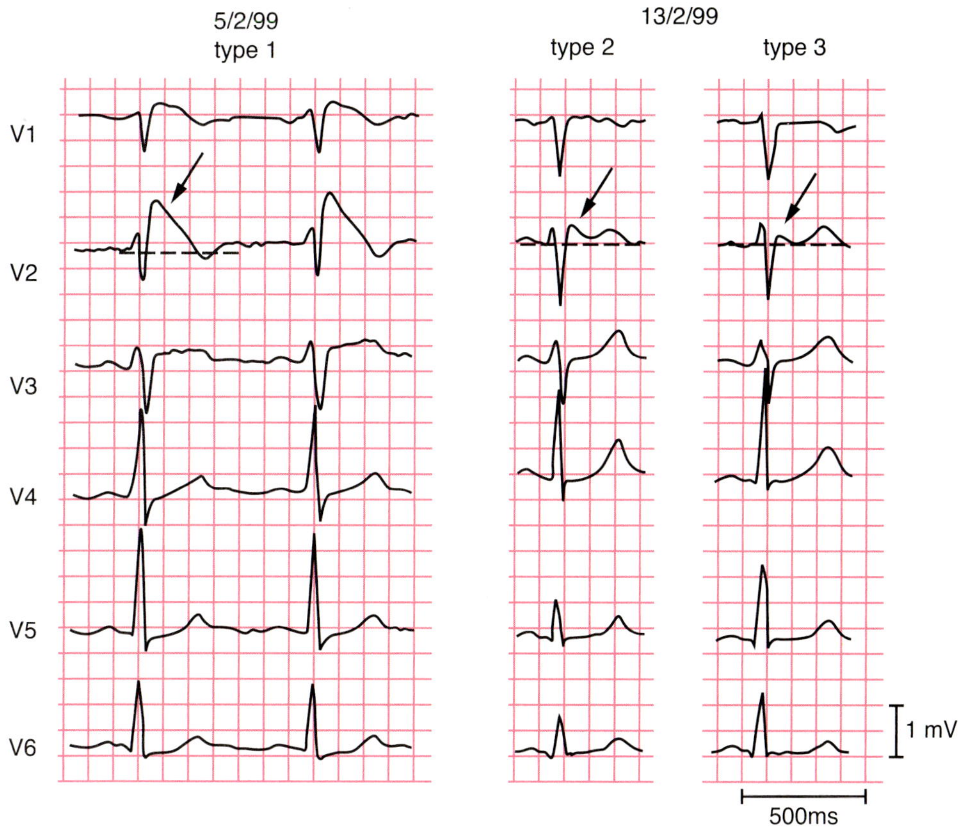

FIGURE 20.3. All three Brugada patterns demonstrated in the same patient. Arrows indicate J wave and the broken lines represent the isoelectric baseline. (Reprinted with permission from Wilde A, Antzelevitch C, Borggrefe M, et al. Proposed diagnostic criteria for the Brugada syndrome: consensus report. *Circulation*. 2002;106:2514-2519.)

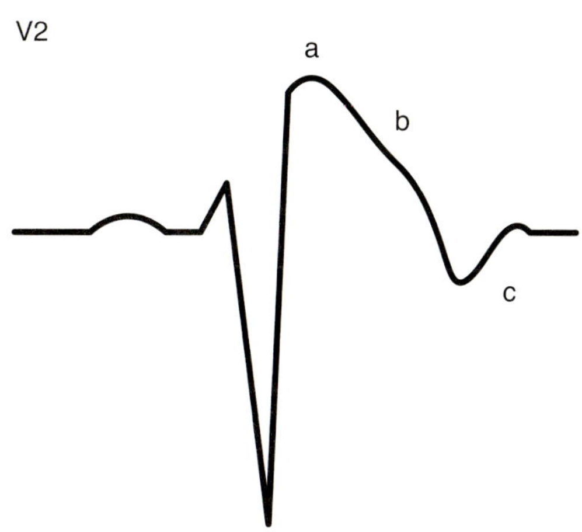

FIGURE 20.4. Electrocardiogram characteristics of the type 1 Brugada pattern: a, J-point elevation >2.0 mm; b, coved downsloping ST segment; and c, T-wave inversion. (Modified with permission from Australian Genetic Heart Disease Registry. Brugada syndrome. Australian Genetic Heart Disease Registry Web site. http://www.heartregistry.org.au/patients-families/genetic-heart-diseases/brugada-syndrome/. Accessed July 26, 2020.)

Arrhythmogenic Right-Ventricular Cardiomyopathy/Dysplasia

Arrhythmogenic right-ventricular cardiomyopathy/dysplasia is a predominantly genetic disorder of the heart muscle characterized pathologically by fibrofatty replacement of the right-ventricular and, occasionally, the left-ventricular myocardium. This myocardial disruption often leads to nonsustained or sustained ventricular arrhythmias and increased risk of SCD.[12-15]

Repolarization abnormalities present early and are sensitive markers of myocardial involvement. In conjunction with depolarization/conduction abnormalities and the presence of ventricular arrhythmias, these ECG findings are part of the diagnostic criteria for arrhythmogenic right-ventricular cardiomyopathy/dysplasia put forth by the European Society of Cardiology that also includes imaging, histology, and family history (**Table 20.4**).[12]

Table 20.4.

2010 Revised ECG-Related Task Force Criteria for Diagnosis of Arrhythmogenic Right-Ventricular Cardiomyopathy/Dysplasia[a]

I. Repolarization Abnormalities
Major
Inverted T waves in right precordial leads (V_1, V_2, and V_3) or beyond in individuals older than 14 years of age (in the absence of complete right-bundle-branch block QRS ≥120 ms) (**Figure 20.5**)
Minor
Inverted T waves in leads V_1 and V_2 in individuals older than 14 years of age (in the absence of complete right-bundle-branch block) or in V_4, V_5, or V_6
Inverted T waves in leads V_1, V_2, V_3, and V_4 in individuals older than 14 years of age in the presence of complete right-bundle-branch block
II. Depolarization/Conduction Abnormalities
Major
Epsilon wave (reproducible low-amplitude signals between end of QRS complex and onset of the T wave) in the right precordial leads (V_1-V_3) (**Figure 20.6**)
Minor
Late potentials by SAECG in ≥1 of 3 parameters in the absence of a QRS duration of ≥110 ms on the standard ECG
Filtered QRS duration (fQRS) ≥114 ms
Duration of terminal QRS, 40 mV (low-amplitude signal duration) ≥38 ms
Root-mean-square voltage of terminal 40 ms ≤20 mV
Terminal activation duration of QRS ≥55 ms measured from the nadir of the S wave to the end of the QRS, including R′, in V_1, V_2, or V_3, in the absence of complete right-bundle-branch block (see **Figure 20.5**)
III. Arrhythmias
Major
Nonsustained or sustained ventricular tachycardia of left-bundle-branch morphology with superior axis (negative or indeterminate QRS in leads II, III, and aVF and positive in lead aVL) (**Figure 20.7**)
Minor
Nonsustained or sustained ventricular tachycardia of RV outflow configuration, left-bundle-branch block morphology with inferior axis (positive QRS in leads II, III, and aVF and negative in lead aVL) or of unknown axis
500 ventricular extrasystoles per 24 hours (Holter)

Abbreviations: ECG, electrocardiogram; RV, right ventricular; SAECG, signal-averaged electrocardiogram.

[a]A definite diagnosis is established by the presence of two major, one major plus two minor, or four minor criteria (from different categories). A borderline diagnosis is established by fulfilling one major and one minor or three minor criteria from different categories. A possible diagnosis is established by the presence of one major or two minor criteria from different categories.[12]

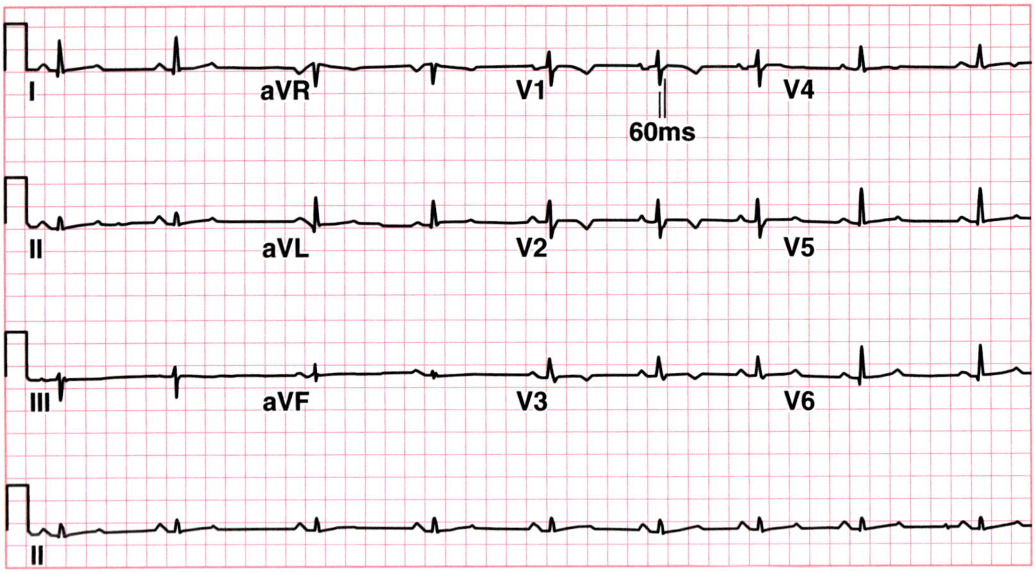

FIGURE 20.5. An electrocardiogram T-wave characteristics of arrhythmogenic right-ventricular cardiomyopathy/dysplasia. T-wave inversion in V_1 through V_4 and prolongation of the terminal activation duration ≥55 ms measured from the nadir of the S wave to the end of the QRS complex in V_1. (From Marcus FI, McKenna WJ, Sherrill D, et al. Diagnosis of arrhythmogenic right ventricular cardiomyopathy/dysplasia: proposed modification of the Task Force Criteria. *Eur Heart J*. 2010;31:806-814. Copyright © 2010 by the European Heart Journal; by permission of Oxford University Press.)

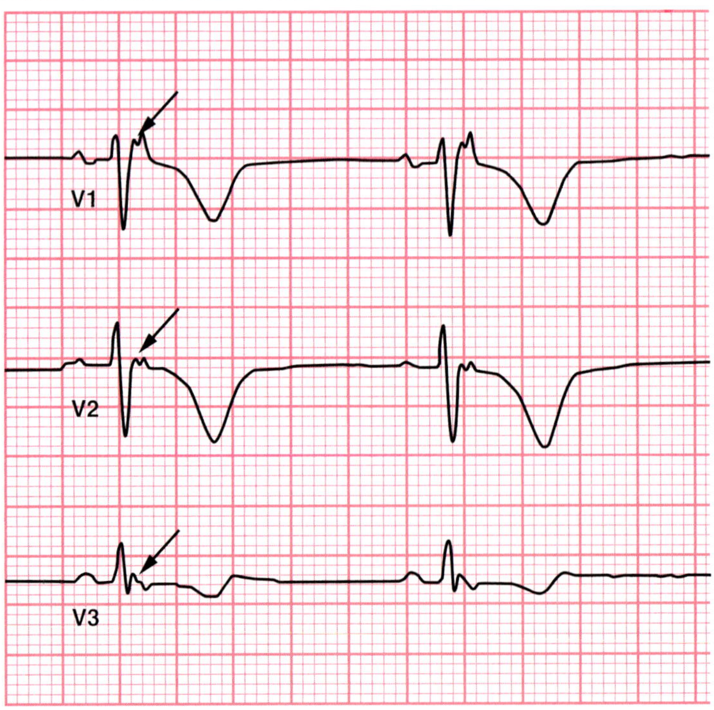

FIGURE 20.6. Electrocardiogram epsilon wave characteristics of arrhythmogenic right ventricular cardiomyopathy/dysplasia. Epsilon wave (arrows) in leads V_1 to V_3. (Modified from Kiès P, Bootsma M, Bax J, Schalij MJ, van de Wall EE. Arrhythmogenic right ventricular dysplasia/cardiomyopathy: screening, diagnosis, and treatment. *Heart Rhythm*. 2006;3[2]:225-234. Copyright © 1983 Elsevier. With permission.)

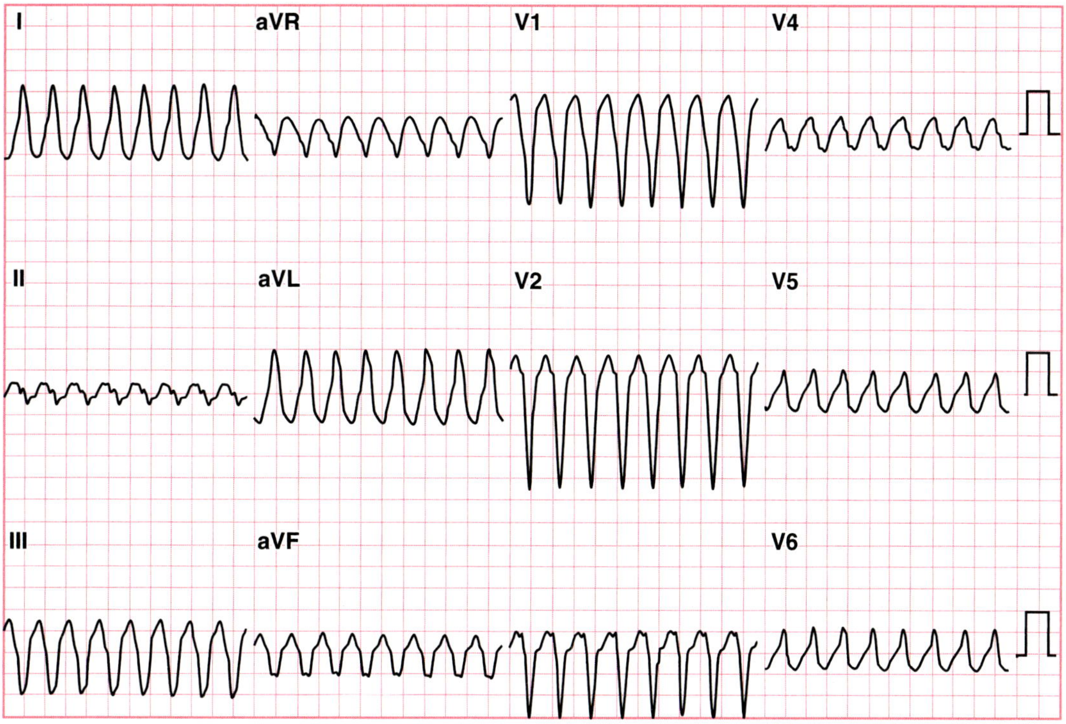

FIGURE 20.7. Left-bundle-branch block/superior axis ventricular tachycardia from a patient with arrhythmogenic right-ventricular cardiomyopathy/dysplasia. (Courtesy of Dr. Kurt S. Hoffmayer and Dr. Melvin M. Scheinman.)

J-wave Syndrome

The pattern on ECG characterized by accentuated J-point elevation at the terminal portion of the QRS and beginning of the ST segment, previously described as early repolarization, is now referred to as the *J-wave pattern*. This pattern is seen in approximately 6% of the general population, but it may be even more prevalent in younger patients, athletes, and persons of African descent. Recently, reports linking this supposedly benign pattern to an increased risk of SCD have garnered much attention.[16,17] Collectively, these studies have demonstrated an increased prevalence of this ECG pattern, defined as ≥0.1 mV J-point elevation in two adjacent inferior or lateral leads with a notching or slurring pattern (**Figure 20.8**),[18] in patients who suffer from idiopathic ventricular fibrillation. When this J-wave pattern occurs with a resuscitated cardiac arrest event, documented ventricular fibrillation or polymorphic ventricular tachycardia (VT), or with a family history of a causative genetic mutation, the terminology *J-wave syndrome* applies.[19]

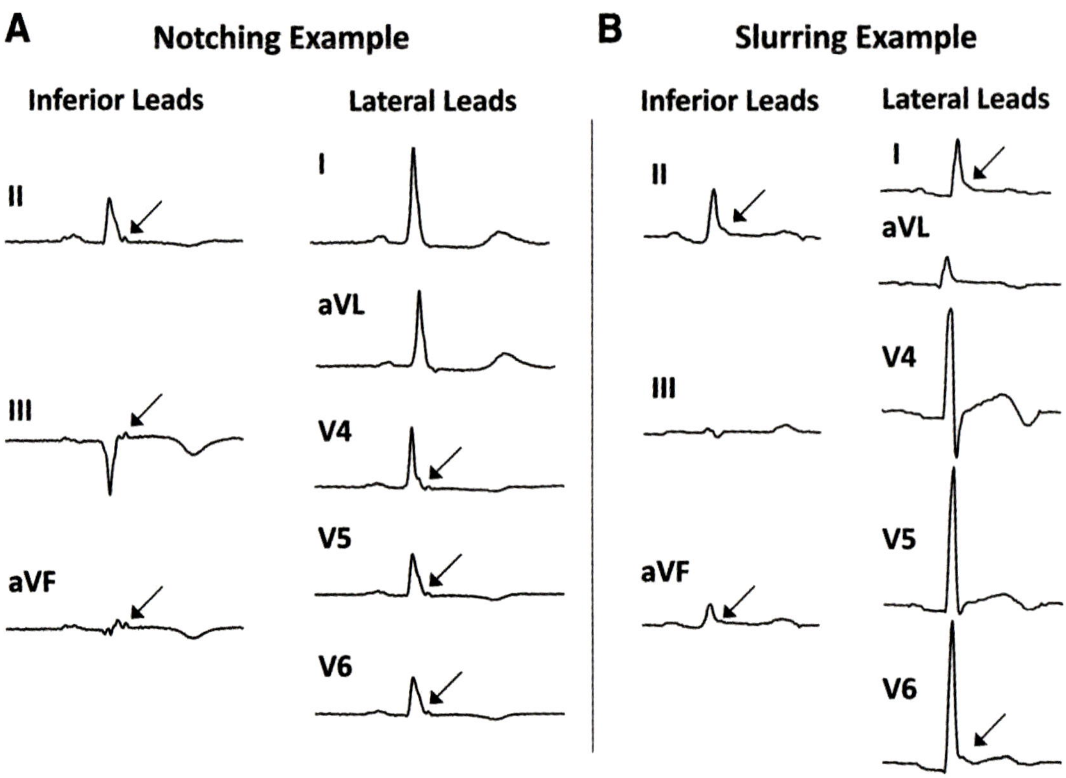

FIGURE 20.8. J-wave patterns on electrocardiogram. **A.** Example of notching pattern (arrows). **B.** Example of slurring pattern (arrows). (Reprinted with permission from Patel RB, Ng J, Reddy V, et al. Early repolarization associated with ventricular arrhythmias in patients with chronic coronary artery disease. *Circ Arrhythm Electrophysiol.* 2010;3:489-495.)

In J-wave syndrome, the J-point elevation and ST-segment changes may be present in only a few ECG leads or globally, suggesting different anatomic locations responsible for each pattern. A classification system has been suggested by Antzelevitch and Yan[20] (**Table 20.5**).

In addition to the location of the J-point or J-wave pattern, Tikkanen et al[21] suggest that including the magnitude of J-point elevation >0.2 mV further increases the risk of sudden death. The direction of the ST segment also appears to be a modifier, with a horizontal or downward direction of the ST segments carrying a 3 times higher risk of arrhythmic death.[22]

Despite these additional criteria, it is extremely important to note that J wave–mediated SCD is extremely rare, and thus, the clinical implications of this finding in an asymptomatic individual are currently unclear.

Table 20.5.

Proposed Classification of J-wave Pattern

	Type 1	Type 2	Type 3
Anatomic location	Anterolateral left ventricle	Inferior left ventricle	Left and right ventricles
Leads displaying J-point or J-wave abnormalities	I, V_4-V_6	II, III, aVF	Global

Catecholaminergic Polymorphic Ventricular Tachycardia

Catecholaminergic polymorphic ventricular tachycardia (CPVT) is an inherited arrhythmia syndrome characterized by a normal ECG in the resting state with characteristic polymorphic or bidirectional ventricular ectopy provoked with exercise or emotional stress. The true prevalence is unknown but estimated to be approximately 1:10,000 in the general population. The clinical course is heterogeneous, but in severely affected patients, mortality can be as high as 50% before the age of 20 years. In one published series, polymorphic or bidirectional VT provoked with exercise in 63% of patients and 82% of the time with provocative epinephrine.[23] Typically, at a certain heart rate threshold above 100 to 130 beats/min, isolated PVCs begin to develop, followed by short bursts of nonsustained VT. Initial PVCs are often relatively late coupled (approximately 400 ms), and frequently of a left-bundle-branch block-like inferiorly directed axis or a RBBB-like superiorly directed axis.[23,24] Electrocardiographic diagnosis is often made with exercise stress testing or in patients who cannot cooperate with exercise stress testing (ie, children) with ambulatory ECG monitoring (**Figure 20.9**).[25]

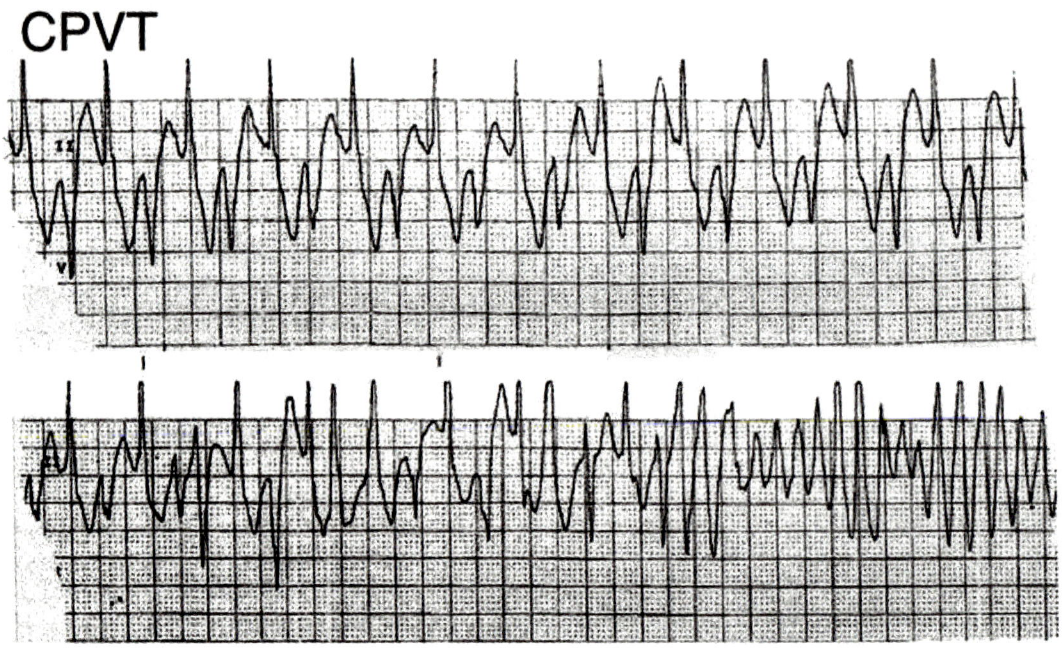

FIGURE 20.9. Bidirectional ventricular tachycardia degenerating into polymorphic ventricular tachycardia and eventually ventricular fibrillation in a patient with catecholaminergic polymorphic ventricular tachycardia (CPVT). (Reprinted from Prystowsky EN, Padanilam BJ, Joshi S, Fogel RI. Ventricular arrhythmias in the absence of structural heart disease. *J Am Coll Cardiol*. 2012;59[20]:1733-1744. Copyright © 2012 Elsevier. With permission.)

CHAPTER 20 SUMMARY ILLUSTRATION

Inherited Arrhythmia Disorders

Genotype*

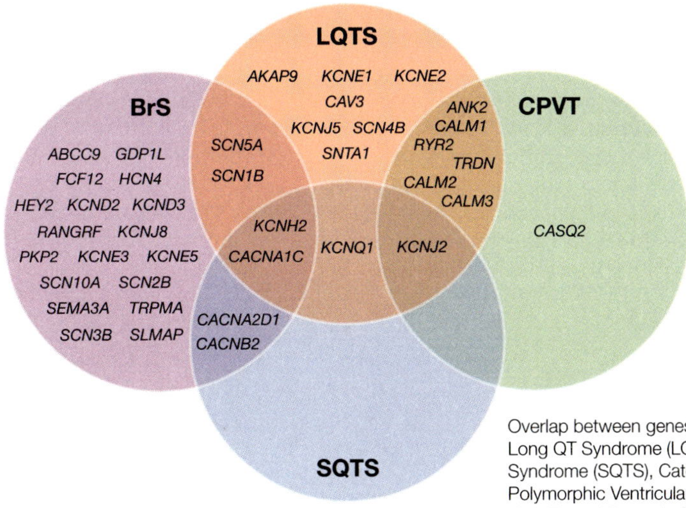

Overlap between genes associated with Long QT Syndrome (LQTS), Short QT Syndrome (SQTS), Catecholaminergic Polymorphic Ventricular Tachycardia (CPVT), and Brugada Syndrome (BrS)

Phenotype

Ion channel disorders
Long QT syndrome
Brugada syndrome**
Short QT syndrome
Catecholaminergic polymorphic VT
Early reoplarization syndrome
Idiopathic VF

Manifestations

Torsade des pointes
Polymorphic VT
Ventricular fibrillation
Sudden death
Atrial fibrillation
Sinus bradycardia
AV block
Heart failure
Abnormal ECG only

*** Note the potential for a gene to have gain of function and cause one condition or loss of function and cause a different condition**
**** Brugada may exhibit RV outflow tract epicardial scar; interplay between ion channels and structural proteins increasingly recognized**

Adapted from Fernandez-Falgueras A, Sarquella-Brugada G, Brugada J, Brugada R, Campuzano O. Cardiac Channelopathies and Sudden Death: Recent Clinical and Genetic Advances. *Biology (Basel)*. 2017 Jan 29;6(1):7.

Glossary

Arrhythmogenic right-ventricular cardiomyopathy/dysplasia: disorder of the heart muscle characterized by fibrofatty replacement of the right or left ventricle.

Brugada pattern: pseudo-RBBB and persistent ST-segment elevation in leads V_1 to V_3.

Brugada syndrome: the clinical syndrome of a Brugada pattern and an increased risk of SCD.

Catecholaminergic polymorphic ventricular tachycardia: the clinical syndrome of exercise or emotion provoked bidirectional or polymorphic VT in an otherwise structurally normal heart.

J-wave pattern: ≥0.1 mV J-point elevation in two adjacent inferior or lateral leads with a notching or slurring pattern.

J-wave syndrome: the clinical syndrome of the J-wave pattern and an increased risk of SCD.

Long QT syndrome: the clinical syndrome of a prolonged QT interval and an increased risk of SCD.

Short QT syndrome: the clinical syndrome of a short QT interval and an increased risk of SCD.

Disclaimer

The views expressed in this manuscript are those of the author and do not reflect the official policy of the Department of Army/Navy/Air Force, Department of Defense, or U.S. Government.

References

1. Moss AJ. Long QT syndrome. *JAMA*. 2003; 289:2041-2044.
2. Camm AJ, Janse MJ, Roden DM, Rosen MR, Cinca J, Cobbe SM. Congenital and acquired long QT syndrome. *Eur Heart J*. 2000;21: 1232-1237.
3. Moss AJ. Measurement of the QT interval and the risk associated with QTc interval prolongation: a review. *Am J Cardiol*. 1993; 72:23B-25B.
4. Priori SG, Schwartz PJ, Napolitano C, et al. Risk stratification in the long-QT syndrome. *N Engl J Med*. 2003;348:1866-1874.
5. Ackerman MJ, Priori SG, Willems S, et al. HRS/EHRA expert consensus statement on the state of genetic testing for the channelopathies and cardiomyopathies: this document was developed as a partnership between the Heart Rhythm Society (HRS) and the European Heart Rhythm Association (EHRA). *Europace*. 2011;13(8):1077-1109.
6. Zareba W. Genotype-specific ECG patterns in long QT syndrome. *J Electrocardiol*. 2006;39(suppl 4):S101-S106.
7. Moss AJ, Zareba W, Benhorin J, et al. ECG T-wave patterns in genetically distinct forms of the hereditary long QT syndrome. *Circulation*. 1995;92:2929-2934.
8. Schwartz PJ, Moss AJ, Vincent GM, Crampton RS. Diagnostic criteria for the long QT syndrome. An update. *Circulation*. 1993;88:782-784.
9. Gollob MH, Redpath CJ, Roberts JD. The short QT syndrome: proposed diagnostic criteria. *J Am Coll Cardiol*. 2011;57:802-812.
10. Wilde AA, Antzelevitch C, Borggrefe M, et al. Proposed diagnostic criteria for the Brugada syndrome. *Eur Heart J*. 2002;23:1648-1654.
11. Brugada P, Brugada J. Right bundle branch block, persistent ST segment elevation and sudden cardiac death: a distinct clinical and electrocardiographic syndrome. A multicenter report. *J Am Coll Cardiol*. 1992;20:1391-1396.
12. Marcus FI, McKenna WJ, Sherrill D, et al. Diagnosis of arrhythmogenic right ventricular cardiomyopathy/dysplasia: proposed modification of the task force criteria. *Eur Heart J*. 2010;31:806-814.
13. Marcus FI. Prevalence of T-wave inversion beyond V1 in young normal individuals and usefulness for the diagnosis of arrhythmogenic right ventricular cardiomyopathy/dysplasia. *Am J Cardiol*. 2005;95:1070-1071.
14. Marcus FI, Abidov A. Arrhythmogenic right ventricular cardiomyopathy 2012: diagnostic challenges and treatment. *J Cardiovasc Electrophysiol*. 2012;23:1149-1153.
15. Cox MG, Nelen MR, Wilde AA, et al. Activation delay and VT parameters in arrhythmogenic right ventricular dysplasia/cardiomyopathy: toward improvement of diagnostic ECG criteria. *J Cardiovasc Electrophysiol*. 2008;19:775-781.
16. Haïssaguerre M, Derval N, Sacher F, et al. Sudden cardiac arrest associated with early repolarization. *N Engl J Med*. 2008;358: 2016-2023.

17. Rosso R, Kogan E, Belhassen B, et al. J-point elevation in survivors of primary ventricular fibrillation and matched control subjects: incidence and clinical significance. *J Am Coll Cardiol.* 2008;52:1231-1238.
18. Patel RB, Ng J, Reddy V, et al. Early repolarization associated with ventricular arrhythmias in patients with chronic coronary artery disease. *Circ Arrhythm Electrophysiol.* 2010;3:489-495.
19. Huikuri HV, Marcus F, Krahn AD. Early repolarization: an epidemiologist's and a clinician's view. *J Electrocardiol.* 2013;46: 466-469.
20. Antzelevitch C, Yan GX. J wave syndromes. *Heart Rhythm.* 2010;7:549-558.
21. Tikkanen JT, Anttonen O, Junttila MJ, et al. Long-term outcome associated with early repolarization on electrocardiography. *New Engl J Med.* 2009;361:2529-2537.
22. Tikkanen JT, Junttila MJ, Anttonen O, et al. Early repolarization: electrocardiographic phenotypes associated with favorable long-term outcome. *Circulation.* 2011;123: 2666-2673.
23. Sy RW, Gollob MH, Klein GJ, et al. Arrhythmia characterization and long-term outcomes in catecholaminergic polymorphic ventricular tachycardia. *Heart Rhythm.* 2011;8(6):864-871.
24. Blich M, Marai I, Suleiman M, et al. Electrocardiographic comparison of ventricular premature complexes during exercise test in patients with CPVT and healthy subjects. *Pacing Clin Electrophysiol.* 2015;38: 398-402.
25. Prystowsky EN, Padanilam BJ, Joshi S, Fogel RI. Ventricular arrhythmias in the absence of structural heart disease. *J Am Coll Cardiol.* 2012;59:1733-1744.

Reference to the South Asian Edition

A. Priori SG, Wilde AA, Horie M, et al. HRS/EHRA/APHRS expert consensus statement on the diagnosis and management of patients with inherited primary arrhythmia syndromes: document endorsed by HRS, EHRA, and APHRS in May 2013 and by ACCF, AHA, PACES, and AEPC in June 2013. *Heart Rhythm.* 2013 Dec;10(12):1932-1963.

21 Implantable Cardiac Pacemakers

BRETT D. ATWATER,
DANIEL J. FRIEDMAN, AND
DALJEET KAUR SAGGU

Basic Concepts of the Implantable Cardiac Pacemaker

Implantable cardiac pacemakers are used for a wide range of cardiac arrhythmias and conduction disorders. Pacemakers are used for the treatment of symptomatic bradyarrhythmias caused by abnormal cardiac impulse formation or conduction.[1] Pacemakers are used in patients with tachyarrhythmias when (1) pharmacologic therapy carries a risk of bradyarrhythmias or more serious arrhythmias or (2) when pacing is required to stop tachyarrhythmias. Pacemakers are combined with the capability of cardiac *defibrillation* in implanted devices for treatment of prior or potential life-threatening ventricular arrhythmias.[2] Pacemakers that pace both cardiac ventricles (biventricular) are used for the treatment of heart failure in patients with reduced and poorly coordinated left-ventricular (LV) contraction associated with severe slowing of interventricular conduction time, usually caused by left-bundle-branch block (LBBB) or right-ventricular (RV) apical pacing.[3]

Figure 21.1A shows the components of a transvenous implantable pacemaker system designed to pace the right atrium and both cardiac ventricles (biventricular pacing). Electronic impulses originate from a *pulse generator* surgically placed subcutaneously in the pectoral area. The pulse generator is connected to transvenous leads with small electrodes mounted at their distal ends. These electrodes are screwed into the endocardial surfaces of the right atrium and right ventricle. The third lead is placed in an epicardial vein to pace the left ventricle.

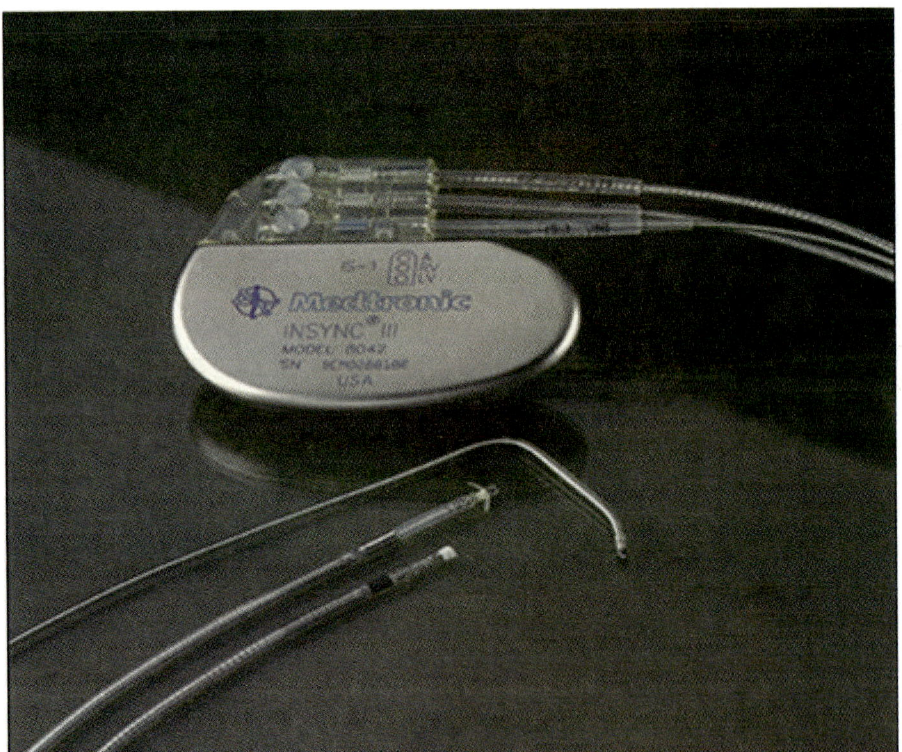

A

FIGURE 21.1. A. *Biventricular pacemaker* with three leads: top lead, coronary sinus (left-ventricular) pacing lead; middle lead, right-ventricular pacing lead; and bottom lead, active fixation pacing lead for the right atrium. *(continued)*

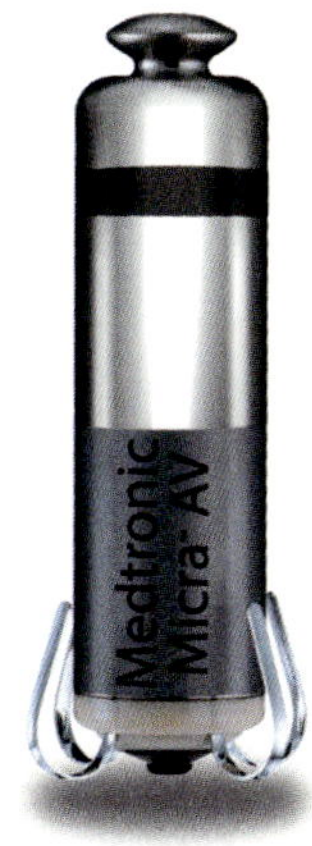

B

FIGURE 21.1. *(continued)* **B.** Leadless pacemaker that incorporate the pulse generator and *pacing electrodes* into a single miniature unit – Micra AV Model MC1AVR1. (© 2020 Medtronic.)

Leadless pacemakers incorporate the pulse generator and *pacing electrodes* into a single miniature unit that is placed entirely within the heart chamber (**Figure 21.1B**; leadless pacemaker picture). Current generation leadless pacemaker devices can sense one or more cardiac chambers and pace the right ventricle to deliver VDD or VVI pacing. See the following text and **Table 21.1** for key to pacemaker identification terminology.

Temporary pacing can be achieved with an external pulse generator connected either to transvenous leads positioned like those for permanent pacing or connected to cutaneous patches. During open-heart surgery, temporary or permanent epicardial electrodes may be placed on the atria or ventricles.

Table 21.1.

The Revised NASPE/BPEG Generic Code

I	II	III	IV	V
Chamber(s) paced	Chamber(s) sensed	Response to sensing	Rate modulation	Multisite pacing
O = none	O = none	O = none	O = none	O = none
A = atrium	A = atrium	T = triggered	R = rate modulation	A = atrium
V = ventricle	V = ventricle	I = inhibited		V = ventricle
D = dual (A + V)	D = dual (A + V)	D = dual (T + I)		D = dual (A + V)

Abbreviation: NASPE/BPEG, North American Society of Pacing and Electrophysiology/British Pacing and Electrophysiology Group.

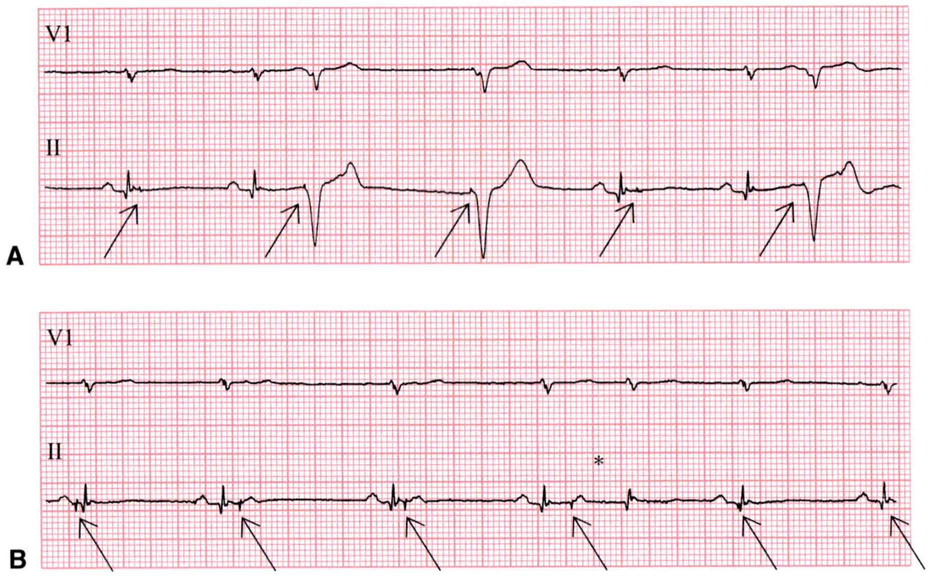

FIGURE 21.2. **A,B.** Fixed-rate ventricular and atrial pacing systems, respectively. Arrows, small pacing artifacts at a rate of 50 beats/min; asterisk, prolonged PR interval.

When an implantable pacemaker delivers stimulation, *pacemaker artifacts* can usually be detected on an electrocardiogram (ECG) recording as positively or negatively directed vertical lines. The pacing stimulus can sometimes be small and not always appreciated in each ECG lead. Pacing artifact preceding a QRS complex indicates ventricular pacing with appropriate capture (**Figure 21.2A**), whereas artifact preceding a P wave indicates atrial pacing with appropriate capture (**Figure 21.2B**). Pacing artifact without a subsequent P wave or QRS complex indicates lack of capture. Occasionally, in a biventricular pacing system, there may be three or even four pacing artifacts seen on ECG. This occurs with atrial pacing followed by ventricular pacing that is programmed with delay between the two or three ventricular pacing locations.

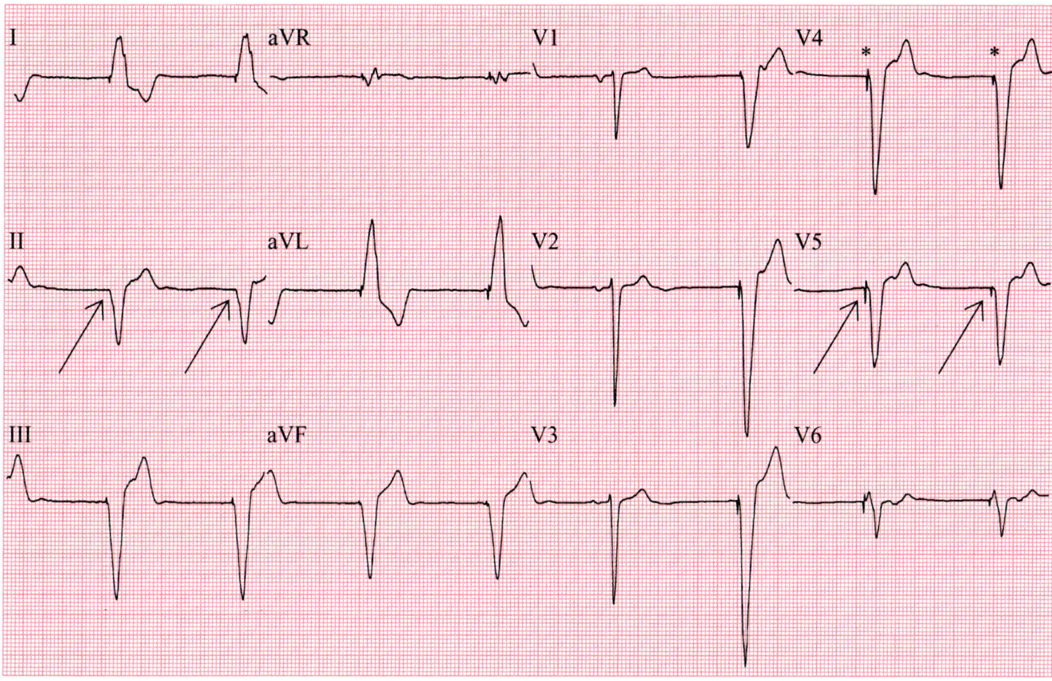

FIGURE 21.3. Arrows, prominent (lead V_5) and absent (lead II) pacing artifacts in different leads; asterisks, varying artifact amplitudes (V_4) characteristic of digital electrocardiogram recordings.

Current pacemakers using narrow-spaced lead electrodes allow pacing with greater efficiency and narrower pulse width (0.4 ms) resulting in less energy use and longer pacemaker battery life. This development makes the artifacts appearing on older generation digital ECG machines smaller and difficult to see (**Figure 21.3**). These older machines sampled the ECG electrical signal only once every 2 to 4 ms (1/1000 of a second). Therefore, if the pacing artifact occurred between samples, it was not displayed. All current generation ECG machines digitize and sample the ECG signal at much higher frequency. The newer ECG machines are better able to recognize pacemaker artifacts and display artificial pacing spikes on the 12-lead ECG in order to permit assessment of pacing function (see **Figure 21.2**).[4,5]

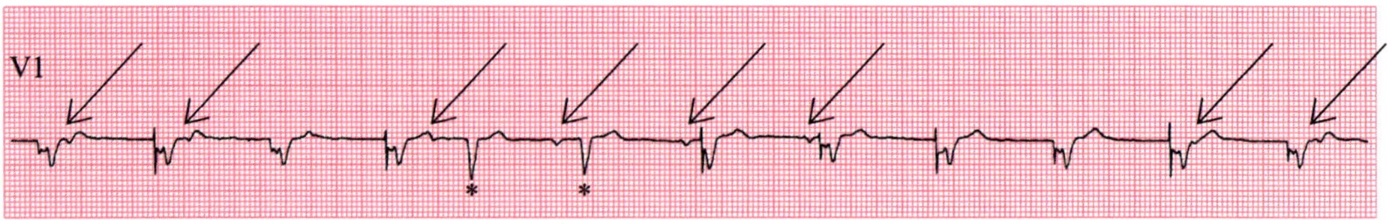

FIGURE 21.4. Ventricular demand pacemaker. Arrows, patient's intrinsic sinus P waves; asterisks, QRS complexes of intrinsic ventricular activation that inhibit impulse generation from the demand pacemaker.

All current implantable pacemakers have a built-in *demand mode* because the rhythm disturbances that require their use may occur intermittently.[2] **Figure 21.4** provides an example of a normally functioning ventricular demand pacemaker. In this mode, the device senses the heart's intrinsic impulses and does not generate impulses while the intrinsic rate exceeds the rate set for the pulse generator. If the intrinsic pacing rate falls below the programmed pacing rate, all cardiac cycles are initiated by the implantable pacemaker, and no evaluation of its sensing function is possible. In this example, the pacemaker cycle length is 840 ms (0.84 s). Intrinsic beats occur in the lead V_1 rhythm strip and are appropriately sensed by the demand pacemaker. Note the prolonged PR interval (0.32 s) required for the first intrinsic ventricular activation. Due to the absence of an atrial lead, atrioventricular (AV) sequential pacing cannot be delivered. This results in retrograde atrial activation (first two and last two P waves on strip) intermingled with sinus P waves and inconsistent PR intervals. This lack of AV synchrony can result in *pacemaker syndrome* and is the reason why an atrial lead is typically implanted in a patient with need for ventricular pacing as long as permanent atrial fibrillation is not present.

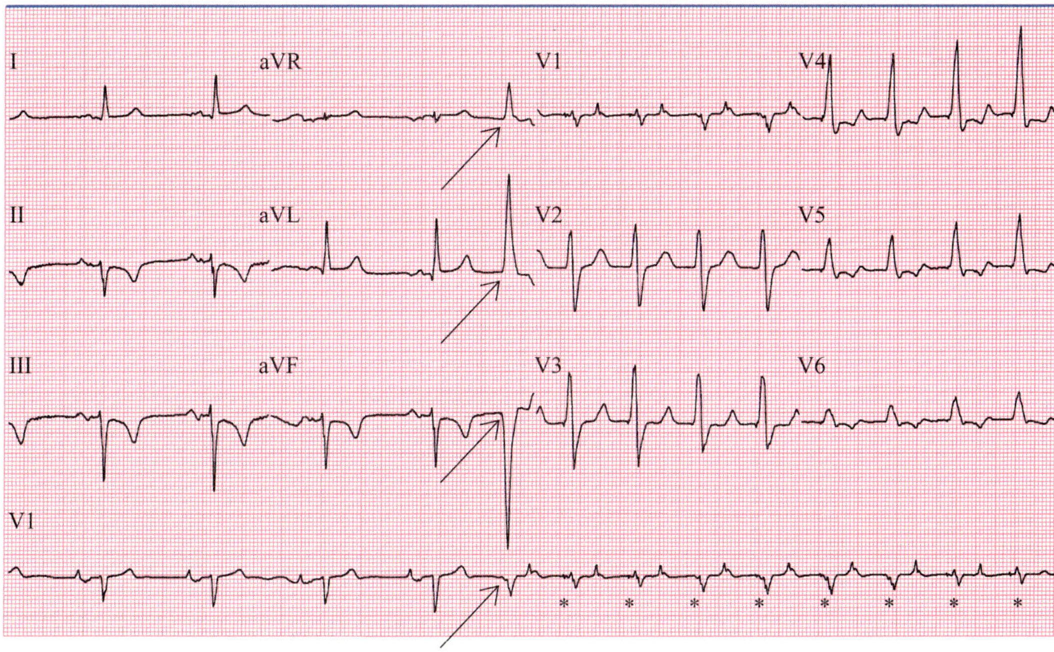

FIGURE 21.5. Arrows, magnet application; asterisks, rapid magnet-induced pacing rate.

If the intrinsic rate is greater than that of the implantable pacemaker, the pacing capability of the demand device may not be detectable on an ECG recording. The activity of the device can only be observed when a bradyarrhythmia occurs or when a magnet is applied (**Figure 21.5**). The magnet converts the pacemaker to *fixed-rate pacing*, disabling sensing function in all pacing channels. The fixed rate is different across pacemaker manufacturers and the pacemaker battery status (**Table 21.2**). Magnet pacing rate on the ECG can be used to identify which brand of pacemaker is implanted and whether the device needs to be replaced for low battery.[6] In the example shown in **Figure 21.5**, the patient's sinus bradycardia is interrupted by magnet application to the *single-chamber* (ventricular) *pacemaker*, causing an increase in the pacemaker rate to 100 beats/min. Note the P waves following the pacemaker-induced QRS complexes, indicating 1:1 ventriculoatrial conduction. Notably, application of a magnet to contemporary transvenous defibrillators (which have pacing capabilities) disables the tachycardia therapies without changing the pacing function.

Table 21.2.

Fixed Rate Pacing Across Pacemaker Manufacturers and Battery Status

	Manufacturer				
Battery Status	Medtronic	Boston Scientific	Abbott Medical	Biotronik	Sorin
Beginning of life	85	100	98.6	90	96
Nearing elective replacement	N/A	90	N/A	N/A	N/A
Elective replacement indicator[a]	65	85	86.3	80	80

Abbreviation: N/A, not applicable.

[a]When battery gets to end of life (below elective replacement indicator), magnet rate becomes unpredictable.

Pacemaker Modes and Dual-Chamber Pacing

The North American Society of Pacing and Electrophysiology (NASPE) Code Committee and the British Pacing and Electrophysiology Group (BPEG) jointly developed the NASPE/ BPEG Generic (NBG) code for artificial pacemakers.[7] This code was revised for modern devices in 2002 and is presented in **Table 21.1**. The code includes three letters to designate the bradycardia functions of a pacemaker, a fourth letter to indicate the pacemaker's programmability and rate modulation, and a fifth letter to indicate the presence of multisite pacing.

The first three letters of the NBG code can be easily remembered by ranking pacemaker functions from most to least important. Pacing is the most important function followed by sensing, and then by the response of the pacemaker to a sensed event. The first letter designates the cardiac chamber(s) that the device paces. The second letter designates the chamber(s) that the device senses. Entries for pacing and sensing include "A" for atrium, "V" for ventricle, "D" for dual (atrium and ventricle), and "O" for none. The third letter in the NBG code designates the response to sensed events. Entries for this third letter include "I" for inhibited, "T" for triggered, "D" for both triggered and inhibited, and "O" for none. The fourth letter describes the presence of rate responsiveness ("R" for the presence and omission of a fourth letter for the absence of rate responsiveness). The fifth letter of the NBG code is seldom used but indicates the presence and location of multisite pacing. Entries for this fifth letter include "O" for none, "A" for atrium, "V" for ventricle, and "D" for dual (atrium and ventricle).

Commonly used pacemaker modes include VVI, AAI, and DDD modes, with VVIR, AAIR, and DDDR designating the rate-modulated modes.[8,9] The VVI pacemakers (see **Figures 21.3-21.5**) pace the ventricle, sense the ventricle, and are inhibited by sensed intrinsic events. The VVI pacemaker has only a single rate (usually called the "minimum rate") to be programmed. By analogy with VVI pacemakers, AAI pacemakers pace the atrium, sense the atrium, and are inhibited by sensed atrial beats. The AAI pacemakers also have only a single programmable rate. Both VVI and AAI pacemakers are "single-chamber" pacemakers; they both pace and sense one cardiac chamber.

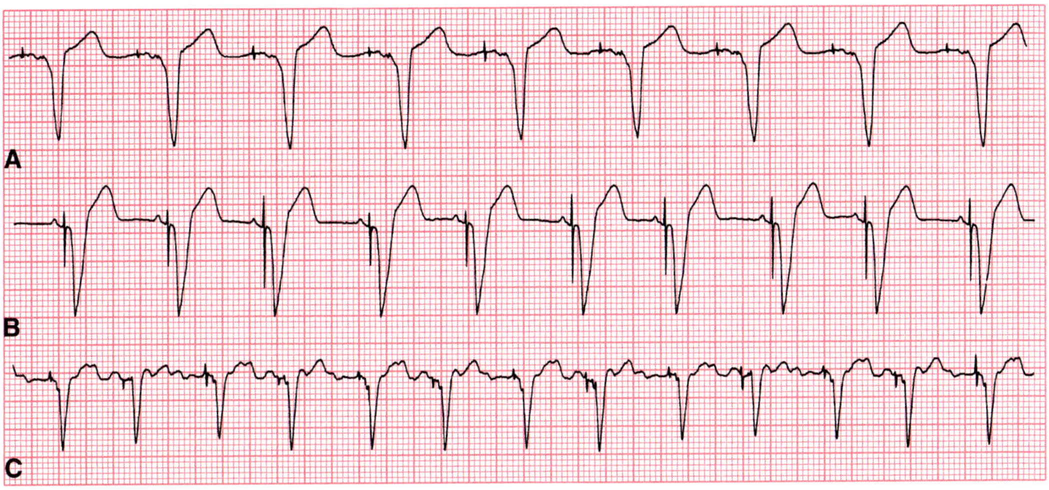

FIGURE 21.6. **A.** Atrial and ventricular minimum-rate-behavior pacing. **B.** Ventricular pacing at the atrially tracked rate with the programmed atrioventricular interval. **C.** Ventricular pacing at varying intervals following sensed atrial flutter waves exhibiting maximum-rate behavior.

The DDD pacemakers are typically *dual-chamber pacemakers*; they pace both the right atrium and right ventricle or both ventricles and sense atrial and ventricular impulses. They are triggered by P waves to pace the ventricle at the programmed AV interval and are inhibited by ventricular sensing not to compete with the patient's underlying rhythm. The DDD pacing varies according to the patient's underlying atrial rate. If the patient's atrial rate is below the minimum tracking rate in the DDD mode, the pacemaker shows "minimum-rate behavior," pacing both the atrium and the ventricle (**Figure 21.6A**). If the sinus rate is above the minimum rate in the DDD mode, the pacemaker tracks atrial activity and paces the ventricle at the programmed AV interval (**Figure 21.6B**). To prevent tracking of rapid atrial rhythms, the DDD pacemaker requires a programmed maximum tracking rate. More rapid atrial rates are sensed, but ventricular pacing is limited to the programmed upper tracking rate ("maximum-rate behavior"; **Figure 21.6C**). If the pacemaker is programmed appropriately, AV intervals following the sensed atrial activity can vary.

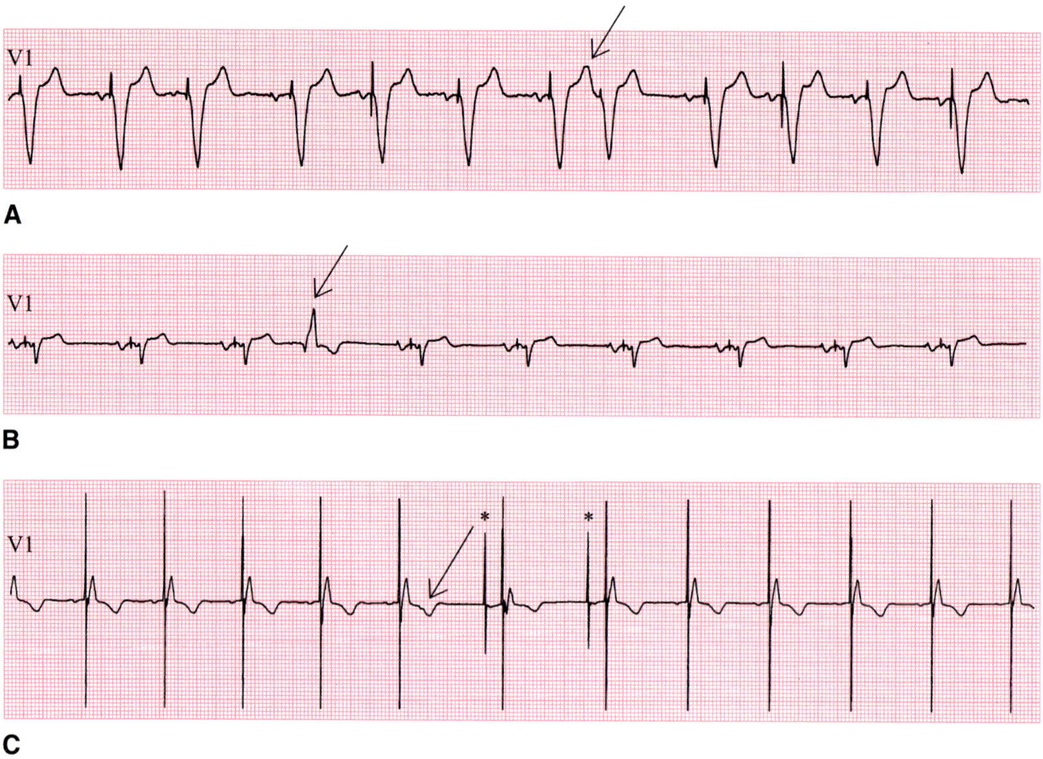

FIGURE 21.7. **A.** Arrow, sensed APB. **B.** Arrow, sensed ventricular premature beat. **C.** Arrow, unsensed atrial premature beat (APB); asterisks, minimum-rate atrioventricular pacing following the APB-induced pause and continuing until intrinsic sinus rhythm exceeds this minimum pacing rate.

Figure 21.7 shows lead V_1 rhythm strips from three patients with syncope owing to intermittent AV block. Displayed are the normal functions of three DDD pacemakers when the atrial rate is above the programmed minimum rate and below the programmed maximal tracking rate of the pacemaker. The DDD pacemaker is best understood by knowing that it approximates normal AV function and conduction and that its function closely approximates normal cardiac physiology. The AV intervals provided by DDD pacemakers may shorten with an increased pacing rate. The DDD pacemaker tracks both sinus arrhythmia and atrial premature beats (APBs; occurring at the peak of a T wave, triggering ventricular pacing; **Figure 21.7A**) and senses and is reset by ventricular premature beats (VPBs; **Figure 21.7B**). The pacemaker may lengthen the AV interval for closely coupled APBs but may not sense very closely coupled APBs when they occur in its atrial refractory period (**Figure 21.7C**). Note the minimum-rate AV pacing following the APB-induced pause and continuing until intrinsic sinus rhythm exceeds this minimum pacing rate in **Figure 21.7C**.

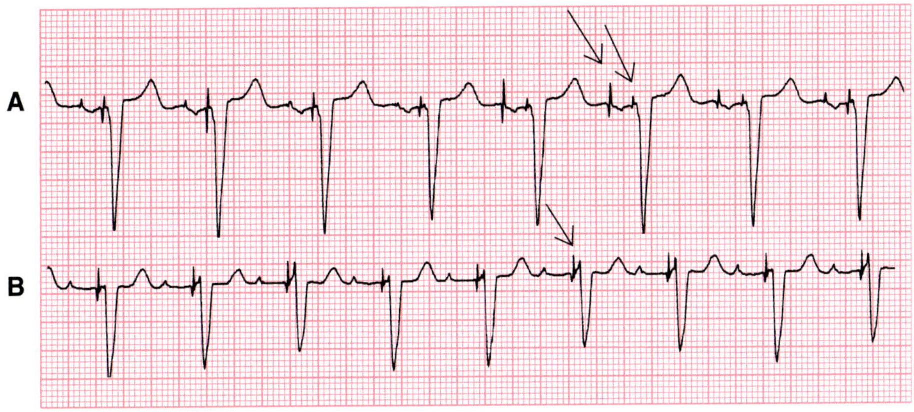

FIGURE 21.8. **A.** Arrows, atrial and ventricular pacing. **B.** Arrow, ventricular pacing tracking a rapid sinus rate.

The VVIR and DDDR pacemakers have the capacity for rate modulation by having their minimum rate automatically increased through an activity sensor. Common sensors include a piezoelectric crystal (activity), accelerometer (body movement), impedance-sensing device (sensing of respiratory rate or minute ventilation), and "closed-loop" simulation. Pacemakers with rate modulation have programmed maximal sensor rates and programmable parameters for sensitivity and rate of response to the sensing parameter.

The DDDR pacing and modulation of the minimum rate through sensor activity is shown in **Figure 21.8A**. Consecutive beats with both atrial and ventricular pacing confirm minimum-rate pacing. The minimum rate has been "modulated" and increased to 84 beats/min as a result of sensor activity (see **Figure 21.8A**). **Figure 21.8B** displays the same pacemaker tracking the same patient's sinus rhythm at a rate faster than that with the sensor-driven pacing shown in **Figure 21.8A**. Note that the sensor has not increased the pacemaker's minimum rate while tracking a rapid sinus rate. Thus, the DDDR pacemaker can increase the rate of ventricular pacing either through an increased rate of atrial pacing driven by the sensor or through sensing of an increased intrinsic sinus rate. Maximal sensor rate and maximal tracking rate may be independently programmed in dual-chamber pacemakers.

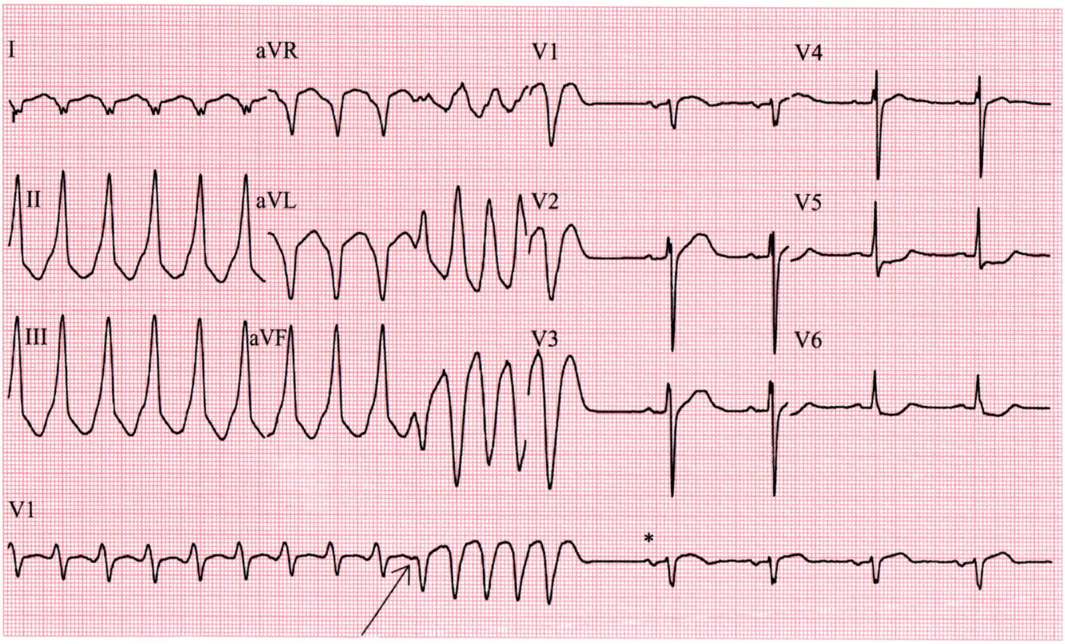

FIGURE 21.9. Arrow, beginning of a five-beat train that terminates the tachycardia; asterisk, return of sinus rhythm.

Pacemaker systems may include antitachycardia pacing (ATP) (**Figure 21.9**), but current practice limits ATP to supraventricular tachyarrhythmias.

The ATP for ventricular tachycardia is usually included in an implantable cardioverter defibrillator (ICD) because of the possibility that ATP may accelerate hemodynamically stable monomorphic ventricular tachycardia to become hemodynamically unstable polymorphic ventricular tachycardia or ventricular fibrillation. As seen in **Figure 21.10**, polymorphic ventricular tachycardia at a rate of 250 beats/min induced by ATP treatment of a stable monomorphic ventricular tachycardia can be successfully terminated with a high-energy ICD shock. Transvenous ICD systems also include all pacing functionality of traditional pacemaker systems to protect against bradyarrhythmias. Current generation subcutaneous ICDs, which have no electrodes within the vasculature, can provide high-output emergency post-ICD shock pacing for temporary bradycardia support. This high-output pacing is painful and places large energy demand on the device battery. As a result, subcutaneous ICDs are not indicated for patients at risk for bradyarrhythmia.

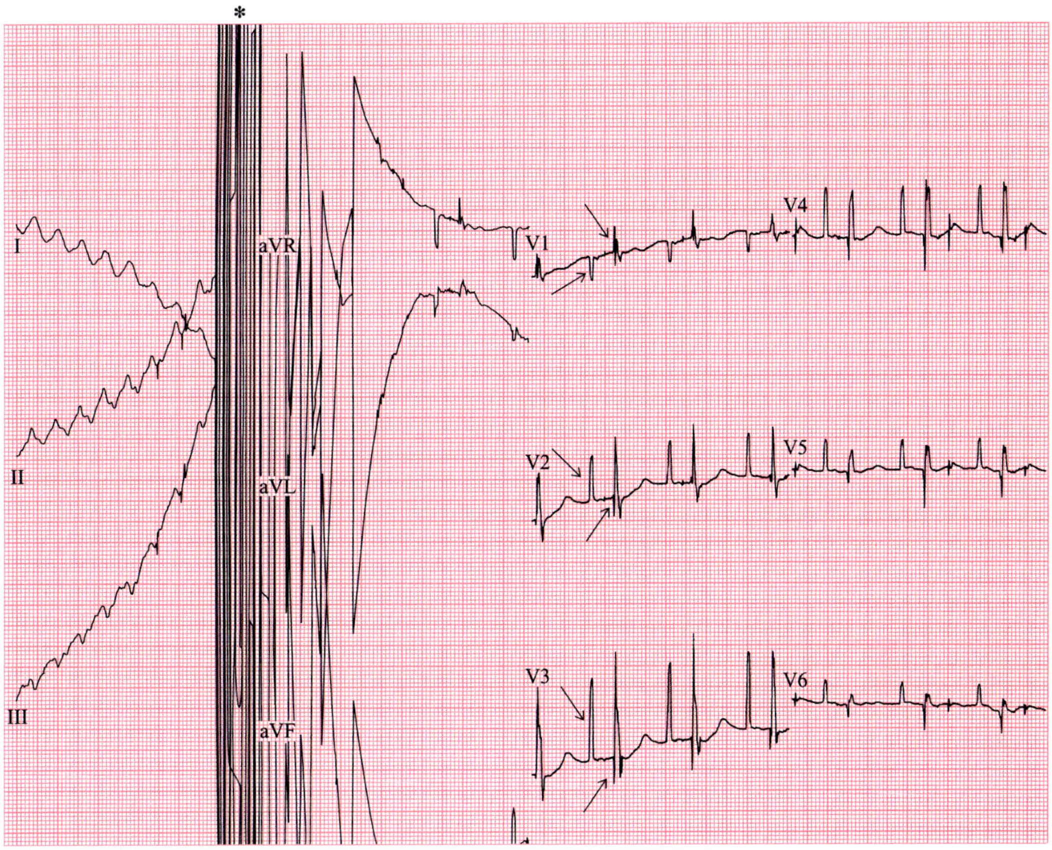

FIGURE 21.10. Asterisk, high-energy implantable cardioverter defibrillator artifact terminating the tachycardia; arrows, return of dual-chamber pacing.

Pacemaker Evaluation

The initial aspect of evaluation of any pacemaker system is the assessment of its pacing and sensing functions. Pacemaker malfunction may manifest as the absence of atrial or ventricular capture after a pacing artifact or under- or *oversensing* of native or external electrical signals.

Figure 21.11 shows the typical appearance of failure of both the pacing and sensing functions of a pacemaker. Pacing artifacts are seen continuing regularly (68 beats/min) without interruption by the patient's intrinsic beats. Furthermore, there are no QRS complexes following most of the pacing spikes. Only a single incidence of ventricular capture occurs. Failure of the sensing function is apparent from the absence of pacemaker inhibition by the patient's intrinsic ventricular beats.

The evaluation of dual-chamber pacing systems must assess both atrial and ventricular capture and sensing.[10,11] **Figure 21.12** demonstrates failure of atrial capture; the ventricular pacing function is intact. Effective atrial sensing is indicated by inhibition of atrial pacing during the first two sinus beats, with ventricular pacing at the sinus rate after the first sensed atrial signal. During the pause after the VPB (third beat), minimum-rate pacing occurs but with failure of atrial capture. Effective ventricular sensing is indicated by inhibition of ventricular pacing after the VPB.

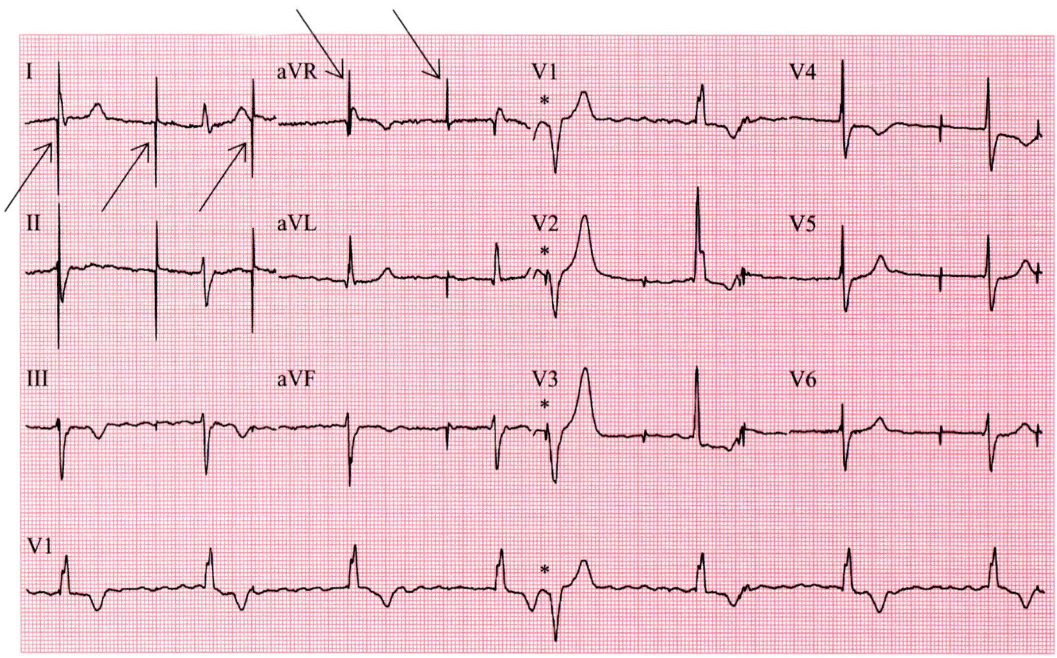

FIGURE 21.11. Arrows, pacing artifacts; asterisks, single instance of ventricular capture by the pacemaker.

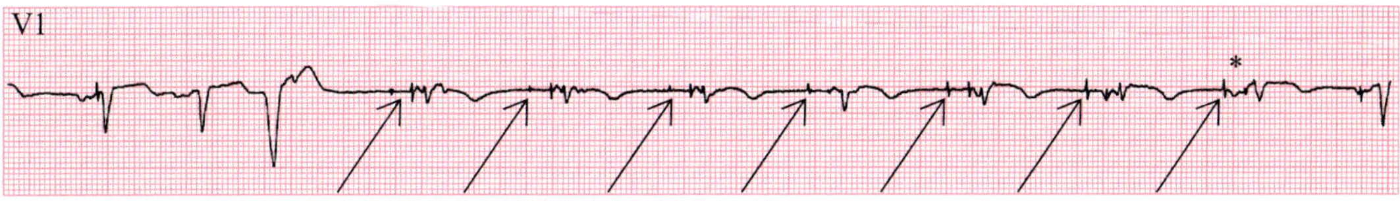

FIGURE 21.12. First six arrows, minimum-rate pacing without atrial capture; asterisk and last arrow, atrial capture by the pacemaker.

Figure 21.13 shows examples of sensing dysfunction: atrial undersensing (**Figure 21.13A**) and ventricular oversensing (**Figure 21.13B,C**). A DDD device was present in **Figure 21.13A,B** and a VVI device in **Figure 21.13C**. In normal DDD pacemaker function, atrial sensing triggers ventricular pacing after the programmed sensed AV delay while ventricular sensing inhibits ventricular pacing and in some cases resets the timer for the next atrial beat. The failure of atrial sensing in **Figure 21.13A** causes failure of the P wave (arrow) to trigger ventricular pacing. **Figure 21.13B** demonstrates ventricular oversensing. In this case, the pacemaker has detected a signal on both the atrial and ventricular channels that is not evident on the surface ECG and inhibited pacing in both channels. This most often occurs as a result of electromagnetic interference. In a device-dependent patient, such oversensing and pacing inhibition may result in syncope or bradycardic arrest. **Figure 21.13C** was obtained in a patient with complete heart block who was programmed VVI. Oversensing results in ventricular pacing inhibition and a long ventricular pause. This oversensing may occur with lead fracture or electromagnetic interference.

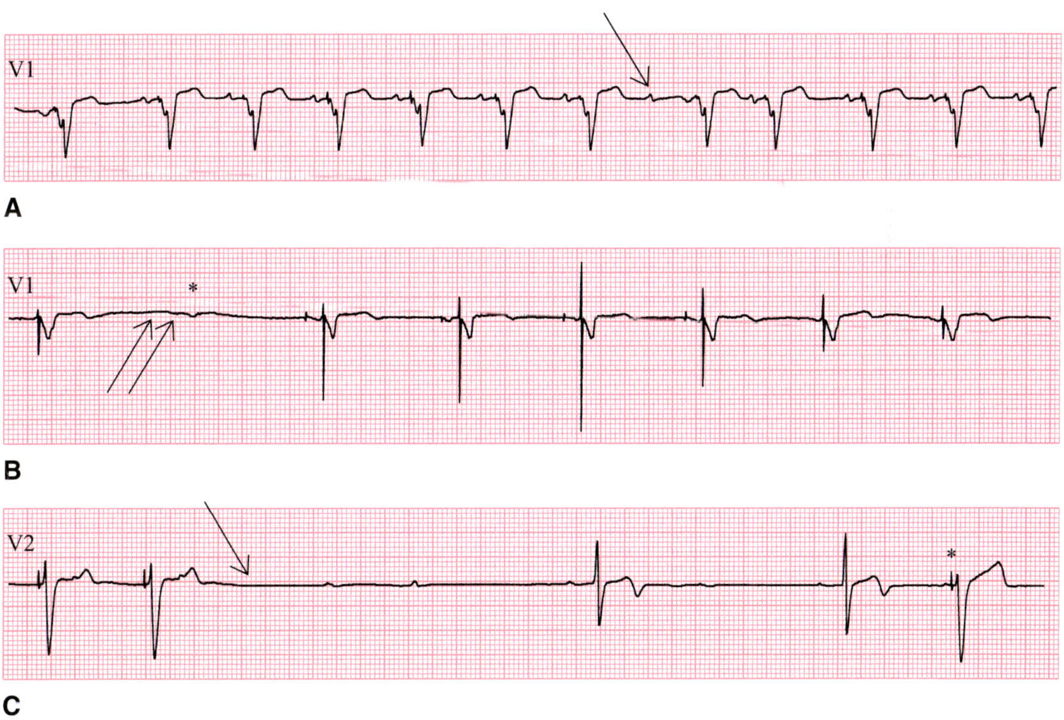

FIGURE 21.13. **A.** Arrow, single undersensed P wave. **B.** Arrows, expected locations of atrial and ventricular pacing artifacts; asterisk, P wave that fails to conduct owing to underlying atrioventricular block. **C.** Arrow, expected location of the next ventricular pacing artifact; asterisk, pacing artifact reappearance.

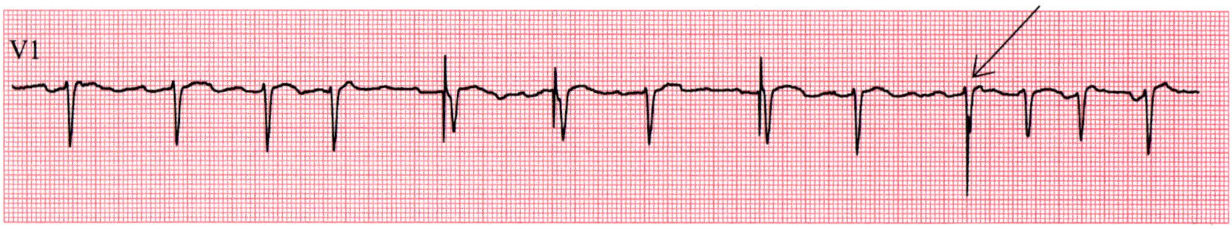

FIGURE 21.14. Arrow, pacemaker artifact 0.04 second into an intrinsic QRS complex.

"Failure to sense" may be incorrectly suspected when the pacing system has not had sufficient time to sense an intrinsic beat.[10,11] This incorrect "failure to sense" occurs when the patient's intrinsic rate is similar to the programmed minimum pacing rate, as in lead V_1 rhythm recording of atrial fibrillation with intermittent slowing and ventricular pacing (**Figure 21.14**). A period of >0.04 second is required for intrinsic activation to reach the pacemaker lead in the RV apex and to be sensed by the pacemaker. The apparent abnormality, in fact, represents normal pacemaker function.

At times, both the pacing and sensing functions of a pacemaker may occur normally in patients with symptoms that are typically associated with pacemaker dysfunction. **Figure 21.15** documents normal function by a VVI pacemaker. Absence of competing intrinsic activity prevents evaluation of the instrument's sensing function. The occurrence of 1:1 retrograde ventricular-to-atrial conduction, however, leads to the possibility that the patient may develop "pacemaker syndrome"[12]—manifest as neck fullness, chest discomfort, and vasovagal syncope caused by atrial dilation produced by the occurrence of atrial contraction during a closed tricuspid valve during ventricular contraction. If 1:1 ventricular-to-atrial conduction occurs with a dual-chamber device, the retrograde P wave can be tracked by the device, prompting ventricular pacing and perpetuation of this cycle resulting in "pacemaker-mediated tachycardia" at the device's upper tracking rate.

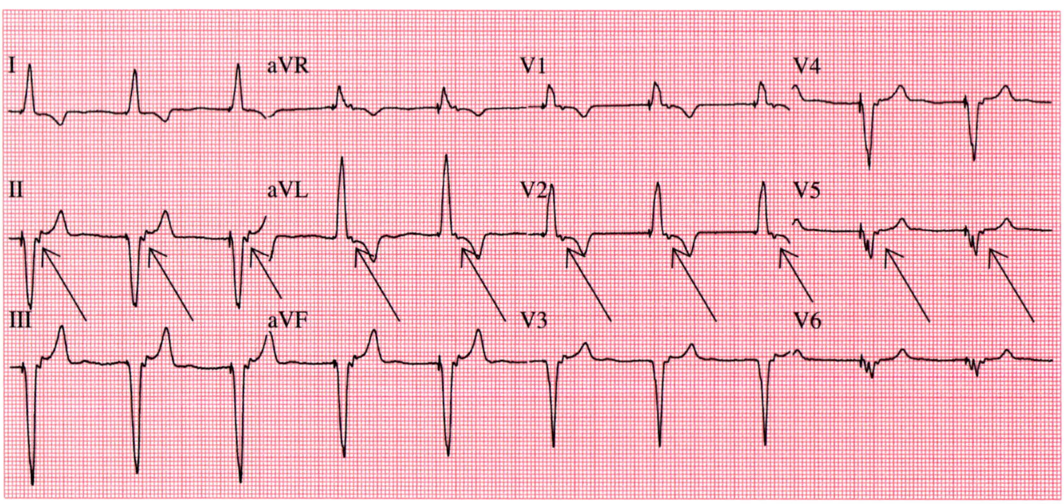

FIGURE 21.15. Arrows, retrograde P waves of 1:1 ventricular-to-atrial conduction.

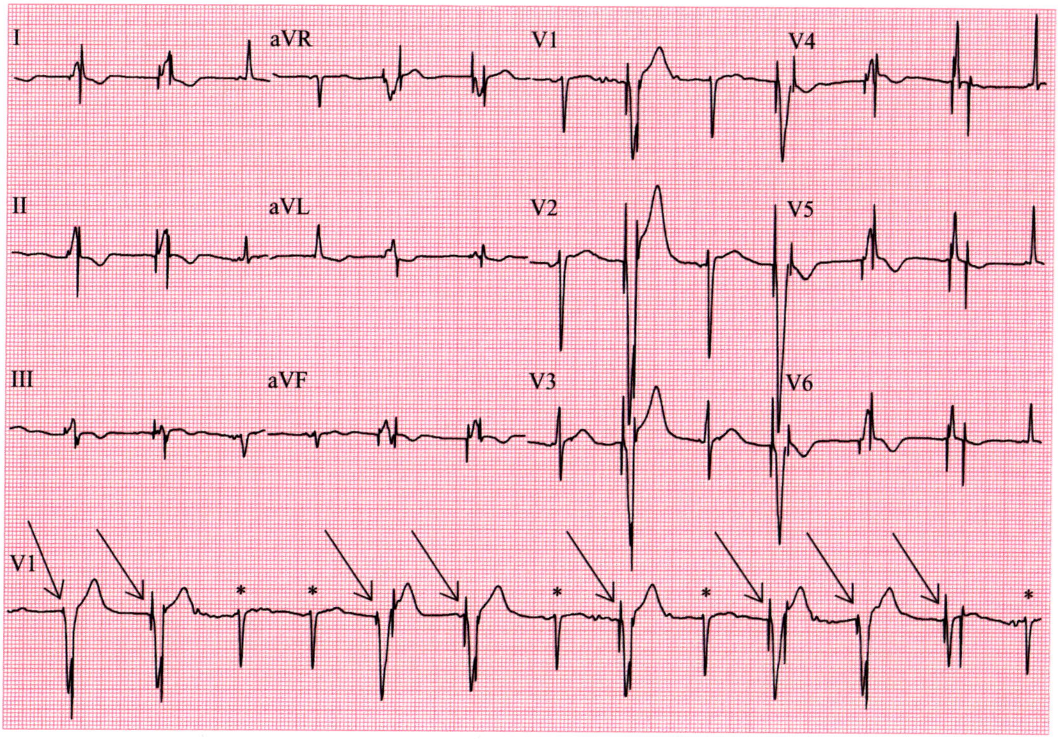

FIGURE 21.16. Arrows, effective ventricular capture by the first of two coupled pacing artifacts; asterisks, intrinsic beats.

In **Figure 21.16**, both the pacemaker's pacing and sensing functions are evident and abnormal. In this case, the abnormality is due to reversal of the atrial and ventricular leads during their connection to the pacemaker during implantation. Ventricular capture by the initial rather than the second of each pair of pacing artifacts suggests that output from the atrial channel causes ventricular capture. The second of each of the pairs is seen occurring either in the QRS complex or in the ST segment of the paced beats. The five intrinsic beats (asterisks) inhibit both the atrial and ventricular channels proving normal sensing function of the P wave (through the ventricular channel) and the R wave (through the atrial channel).

Myocardial Location of the Pacing Electrodes

The spread within the heart of the wavefronts of depolarization from a pacemaker depends on the location of the stimulating electrode. Currently, most endocardial electrodes are positioned near the RV apex. This location of the RV pacing electrode produces sequential RV and then LV activation and therefore an LBBB pattern on lead V_1 of the ECG. As activation proceeds from the RV apex toward the base, the frontal axis is superiorly directed, producing extreme left-axis deviation (**Figure 21.17A**). Endocardial electrodes placed in the RV outflow tract produce activation beginning at the base and directed inferiorly. The frontal axis is then inferiorly directed (**Figure 21.17B**).

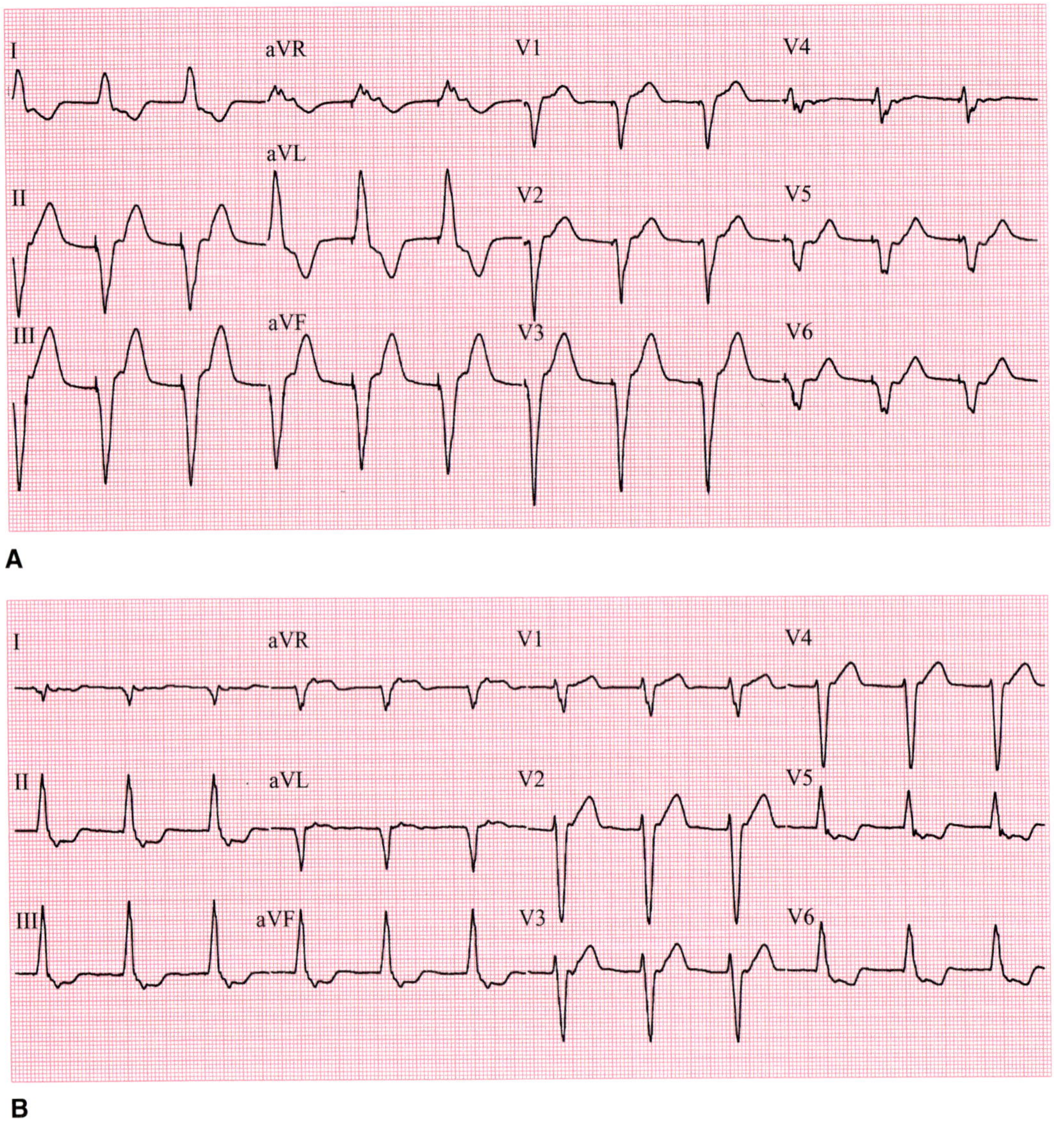

FIGURE 21.17. **A.** Right-ventricular apex pacing. **B.** Right-ventricular outflow tract pacing.

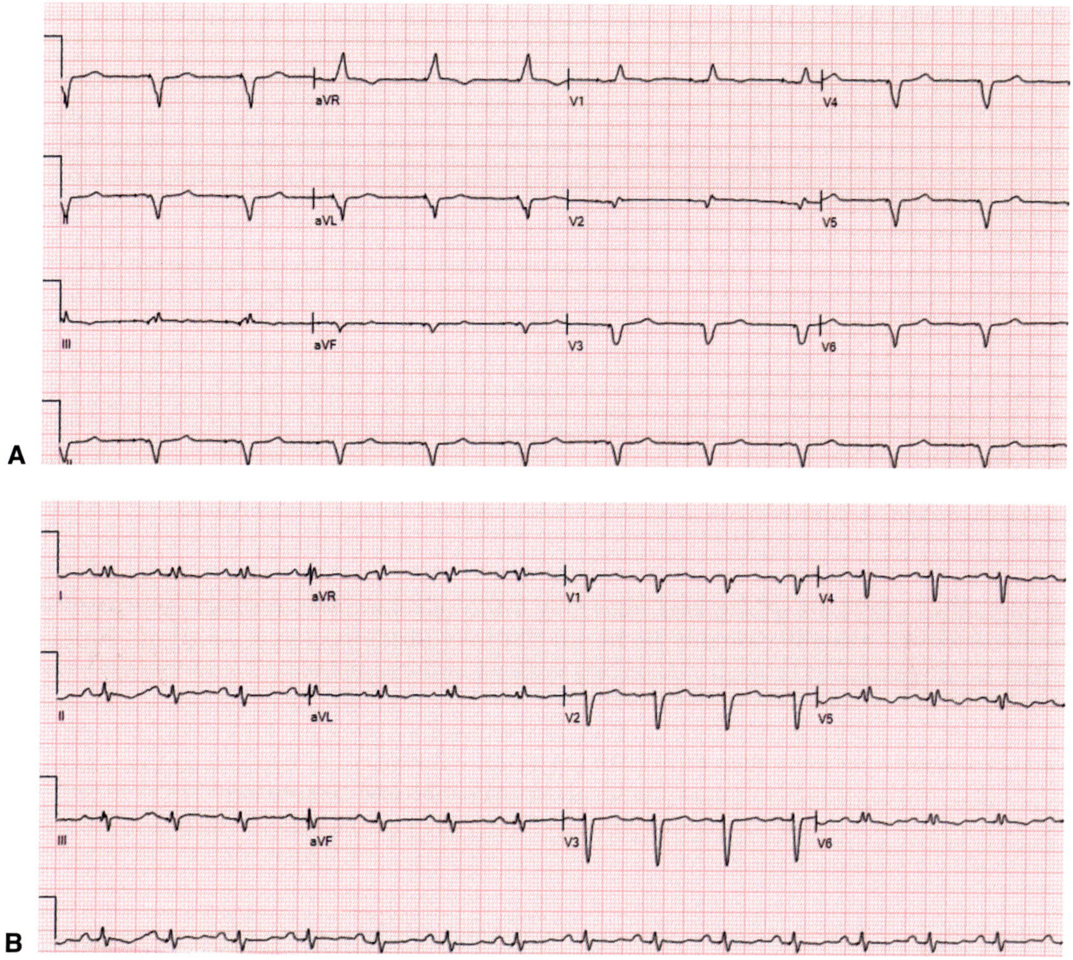

FIGURE 21.18. **A.** Traditional cardiac resynchronization therapy is delivered with pacing of both the right and left ventricles and is characterized by an R wave in V_1 and an initial Q wave in I. **B.** Cardiac resynchronization therapy can also be delivered with left-ventricular–only pacing where the left-ventricular pacing stimulus is timed to coincide with intrinsic activation of the right bundle, which can result in a narrow, more "normal"-appearing QRS complex.

The LV epicardial electrodes or electrodes placed in the distal coronary sinus pace the left ventricle. This distal coronary sinus pacing location produces sequential LV then RV activation and therefore a right-bundle-branch block (RBBB) pattern in lead V_1. *Cardiac resynchronization therapy* (CRT) has traditionally been delivered by pacing from the RV apex and a posterior/lateral branch of the coronary sinus (**Figure 21.18A**; CRT-only pacing). This posterolateral coronary sinus branch pacing produces a fusion RV-/LV-paced wavefront, usually with narrowing of the QRS complex. Biventricular pacing can be identified on a 12-lead ECG by the presence of an R wave in lead V_1 and an initial negative than positive deflection in lead I. Newer CRT devices allow for the LV pacing stimulus to be delivered at the time of conduction down the right bundle allowing for more physiologic activation of the right ventricle and septum. This type of "LV-only" pacing (**Figure 21.18B**) can result in a narrower QRS complex compared to traditional CRT pacing.

Special Algorithms to Avoid Right-Ventricular Pacing

Although the majority (86%) of implanted pacemakers are programmed DDD, the frequency of atrial and ventricular pacing on the ECG should vary greatly between subjects based on whether their indication for pacing is sick sinus syndrome, AV block, bundle branch block with heart failure, or a combination of these. The Dual Chamber and VVI Implantable Defibrillator study demonstrated shorter survival free of heart failure–related hospitalization in patients with a history of heart failure who were paced on DDD mode with RV lead placement.[13] The Mode Selection Trial (MOST) study comparing VVI and DDD pacing found that frequent RV (>40%-50%) pacing was deleterious and increased mortality and heart failure admissions when compared with sinus rhythm.[14] Consequently, manufacturers have developed new algorithms to provide minimal use of ventricular pacing in dual-chamber pacemakers and defibrillators with RV leads.

Algorithms used in modern dual-chamber pacemakers and defibrillators can recognize and test for periodic return of intrinsic AV conduction in patients with intermittent second- or third-degree AV block (**Figure 21.19**). Three atrial pacing artifacts are followed by paced P waves, a long AV interval (previously lengthened by the pacemaker to promote intrinsic conduction), with a pacemaker spike superimposed on the QRS (see **Figure 21.14**). Following the fourth atrial paced beat, ventricular pacing is suspended for a single cycle and no QRS is seen. The pacemaker algorithm allows a single "dropped" QRS before resuming both atrial and ventricular pacing with a short AV interval.

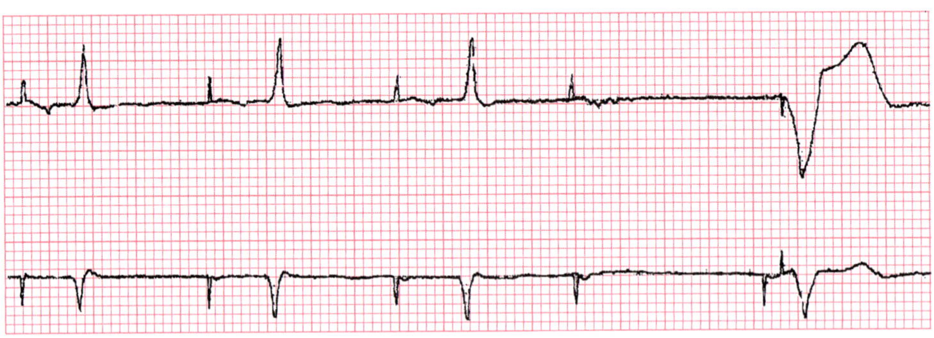

FIGURE 21.19. Dual-chamber pacemaker algorithm to minimize ventricular pacing. Three atrial pacing artifacts are followed by paced P waves, a long atrioventricular interval (previously lengthened by the pacemaker to promote intrinsic conduction), with a pacemaker spike superimposed on the QRS (see **Figure 21.14**). Following the fourth atrial paced beat, ventricular pacing is suspended for a single cycle and no QRS is seen. The pacemaker algorithm allows a single "dropped" QRS before resuming both atrial and ventricular pacing with a short atrioventricular interval.

Cardiac Resynchronization Therapy

The left of **Figure 21.20** illustrates lead placement for biventricular pacing used for CRT. In patients without chronic atrial arrhythmias, a right-atrial lead is positioned in the appendage or lateral wall of the atrium. The RV lead is usually placed at the RV apex but may be positioned in the outflow tract. A transvenous LV lead is inserted through the coronary sinus and advanced to epicardial veins. Optimal position of the LV pacing lead is usually in the lateral wall, midway between the base and LV apex for most patients. The right of **Figure 21.20** illustrates the separately programmable RV and LV pacing pulses of a CRT device.

More than one in three patients with heart failure have an underlying LBBB, which contributes to poor LV function by causing delayed contraction of the lateral LV wall, resulting in *dyssynchrony* between septal and free wall contraction. The ECG is important in selecting patients most likely to benefit from CRT and in improving site selection of the LV lead by recognizing areas of LV scar. Patients most likely to benefit from CRT are those with LBBB and a QRS duration greater than 140 ms for males and 130 ms for females.[15] Forty percent of patients with LBBB with QRS duration of 120 ms have underlying LV dyssynchrony. Seventy percent of those with LBBB and QRS width of >150 ms have LV dyssynchrony.[3] Controlled studies show improved LV function, exercise performance, and ejection fraction, and reduced LV diastolic size (reversal of remodeling) in the majority of patients treated with CRT who have LBBB and QRS prolongation. Randomized trials in patients with heart failure have shown reduction of symptoms, improved functional capacity, fewer hospitalizations for heart failure, and increased survival.[16-19] However, up to 30% may fail to benefit from CRT.

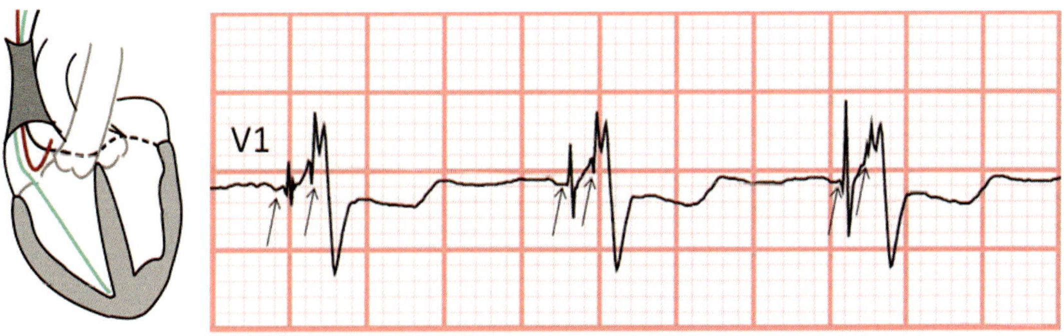

FIGURE 21.20. Biventricular pacing. Left, schematic showing atrial, right-ventricular, and left-ventricular lead positions; right, rhythm strip showing two pacing impulses for each QRS, with an interval between pacing of the left and right ventricles. Arrows show the two pacing pulses for each QRS. This interval may be adjusted to optimize ventricular function for CRT.

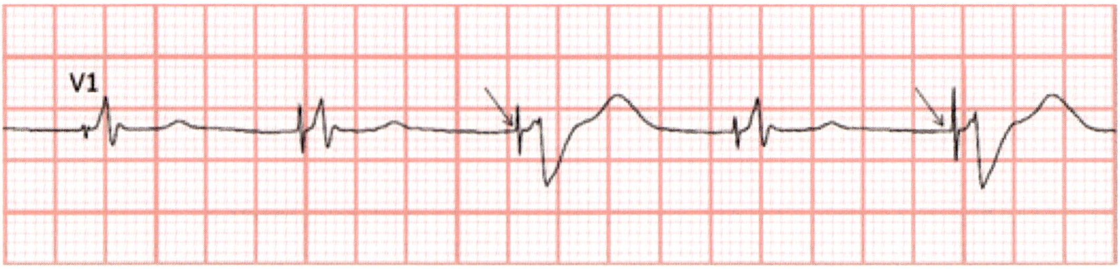

FIGURE 21.21. Biventricular pacing at follow-up. Arrows illustrate intermittent loss of left-ventricular capture evidenced by loss of the right-bundle-branch block pattern.

The ECG has a major role in follow-up of CRT patients for optimization of AV and RV-LV intervals and to verify adequate capture of both the RV and LV.[20] **Figure 21.21** shows intermittent capture of the LV as shown by loss of the R-wave amplitude on the beats marked with the arrows. This intermittent capture should be corrected by increasing the pacing energy for the LV electrode or switching to a different LV pacing electrode.

Although CRT was developed to treat patients with QRS prolongation and moderate to severe LV dysfunction, it is now also commonly used to prevent RV pacing-induced cardiomyopathy in patients with even mildly reduced ejection fraction.

Physiologic Ventricular Pacing—His-Bundle Pacing

Dual-chamber RV pacing will continue to have a role in patients with intermittent bradyarrhythmias or intermittent AV block and normal LV function. The RV pacing burden >20%, male sex, and a native QRS duration >115 ms have been associated with an increased risk of developing pacemaker-induced heart failure from RV apical pacing,[21] but more data are needed to better identify those patients at highest risk for heart failure development in response to RV pacing.

Pacing-induced dyssynchrony and subsequent development of pacing-induced heart failure can be avoided if the ventricular lead is positioned to pace the specialized conduction system rather than the RV apex. The His-bundle deflection can be identified and localized on the intracardiac electrogram obtained from the ventricular pacing lead (**Figure 21.22**), and the lead can be permanently anchored in this location. In many cases of AV block, the level of block is in the AV node or proximal His bundle and can be bypassed by positioning the lead distal to the level of block. His-bundle pacing can also be used to correct underlying LBBB or RBBB in 70% to 90% of patients.[22] His-bundle pacing may prove useful as an alternative to biventricular pacing for the delivery of CRT. The summary illustration depicts the anatomic locations for the most common types of ventricular pacing, including physiologic His pacing.

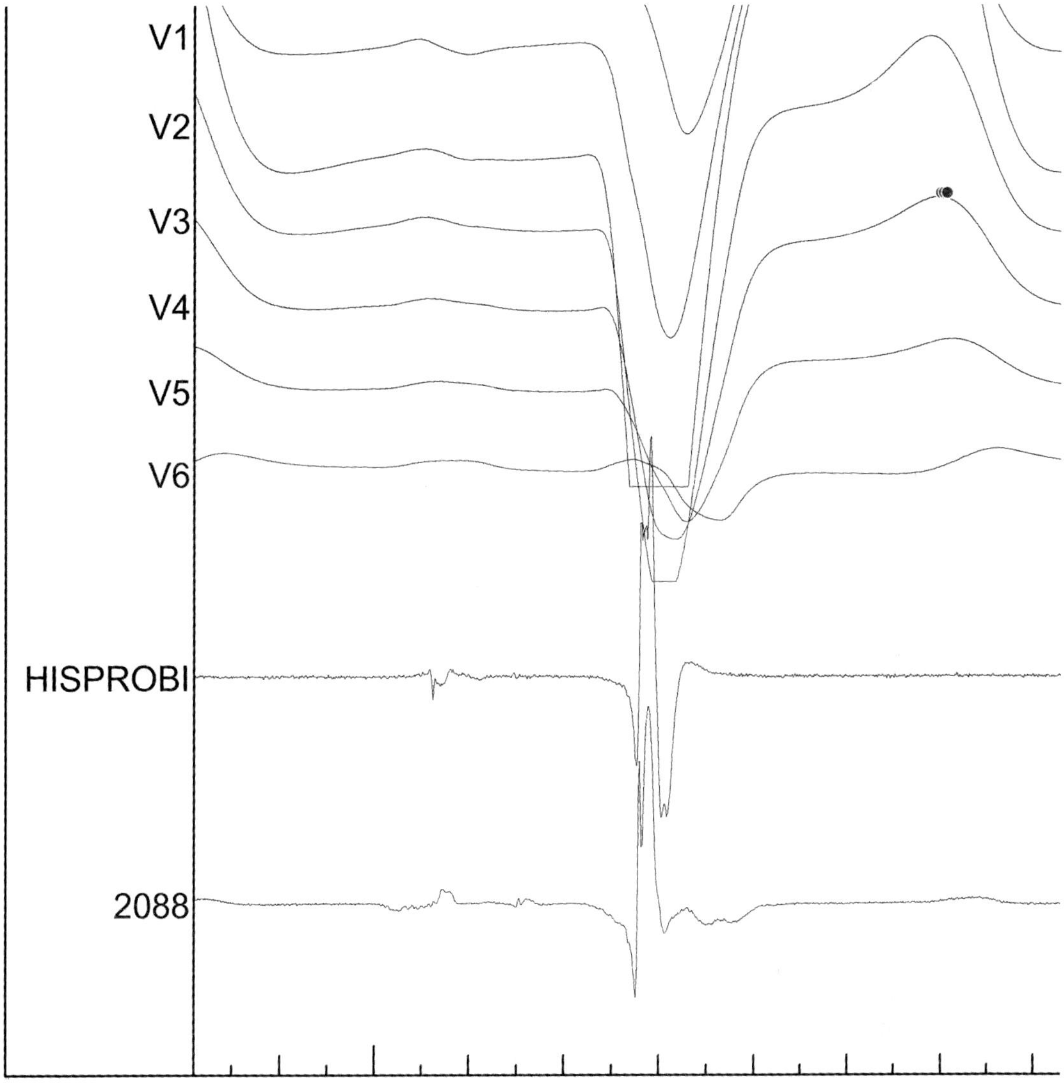

FIGURE 21.22. The His bundle can be located using electrogram mapping. The His bundle creates a distinct signal.

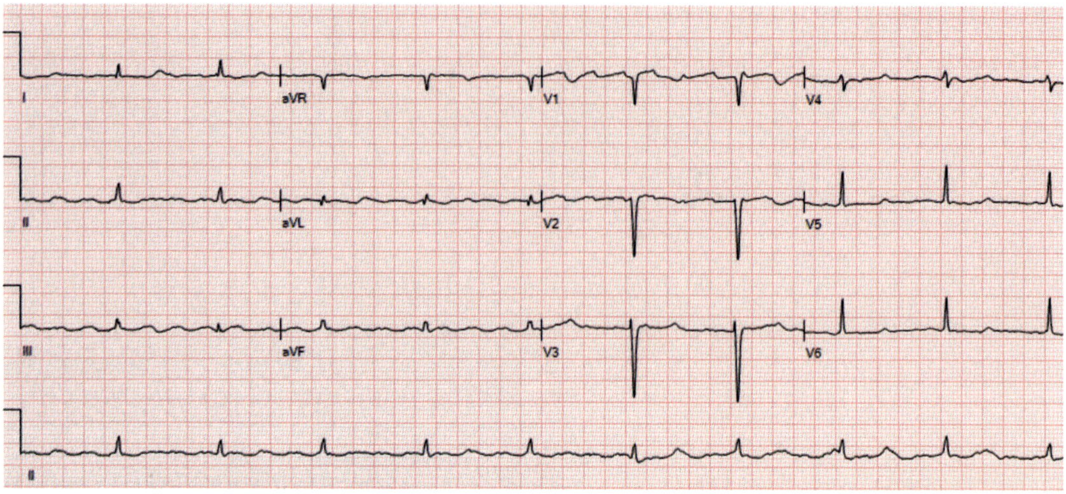

A

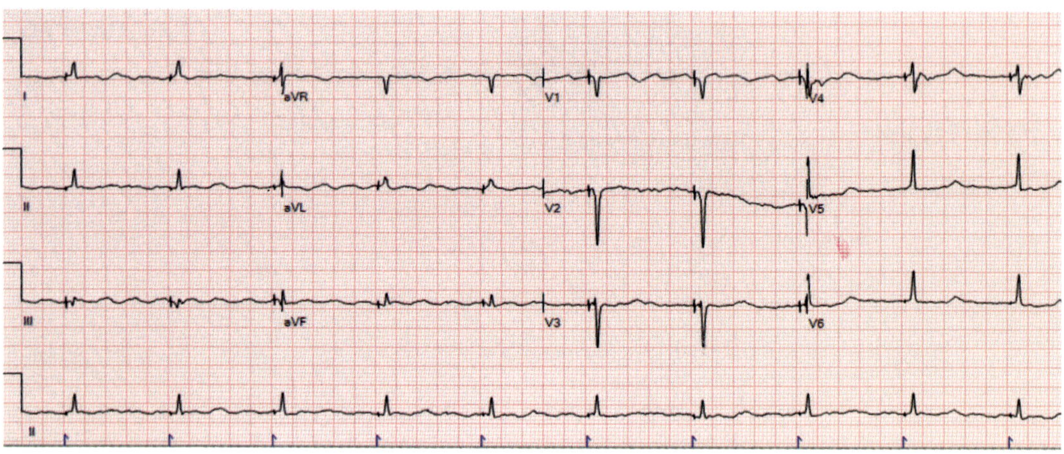

B

FIGURE 21.23. Intrinsic conduction on 12-lead electrocardiogram (**A**) and His-bundle paced 12-lead electrocardiogram (**B**). Note the isoelectric interval between the His-bundle pacing spike and QRS onset and the identical QRS morphology between the native and paced QRS complexes. These features are characteristic of successful selective His-bundle capture from a lead positioned above the tricuspid valve.

His-bundle pacing can occur with selective capture of the His bundle, usually obtained when the pacing lead is positioned above the tricuspid valve (**Figure 21.23**) or with non-selective capture usually obtained when the pacing lead is positioned below the tricuspid valve (**Figure 21.24**). Selective His-bundle capture can be identified on a 12-lead ECG by a pacing artifact from the ventricular channel followed by an isoelectric interval of at least 30 ms, followed by a QRS complex identical in appearance to beats with native conduction. Nonselective capture can be identified by a pacing stimulus followed immediately by a QRS complex that demonstrates initial slurring followed 30 to 40 ms later by a sharp QRS complex with rapid terminal forces. Nonselective His-bundle paced complexes have an appearance similar to preexcited conduction when an anteroseptal accessory pathway is present (see Chapter 19).

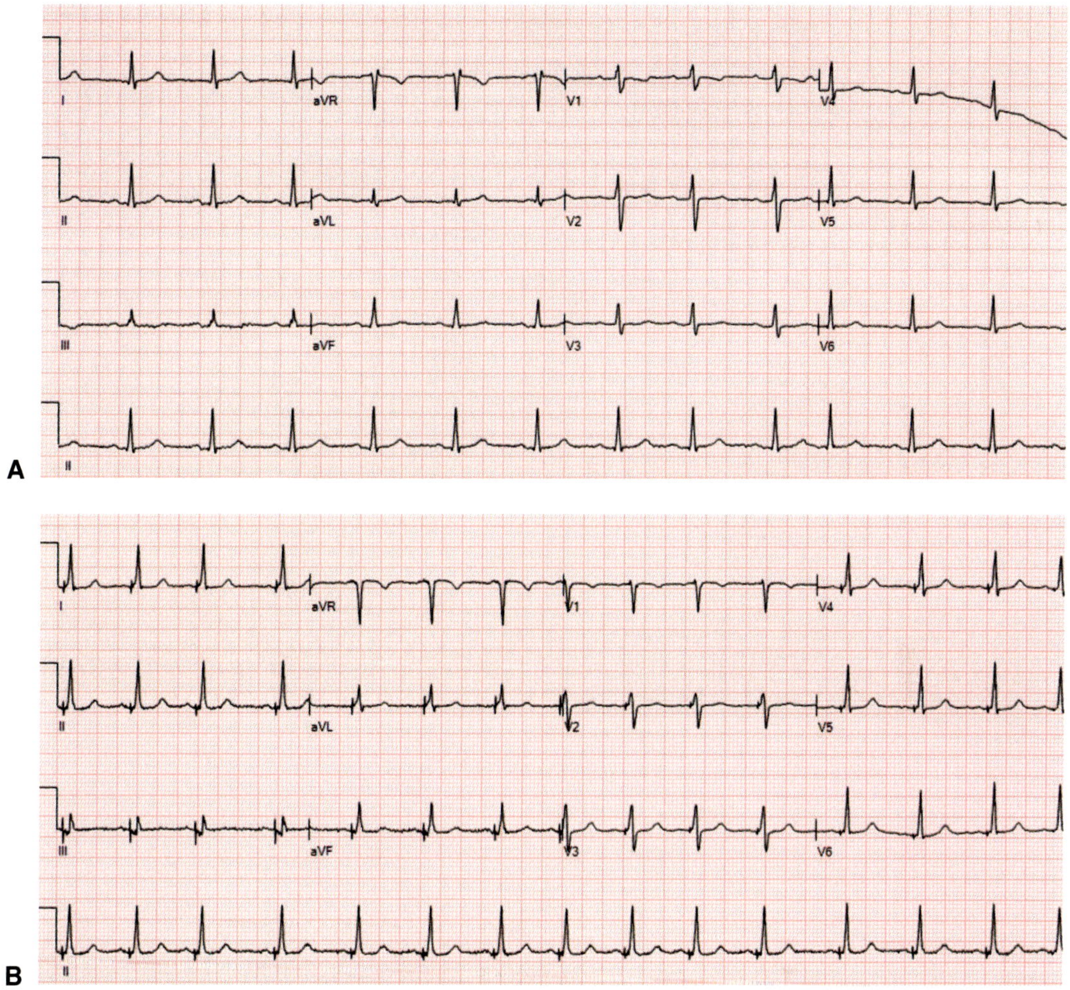

FIGURE 21.24. Intrinsic conduction on 12-lead electrocardiogram (**A**) and His-bundle paced 12-lead electrocardiogram (**B**). Note the lack of isoelectric interval between the His-bundle pacing spike and QRS onset and the "delta wave" appearance to the QRS onset created by capture of right-ventricular myocardium surrounding the His bundle. Approximately 40 to 60 ms after the pacing spike, the QRS complex becomes identical to intrinsic rhythm. These features are characteristic of successful nonselective His-bundle capture from a lead positioned just below the tricuspid valve.

CHAPTER 21 SUMMARY ILLUSTRATION

Alternative pacing sites to mimic physiological pacing

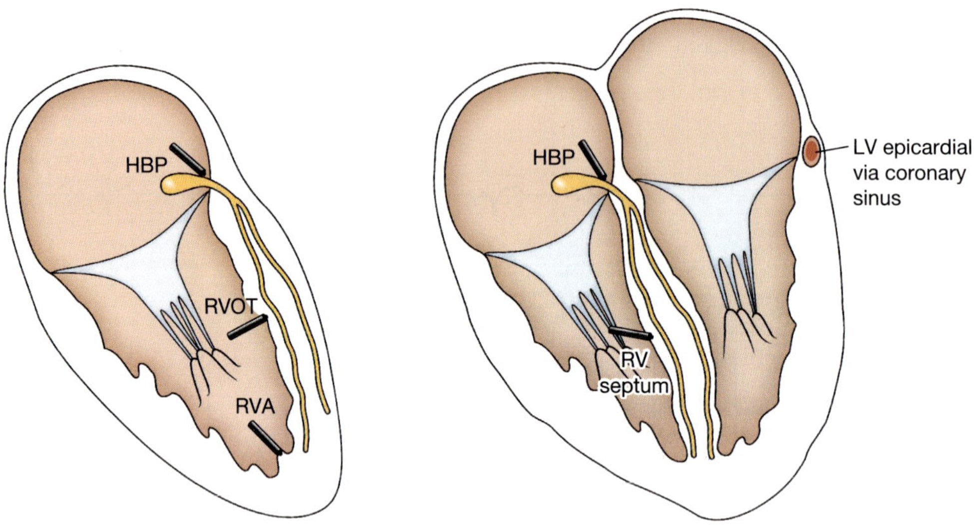

Abbreviations: HBP, His bundle pacing; LV, left ventricle; RV, right ventricle; RVA, right ventricular apex; RVOT, right ventricular outflow tract.

Glossary

Biventricular pacemaker: a pacemaker that paces both the right and left ventricles. Atrial pacing is also included unless the patient has chronic atrial arrhythmias that would prevent atrial pacing or tracking.

Cardiac resynchronization therapy: use of biventricular pacing or His-bundle pacing to synchronize ventricular activation and contraction.

Defibrillation: termination of either atrial or ventricular fibrillation by an extrinsic electrical current.

Demand mode: a term describing an implantable pacemaker system with the ability to sense and be inhibited by intrinsic cardiac activity.

Dual-chamber pacemaker: a pacemaker that includes both atrial and ventricular pacing.

Dyssynchrony: loss of the normal synchronous mechanical contraction of the ventricular walls. The classic mechanical dyssynchrony with LBBB or RV pacing includes early activation and contraction of the septal LV wall with LV free wall stretching followed later by LV free wall contraction with LV septal bounce.

Fixed-rate pacing: pacing with the capability only to generate an electrical impulse without sensing the heart's intrinsic rhythm or varying the rate using physiologic sensors.

Implantable cardiac pacemakers: devices capable of sensing native electrical impulses and/or generating electrical impulses and delivering them to the myocardium to stimulate mechanical contraction.

Oversensing: abnormal function of an implantable pacemaker in which electrical signals other than those created by the myocardium in the chamber of interest are sensed and inhibit or trigger impulse generation.

Pacemaker artifacts: high-frequency signals appearing on an ECG and representing impulses generated by an implanted pacemaker.

Pacemaker syndrome: a constellation of symptoms including neck fullness, light-headedness, and occasionally vasovagal syncope caused by retrograde conduction of ventricular-paced beats.

Pacing electrodes: electrodes that, when connected to a pacemaker generator, are designed to transmit electrical impulses to the myocardium. In pacing systems with sensing capability, these electrodes also transmit the intrinsic impulses of the heart to the pacemaker.

Pulse generator: a device that contains a battery, ports for connection of pacing leads, and a computer processor that produces electrical impulses as the key component of an implantable pacing system.

Single-chamber pacemaker: a pacemaker with one lead pacing and sensing one cardiac chamber.

Acknowledgment

We gratefully acknowledge the past contributions of the previous edition's author, Dr. Galen S. Wagner, as portions of that chapter were retained in this revision.

References

1. Ellenbogen KA, Wood MA, eds. *Cardiac Pacing and ICDs*. 5th ed. Hoboken, NJ: Wiley-Blackwell; 2008.
2. Hayes DL, Asirvatham SJ, Friedman PA, eds. *Cardiac Pacing, Defibrillation and Resynchronization: A Clinical Approach*. 3rd ed. Hoboken, NJ: Wiley-Blackwell; 2013.
3. Tracy CM, Epstein AE, Darbar D, et al. 2012 ACCF/AHA/HRS focused update of the 2008 guidelines for device-based therapy of cardiac rhythm abnormalities: a report of the American College of Cardiology Foundation/American Heart Association Task Force on Practice Guidelines and the Heart Rhythm Society. *Circulation*. 2012;126:1784-1800.
4. Ricke AD, Swiryn S, Bauernfeind RA, Conner JA, Young B, Rowlandson GI. Improved pacemaker pulse detection: clinical evaluation of a new high-bandwidth electrocardiographic system. *J Electrocardiol*. 2011;44:265-274.
5. Jennings M, Devine B, Lou S, Macfarlane PW. Enhanced software based detection of implanted cardiac pacemaker stimuli. *Computers Cardiol*. 2009;36:833-836.
6. Jacob S, Panaich SS, Maheshwari R, Haddad JW, Padanilam BJ, John SK. Clinical applications of magnets on cardiac rhythm management devices. *Europace*. 2011;13:1222-1230.
7. Bernstein AD, Camm AJ, Fletcher RD, et al. The NASPE/BPEG generic pacemaker code for antibradyarrhythmia and adaptive-rate pacing and antitachyarrhythmia devices. *Pacing Clin Electrophysiol*. 1987;10(4, pt 1):794-799.

8. Greenspon AJ, Patel JD, Lau E, et al. Trends in permanent pacemaker implantation in the United States from 1993 to 2009: increasing complexity of patients and procedures. *J Am Coll Cardiol.* 2012;60:1540-1545.
9. Mond HG, Proclemer A. The 11th world survey of cardiac pacing and implantable cardioverter-defibrillators: calendar year 2009—a World Society of Arrhythmia's project. *Pacing Clin Electrophysiol.* 2011;34:1013-1027.
10. Castellanos A Jr, Agha AS, Befeler B, Castillo CA, Berkovits BV. A study of arrival of excitation at selected ventricular sites during human bundle branch block using close bipolar catheter electrodes. *Chest.* 1973;63:208-213.
11. Vera Z, Mason DT, Awan NA, Hiliard G, Massumi RA. Lack of sensing by demand pacemakers due to intraventricular conduction defects. *Circulation.* 1975;51:815-822.
12. Ausubel K, Boal BH, Furman S. Pacemaker syndrome: definition and evaluation. *Cardiol Clin.* 1985;3:587-594.
13. Wilkoff BL, Cook JR, Epstein AE, et al; for DAVID Trial Investigators. Dual-chamber pacing or ventricular backup pacing in patients with an implantable defibrillator: the Dual Chamber and VVI Implantable Defibrillator (DAVID) trial. *JAMA.* 2002;288:3115-3123.
14. Sweeney MO, Hellkamp AS, Ellenbogen KA, et al. Adverse effect of ventricular pacing on heart failure and atrial fibrillation among patients with normal baseline QRS duration in a clinical trial of pacemaker therapy for sinus node dysfunction. *Circulation.* 2003;23:2932-2937.
15. Straus DG, Selvester RH, Wagner GS. Defining left bundle branch block in the era of cardiac resynchronization therapy. *Am J Cardiol.* 2011;107:927-934.
16. Abraham WT, Fisher WG, Smith AL, et al. Cardiac resynchronization in chronic heart failure. *N Engl J Med.* 2002;346: 1845-1853.
17. Bristow MR, Saxon LA, Boehmer J, et al. Cardiac-resynchronization therapy with or without an implantable defibrillator in advanced chronic heart failure. *N Engl J Med.* 2004;350:2140-2150.
18. Moss AJ, Hall WJ, Cannom DS, et al. Cardiac resynchronization therapy for the prevention of heart-failure events. *N Engl J Med.* 2009;361:1329-1338.
19. Cleland JG, Daubert JC, Erdmann E, et al. The effect of cardiac resynchronization on morbidity and mortality in heart failure. *N Engl J Med.* 2005;352:1539-1549.
20. Mullens W, Grimm RA, Verga T, et al. Insights from a cardiac resynchronization optimization clinic as part of a heart failure disease management program. *J Am Coll Cardiol.* 2009;53:765-773.
21. Kiehl EL, Makki T, Kumar R, et al. Incidence and predictors of right ventricular pacing-induced cardiomyopathy in patients with complete atrioventricular block and preserved left ventricular systolic function. *Heart Rhythm.* 2016;13(12):2272-2278.
22. Huang W, Su L, Wu S, et al. Long-term outcomes of His bundle pacing in patients with heart failure with left bundle branch block. *Heart.* 2019;105(2):137-143.

Index

Page numbers followed by "f" indicate figures; page numbers followed by "t" indicate tables

C

D

M

N

Q

R

T

U

V

W

X